15 Update in Intensive Care and Emergency Medicine

Edited by J.L.Vincent

J. J. Marini C. Roussos (Eds.)

Ventilatory Failure

With 179 Figures and 59 Tables

Springer-Verlag
Berlin Heidelberg New York
London Paris Tokyo
Hong Kong Barcelona
Budapest

Series Editor

Prof. Dr. Jean Louis Vincent
Clinical Director, Department of Intensive Care, Erasme Hospital
Free University of Brussels, Route de Lennik 808
1070 Brussels, Belgium

Volume Editors

Prof. Dr. J. J. Marini
St. Paul-Ramsey Medical Center, 640 Jackson Street
St. Paul, MN 55101-2595, USA

Prof. Dr. C. Roussos
Department of Critical Care, Evangelismos Hospital
45, Ipsilandou Street, Athens 11521, Greece

ISBN-13 : 978-3-642-84556-7
e-ISBN-13 : 978-3-642-84554-3
DOI : 10.1007 / 978-3-642-84554-3

Library of Congress Cataloging-in-Publication Data
Ventilatory failure / edited by J. J. Marini and C. Roussos.--(Update in intensive care and emergency medicine; 15) Includes bibliographical references and index. ISBN 3-540-54297-3 (alk. paper).--ISBN (invalid) 0-387-54297-3 (alk. paper) 1. Respiratory insufficiency. I. Marini, John J. II. Roussos, Charis, 1942- . III. Series. [DNLM: 1. Respiratory Insufficiency. 2. Respiratory Therapy--instrumentation. 3. Ventilators, Mechanical. W1 UP66H v. 15 / WF 140 V465] RC776.R4V45 1991 616.2--dc20 DNLM/DLC

Typesetting and printing: Zechnersche Buchdruckerei, D-6720 Speyer

19/3130-5 4 3 2 1 0 – Printed on acid-free paper

Contents

List of Contributors

Aubier, M.
Department of Pulmonary Medicine, INSERM U 226, 46 rue Henri Huchard, Paris 75018, France

Barbera, J.A.
Department of Pulmonary Medicine, Hospital Clinic, Villarroel 170, Barcelona 08036, Spain

Benito, S.
Department of Critical Care, Hospital de la Santa Creu i Saint Pau, Avda Sant Antoni Ma Claret 167, Barcelona 08025, Spain

Brandi, G.
Institute of Human Physiology, University of Padova, Padova, Italy

Branthwaite, M.A.
Department of Thoracic Medicine, Royal Brompton Hospital, Sydney Street, London SW3 6NP, United Kingdom

Brazzi, L.
Department of Intensive Care, Nuovo Ospedale San Gerardo, Via G. Donizetti 106, Monza (MI) 20052, Italy

Brochard, L.
Department of Intensive Care, Henri Mondor Hospital, 51 Av du Maréchal de Lattre de Tassigny, 94010 Créteil, France

Celli, B.
Department of Pulmonary Medicine, Veterans Affairs Medical Center, 150 South Huntington Avenue, Boston, MA 02130, USA

Criner, G.J.
Division of Pulmonary and Critical Care, Temple University Hospital, 3401 N Broad Street, Philadelphia, PA 19140, USA

Decramer, M.
Respiratory Division, University Hospital, Weligerveld 1, 3212 Pellenberg, Belgium

Elliott, M.W.
Department of Thoracic Medicine, Royal Brompton Hospital, Sydney Street, London SW3 6NP, United Kingdom

Estenne, M.
Department of Pulmonary Medicine, Erasme University Hospital, Route de Lennik 808, Brussels 1070, Belgium

Eveloff, S.E.
Department of Pulmonary Medicine, Memorial Hospital, Pawtucket, Rhode Island 02860, USA

Fitting, J.W.
Division of Pulmonary Medicine, C.H.U. Vaudois, Lausanne 1011, Switzerland

Gattinoni, L.
Department of Intensive Care, Nuovo Ospedale San Gerardo, Via G. Donizetti 106, Monza (MI) 20052, Italy

Gaultier, C.
Laboratory of Physiology, A. Béclère Hospital, 157 rue de la Porte de Trivaux, Clamart 92141, France

Gottfried, S.B.
Meakins-Christie Laboratories and Department of Respiratory and Critical Care Medicine, Montreal General Hospital, 1650 Cedar Avenue, Montreal, Quebec, Canada H3G 1A4

Hagan, B.M.
Department of Thoracic and Critical Care, Mayo Clinic, 200 First Street SW, Rochester, MN 55905, USA

Hubmayr, R.D.
Department of Thoracic and Critical Care, Mayo Clinic, 200 First Street SW, Rochester, MN 55905, USA

Kelsen, S.G.
Division of Pulmonary and Critical Care, Temple University Hospital, 3401 N Broad Street, Philadelphia, PA 19140, USA

Lakynthinos, S.
Department of Critical Care, Evangelismos Hospital, 45 Ipsilandou Street, Athens 11521, Greece

McCool, F.D.
Department of Pulmonary Medicine, Memorial Hospital, Pawtucket, Rhode Island 02860, USA

Mancebo, J.
Department of Critical Care, Hospital de la Santa Creu i Saint Pau, Avda Sant Antoni Ma Claret 167, Barcelona 08025, Spain

Marini, J.J.
Department of Pulmonary/Critical Care, St Paul-Ramsey Medical Center, 640 Jackson Street, St Paul, Minnesota, MN 55101-2595, USA

Milic-Emili, J.
Meakins-Christie Laboratories and Department of Physiology, McGill University, 3626 St Urbain Street, Montreal, Quebec H2X 2P2, Canada

Mortensen, J.D.
CardioPulmonics Inc, 5060 West Amelia Earhart Drive, Salt Lake City, Utah 84116, USA

Pesenti, A.
Department of Intensive Care, Nuovo Ospedale San Gerardo, Via G. Donizetti 106, Monza (MI) 20052, Italy

Pingleton, S.K.
Division of Pulmonary Medicine, University of Kansas Medicine Center, 39th and Rainbow Blvd, Kansas City, Kansas 66103, USA

Polese, G.
Department of Internal Medicine, University of Verona, Verona 37126, Italy

Roca, J.
Department of Pulmonary Medicine, Hospital Clinic, Villarroel 170, Barcelona 08036, Spain

Rochester, D.F.
Division of Pulmonary and Critical Care, University of Virginia, Health Sciences Center, Charlottesville, VA 22908, USA

Rodriguez-Roisin, R.
Department of Pulmonary Medicine, Hospital Clinic, Villarroel 170, Barcelona 08036, Spain

Rossi, A.
Respiratory Division, Ospedale Civile Maggiore ULSS 25, Piazzale Stefani 1, Verona 37126, Italy

Rouby, J.J.
Department of Intensive Care, G.H. Pitié-Salpêtrière, 83 Blvd de l'Hôpital, Paris 75013, France

Roussos, C.
Department of Critical Care, Evangelismos Hospital, 45 Ipsilandou Street, Athens 11521, Greece

Sexauer, W.P.
Division of Pulmonary and Critical Care, Temple University Hospital, 3401 N Broad Street, Philadelphia, PA 19140, USA

Simonds, A.K.
Department of Thoracic Medicine, Royal Brompton Hospital, Sydney Street, London SW3 6NP, United Kingdom

Slutsky, A. S.
Division Respiratory Medicine, Mount Sinai Hospital, 600 University Avenue Room 656A, Toronto, Ontario, Canada M6C 3G4

Tobin, M. J.
Division of Pulmonary and Critical Care, Hines Veterans Affairs Hospital, Hines, IL 60142, USA

Vallverdu, I.
Department of Critical Care, Hospital de la Santa Creu i Saint Pau, Avda Sant Antoni Ma Claret 167, Barcelona 08025, Spain

Younes, M.
Respiratory Hospital, Health Sciences Center, 810 Sherbrook Street Room RS-307, Winnipeg, Manibota, Canada R3A 1R8

Abbreviations

ARDS	Adult respiratory distress syndrome
ARF	Acute respiratory failure
CMV	Control mode ventilation
CNEP	Continuous negative extrathoracic pressure
CNPV	Continuous negative pressure ventilation
CNS	Central nervous system
CO	Cardiac output
COPD	Chronic obstructive pulmonary disease
CPAP	Continuous positive airway pressure
CPPV	Conventional positive pressure ventilation
CSF	Cerebrospinal fluid
CVP	Central venous pressure
$ECCO_2R$	Extracorporeal CO_2 removal
EMG	Electromyogram
FRC	Functional residual capacity
FVC	Forced vital capacity
HFJV	High frequency jet ventilation
ICU	Intensive care unit
IMV	Intermittent mandatory ventilation
IPPV	Intermittent positive pressure ventilation
IRV	Inverse ratio ventilation
MIP	Maximal inspiratory pressure
MV	Mechanical ventilation
$PaCO_2$	Partial pressure of carbon dioxide in arterial blood
PaO_2	Partial pressure of oxygen in arterial blood
PAP	Pulmonary artery pressure
PDi	Maximal transdiaphragmatic pressure
PEEP	Positive end-expiratory pressure
PEEPi	Intrinsic PEEP
PS	Pressure support
PTI	Pressure time index

$P\bar{v}O_2$	Mixed venous oxygen tension
PVR	Pulmonary vascular resistance
RV	Residual volume
SIMV	Synchronized intermittent mandatory ventilation
TLC	Total lung capacity
VA/Q	Ventilation-perfusion ratio
VC	Vital capacity
VD	Dead space
VE	Minute ventilation
VO_2	Oxygen consumption
VT	Tidal volume
WOB	Work of breathing

Ventilatory Failure: An Overview

D.F. Rochester

Introduction

Ventilatory failure is defined as a state or condition in which the partial pressure of carbon dioxide in arterial blood ($PaCO_2$) is consistently elevated. It is generally accepted that the normal range of $PaCO_2$ is 35 to 45 torr, in the awake subject at or near sea level. Therefore, one would not make a diagnosis of ventilatory failure unless the $PaCO_2$ were consistently above 45 torr. The acceptable upper limit of $PaCO_2$ might be higher during sleep, and lower if the person lived at altitude. Another way to think about ventilatory failure is to consider how much effort is required to maintain a normal, metabolically appropriate $PaCO_2$. Thus, a state of ventilatory failure can also be said to exist if a patient can maintain an acceptable $PaCO_2$ only with extreme dyspnea, or with mechanical ventilatory assistance.

The act of breathing is performed by the respiratory system, which is comprised of a collection of organs which subserve the various functions needed for breathing and gas exchange. This system functions in an integrated fashion, in health and in disease. Thus, one must understand the syndromes of acute and chronic ventilatory failure in terms of the interactions among the different parts of the respiratory system, with particular emphasis on the respiratory muscles, the ventilatory control, the pattern of breathing and the efficiency of gas exchange.

This overview addresses the hypotheses

1. that the respiratory system response to excessive loading is to reduce the tidal volume in order to minimize perceived effort; and
2. that the reduction in tidal volume is the final common pathway to ventilatory failure in a variety of unrelated clinical conditions, including obstructive disease of the airways, thoracic restrictive disorders, neuromuscular disease and other forms of respiratory muscle weakness.

The Process of Normal Breathing

The Respiratory Muscles

Respiratory muscle groups. Normal breathing depends on the appropriate actions of both upper and lower groups of respiratory muscles. The upper airway muscles open the upper airway prior to inspiration, and maintain its caliber as inspiration proceeds. The principal upper airway muscles are the tongue, muscles of the palate and pharynx, and adductors of the vocal cords. The lower respiratory muscles are responsible for delivery of fresh air to the gas exchange apparatus. They are subdivided into those which are primarily inspiratory in action, and those which are primarily expiratory. The principal inspiratory muscles are the diaphragm, the parasternal intercostal, scalene and sternocleidomastoid muscles. The principal expiratory muscles are the external and internal abdominal obliques, the transversus abdominis and the transversus thoracic muscles.

Among the inspiratory muscles, the diaphragm is best suited to displace volume when it contracts. The diaphragm has long muscle fibers, and it can shorten as much as 40% between full expiration (residual volume, RV) and full inspiration (total lung capacity, TLC) in both animals and humans [1, 2]. It appears that the diaphragm is responsible for most of the tidal volume, when the subject is at or near the normal breathing position (functional residual capacity, FRC). However, even during quiet breathing at FRC, other inspiratory and expiratory muscle groups contribute to the ventilatory effort [3]. At higher lung volumes the contribution of the diaphragm to the tidal volume is much less [4] whereas the contribution of other inspiratory muscles such as the parasternal intercostals, the scalenes and the sternomastoids is greatly increased.

Interactions among respiratory muscles. There are important interactions among the respiratory muscles, which strive to maintain an appropriate level of minute ventilation in spite of potential impediments to breathing. Simply changing from the supine to the erect position recruits the expiratory abdominal and inspiratory parasternal and scalene muscles [5]. This serves two purposes. Gravity causes the diaphragm to descend and shorten, thereby incurring some mechanical disadvantage. The increase in tonic and phasic activity of the abdominal muscles helps to maintain the diaphragm at a more effective operating length, while increased activity of the parasternal intercostal and scalene muscles helps to maintain the tidal volume, despite the reduction in the contribution of the diaphragm.

The respiratory muscles are also rapidly recruited by any event that increases the effort required to breathe, such as physical exercise, an increase in airway resistance consequent to external breathing apparatus or breathing under hyperbaric conditions, and by breathing at a higher than normal lung volume. Thus, recruitment of both inspiratory and expiratory muscles is not only a normal phenomenon, but also a commonplace one.

Respiratory muscle endurance and energy expenditure. Normal breathing requires very little effort. The energy expended by the respiratory muscles during quiet breathing is less than 2% of the resting energy expenditure of the whole body. During inspiratory resistive breathing, the respiratory muscle energy expenditure is much higher, and it is proportional to inspiratory work [6]. This means that for a constant tidal volume, the energy cost of breathing is directly proportional to the pressure needed to inspire the breath (Pbreath).

The endurance of the inspiratory muscles can be assessed by determining the inspiratory pressure-time index (PTI). This has two components: the fractional duration of inspiration (Ti/Ttot), and the ratio of the pressure required to inspire a breath (Pbreath) to the maximal inspiratory pressure (PImax). The PTI is the prod-

Table 1. Calculation of the pressure-time index (PTI)

Pbreath	= Pressure needed to inspire a breath
PImax	= Maximal inspiratory pressure
Ti	= Duration of inspiration
Ttot	= Duration of whole breath
PTI	= (Pbreath/PImax) × (Ti/Ttot)

uct of these two ratios (Table 1). Since Ti/Ttot is relatively constant, changes in PTI are generally the result of changes in Pbreath/PImax.

The PTI reflects the force and duration of inspiratory muscle contraction. During normal quiet breathing, Pbreath is −5 cm H_2O, and Ti/Ttot is 0.4. In normal subjects, PImax is typically about −100 cm H_2O. Therefore, Pbreath/PImax is approximately 0.05, and PTI is 0.02 during quiet breathing. These values are consistent with the low energy cost of breathing.

Pbreath can be increased by inspiring through an inspiratory flow resistive load, and Ti/Ttot can be varied by having the subject follow a prescribed pattern of breathing. In experiments in which PTI was increased by changing either Pbreath or Ti/Ttot, it was found that normal subjects will develop inspiratory muscle fatigue whenever the PTI exceeds a threshold value of 0.15 [7]. However, overt inspiratory muscle fatigue does not appear instantaneously. It takes over an hour for overt fatigue to develop when the PTI is at the threshold level. When the PTI is greater than 0.3, severe fatigue will ensue within minutes.

The ratio Pbreath/PImax is also directly related to the perception of added ventilatory loads [8]. Although load perception and dyspnea are not the same, there is growing evidence that an increase in Pbreath/PImax is important in the generation of the sensation of dyspnea, especially when mechanical impediments to breathing, muscle weakness or combinations of these increase the effort needed to maintain an adequate tidal volume.

Ventilatory Control

Nature of the control system. The control system, located in the brain stem, has been described as a central pattern generator [9, 10]. The controller, which generates the respiratory rhythm, receives and integrates multiple inputs, both from the periphery and from other parts of the central nervous system [11]. The output of the central pattern generator is distributed to the respiratory muscles, which shorten, displace volume and generate respiratory pressures. The relationship between neural drive on the one hand, and inspiratory pressure or inspired volume on the other, is often referred to as "coupling" of drive to inspiratory pressure generation or volume displacement.

Assessment of control. The volume displaced by the shortening of the respiratory muscles is the tidal volume (VT), and the final, common pathway for expression of ventilatory drive is the minute ventilation (VE). This is usually calculated as the product of respiratory frequency (f) and VT, but Milic-Emili et al. [12] showed that it is more useful in assessing ventilatory control to express minute ventilation as the product of the mean inspiratory flow rate (VT/Ti) and the fractional duration of inspiration (Ti/Ttot). The first term reflects neural drive to the inspiratory muscles, whereas the second term reflects timing. Minute ventilation can be altered by changes in either variable alone, or as is usually the case, changes in both drive and timing together.

Another measure of ventilatory drive is the mouth occlusion pressure measured 0.1 sec after the onset of inspiration (P0.1). When the airway is occluded just prior to the onset of inspiration, the pressure fall in the first 100–200 millisec reflects the level of neural drive that was present for the corresponding part of the previous non-occluded breath [12]. When ventilatory drive is increased, the P0.1 increases faster than VT/Ti, because impedance to flow is higher at the higher flow rates. Thus the relation between these two indices of ventilatory drive is curvilinear.

The Pattern of Breathing and Gas Exchange

The normal pattern of breathing. The pattern of breathing is affected by the means to measure it, especially in resting normal subjects. Results of measurements made using face masks, magnetometers or respiratory inductance plethysmography differ from those obtained spirometrically, probably because the mouth piece and nose clip significantly alter the pattern of breathing. Typically, the non-spirometric methods yield somewhat lower values for VT and VT/Ti, and higher values of f, but Ti/Ttot is unchanged [13–16].

The process of ventilation requires alternate ingress and egress of air, which must pass through a conducting system to the gas exchange surface, and back. Therefore, part of each VT must be dead space (VD). Normally, the ratio VD/VT is about 0.3 at rest, and it falls to 0.2 when VT is increased by physical exercise. Put another way, in the normal subject at rest approximately 30% of VE is dead space ventilation, leaving 70% of VE for alveolar ventilation. This distribution of ventilation, combined with the normal pattern of breathing, maintains $PaCO_2$ at its normal value of 40 torr.

The efficiency of gas exchange. As an alternative to determining VD/VT, one may quantify the efficiency of gas exchange by calculating VE40 which is defined as the level of VE needed to attain the normal $PaCO_2$ of 40 torr (Table 2). The advantage

Table 2. Calculating the efficiency of gas exchange

VTsb	= Spontaneous breathing tidal volume
fsb	= Spontaneous respiratory rate
VEsb	= Spontaneous breathing minute ventilation
$PaCO_2sb$	= Spontaneous breathing $PaCO_2$
VE40	= VEsb × ($PaCO_2sb$/40)
RR40	= VE40/VTsb

of this approach is that one can utilize for the calculation of VE40 the VE and $PaCO_2$ measured under clinical circumstances, as for example while the patient is being mechanically ventilated. An increase in VE40 usually reflects an increase in VD/VT, but it could also reflect an increased CO_2 production.

Even greater insight is provided by evaluating the ratio VE40/VTsb, where VTsb is the size of the tidal volume measured during spontaneous quiet breathing. The units of VE40/VTsb are breaths/minute. Thus the ratio VE40/VTsb can be thought of as "RR40", or the respiratory rate needed to achieve a $PaCO_2$ of 40 torr, given the dead space or wasted ventilation, the CO_2 production, and the size of the spontaneous breathing VT. In normal subjects at rest, RR40 is normally 12–17 breaths/min, both at rest and during mild activity. Values in excess of 20 breaths/min at rest are almost certainly abnormal.

The advantage of using RR40 is that it incorporates the pattern of breathing into evaluation of the efficiency of gas exchange. This is important because the pattern of breathing reflects the integrated response of the respiratory controller to multiple signals, including metabolic rate, the mechanics of the respiratory system, and the integrity of the respiratory muscles.

Clinical Causes of Ventilatory Failure

Increased Effort of Breathing

The effort required to breathe is reflected by the pressure (Pbreath) needed to inspire a given VT. When Pbreath is increased, both the work of breathing (mean Pbreath × VT) and the pressure-time index (PTI) are increased. It is important to realize that Pbreath depends not only on lung and chest wall mechanics, but also on the size of VT and the inspiratory flow rate. Thus, the effort required to breathe can be increased by a reduction of lung and/or chest wall compliance, an increase in upper or lower airway resistance, an increase in VE or inspiratory flow rate, and by combinations of all these factors.

Almost all of the conditions that predispose to CO_2 retention (Table 3) are characterized either by increasing the effort required to breathe, or by respiratory muscle weakness. Disorders which increase the effort required to breathe include:

Table 3. Disorders which predispose to ventilatory failure

Obstructive diseases of the lower airways
Upper airway obstruction, including obstructive sleep apnea (OSA)
Restrictive disorders of the chest wall
Obesity hypoventilation syndrome (OHS)
Neuromuscular diseases with respiratory muscle involvement
Other causes of respiratory muscle weakness
Sedative, tranquilizing or narcotic drugs
Central alveolar hypoventilation (Ondine's curse)
Combinations of the above

a) those which reduce pulmonary compliance,
b) those which impede the motion of the chest wall, and
c) those which increase the resistance to airflow.

Restrictive pulmonary diseases such as pulmonary fibrosis generally do not cause hypercapnic respiratory failure. When CO_2 retention occurs in extensive pulmonary edema, it is much more likely to be the result of impaired gas exchange (large shunt, fluid in airways) than the restriction of lung motion. The restrictive diseases of the chest wall which are most often associated with ventilatory failure are kyphoscoliosis, chest deformity secondary to thoracoplasty or fibrothorax, and flail chest. What these disorders have in common is that the abnormal mechanics of the chest wall are responsible for the ventilatory impairment.

In the obesity hypoventilation syndrome (OHS) it is likely that several mechanisms contribute to hypercapnia. Morbid obesity restricts the chest wall, but upper airway obstruction and abnormal control of breathing are also features of OHS. With the recognition of the obstructive sleep apnea syndrome (OSA), it has been appreciated that both obstructive and central apnea play major roles in the pathogenesis of ventilatory failure, in OHS as well as OSA, and that there is a marked degree of overlap between the OHS and OSA syndromes. In addition to these disorders, one may encounter ventilatory failure from other forms of upper airway obstruction, such as tracheal stenosis secondary to intubation and mechanical ventilation.

By far the commonest cause of ventilatory failure is severe obstructive disease of the intrapulmonary or lower airways. Although CO_2 retention is an occasional complication of acute asthma attack, hypercapnia occurs much more frequently in chronic obstructive pulmonary disease (COPD). Indeed, most of the published data concerning the pathophysiology of ventilatory failure have been obtained from patients with COPD. Perhaps this is because COPD affects breathing in multiple ways, including severe impairment of gas exchange, a marked increase in the effort required to breathe, a concomitant increase in VE, severely compromised inspiratory muscle function and an altered pattern of breathing.

Respiratory Muscle Weakness

Respiratory muscle weakness is as common in chronically or critically ill patients as it is in neuromuscular disease. The leading causes (Table 4) are mechanical disadvantage to inspiratory muscles in obstructive lung disease, undernutrition, sepsis [17–19], and a variety of electrolyte and other deficiencies [20–22]. In order for

Table 4. Respiratory muscle weakness in ventilatory failure

Mechanical disadvantage from increased lung volume
Malnutrition, metabolic disarray
Electrolyte imbalance, acidosis, hypoxia
Shock, trauma, sepsis, neoplasm

respiratory muscle weakness alone to cause CO_2 retention, respiratory muscle strength must be less than one-third normal [23]. More frequently, respiratory muscle weakness is not the sole cause of hypercapnia, but serves as an important co-factor with impaired gas exchange and altered control of breathing.

Decreased Ventilatory Drive

It is readily apparent that a reduction in the neural drive to breathe can cause ventilatory failure. This is most likely to result from excessive use of drugs that are known to depress the "respiratory center", such as opiates, barbiturates and tranquilizers. However, drive may also be reduced by an elevation of serum bicarbonate, consequent to metabolic alkalosis or the renal response to hypercapnia [24]. The syndrome of primary alveolar hypoventilation or "Ondine's Curse" is a rare cause for hypercapnic respiratory failure [25]. It sometimes occurs in diffuse muscle diseases [23].

Combinations of Factors

The clinician should bear in mind that even if a single major clinical "cause" of ventilatory failure has been identified, more often than not several mechanisms for CO_2 retention are operative. For example, respiratory muscle weakness, upper airway obstruction and narcotic, sedating or tranquilizing drugs are often important co-factors in the pathogenesis of ventilatory failure, adding to the effects of the underlying COPD, obesity, thoracic restriction or ARDS.

Pathophysiology of Ventilatory Failure

The Respiratory Muscles

Mechanical disadvantage. Inspiratory muscle function is seriously impaired in acute asthma and COPD, owing to the mechanical disadvantage conferred by hyperinflation of the lung. Acutely increasing the lung volume from FRC to TLC reduces maximal inspiratory pressures and diaphragmatic force by approximately 50% [1, 2]. Maximal inspiratory and transdiaphragmatic pressures are also reduced at high lung volumes when hyperinflation is chronic [26–32]. However, at lung volumes equivalent to normal TLC, the transdiaphragmatic pressure responses to phrenic nerve stimulation are higher in the hamster or human with COPD than in the corresponding normal subject [33, 34].

The contractile force of the chronically shortened diaphragm can be restored by sarcomere adaptation [35, 36], and this could partially explain the improvement in transdiaphragmatic pressure at high lung volumes. Other factors must also be operative, probably including a change in the relative compliances of the rib cage and abdomen from the normal to the chronically hyperinflated subject.

Perhaps a more important issue is what effect acute or chronic hyperinflation has on the shortening capacity of the diaphragm, and therefore, on the diaphragm's capacity to displace volume. Unfortunately, there are no data relating to this point. It is likely that both the relative and the absolute degree of active shortening are reduced by the passive shortening which accompanies acute hyperinflation. With chronic hyperinflation and sarcomere adaptation, one would expect that the relative active shortening capacity would be restored to normal. That is, the muscle would be able to shorten to 60–70% of its optimal resting length. However, because the whole muscle is now shorter, the loss of sarcomeres would cause the absolute shortening to be about 15% less than normal (calculated from the hamster data) [35, 36]. This effect would be added to passive shortening of about 15%, so that the overall impairment of shortening capacity could be 30% or more.

Asynchrony and dyspnea. The increase in ventilatory drive in COPD is accompanied by increased recruitment of upper airway muscles and respiratory muscles in the neck, rib cage and abdomen [32]. This gives rise to physical signs such as flaring of the alae nasi, obvious inspiratory contraction of the sternocleidomastoid muscles, and asynchronous movements of the rib cage and abdomen. These features are especially characteristic of COPD patients who are markedly hyperinflated [37]. Chest-abdomen asynchrony also develops during trials of weaning from mechanical ventilation, and may be a poor prognostic sign [38, 39].

Chest-abdomen asynchrony was at one time considered to be evidence of diaphragmatic fatigue, because paradoxical inward movement of the abdomen is characteristic of bilateral diaphragmatic paralysis, and chest-abdomen asynchrony during weaning trials is associated with the electromyographic power spectral alterations which accompany fatigue [39]. Moreover, Roussos et al. observed that normal subjects who were made to inspire through severe flow-resistive loads exhibited rhythmic alternation in the contribution of the diaphragm and the neck-rib cage inspiratory muscles [40]. Subsequently, Tobin et al. showed that chest-abdomen asynchrony during weaning or inspiratory flow-resistive loading is a response to the increased ventilatory load [41], but it does not necessarily imply that the inspiratory muscles have become fatigued.

Hyperinflation and excessive use of the neck inspiratory muscles are also associated with dyspnea and tachypnea in COPD [29, 42]. This is related to dynamic compression of the airways [43]. Tachypnea contributes to hyperinflation because the increased respiratory rate causes a new inspiration to start before the respiratory system can achieve its relaxation volume at the end of the preceding expiration. Thus, there is a dynamic as well as a passive component to the hyperinflation, which indicates that expiratory flow limitation increases the workload of the inspiratory muscles.

The pattern of spontaneous breathing chosen by COPD patients is one that minimizes dyspnea. Bellemare and Grassino [28] found that patients with COPD had a high but non-fatiguing level of the pressure-time index (PTI) at rest. When these patients were encouraged to breathe slowly and deeply, the PTI increased to potentially fatiguing levels. When Pbreath of other COPD patients was increased by external inspiratory flow-resistive loads or acute bronchoconstriction, they experienced dyspnea, a reduction in VT and CO_2 retention [31]. There was a significant inverse relationship between the size of VT and the degree of CO_2 retention.

Weakness and ventilatory failure. In patients with COPD, inspiratory muscle weakness without expiratory muscle weakness can be explained by the mechanical disadvantage alone [30]. When the expiratory muscles are involved, it is a sign of generalized muscle weakness, and PImax is much lower than can be explained by mechanical disadvantage alone. In any case, when PImax is less than 50% of normal, there is a significant inverse relationship between $PaCO_2$ and PImax [30]. The relationship between $PaCO_2$ and PImax in COPD patients parallels that seen in patients with proximal myopathies [23], but at any level of PImax, $PaCO_2$ is higher in patients with COPD. Not surprisingly, the most severe respiratory muscle weakness is found in COPD patients with acute respiratory failure [21, 44–46].

Respiratory muscle weakness contributes to ventilatory failure in kyphoscoliosis and obesity as well as in neuromuscular disease and COPD. Lisboa et al. [47] found an inverse relationship between PImax and $PaCO_2$ in patients with kyphoscoliosis, that was similar to that in patients with COPD [30]. The $PaCO_2$ was correlated with respiratory system elastance and age [48], but not with the angle of the kyphoscoliosis [47, 48]. The development of chronic hypercapnia in the older patients is consistent with slowly developing muscle weakness. In the OHS, respiratory muscle weakness also appears to contribute to CO_2 retention. Respiratory muscle strength was 63% normal in patients with OHS, as compared with 108% predicted in simple obesity [49], and CO_2 retention was manifest when the respiratory muscle strength was less than 70% predicted.

Fatigue and ventilatory failure. In order for normal subjects to develop inspiratory muscle fatigue, they must maintain a fixed, fatiguing pattern of breathing [7]. Prior to the onset of overt fatigue, manifestations of altered contractility are apparent, including changes in the electromyogram power spectrum (decrease in centroid frequency or fall in High/Low ratio) and slowing of relaxation [50]. This kind of inspiratory muscle or diaphragmatic fatigue has no effect on the breathing pattern of normal subjects [51].

Patients with COPD can also be made to adopt a fatiguing pattern of breathing [28], but this is not their spontaneous pattern of breathing. Moreover, overt inspiratory muscle fatigue was present in less than 10% of patients with severe lung disease who were admitted to hospital because of breathlessness [52]. These findings are evidence against the hypothesis that ventilatory failure is caused by respiratory muscle fatigue.

Additional evidence comes from studies of patients during attempts to wean from mechanical ventilation. Patients who fail weaning trials often exhibit the fall in the electromyographic High/Low ratio [39, 53] as well as asynchronous movements of the chest, abdomen or diaphragm [38, 39, 44]. A reduction in maximal inspiratory or transdiaphragmatic pressure [44] may reflect a reduction in ventilatory drive [54], rather than fatigue. Since the electromyographic phenomena and chest-abdomen asynchrony precede overt fatigue [41, 50], perhaps these findings should be interpreted to mean that patients who are failing weaning trials are in a potentially fatiguing pattern of breathing, rather than experiencing overt inspiratory muscle fatigue.

In like fashion, severe inspiratory flow resistive loading alone does not cause diaphragmatic fatigue in the spontaneously breathing animal, even after ventilatory failure has occurred [55, 56]. Diaphragmatic fatigue can be induced in experimental animals, but it requires a combination of inspiratory flow-resistive loading, abdominal binding and/or stimulation of the phrenic nerves [56]. With such strenuous interventions, there is also biochemical evidence of diaphragmatic fatigue, including glycogen depletion and lactate accumulation in the muscle tissue, which are not seen with flow-resistive loading alone.

Control of Breathing

Typical values for indices of ventilatory drive and timing, in disorders which predispose to ventilatory failure and in normal subjects, are summarized in Table 5. Drive is normal in eucapnic obese patients [57, 58] and patients with neuromuscular disease [59]. By way of contrast, ventilatory drive is about twice normal in chronic obstructive pulmonary disease (COPD), and it is even higher in the presence of hypercapnia [26, 60–64]. The increase in drive is most evident in the P0.1, with VT/Ti increasing only slightly because of the impedance to flow [26]. By far the highest values of P0.1 are found in acute respiratory failure. It should be noted that these data are from COPD patients [44, 45, 53, 65] and might not apply to other patients in acute respiratory failure from other causes such as muscle weakness alone or restrictive chest wall disease.

Ti/Ttot is normal in neuromuscular disease, eucapnic obese patients, and eucapnic COPD patients (Table 5). However, in COPD patients who are chronically hypercapnic or in acute respiratory failure, Ti/Ttot falls by 10–15%. This partly offsets the increase in Pbreath consequent to elevated airway resistance and/or lowered compliance. That is, the reduction in Ti/Ttot prevents the pressure-time index from rising too high, and thereby minimizes the probability of inspiratory muscle fatigue.

Table 5. Ventilatory timing and drive

Group*	Ti/Ttot	VT/Ti (ml/sec)	P0.1 (cm H_2O)	P0.1/(VT/Ti) (cm H_2O/l/sec)
NL	0.41	330	1.3	2.9
OB	0.39	490	1.9	3.9
NMD	0.43	325	1.5	4.6
COPD EC	0.37	530	3.8	6.9
COPD HC	0.35	500	4.0	7.0
COPD ARF	0.34	540	7.2	13.5

* *NL* = Normal Subjects [13–16, 26, 60], *OB* = Obesity [57, 58], *NMD* = Neuromuscular Disease [59], *COPD* = Chronic Obstructive Pulmonary Disease [26, 60–64]. *EC* = Eucapnic, *HC* = Chronically Hypercapnic, *ARF* = Acute Respiratory Failure [44, 45, 52, 64].

The Pattern of Breathing and Efficiency of Gas Exchange

Pattern of spontaneous breathing. The spontaneous breathing patterns of normal subjects and patients with obesity, kyphoscoliosis, COPD and acute respiratory failure are summarized in Table 6. f, VT and VE are normal in the eucapnic patients with obesity or COPD. In patients with neuromuscular disease and kyphoscoliosis, f is higher and VT is lower than in normal subjects. Note that hypercapnic patients with kyphoscoliosis or COPD exhibit higher respiratory rates and smaller tidal volumes than their eucapnic peers, but that the reciprocal changes in f and VT operate to maintain VE approximately the same in eucapnic and hypercapnic patients.

Efficiency of gas exchange. The efficiency of gas exchange is summarized in Table 7. The hypothetical level of minute ventilation needed to achieve a $PaCO_2$ of 40 torr (VE40) is elevated in all COPD patients. In both kyphoscoliosis and COPD, VE40 is higher in the hypercapnic patients than in the eucapnic patients. By relating

Table 6. The pattern of breathing

Group*	$PaCO_2$ (torr)	f (br/min)	VT (ml)	VT (ml/kg)	VE (l/min)
NL	38	15.7	490	7.9	7.8
OB	37	15.8	730	5.6	11.4
NMD	43	23.4	360	6.0	8.4
KS EC	39	16.6	430	9.3	6.5
KS HC	52	21.6	300	6.0	6.5
COPD EC	40	17.8	660	10.3	11.3
COPD HC	50	20.9	540	8.5	10.8
COPD ARF	54	27.9	410	6.3	11.3

* KS = Kyphoscoliosis [47, 48]. Other groups as in Table 5.

Table 7. The efficiency of gas exchange

Group	VE40* (l/min)	VE40* (ml/kg/min)	RR40* (br/min)
NL	7.8	110	14.0
OB	10.7	80	14.6
NMD	9.0	150	25.0
KS EC	6.3	140	16.1
KS HC	8.4	160	28.2
COPD EC	11.2	170	16.9
COPD HC	13.4	210	25.1
COPD ARF	15.2	240	37.8

* VE40 and RR40 are the minute ventilation and respiratory rate, respectively, needed to attain a $PaCO_2$ of 40 torr, given VD, CO_2 production and size of the spontaneous tidal volume. Groups as in Table 5.

VE40 to body weight, one can see that VE40 is elevated in kyphoscoliosis as well as COPD, reflecting the documented increases in VD/VT in these disorders [48, 61]. Owing to the severe ventilation-perfusion mismatch, VE40/kg is more than twice normal in acutely and chronically hypercapnic COPD patients.

Perhaps the best way to assess overall gas exchange is to utilize RR40, which is the respiratory rate needed to achieve a $PaCO_2$ of 40 torr, given the size of the spontaneous VT, VD and CO_2 production. The RR40 is normal in obesity and in eucapnic patients with kyphoscoliosis or COPD. However, RR40 is twice normal in patients with neuromuscular disease, and in hypercapnic patients with kyphoscoliosis or COPD. The increase in RR40 is the result of an increase in VD/VT, largely because of the small VT in neuromuscular disease and kyphoscoliosis, and because of the ventilation-perfusion imbalance in COPD. The highest values of RR40 are found in COPD patients with acute respiratory failure, in part because gas exchange is worse, and in part because VT is smaller.

Summary of Patient Data

Hypercapnic patients with COPD are more dyspneic, and they exhibit rapid, shallow breathing. Dyspnea and tachypnea are frequently accompanied by increased use of muscles in the upper airway, neck and abdomen, as well as asynchronous movements of the chest and abdomen. Hypercapnic COPD patients have a high ventilatory drive, a high inspiratory pressure-time index, weak inspiratory muscles and extremely inefficient gas exchange.

To some extent, these abnormalities are also present in kyphoscoliosis, obesity and neuromuscular disease. The pressure-time index (PTI) is increased in kyphoscoliosis and obesity, and gas exchange is inefficient in kyphoscoliosis. In neuromuscular disease Pbreath is normal, but PTI is high owing to severe muscle weakness. The efficiency of CO_2 gas exchange is near normal in obesity, kyphoscoliosis and neuromuscular disease, provided VT is well maintained. The one thing that hypercapnic patients with COPD, kyphoscoliosis, obesity and neuromuscular disease share in common is the rapid, shallow pattern of breathing.

Mechanism of the Reduction in Tidal Volume

Dyspnea and Ventilatory Load

In asthma and COPD, dyspnea and tachypnea may arise from several sources, including inflammation or dynamic compression of the airways, increased neural drive to the respiratory muscles, and an increase in the ratio Pbreath/PImax. Dyspnea consequent to an increase in Pbreath/PImax is also present in neuromuscular and thoracic restrictive diseases. In each case, the result is an increase in neural drive with concomitant alteration in timing.

Asthma and COPD impose a unique type of ventilatory load. Younes [66] has emphasized that the static properties of the respiratory system in COPD offer only modest increases in elastic and flow-resistive work. Thus, the principal effect of passive hyperinflation is the mechanical disadvantage to the diaphragm. However, a more important problem is dynamic hyperinflation which imposes additional elastic and threshold loads on the inspiratory muscles, while simultaneously making their mechanical disadvantage even worse. Computer modelling experiments suggest that dynamic hyperinflation increases with neural drive, and that it limits the tidal volume so that VE cannot be increased by increasing respiratory rate [66].

Interaction between Pressure-time Index and Gas Exchange

Recently, we studied patients recovering from acute respiratory failure, in an attempt to assess which variables might best define the ventilatory capacity needed to wean from mechanical ventilation [67]. We calculated a modified pressure-time index (PTI), based on ventilator pressure and VT, and the patient's spontaneous VT (VTsb). We estimated VE40 from VE and $PaCO_2$ measured during mechanical ventilation, and related VE40 to the pattern of spontaneous breathing, using the ratio VE40/VTsb to obtain RR40.

The results are summarized in Table 8. PImax was somewhat lower in patients who failed the weaning trial, but Pbreath was approximately the same in patients who failed as in patients who succeeded. As a result, Pbreath/PImax and PTI were somewhat higher in the weaning failure group. This group also had somewhat higher values of VE40 and f40. Neither PTI nor RR40 was useful as a predictive test, owing to the extensive overlap of values in patients who failed and those who succeeded in weaning. By way of contrast, a weaning index which was calculated as the product of PTI and RR40 clearly separated the two groups [67], and was 95% successful in predicting weaning failure (high weaning score) or weaning success (low weaning score).

We concluded from these observations that patients who failed weaning trials lowered their Pbreath and Pbreath/PImax by reducing their VT. The advantages of this response are minimization of dyspnea and less the potential for inspiratory muscle fatigue. The disadvantage is that the small VT predisposes to CO_2 retention, especially when VE40 is high.

Table 8. Data from weaning trials. (From [67])

Variable	Weaned	Not weaned
PImax (cm H_2O)	−49	−35
Pbreath (cm H_2O)	15	13
Pbreath/PImax	0.31	0.39
VE40 (ml/kg/min)	136	185
VTsb (ml/kg)	5.9	4.8
RR40 (breath/min)	25	42
Weaning index	16.0	7.1

Effects of Vagotomy Plus Inspiratory Resistive Load

The results of a study in which ventilatory loading was combined with vagotomy [55] support the conclusions drawn from the weaning trials. When anesthetized dogs were made to inspire through a severe inspiratory flow-resistive load, their VT fell abruptly. The respiratory rate gradually increased so that VE was restored to control levels, but the animals became mildly hypercapnic. At this point, with the inspiratory resistance still in place, both vagus nerves were severed. This caused an abrupt fall in respiratory rate and an immediate large increase in tidal volume, and $PaCO_2$ returned to normal.

Ventilatory drive was increased in these animals, and there was no evidence of diaphragmatic fatigue. More importantly, the fact that the dogs were able to inspire a larger than normal VT through the inspiratory resistance after bilateral cervical vagotomy, indicates that the fall in tidal volume when the load was first applied was mediated by mechanisms other than inspiratory muscle failure. That is, the animals could inspire a normal or increased tidal volume, but would not.

Unifying Hypothesis

The common feature of ventilatory failure, regardless of the clinical setting, is the reduction in VT. This is partly due to dynamic mechanical limitation, especially in COPD. Yet in all the disorders that predispose to ventilatory failure, VT is reduced for other than purely mechanical reasons. The most likely candidate is the perception of dyspnea, effort or respiratory distress. Factors contributing to this sensation include ventilatory flow-resistive or elastic loads, mechanical disadvantage to inspiratory muscles and muscle weakness, in any combination that increases Pbreath/PImax.

The data from patients undergoing trials of weaning from mechanical ventilation are consistent with the results of the inspiratory resistive loading study in animals. That is, when Pbreath/PImax is too high, the response is to limit Pbreath by curtailing VT. Respiratory muscle weakness contributes significantly to the increase in Pbreath/PImax, but when patients or experimental animals breathe spontaneously, they seldom develop inspiratory muscle fatigue. When the efficiency of pulmonary gas exchange is near normal, as in neuromuscular disease, the small tidal volume is well tolerated, but when the efficiency of gas exchange is abnormal, as in COPD, even modest reductions in tidal volume lead to CO_2 retention.

Conclusion

The pathogenesis of ventilatory failure has therapeutic implications. Obviously, airway inflammation and bronchospasm should be treated optimally. In addition, when inspiratory muscle weakness major contributes to the sense of respiratory distress, then everything possible should be done to improve respiratory muscle function. Training regimens should be devised which focus on increasing the shortening capacity of the inspiratory muscles, as well as their strength and endurance.

It might even be advantageous to include biofeedback techniques to help suppress unpleasant respiratory sensation. In any case, it is worth exploring ways to shift from a "won't do" to a "can do" mode of breathing in ventilatory failure.

References

1. Braun NMT, Arora NS, Rochester DF (1982) The force-length relationship of the normal human diaphragm. J Appl Physiol 53:405–412
2. Farkas GA, Decramer M, Rochester DF, De Troyer A (1985) Contractile properties of intercostal muscles and their functional significance. J Appl Physiol 59:528–535
3. De Troyer A, Estenne M (1988) Functional anatomy of the respiratory muscles. Clin Chest Med 9:175–193
4. Rochester DF, Farkas GA, Lu J-Y (1987) Contractility of the in situ human diaphragm: assessment based on dimensional analysis. In: Sieck GS, Gandevia SC, Cameron WE (eds) Respiratory muscles and their neuromotor control. Neurology and Neurobiology, Vol. 26, Alan R. Liss, New York, pp 327–336
5. Druz WS, Sharp JT (1981) Activity of the respiratory muscles in upright and recumbent humans. J Appl Physiol 51:1552–1561
6. Collett PW, Perry C, Engel LA (1985) Pressure-time product, flow and oxygen cost of resistive breathing in humans. J Appl Physiol 58:1263–1272
7. Bellemare F, Grassino A (1982) Effect of pressure and timing on human diaphragm fatigue. J Appl Physiol 53:1190–1195
8. Killian KJ, Jones NL (1988) Respiratory muscles and dyspnea. Clin Chest Med 9:237–248
9. Von Euler C (1983) On the central pattern generator for the basic breathing rhythmicity. J Appl Physiol 55:1647–1659
10. Sears TA (1990) Central rhythm and pattern generation. Chest 97:45S–51S
11. Cherniack NS (1990) The central nervous system and respiratory muscle coordination. Chest 97:52S–57S
12. Milic-Emili J, Grassino AE, Whitelaw WA (1981) Measurement and Testing of Respiratory Drive. In: Hornbein TF (ed) Regulation of breathing, Vol. 17, Lung Biology in Health and Disease, Lenfant C (ed), Marcel Dekker, New York, pp 675–743
13. Gilbert R, Auchincloss JH Jr, Brodsky J, Boden W (1972) Changes in tidal volume, frequency and ventilation induced by their measurement. J Appl Physiol 33:252–254
14. Hirsch JA, Bishop B (1982) Human breathing patterns on mouthpiece or face mask during air, CO_2 or low O_2. J Appl Physiol 53:1281–1290
15. Tobin MJ, Chadha TS, Jenouri G, Birch SJ, Gazeroglu HB, Sackner MA (1983) Breathing patterns 1. Normal subjects. Chest 84:202–205
16. Loveridge B, West P, Anthonisen NR, Kryger MH (1984) Breathing patterns in patients with chronic obstructive pulmonary disease. Am Rev Respir Dis 130:730–733
17. Hussain SNA, Sinkus G, Roussos C (1985) Respiratory muscle fatigue: a cause of ventilatory failure in septic shock. J Appl Physiol 58:1802–1808
18. Boczkowski J, Dureuil B, Branger C, et al (1988) Effects of sepsis on diaphragmatic function in rats. Am Rev Respir Dis 138:260–265
19. Drew JS, Farkas GA, Pearson RD, Rochester DF (1988) Effects of a chronic wasting infection on skeletal muscle size and contractile properties. J Appl Physiol 64:460–465
20. Kelly SM, Rosa A, Field S, Coughlin M, Shizgal HM, Macklem PT (1984) Inspiratory muscle strength and body composition in patients receiving total parenteral nutrition therapy. Am Rev Respir Dis 130:33–37
21. Aubier M, Murciano D, Lecocguic Y, et al (1985) Effect of hypophosphatemia on diaphragmatic contractility in patients with acute respiratory failure. N Engl J Med 313:420–424
22. Janssens S, Decramer M (1989) Corticosteroid-induced myopathy and the respiratory muscles. Report of two cases. Chest 95:1160–1162
23. Braun NMT, Arora NS, Rochester DF (1983) Respiratory muscle and pulmonary function in polymyositis and other proximal myopathies. Thorax 38:616–623

24. Goldring RM, Turino GM, Heinemann HO (1971) Respiratory-renal adjustments in chronic hypercapnia in man. Am J Med 51:772–784
25. Wolkove N, Altose MD, Kelsen SG, Cherniack NS (1980) Respiratory control abnormalities in alveolar hypoventilation. Am Rev Respir Dis 122:163–167
26. Gorini M, Spinelli A, Ginanni R, Duranti R, Gigliotti F, Scano G (1990) Neural respiratory drive and neuromuscular coupling in patients with chronic obstructive pulmonary disease (COPD). Chest 98:1179–1186
27. Decramer M, Demedts M, Rochette F, Billiet L (1980) Maximal respiratory pressures in obstructive lung disease. Bull Europ Physiopath Resp 16:479–490
28. Bellemare F, Grassino A (1983) Force reserve of the diaphragm in patients with chronic obstructive pulmonary disease. J Appl Physiol 55:8–15
29. O'Neill S, McCarthy DS (1983) Postural relief of dyspnoea in severe chronic airflow limitation: relationship to respiratory muscle strength. Thorax 38:595–600
30. Rochester DF, Braun NMT (1985) Determinants of maximal inspiratory pressure in chronic obstructive pulmonary disease. Am Rev Respir Dis 132:42–47
31. Oliven A, Kelsen SG, Deal EC Jr, Cherniack NS (1985) Respiratory pressure sensation. Relationship to changes in breathing pattern and PCO_2 during acute increase in airway resistance in patients with chronic obstructive pulmonary disease. Am Rev Respir Dis 132:1214–1218
32. Martinez FJ, Couser JI, Celli BR (1990) Factors influencing ventilatory muscle recruitment in patients with chronic airflow obstruction. Am Rev Respir Dis 142:276–282
33. Oliven A, Supinski GS, Kelsen SG (1986) Functional adaptation of diaphragm to chronic hyperinflation in emphysematous hamsters. J Appl Physiol 60:225–231
34. Similowski T, Yan S, Gauthier AP, Macklem PT, Bellemare F (1990) Contractile properties of the human diaphragm during chronic hyperinflation. Am Rev Respir Dis 141:A166
35. Supinski GS, Kelsen SG (1982) Effect of elastase-induced emphysema on the force-generating ability of the diaphragm. J Clin Invest 70:978–988
36. Farkas GA, Roussos C (1983) Diaphragm in emphysematous hamsters: sarcomere adaptability. J Appl Physiol 54:1635–1640
37. Sharp JT, Goldberg NB, Druz WS, Fishman HC, Danon J (1977) Thoracoabdominal motion in chronic obstructive pulmonary disease. Am Rev Respir Dis 115:47–56
38. Cohen C, Zagelbaum G, Gross D, Roussos C, Macklem PT (1982) Clinical manifestations of inspiratory muscle fatigue. Am J Med 73:308–316
39. Tobin MJ, Guenther SM, Perez W, et al (1987) Konno-Mead analysis of rib cage-abdominal motion during successful and unsuccessful trials of weaning from mechanical ventilation. Am Rev Respir Dis 135:1320–1328
40. Roussos C, Fixley M, Gross D, Macklem PT (1979) Fatigue of the inspiratory muscles and their synergic behaviour. J Appl Physiol 46:897–904
41. Tobin MJ, Perez W, Guenther SM, Lodato RF, Dantzker DR (1987) Does rib cage-abdominal paradox signify respiratory muscle fatigue? J Appl Physiol 63:851–860
42. Ward ME, Eidelman D, Stubbing DG, Bellemare F, Macklem PT (1988) Respiratory sensation and pattern of respiratory muscle activation during diaphragm fatigue. J Appl Physiol 65:2181–2189
43. O'Donnell DE, Sanii R, Anthonisen NR, Younes M (1987) Effect of dynamic airway compression on breathing pattern and respiratory sensation in severe chronic obstructive pulmonary disease. Am Rev Respir Dis 135:912–918
44. Pourriat JL, Lamberto C, Hoang PH, Fournier JL, Vasseur B (1986) Diaphragmatic fatigue and breathing pattern during weaning from mechanical ventilation in COPD patients. Chest 90:703–707
45. Sassoon CSH, Te TT, Mahutte CK, Light RW (1987 Airway occlusion pressure. An important indicator for successful weaning in patients with chronic obstructive pulmonary disease. Am Rev Respir Dis 135:107–113
46. Tobin MJ, Perez W, Guenther SM, et al (1986) The pattern of breathing during successful and unsuccessful trials of weaning from mechanical ventilation. Am Rev Respir Dis 134:1111–1118
47. Lisboa C, Moreno R, Fava M, Ferretti R, Cruz E (1985) Inspiratory muscle function in patients with severe kyphoscoliosis. Am Rev Respir Dis 132:48–52

48. Kafer ER (1976) Idiopathic scoliosis. Gas exchange and the age dependence of arterial blood gases. J Clin Invest 58:825–833
49. Arora NS, Rochester DF (1979) Respiratory muscle function in obesity and obesity-hypoventilation syndrome. Clin Research 27:394
50. Esau SA, Bellemare F, Grassino A, Permutt S, Roussos C, Pardy RL (1983) Changes in relaxation rate with diaphragmatic fatigue in humans. J Appl Physiol 54:1353–1360
51. Mador MJ, Acevedo FA (1991) Effect of inspiratory muscle fatigue on breathing pattern during inspiratory resistive loading. J Appl Physiol 70:1627–1632
52. Efthimiou J, Fleming J, Spiro SG (1987) Sternocleidomastoid muscle function and fatigue in breathless patients with severe respiratory disease. Am Rev Respir Dis 136:1099–1105
53. Murciano D, Boczkowski J, Lecocguic Y, Milic Emili J, Pariente R, Aubier M (1988) Tracheal occlusion pressure: A simple index to monitor respiratory muscle fatigue during acute respiratory failure in patients with chronic obstructive pulmonary disease. Ann Intern Med 108:800–805
54. Truwit JD, Lamb VJ, Marini JJ (1989) Validation of a technique to assess maximal inspiratory pressure in poorly cooperative patients. Am Rev Respir Dis 139:A98
55. Adams JM, Farkas GA, Rochester DF (1988) Vagal afferents, diaphragm fatigue and inspiratory resistance in the anesthetized dog. J Appl Physiol 64:2279–2286
56. Ferguson GT, Irvin CG, Cherniack RM (1990) Relationship of diaphragm glycogen, lactate, and function to respiratory failure. Am Rev Respir Dis 141:926–932
57. Sampson MG, Grassino A (1983) Neuromechanical properties in obese patients during carbon dioxide rebreathing. Am J Med 75:81–90
58. Burki NK, Baker RW (1984) Ventilatory regulation in eucapnic morbid obesity. Am Rev Respir Dis 129:538–543
59. Baydur A (1991) Respiratory muscle strength and control of ventilation in patients with neuromuscular disease. Chest 99:330–338
60. Sorli J, Grassino A, Lorange B, Milic-Emili J (1978) Control of breathing in patients with chronic obstructive lung disease. Clin Sci Molec Med 54:295–304
61. Javaheri S, Blum J, Kazemi H (1981) Pattern of breathing and carbon dioxide retention in chronic obstructive lung disease. Am J Med 71:228–234
62. Parot S, Miara B, Milic-Emili J, Gautier H (1982) Hypoxemia, hypercapnia and breathing pattern in patients with chronic obstructive pulmonary disease. Am Rev Respir Dis 126:882–886
63. Tobin MJ, Chadha TS, Jenouri G, Birch SJ, Gazeroglu HB, Sackner MA (1983) Breathing patterns 2. Diseased subjects. Chest 84:286–294
64. Loveridge B, West P, Kryger MH, Anthonisen NR (1986) Alteration in breathing pattern with progression of chronic obstructive pulmonary disease. Am Rev Respir Dis 134:930–934
65. Aubier M, Murciano D, Fournier M, Milic-Emili J, Pariente R, Derenne JP (1980) Central respiratory drive in acute respiratory failure of patients with chronic obstructive pulmonary disease. Am Rev Respir Dis 122:191–199
66. Younes M (1990) Load responses, dyspnea and respiratory failure. Chest 97:59S–68S
67. Jabour ER, Rabil DM, Truwit JD, Rochester DF (1991) Evaluation of a new weaning index, based on inspiratory effort, gas exchange, and tidal volume. Am Rev Respir Dis (in press)

Extrapulmonary and Intrapulmonary Determinants of Pulmonary Gas Exchange

R. Rodriguez-Roisin, J. Roca, and J.A. Barbera

Introduction

In order to best manage patients with respiratory failure in both the intensive and the medical care setting, proper assessment of pulmonary gas exchange is crucial. Arterial blood respiratory gases (O_2 and CO_2) and acid-base status are the directly measurable variables used by most clinicians for this purpose. However, while respiratory gases have become increasingly easy to obtain in recent years, their interpretation has become also progressively more difficult, especially in the intensive care setting. This is because of deepening awareness that factors other than intrapulmonary abnormalities can alter arterial PO_2 and PCO_2. Ideally, it would be of great practical interest to clinicians to handle respiratory blood gas measurements as an index of the state of the lungs, such that improved or impaired results could be equated to improve or impair lung function, respectively. The situation is that arterial PO_2 and PCO_2 reflect not only the state of the lung, at least as a gas exchanger, and thereby their intrapulmonary determinants (i.e. ventilation-perfusion ($\dot{V}_A/\dot{Q}$) mismatch, intrapulmonary shunt and alveolar-end-capillary diffusion limitation for oxygen) but also the conditions under which the lung is operating, namely the composition of inspired gas and mixed venous blood, i.e. their extrapulmonary factors.

This chapter will focus essentially on the pathophysiologic determinants of arterial PO_2 and PCO_2 in the light of the results obtained with the multiple inert gas elimination technique, in order to provide a solid framework for the proper interpretation of the interplay of the extra- and intrapulmonary factors determining respiratory gases. This analysis is exclusively addressed to conditions characterized by hypercapnic respiratory failure, henceforth called *ventilatory failure,* more specifically caused by chronic obstructive pulmonary disease (COPD).

Physiological Background

Table 1 shows the three intrapulmonary factors that may contribute individually or combinedly to hypoxemia and hypercapnia as well as the nine extrapulmonary factors that, either directly or indirectly (through their effect on mixed venous oxygen tension ($P\bar{v}O_2$)), can also influence arterial PO_2 and $PaCO_2$. It is important here to emphasize the key role of $P\bar{v}O_2$ and how extrapulmonary factors (other than inspired PO_2 and total ventilation) may contribute to reduce PaO_2 through the effects on $P\bar{v}O_2$. In this regard, a diminished $P\bar{v}O_2$ may result from a low cardiac output, an increased oxygen uptake, and/or a decreased blood oxygen content due to several alterations in the principal factors modulating the oxyhemoglobin dissociation curve [1].

Factors Governing PO_2

The most prominent clinical intrapulmonary factor determining the pathophysiology of hypoxemia in ventilatory failure caused by COPD is undoubtedly abnormal $\dot{V}_A/\dot{Q}$ relationships [2, 3]. Although shunt may also have some relevance in modulating hypoxemia, particularly when COPD patients suffer from acute respiratory failure and have retained secretions and abundant mucus plugging [4] or when there is a reopening of *foramen ovale,* its amount is by and large small [2, 3]. By contrast, the role played by diffusion limitation for oxygen in COPD is almost negligible [5].

The PO_2 and PCO_2 values in any alveolar unit and hence the end-capillary PO_2 and PCO_2 of each lung are basically determined by the composition of the inspired gas, the composition of mixed venous blood and, even more importantly, by the ratio of gas flow (ventilation) to blood flow (perfusion) ($\dot{V}_A/\dot{Q}$) of the unit. The $\dot{V}_A/\dot{Q}$ ratio may vary from completely unventilated but perfused units (0 = shunt) to completely unperfused but ventilated units (∞ = dead space). While breathing room air, lung units with very low $\dot{V}_A/\dot{Q}$ ratios (not completely unventilated) have alveolar gas tensions very close to mixed venous blood values such that they behave very similarly to shunt from a gas exchange standpoint. As the $\dot{V}_A/\dot{Q}$ ratio increases above 0.1, while end-capillary PO_2 increases rapidly, $PaCO_2$ also falls rapidly. Arterial blood saturates fully approaching the $\dot{V}_A/\dot{Q}$ ratio of 1.0, but it is of note that once the $\dot{V}_A/\dot{Q}$ ratio is above 1.0, the end-capillary PO_2 increases progressively as long as the $\dot{V}_A/\dot{Q}$ ratios increase until reaching inspired gas levels. However, this has little effect on the transfer of O_2 due to the alinear (sigmoid) shape of the oxyhemoglobin dissociation curve. Likewise, the $PaCO_2$ will approach the inspired gas composition as long as the $\dot{V}_A/\dot{Q}$ ratios continue to increase. Because of the more linear characteristics of the CO_2 hemoglobin dissociation curve, the lung units with high $\dot{V}_A/\dot{Q}$ ratios will continue to be progressively useful for CO_2 output. The distributions of $\dot{V}_A/\dot{Q}$ ratios are crucial in determining the levels of PaO_2 and $PaCO_2$. Thus, in the presence of acute or chronic pulmonary disease, $\dot{V}_A/\dot{Q}$ distributions use to become markedly abnormal such that it is common to see areas of low and/or high $\dot{V}_A/\dot{Q}$ ratios and different patterns of $\dot{V}_A/\dot{Q}$ distributions (bimodal bloodflow and/or ventilation distributions) [1].

During acute exacerbation of COPD, several abnormal $\dot{V}_A/\dot{Q}$ distributions have been documented [3]. These are, however, qualitatively similar to what is seen in less severe clinical forms of COPD [2]. Not uncommonly, a combined bimodal pattern including the bloodflow distribution and also the ventilation distribution may be one of the most representative $\dot{V}_A/\dot{Q}$ abnormalities. This means that a large proportion of bloodflow is perfusing lung units with low or very low $\dot{V}_A/\dot{Q}$ ratios; likewise, a large proportion of ventilation is diverted to lung units with high or very high $\dot{V}_A/\dot{Q}$ ratios. In other occasions, however, COPD patients show a bimodal blood flow distribution together with a broadly unimodal ventilation curve; and *vice versa,* the bimodal pattern is disclosed sometimes at the level of the alveolar ventilation distribution alone, whereas the bloodflow pattern is abnormally broader only. Units with low $\dot{V}_A/\dot{Q}$ ratios are likely to represent regions subtended by airways partially blocked by mucus secretions, smooth muscle hypertrophy, bronchospasm, distortion or some combination of these abnormalities. By contrast, lung units with high $\dot{V}_A/\dot{Q}$ ratios are likely produced by continued ventilation of regions of alveolar destruction, which presumably greatly reduce blood flow in these areas, hence leading to units with high $\dot{V}_A/\dot{Q}$ ratios. Conceivably, they represent emphysematous regions where destruction of the alveolar walls results in the loss of the vascular cross-sectional areas [2]. Alternatively, it is considered that the relative small amounts of shunt are due to the efficiency of collateral ventilation in maintaining alveolar ventilation beyond obstructed airways.

Among the extrapulmonary factors determining arterial PO_2, the most relevant from the clinical standpoint (in *italics* in Table 1) are inspired PO_2, total (overall) ventilation, cardiac output (CO) and oxygen uptake. Total (overall) ventilation is considered an extrapulmonary factor because it is primarily the result of tidal volume (less series dead space – dead space common to more than one $\dot{V}_A/\dot{Q}$ unit –) times frequency, which are set by extrapulmonary breathing control mechanisms [1]. Although important from a physiological viewpoint, hemoglobin concentration, body temperature, acid-base status and position of the oxyhemoglobin dissociation curve (e.g. a characterized by P_{50}) do less influence PaO_2.

Regarding the effects of inspired O_2 fraction in the presence of $\dot{V}_A/\dot{Q}$ mismatching, arterial PO_2 is very sensitive to this extrapulmonary factor as opposed to the situation where shunt is the predominant mechanism of hypoxemia [6]. In fact, inspired PO_2 is very little effective to increasing the alveolar PO_2 of lung units with very low $\dot{V}_A/\dot{Q}$ ratios (although not completely unventilated) such that substantial levels of inspired oxygen fraction are needed to improve PaO_2. Thus, it has been shown that fully saturating PaO_2 in the presence of moderate to severe $\dot{V}_A/\dot{Q}$ abnormalities requires to increase FiO_2.

By using multicompartments lung model, West [7] was able to show that increases in overall ventilation have a powerful effect on gas exchange when $\dot{V}_A/\dot{Q}$ distributions are normal, PaO_2 increasing and $PaCO_2$ decreasing. However, when

Table 1. Factors modulating PO_2 and PCO_2

Intrapulmonary	Extrapulmonary
1) *Ventilation-perfusion mismatching**	1) *Inspired oxygen fraction*
2) *Intrapulmonary shunt*	2) *Overall ventilation*
3) Alveolar – endcapillary diffusion limitation	3) *Cardiac output*
	4) *Oxygen uptake*
	5) Hemoglobin
	6) Temperature
	7) Acid-base Status
	8) P_{50}
	9) Carbon dioxide production

* In *italics*: the most relevant

$\dot{V}_A/\dot{Q}$ distributions are abnormal, this is usually accompanied by an increase in $PaCO_2$ (other factors being equal) which is rapidly brought down to normal values by an increase in ventilation. Interestingly, PaO_2 also increases with further increases in ventilation, although when $\dot{V}_A/\dot{Q}$ distributions are impaired, normal values cannot be regained easily. Yet, with further increases in ventilation, there is little effect on the PO_2. Since increasing $\dot{V}_A/\dot{Q}$ mismatch reduces the transfer of O_2 and CO_2, it might be expected that this situation will lead always to both hypoxemia and hypercapnia. However, small increases in $PaCO_2$ may activate chemoreceptor, thus causing hyperventilation as long as the ventilatory system works appropriately and the patient is able to respond. This increased ventilation distributed to well ventilated areas will increase their $\dot{V}_A/\dot{Q}$ ratios causing a raise in end-capillary PO_2 and a fall in PCO_2. When the ability to increase ventilation is exceeded by the degree of $\dot{V}_A/\dot{Q}$ mismatching, there is an increase in $PaCO_2$. Maintaining a relatively increased minute ventilation effectively prevents simultaneous increases in the levels of $PaCO_2$ provided that there is no parallel increase in the work of breathing [8]. In patients who cannot maintain a high rate of ventilation due to the increased work of breathing, and in those whose respiratory drive increases slightly when $PaCO_2$ is high, hypercapnia can ensue.

There are three potential ways in which CO may influence pulmonary gas exchange [9]. The most influential one is through the effect on the O_2 content of the mixed venous blood. This may occur directly through changes in CO and its effect on arterial-venous O_2 difference, by failure of the cardiovascular system (cardiac output) to respond to changes in O_2 delivery (CO x arterial O_2 content) with reduction in the extraction fraction of oxygen (O_2 consumption/O_2 delivery). A second way in which CO may alter pulmonary gas exchange is by modifying the transit time of the red blood cell spent in the pulmonary capillary. If CO increases, then the transit time decreases, such that abnormal gas exchange due to incomplete alveolar end-capillary equilibration may, at least in theory, occur. However, this is only possible when there is a combined diffusion limitation for oxygen, as it happens in idopathic pulmonary fibrosis not only during exercise but also under resting conditions [10]. A third way by which CO may alter pulmonary gas exchange is by redistributing pulmonary bloodflow within the lungs. Alterations in bloodflow may be achieved by different ways. One way is through the well-known, although poorly understood, positive association between intrapulmonary shunt and CO, such that shunt fraction increases when CO raises, and *vice versa* [11, 12]. Another way may also be acheived by modification in the pulmonary vascular tone. The latter is basically sensed by the levels of alveolar oxygen tension, the major determinant of pulmonary vascular resistance. However, $P\bar{v}O_2$ may also play a key role influencing pulmonary vascular tone through an, as yet, undetermined pathway [13, 14]. Finally, increases and decreases in intracardiac and intrapulmonary artery pressures may also lead to redistribution of pulmonary blood flow [9].

Changes in oxygen consumption may represent another way of modulating the levels of PaO_2. By using a lung model essentially characterized by $\dot{V}_A/\dot{Q}$ mismatching, Wagner [15] has shown that changes in oxygen utilization have marked effects on PaO_2. Thus, a 10% change in O_2 uptake can alter PaO_2 by 10 mm Hg in either direction. This is in contrast with what happens when the major mechanism of hypoxemia is intrapulmonary shunt, where arterial PO_2 is less more sensitive to a change in oxygen uptake. This is explained by the shape of the oxyhemoglobin dissociation curve. Thus, when PaO_2 lies on the flat (top) part of the oxyhemoglobin curve, as it happens under the conditions of $\dot{V}_A/\dot{Q}$ inequality, changes in PaO_2 are much larger than when it falls in the steep part of the curve, where the effects on PaO_2 are more reduced.

Factors Modulating PCO_2

From a clinical standpoint, three major factors can modulate the levels of $PaCO_2$ (Table 1). One corresponds to an intrapulmonary factor, i.e. $\dot{V}_A/\dot{Q}$ inequality, already alluded to above. The other three are extrapulmonary factors, namely overall ventilation, changes in acid-base status and carbon dioxide production [16].

Among alterations in overall ventilation, abnormalities in respiratory mechanics, namely respiratory muscle fatigue, abnormal neuromuscular function and/or structural changes in the chest wall, and changes in the control of ventilation, emerge as the two major extrapulmonary factors. Changes in overall ventilation may be produced by quantitative or qualitative abnormalities in the breathing pattern, increases in dead space, or both. A decrease in alveolar ventilation is always associated with an increase in $PaCO_2$. Hypercapnia due to metabolic alkalosis can be also contemplated, to some extent, as a condition which is accompanied by a depression in the ventilatory control system with normal lungs. Finally, changes in the metabolic rate (CO_2 output) due to alterations in the level of activity, fever, disease or carbohydrate metabolism (for instance, high glucose loads during parenteral nutrition) may be major causes of hypercapnia. Usually, if the lungs are normal, ventilation increases simultaneously and, therefore, the retention of carbon dioxide is prevented. Patients with lung disorders, unable to increase appropriately their degree of ventilation, may show hypercapnia.

Methods for Measuring $\dot{V}_A/\dot{Q}$ Inequality

Topographical radioactive tracers have long been available to the clinician and are quite useful for specific clinical conditions (i.e. pulmonary embolism). Yet, their use in generalized pulmonary disease such as chronic obstructive pulmonary disease, usually underestimates the degree of $\dot{V}_A/\dot{Q}$ inequality actually present. Isotopic approaches only give relative $\dot{V}_A/\dot{Q}$ distribution because the global $\dot{V}_A/\dot{Q}$ relationship is assumed to be equal to one.

Alternatively, the respiratory gases are also too insensitive for accurate assessment of the degree of $\dot{V}_A/\dot{Q}$ mismatching actually present, hence leading to underestimation of the $\dot{V}_A/\dot{Q}$ inequality. Furthermore, the classical tools based upon these respiratory, physiologic gases such as venous admixture breathing room air ($\dot{Q}_S/\dot{Q}_T$) or 100% O_2 breathing (shunt), physiological dead space (V_D/V_T) or alveolar-arterial O_2 pressure difference ($AaPO_2$), are all "as if" indicators of the underlying degree of $\dot{V}_A/\dot{Q}$ heterogeneity. However, all these approaches are simple estimates based upon simple two-compartment models of the lung and yield very limited and simplified "as if" models of what must be very complex changes in disease [1, 17]. Consequently, they are difficult to interpret in terms of actual pulmonary pathophysiology. In addition, they are highly dependent upon the composition of mixed venous PO_2, only available if a pulmonary catheter is in place. Finally, all these variables are also very sensitive to the most determinant extrapulmonary factors (such as inspired PO_2, minute ventilation, CO or oxygen consumption). When one or more of these four parameters is altered, and this often happens in the clinical care setting, modifications in the variables will occur even if the intrapulmonary factors regulating respiratory blood gases remain essentially unchanged. West [7] has shown that while increases in overall ventilation will increase the physiological dead space and decrease the venous admixture, increases in total bloodflow have an opposite effect.

By contrast, the multiple inert gas elimination technique represents a major breakthrough in our understanding of the role of $\dot{V}_A/\dot{Q}$ inequality in pulmonary disease [18, 19]. This technique gives a detailed picture of distributions (quantities) of pulmonary perfusion and alveolar ventilation. And it does so without inflicting by itself perturbation to pulmonary circulation. It allows a more complete analysis of the changes induced by oxygen on the distribution of $\dot{V}_A/\dot{Q}$ ratios, since the tracer nature of the method does not alter pulmonary gas exchange.This should be contrasted with the more traditional approaches in which there is evidence that breathing high concentrations of inspired O_2 will either release hypoxic pulmonary vasoconstriction, or induce reabsorption atelectasis, or both [20–22]. The principles governing the inert gas approach are based on mass balance equations under steady state conditions for gas exchange in the lungs and the peripheral tissues [1]. According to this, it was shown that the uptake (retention) ($Pc'/P\bar{v}$) or elimination (or excretion) ($PA/P\bar{v}$) of an inert gas in any homogenous area of the lung is given by the following equation,

$$Pc'/P\bar{v} = PA/P\bar{v} = \lambda/(\lambda + \dot{V}_A/\dot{Q})$$

where Pc', $P\bar{v}$, and PA correspond to end-capillary, mixed venous and alveolar partial pressures, respectively, and λ to the blood gas partition coefficient or solubility.

After infusing 5% dextrose solution of a mixture of 6 gases into a peripheral vein at a rate of 3–5 ml/min for about 30 min to ensure an adequate steady-state, samples of arterial and mixed venous blood and mixed expired gas are simultaneously collected. If a pulmonary catheter is not in place, mixed venous inert gas levels can also be calculated by mass balance from arterial and mixed expired samples using the CO measured by indocyanine green. For each infused gas, the ratio of arterial to mixed venous concentration (or retention) or mixed expired to mixed venous concentration (or excretion) is calculated and retention-solubility and excretion-solubility curves are drawn, which are fingerprints of a particular distribution of pulmonary perfusion and of alveolar ventilation, respectively. These are the basic aspects of the methodology of the inert gas approach. Both distributions are unimodal, namely symmetrical, well centered about a $\dot{V}_A/\dot{Q}$ ratio of 1.0, and with little dispersion (narrowness) on each curve. With the latter, shunt (below a $\dot{V}_A/\dot{Q}$ ratio of 0.005) is absent in healthy individuals as the inert gas concentrations remain unaltered in both the bronchial and the besian veins; likewise, inert dead space (above a $\dot{V}_A/\dot{Q}$ ratio of 100) is also slightly lower than that traditionally measured with the Bohr's formula.

Clinical Implications

Influence of Cardiac Output and Ventilation

Torres et al. [23] studied $\dot{V}_A/\dot{Q}$ inequalities in 8 patients with COPD during mechanical ventilation and also during weaning (spontaneous breathing) from mechanical ventilation required for acute respiratory failure (Fig. 1). While there were no differences in most of the pulmonary and systemic hemodynamic parameters between the two conditions studied, CO increased significantly when patients were removed from the ventilator. Interestingly, while neither PaO_2 non $AaPO_2$ and venous admixture showed significant changes between the two conditions, both $P\bar{v}O_2$ and O_2 delivery increased significantly when patients were removed from mechanical ventilation. Oxygen uptake (calculated through the Fick principle) did not change. Another important finding at spontaneous breathing was that while minute ventilation remained essentially unchanged, respiratory frequency increased and tidal volume fell significantly. In other words, the efficiency of breathing fell such that $PaCO_2$ increased and pH decreased also significantly. Substantial alterations in low $\dot{V}_A/\dot{Q}$ areas (i.e. increase in the percentage of bloodflow to these regions) were shown during spontaneous ventilation. Moreover, both the dispersion of ventilation and one of the overall indices of $\dot{V}_A/\dot{Q}$ heterogeneity (so called, DISP R–E*)

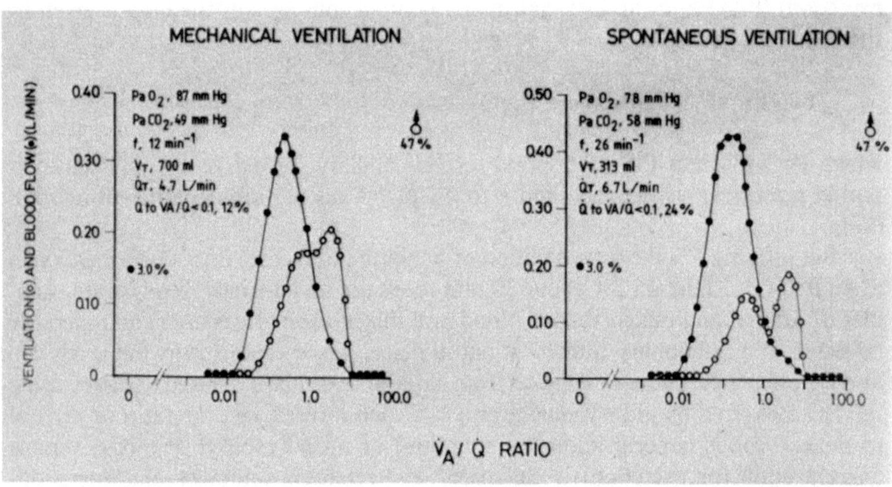

Fig. 1. $\dot{V}_A/\dot{Q}$ distributions (closed symbols = bloodflow; open symbols = alveolar ventilation) corresponding to Patient 7 from [23]. At mechanical ventilation *(left panel)*, both distributions were broadly unimodal, whereas following removal from ventilator *(right panel)* ventilation distribution was bimodal. Note that both the respiratory blood gases and the breathing pattern worsened, while cardiac output ($\dot{Q}_T$) and the amount of bloodflow to low $\dot{V}_A/\dot{Q}$ units (below 0.1) increased substantially. Shunt (closed circle alone, 3.0% of $\dot{Q}_T$) and dead space (open circle alone, 47% of $\dot{V}_E$) remained unchanged (From [23] with permission)

increased (worsened) significantly. The variable DISP R–E* is an overall index of heterogeneity of lung function and represents the combined dispersion of both bloodflow and ventilation distributions [24]. It corresponds to the root mean square difference between retentions (R) and excretions (E) after correcting for series dead space (using acetone data). By contrast, shunt, the dispersion of bloodflow, and inert dead space remained essentially unchanged.

These results show that patients with COPD, during spontaneous ventilation after removal from mechanical ventilation, further worsened $\dot{V}_A/\dot{Q}$ mismatch. This worsening can be explained by alterations in breathing pattern and also by changes in CO. It is of note that dispersion of pulmonary bloodflow did not increase despite the increase in perfusion observed in low $\dot{V}_A/\dot{Q}$ areas during spontaneous ventilation, since the $\dot{V}_A/\dot{Q}$ distributions shifted to the left because of a reduction in overall $\dot{V}_A/\dot{Q}$ ratio. Yet, neither the PaO_2 nor the $AaPO_2$ underwent major changes, indicating that respiratory blood gas measurements may not sufficiently reflect changes in $\dot{V}_A/\dot{Q}$ relationships because other factors, such as minute ventilation and CO were influencing pulmonary gas exchange in this clinical setting. Indeed, CO increased substantially after cessation of mechanical ventilation because of a concomitant increase in venous return. The importance of the latter and other hemodynamic changes has been stressed by Lemaire et al. [25] during unsuccessful weaning in patients with COPD. Additional factors contributing to respiratory weaning failure could be myocardial infarction and left ventricular failure, due to abrupt alterations in venous return. According to Permutt [26], an increase of gastric pressure during spontaneous ventilation with subsequent increased splanchnic flow could be also an additional pathogenetic mechanism. Simultaneously, there were increases in $P\bar{v}O_2$ and O_2 delivery due to the increase in CO (extrapulmonary factor). The resulting beneficial effect of the latter on PaO_2 , thus, was offset by the impairment in PaO_2 due to further worsening of $\dot{V}_A/\dot{Q}$ relationships (increased dispersion of ventilation, intrapulmonary factor), enhanced (decreased overall $\dot{V}_A/\dot{Q}$ ratio) in turn by a concomitant less efficient breathing pattern (increased respiratory frequency and decreased tidal volume, extrapulmonary factor) (Fig. 2). Inter-

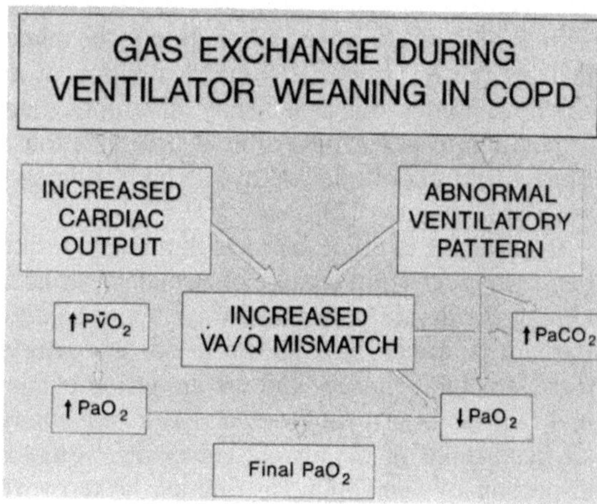

Fig. 2. During weaning, $\dot{V}_A/\dot{Q}$ mismatch (intrapulmonary factor) worsened due to both an increase in cardiac output (extrapulmonary factor) and a less efficient breathing pattern (increased frequency and decreased tidal volume, extrapulmonary factor). As a result, PaO_2 decreased and $PaCO_2$ increased. Concomitantly, increased cardiac output increased PaO_2 through an increase in $P\bar{v}O_2$, other things being equal. Overall, the final PaO_2 may be influenced in either direction or remain unaltered according to the respective roles played by all these factors

estingly, in this particular setting, the qualitative alterations in minute ventilation had a powerful effect on pulmonary gas exchange. The finding that the dispersion of ventilation was one of the most significant altered $\dot{V}_A/\dot{Q}$ variables, together with the overall index of $\dot{V}_A/\dot{Q}$ heterogeneity, suggests that maldistribution of ventilation may play a key role in the worsening of $\dot{V}_A/\dot{Q}$ mismatch during weaning. By contrast, inert dead space did not play any role.

During 100% O_2 breathing, there was a significant increase in $\dot{V}_A/\dot{Q}$ mismatching, specifically the distribution of pulmonary bloodflow and the percentage of bloodflow to low $\dot{V}_A/\dot{Q}$ areas worsened (increased), regardless the breathing conditions of the patient. Although pulmonary artery pressure did not vary nor pulmonary vascular resistance, the increase of a more sensitive parameter such as the dispersion of perfusion alone suggests release or inhibition of hypoxic pulmonary vasoconstriction and reflects a measurable level of hypoxic vascular response. Interestingly, during spontaneous ventilation and mechanical ventilation, administration of 100% O_2 did not increase significantly pulmonary shunting. The absence of changes in shunt indicates that reabsorption atelectasis did not occur probably because of the efficiency of collateral ventilation, as it has been shown in other acute and chronic lung disorders [22]. Similar results have been shown by Castaing et al. [27] in patients with advanced COPD suffering from chronic ventilatory failure when treated with low inspired PO_2. More specifically, there was a significant moderate increase in inert dead space and an increase in the percentage of bloodflow to areas with low $\dot{V}_A/\dot{Q}$ units, hence, suggesting inhibition of hypoxic pulmonary vasconstriction.

More recently, to investigate the time-course and pattern of $\dot{V}_A/\dot{Q}$ relationships, Ferrer et al. [28] have studied sequentially 10 patients with acute hypercapnic respiratory failure not receiving mechanical ventilation (Fig. 3). It is of note that most of the respiratory and inert gas data improved one month following the initial episode. More specifically, PaO_2 increased and $PaCO_2$ decreased and both the dispersion of alveolar ventilation and one of the overall indices of $\dot{V}_A/\dot{Q}$ heterogeneity decreased (improved) significantly. Furthermore, there was a significant relationship between the improvement in the dispersion of ventilation distribution and that of FEV_1, one of the best functional descriptors of the degree of airway obstruction. This suggests, therefore, that some of the $\dot{V}_A/\dot{Q}$ abnormalities observed in patients with COPD with ventilatory failure may be related to reversible functional abnormalities related, in part, to maldistribution of ventilation (namely, bronchoconstriction, edema, mucus plugging, air trapping and, also, intrinsic or auto-PEEP) in addition to other irreversible structural lesions, such as airways (inflammation, fibrosis and smooth muscle hypertrophy, among other major lesions) and emphysema abnormalities [29].

By using the multiple inert gas elimination technique in patients with mild COPD before lung resection because of a small localized neoplasm and subsequently determining the degree of small airways abnormalities and of pathologic emphysema. Barberà et al. [29] have shown in our laboratory significant correlations between these structural changes and the dispersion of bloodflow and ventilation. Accordingly, it has been hypothesized that a non-homogeneous distribution of inspired air, as a result of the airway narrowing, would be at the origin of the increased dispersion of ventilation distribution. Alternatively, the loss of alveolar attach-

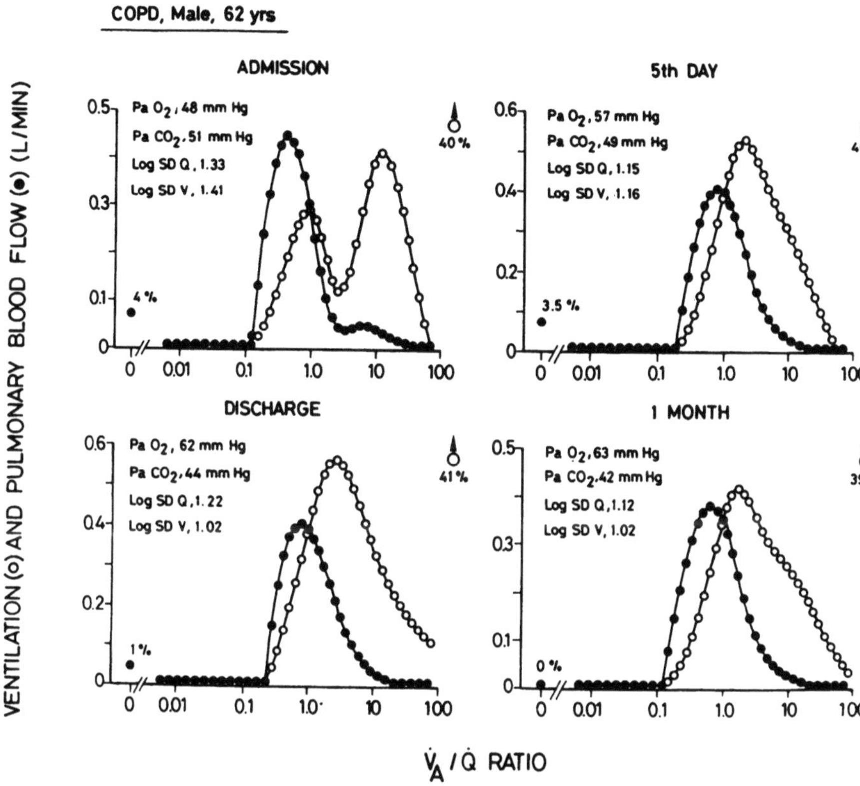

Fig. 3. $\dot{V}_A/\dot{Q}$ distributions of a representative patient from [28]. Note the improvement in PaO_2 and $PaCO_2$ paralleled by an improvement in both the distributions of ventilation (log SD V) and perfusion (log SD Q). Both distributions denote a severe underlying $\dot{V}_A/\dot{Q}$ inequality on admission. Note also that the bimodel ventilation distribution on admission disappeared at Day 5. Although modestly, shunt (4% of $\dot{Q}_T$, on admission) decreased, whereas dead space (40% of $\dot{V}_E$) remained essentially unchanged throughout the period of study (For symbols, see Fig. 1)

ments of bronchiolar walls observed in pulmonary emphysema may result in both distortion and narrowing of the lumen of bronchioles. The latter may cause reduced alveolar ventilation in the dependent alveolar units, which will produce lung units with continued bloodflow and thus low $\dot{V}_A/\dot{Q}$ ratios. This abnormality in $\dot{V}_A/\dot{Q}$ relationships would become more evident in the bloodflow curve, as an increased dispersion of perfusion. In addition, emphysema was related to abnormalities of ventilation distribution. The latter may be related, at least in part, to the loss of pulmonary capillary network associated to alveolar destruction of emphysematous spaces (namely, wasted ventilation). This would lead in turn to the development of lung units with high $\dot{V}_A/\dot{Q}$ ratios, and hence to increased dispersion of ventilation. Accordingly, the bimodal ventilation distribution alluded to before [2, 3] would be an extension of this phenomenon likely reflecting large areas of destroyed parenchyma.

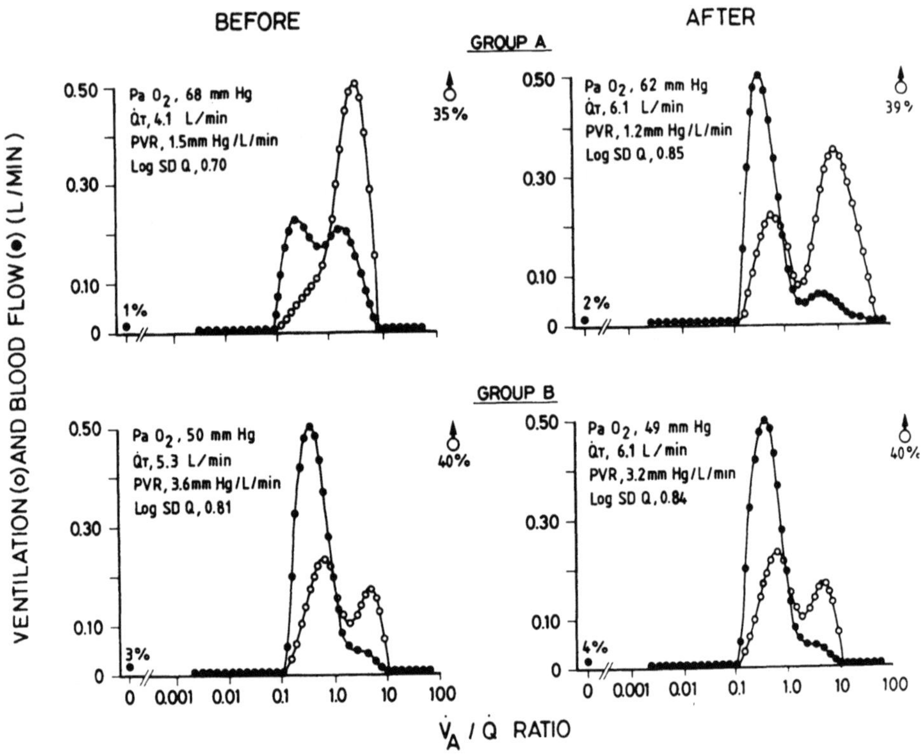

Fig. 4. $\dot{V}_A/\dot{Q}$ distributions corresponding to 2 representative patients from [30]. *Top, Group A:* Note that, after terbutaline, this patient *(right panel)* disclosed bimodal distributions clearly, decreased both PaO_2 and pulmonary vascular resistance (PVR), increased $\dot{Q}_T$, and increased (worsened) log SD Q. Shunt and dead space remained essentially unchanged. *Bottom, Group B:* By contrast, this other patient (with worse overall lung function at baseline) did not show changes in any of the variables after the bronchodilator was given (For symbols and abbreviations, see Fig. 1 and 3) (From [30] with permission)

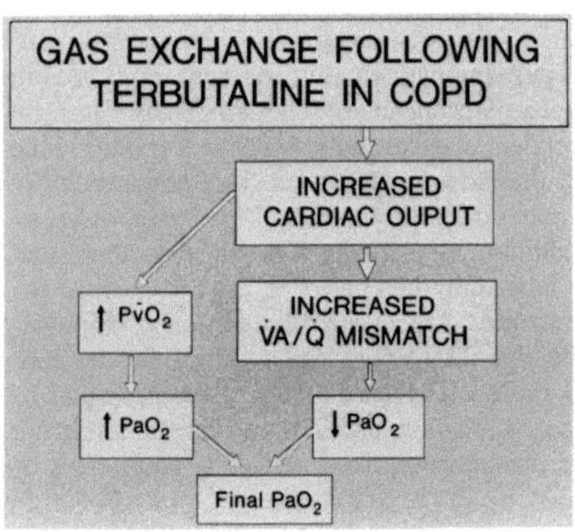

Fig. 5. During terbutaline infusion, cardiac output (extrapulmonary factor) increased which, in turn, further worsened $\dot{V}_A/\dot{Q}$ inequality (intrapulmonary factor) which decreases PaO_2. Note that PaO_2 fell despite the concomitant increase in PaO_2, through an increase in $P\bar{v}O_2$

Influence of Pulmonary Vascular Tone

Ringstedt et al. [30] studying 6 stable mixed-type COPD patients (according to Burrows et al.'s classification [31]) with mild ventilatory failure spontaneously breathing before and 1 h after a continuous intravenous terbutaline (β_2-agonist bronchodilator, 5 μg/min), were able to further explore the importance and possible role of the pulmonary vascular tone in modulating gas exchange in these patients (Fig. 4, top: Group A). Following terbutaline, there were significant increases in CO coupled with an accompanying partial vasodilatation (systemic blood pressure and pulmonary vascular resistance significantly decreased). In addition, PaO_2 decreased and $P\bar{v}O_2$ and O_2 delivery increased significantly, whereas $PaCO_2$ remained unchanged. Moreover, $\dot{V}_A/\dot{Q}$ mismatching further worsened, as assessed by an increase in perfusion to low $\dot{V}_A/\dot{Q}$ areas and also in the dispersion of bloodflow. Although FEV_1 and minute ventilation increased, these increments were not significant. Thus, the $\dot{V}_A/\dot{Q}$ worsening (intrapulmonary factor) could have resulted either from an increased dispersion of pulmonary bloodflow or from a decrease in the overall ventilation to bloodflow ratio (not efficiently counterbalanced by the concomitant modest increased minute ventilation), or both, due to the increase in CO (extrapulmonary factor).

This decrease in the overall $\dot{V}_A/\dot{Q}$ ratio indicates a parallel shift towards lower $\dot{V}_A/\dot{Q}$ ratios, hence suggesting homogenously decreased pulmonary vascular tone. By contrast, the increase in the dispersion of bloodflow may result from a regional, localized reduction in regional vascular tone. Conceivably, both mechanisms were present following the administration of the β_2 agonist. The concomitant significant increase in $P\bar{v}O_2$ may have also contributed to further worsen $\dot{V}_A/\dot{Q}$ mismatch by releasing hypoxic pulmonary vasoconstriction. However, from these data it is not possible to differentiate between an increased CO, hence provoking an increase in the amount of dispersion of pulmonary bloodflow, or a reduction in pulmonary vascular tone. In fact, part of the decrease observed in pulmonary vascular resistance (PVR) in this group of COPD patients without a concomitant decreased pulmonary artery pressure (PAP), could represent both recruitment and possibly also distention of pulmonary vessels. Under these circumstances, PaO_2 decreased without associated changes in $PaCO_2$.

By contrast, in another group of 6 similar type COPD patients with more airflow obstruction (worse spirometric indices), more abnormal gas exchange (more hypoxemia and more hypercapnia), and also with both higher PAP and PVR values, CO increased significantly with a small but not significant reduction in PAP nor in PVR (Fig. 4, bottom: Group B). Likewise, minute ventilation increased modestly but significantly without accompanying changes in the degree of airflow obstruction (i.e. FEV_1 and FVC). Interestingly, $P\bar{v}O_2$ increased significantly but not O_2 delivery. Yet, respiratory arterial blood gases did not change, neither did the underlying $\dot{V}_A/\dot{Q}$ abnormalities. Consequently, despite a substantial increase in CO, pulmonary gas exchange remained essentially unchanged as opposed to Group A.

In summary, despite the fact that terbutaline caused a similar increase in CO and, consequently, in $P\bar{v}O_2$ in all patients, those patients with worse lung function (more severe airways obstruction, higher pulmonary hypertension, and worse pulmonary gas exchange, Group B) at baseline did not modify their gas exchange data following administration of terbutaline. By contrast, those individuals with a better overall lung function (Group A) demonstrated a worsening in $\dot{V}_A/\dot{Q}$ relationships and therefore in PaO_2. It is of note that the patients of Torres et al. [23] showed the same degree of pulmonary hypertension than the Group B (with worse basal lung function to begin with). Although the reasons for the discrepancy between Groups A and B in Ringstedt et al.'s study [30] need as yet to be elucidated, these authors concluded that hypoxic vascular response could have played probably a "pivotal" role in modulating the behavior of pulmonary gas exchange before and after the administration of the bronchodilator. Thus, the patients with more severe COPD could have weaker or even absent hypoxic vascular response. As a result, there was no effect at all following terbutaline. This lack of hypoxic vascular response in advanced severe COPD could be related to either severe chronically established alveolar hypoxia and/or to structural changes in the pulmonary circulation coupled with areas of parenchymal destruction due to emphysema, or both. This contention could be still consistent with Torres et al. data [23], whose patients did show a measurable level of hypoxic vascular response as assessed by the use of inert gas indices only (but not according to conventional hemodynamic measurements). This would be in keeping with the concept that the progressive increase of PVR seen in advanced COPD not only is due to irreversible structural vascular lesions but also includes a reversible vasoconstrictive component [32]. In fact, PAP was slightly but significantly reduced and PVR showed also a trend to decrease in the patients with worse lung function (Group B) in Ringstedt et al. study. However, despite using the inert gas approach in the latter study, the effects of 100% O_2 breathing were not explored, which precludes therefore to make useful comparisons between both studies. A recent study of Barberà et al. [33], investigating the influence of the structure of pulmonary arteries and the contribution of the hypoxic vascular response in preserving an adequate matching of ventilation and bloodflow in a series of patients with mild COPD prior to lobectomy for solitary lesions, seems to be consistent with these concepts. These authors showed that patients with low pulmonary vascular reactivity, as assessed by the inert gas technique, had a significantly greater degree of intimal and muscular hypertrophy in small arteries than those with a high hypoxic vascular response. Furthermore, there was a significant relationship between these vascular abnormalities and the degree of inflammation in the peripheral airways. Conceivably, the inflammatory process that takes place in the small airways may play a key role in the development of mechanisms that lead to intimal fibrosis in the pulmonary arteries.

Another good example of the influence of pulmonary vascular tone combined with a concomitant increase in CO is given by the use of oral nifedipine in a short series of patients with chronic respiratory failure [34]. After one hour of drug administration, there was a reduction in mean systemic arterial pressure and also in systemic vascular resistance by 16 and 36%, respectively. While CO increased by 29%, PVR decreased by 28% without accompanying changes in PAP. At the same time, PaO_2 decreased and there was further deterioration in the underlying $\dot{V}_A/\dot{Q}$ showing a redistribution of bloodflow to areas with low $\dot{V}_A/\dot{Q}$ units and an increased dispersion in the distribution of pulmonary perfusion. These changes suggest partial release of hypoxic pulmonary vasoconstriction and represents, in part, a real concern regarding the use of vasodilating drugs for the therapy of pulmonary vasonconstriction due to COPD. Later, similar results were shown by Agustí et al. [5] in a group of COPD patients with mildly abnormal blood gases and less severe disease. In another study, Brate et al. [35] used felodipine, a calcium antagonist vasodilator, as an adjuvant to long-term oxygen therapy in patients with advanced COPD and chronic respiratory failure. Short-term infusion of felodipine produced similar pulmonary gas exchange alterations to the two previous studies [5, 34], explained also by a reduction of hypoxic vasoconstriction. Interestingly, while long-term oral administration of the same drug over a period of several weeks induced hemodynamic changes similar to those produced during oral therapy, there was no further worsening in $\dot{V}_A/\dot{Q}$ mismatch. Although the mechanisms need as yet to be elucidated, it was speculated that a redistribution of ventilation to areas with low $\dot{V}_A/\dot{Q}$ units receiving simultaneously an increased amount of bloodflow could be the most likely explanation. Interestingly, a recent study by Reyes et al. [36] has shown that intravenous administration of aminophylline during one hour to patients with COPD during recovery from ventilatory failure produced no change on forced spirometry, ventilation, hemodynamics or the $\dot{V}_A/\dot{Q}$ distribution. This is of interest since traditionally aminophylline has been considered a drug which might release hypoxic pulmonary vasoconstriction, even when given at therapeutic range.

There have been two other studies in patients with COPD and different degrees of ventilatory respiratory failure in which, by investigating the effects of oral almitrine (1.5 mg/kg), a peripheral chemoreceptor, the influence of pulmonary vascular tone played a key role in improving pulmonary gas exchange. In the first report, Mélot et al. [37] (Fig. 6) studied a series of 6 patients breathing spontaneously, 4 of them with hypercapnic respiratory failure, and demonstrated that respiratory blood gases improved significantly. Concomitantly, the underlying $\dot{V}_A/\dot{Q}$ mismatching improved also significantly. The only associated significant hemodynamic change

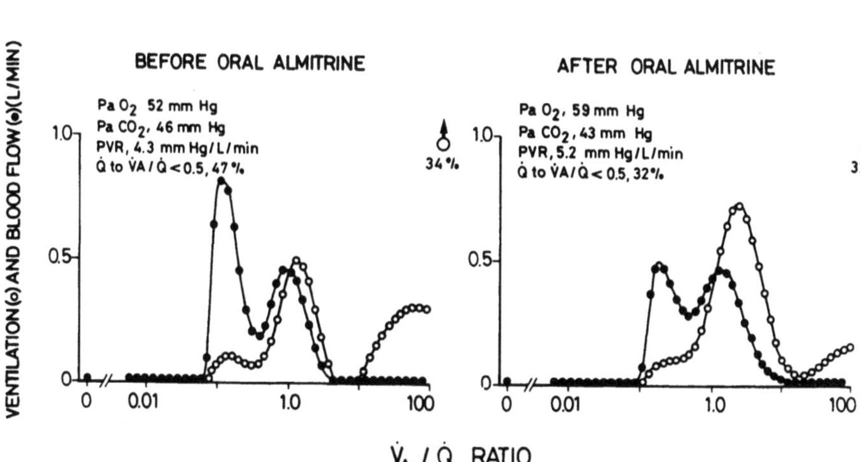

Fig. 6. $\dot{V}_A/\dot{Q}$ distributions of a representative patient before and after almitrine from [38]. Note that PaO_2 increased and $PaCO_2$ decreased together with a modest increase in PVR after the drug was given *(right panel)*. Similarly, there was a significant redistribution of bloodflow from areas with low $\dot{V}_A/\dot{Q}$ units (below 0.5) to those with normal $\dot{V}_A/\dot{Q}$ ratios (From [38] with permission)

was a modest increase in PVR without increases in PAP. In the second study, Castaing et al. [38] studied 9 patients who required mechanical ventilation because of severe respiratory failure. Conventional and inert gas exchange indices improved significantly together with a small but significant decrease in both CO (but not in $P\bar{v}O_2$) and a mild increase in PVR. In both studies, there was essentially a redistribution of pulmonary bloodflow from regions of low $\dot{V}_A/\dot{Q}$ units to areas with normal $\dot{V}_A/\dot{Q}$ ratios (intrapulmonary factor) (Fig. 7). It was suggested that the enhancement of hypoxic pulmonary vasoconstriction (i.e. increased pulmonary vascular tone, extrapulmonary factor) as assessed by a slight increase in pulmonary vascular resistance, was at the origin of the overall improvement in pulmonary gas exchange.

More recently, our group has investigated the short term effects of fenoterol, a selective β_2-agonist, given by inhalation, among other bronchodilators, in a double-blind, placebo-controlled study in a series of 24 patients with advanced COPD and mild to moderate abnormal blood gases [39]. It was shown that fenoterol decreased PaO_2 (mean -7 mm Hg) and increased CO (mean +22%). Moreover, there was further worsening in the dispersion of pulmonary bloodflow compared to the lack of changes following the other interventions. Although pulmonary hemodynamics were not measured, it may be suggested that the pulmonary vascular tone was probably decreased, hence inducing further $\dot{V}_A/\dot{Q}$ mismatch and more arterial hypoxemia, despite the simultaneous increase in CO. Probably, the beneficial effect of the increased $P\bar{v}O_2$ was not sufficiently powerful to offset the deleterious effect of the decreased pulmonary vascular tone on $\dot{V}_A/\dot{Q}$ mismatch. The final result was that arterial hypoxemia ensued. These results contrast with the effects of intravenous salbutamol given to patients with acute severe asthma [40] in whom PaO_2 remained unchanged despite similar changes in CO and $\dot{V}_A/\dot{Q}$ inequalities. This suggests that fenoterol has a direct effect on the pulmonary vascular wall, which decreases the vascular tone. Very recently, it has been shown that at doses based on those used in clinical practice, fenoterol causes more adverse effects (namely car-

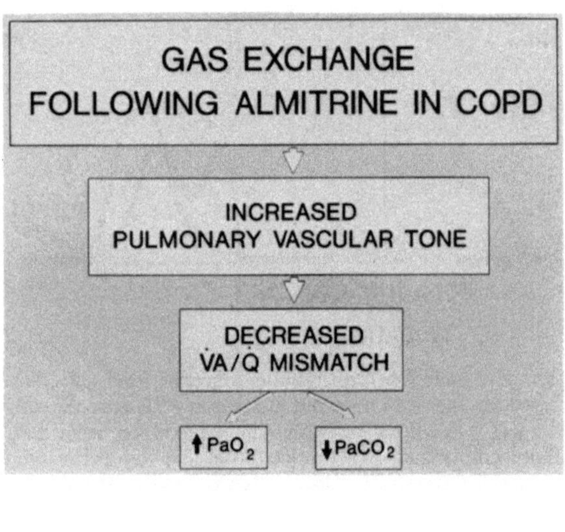

Fig. 7. During almitrine, both the increased pulmonary vascular pressures and pulmonary vascular resistance, which strengthen the pulmonary vascular tone (extrapulmonary factor), play a beneficial role on pulmonary gas exchange by improving the underlying degree of $\dot{V}_A/\dot{Q}$ mismatch (intrapulmonary factor). As a result respiratory gases (O_2 and CO_2) improve

diac, metabolic and systemic) than salbutamol or terbutaline in patients with mild asthma [41]. The most likely explanation is that fenoterol has been marketed at a higher dose than the other two conventional β_2-agonists, despite having *in vitro* the same potency than isoproterenol; furthermore, it is suggested that fenoterol may be less selective for β_2 receptors.

Influence of Oxygen Uptake and ventilation

Lemaire et al. [25] studied carefully the hemodynamic effects of rapid weaning from mechanical ventilation in 15 patients with severe advanced COPD and pre-existing cardiovascular disease. Although inert gas exchange data were not measured, it is of interest to note that there was a significant impairment in both PaO_2 and $PaCO_2$ together with an increase in CO and the presence of significant deleterious hemodynamic events. Interestingly, oxygen uptake increased significantly; unfortunately, measurements of breathing pattern were not documented. The important conclusion that can be drawn from this study, however, is that the increased metabolic (extrapulmonary factor) demands of these patients could have influenced negatively the final PaO_2, thus overwhelming the beneficial effects on the latter variable produced by the accompanying increase in CO (extrapulmonary factor). According to our experience, the underlying $\dot{V}_A/\dot{Q}$ relationships (intrapulmonary factor, not measured) should have worsened. The latter variable, possibly with an expected less efficient breathing pattern could have also contributed to further worsen respiratory blood gases (decreased PaO_2 and increased $PaCO_2$), just as they did in our patients [23]. Interestingly, Annat et al. [42] also showed in 8 COPD patients during weaning from mechanical ventilation to both continuous positive pressure ventilation and inspiratory pressure support ventilation, increases in both oxygen consumption and decreases in minute ventilation. In addition there was a marked increment in $PaCO_2$ without changes in PaO_2. Conceivably, the concomitant increase in CO (not measured) would be at the origin of the results of arterial blood gases. An increased CO would have raised mixed venous PO_2, thus counterbalancing the combined deleterious effects on PaO_2 of both the reduced ventilation and the increased oxygen uptake. Just as with the study of Lemaire et al. [25], the increase in oxygen uptake was one of the most outstanding findings compared to the work of Torres et al. [23]. The absence of an increased oxygen consumption in the latter study may be, however, perfectly explained by the large variability of CO measurements with the thermodilution technique in the clinical setting, used to calculate oxygen uptake through the Fick principle. Furthermore, in the experimental setting, the Fick method can underestimate oxygen consumption measured at the mouth because bronchial and thebesian veins empty into the systemic circulation such that the oxygen consumed by parts of the lung and the heart may not be reflected necessarily in the Fick measurement [43, 44]. In brief, it is considered that oxygen consumption measured from the mixed expired samples at the mouth is more accurate than that calculated from the CO and the arterial-mixed venous oxygen contents. Although the differences between each measurement are not statistically significant, it has been shown that their correlation is relatively weak [45].

Alternatively, in Annat et al. study [42] the outstanding influence of a decreased overall ventilation in worsening pulmonary gas exchange needs also to be emphasized.

Conclusion

In summary, taken all together, these findings highlight the key role played by the interplay of extrapulmonary and intrapulmonary factors governing pulmonary gas exchange in COPD patients with ventilatory failure under different clinical conditions. According to their respective role, respiratory blood gases may be influenced in either direction, or remain unaltered in different clinical settings. In these patients, $\dot{V}_A/\dot{Q}$ mismatching emerges undoubtedly as the principal intrapulmonary determinant of pulmonary gas exchange, being the role of shunt almost negligible. In addition, the contribution of CO and overall ventilation among other predominantly extrapulmonary factors may play a key role in modulating the observed arterial respiratory gases. The influence of CO and total ventilation need to be particularly highlighted since each of them is able to offset the effects of changes on PaO_2 and $PaCO_2$ produced by further worsening in $\dot{V}_A/\dot{Q}$ mismatch *per se*. The important message for the clinician though is that arterial blood gas measurements may be totally insensitive to properly reflect the alterations operating at the level of the extrapulmonary and intrapulmonary determinants of pulmonary gas exchange.

References

1. Rodriguez-Roisin R, Wagner PD (1989) Clinical relevance of ventilation-perfusion inequality determined by inert gas elimination. Eur Respir J 3:469–482
2. Wagner PD, Dantzker DR, Dueck R, Clausen JL, West JB (1977) Ventilation-perfusion inequality in chronic obstructive pulmonary disease. J Clin Invest 59:203–216
3. Dantzker DR (1984) Gas exchange. In: Montenegro HD (ed) Chronic obstructive pulmonary disease. Churchill Livingstone, Edinburgh, pp 141–160
4. Glauser FL, Pollaty RC, Sessler CN (1988) Worsening oxygenation in the mechanically ventilated patient. Causes, mechanisms, and early detection. Am Rev Respir Dis 138:458–465
5. Agustí AGN, Barberà JA, Roca J, Wagner PD, Guitart R, Rodriguez-Roisin R (1990) Hypoxic pulmonary vasoconstriction and gas exchange in chronic obstructive pulmonary disease. Chest 97:268–275
6. Dantzker DR (1987) Ventilation-perfusion inequality in lung disease. Chest 91:749–754
7. West JB (1969) Ventilation-perfusion inequality and overall gas exchange in computer lung models of the lung. Respir Physiol 7:88–110
8. West JB (1971) Causes of carbon dioxide retention in lung disease. N Engl J Med 284:1232–1236
9. Dantzker DR (1983) The influence of cardiovascular function on gas exchange. Clin Chest Med 4:149–159
10. Agustí AGN, Roca J, Gea J, Wagner PD, Xaubet A, Rodriguez-Roisin R (1991) Mechanisms of gas exchange impairment in idiopathic pulmonary fibrosis. Am Rev Respir Dis 143:219–225

11. Lynch JP, Mhyre JG, Dantzker DR (1979) Influence of cardiac output on intrapulmonary shunt. J Appl Physiol 46:315–321
12. Breen PH, Schumacker PT, Hedenstierna G, Ali J, Wagner PD, Wood LDH (1982) How does increased cardiac output increase shunt in pulmonary edema. J Appl Physiol 53:1487–1495
13. Hyman AL, Higashida RT, Spannhake EW, Kadowitz PJ (1981) Pulmonary vasoconstrictor responses to graded decreases in precapillary blood PO_2 in intact-chest cat. J Appl Physiol 51:1009–1016
14. Benumof JL, Pirlo AF, Johanson I, Trousdale FR (1981) Interaction of $P\bar{v}O_2$ with P_AO_2 on hypoxic pulmonary vasoconstriction. J Appl Physiol 51:871–874
15. Wagner PD (1982) Ventilation-perfusion inequality in catastrophic lung disease. In: Prakash O (ed) Applied physiology in clinical respiratory care. Martinus Nijhoff, The Hague, pp 363–379
16. Weinberger SE, Schwartzstein RM, Weiss JW (1989) Hypercapnia. N Engl J Med 321:1223–1231
17. Wagner PD, Rodriguez-Roisin R (1991) Clinical advances in pulmonary gas exchange. Am Rev Respir Dis (in press)
18. Wagner PD, Saltzman HA, West JB (1974) Measurements of continuous distributions of ventilation-perfusion ratios: theory. J Appl Physiol 36:588–599
19. Evans JW, Wagner PD (1977) Limits on $\dot{V}_A/\dot{Q}$ distributions from analysis of experimental inert gas elimination. J Appl Physiol 42:889–898
20. Briscoe WA, Cree EM, Filler J, Houssay HEJ, Cournand A (1960) Lung volume, alveolar ventilation and perfusion interrelationships in chronic pulmonary emphysema. J Appl Physiol 15:785–795
21. Dantzker DR, Wagner PD, West JB (1975) Instability of lung units with low $\dot{V}_A/\dot{Q}$ ratios during O_2 breathing. J Appl Physiol 38:886–895
22. Rodriguez-Roisin R, Ballester E, Roca J, Torres A, Wagner PD (1989) Mechanisms of hypoxemia in patients with status asthmaticus requiring mechanical ventilation. Am Rev Respir Dis 139:732–739
23. Torres A, Reyes A, Roca J, Wagner PD, Rodriguez-Roisin R (1989) Ventilation-perfusion mismatching in chronic obstructive pulmonary disease during ventilator weaning. Am Rev Respir Dis 14:1246–1250
24. Gale GE, Torre-Bueno JR, Moon RE, Saltzman HA, Wagner PD (1985) Ventilation-perfusion inequalities in normal humans during exercise at sea level and simulated altitude. J Appl Physiol 58:978–988
25. Lemaire F, Teboul JL, Cinotti L, et al (1988) Acute left ventricular dysfunction during unsuccessful weaning from mechanical ventilation. Anesthesiology 69:171–179
26. Permutt S (1988) Circulatory effects of weaning from mechanical ventilation: the importance of transdiaphragmatic pressure. Anesthesiology 69:157–160
27. Castaing Y, Manier G, Guénard H (1985) Effect of 26% oxygen breathing on ventilation and perfusion distribution in patients with COPD. Bull Eur Physiopathol Respir 21:17–23
28. Ferrer A, Roca J, Barberà JA, Agustí AGN, Wagner PD, Rodriguez-Roisin R (1990) Evolution of ventilation-perfusion mismatch during exacerbations of chronic obstructive pulmonary disease (abstract). Eur Respir J 3 (Suppl 10):101S
29. Barberà JA, Remirez J, Roca J, Wagner PD, Sánchez-Lloret J, Rodriguez-Roisin R (1990) Lung structure and gas exchange in mild chronic obstructive pulmonary disease. Am Rev Respir Dis 141:895–901
30. Ringstedt CV, Eliasen K, Andersen JB, Heslet L, Qvist J (1989) Ventilation-perfusion distributions and central hemodynamics in chronic obstructive pulmonary disease. Chest 96:976–983
31. Burrows B, Fletcher CM, Heard BE, Jones NL, Wootliff JS (1966) The emphysematous and bronchial types of chronic airways obstruction: a clinicopathological study of patients in London and Chicago. Lancet 1:830–835
32. Dawson CA, Grimm DJ, Linchan JH (1978) Influence of hypoxia on the longitudinal distribution pulmonary vascular resistance. J Appl Physiol Respir Environ Exercise Physiol 44:493–498

33. Barberà JA, Riverola A, Ramirez J, et al (1990) Pulmonary vascular structure and ventilation-perfusion relationships in patients with mild COPD (abstract). Eur Respir J 3 (Suppl 10): 184S
34. Mélot C, Hallemans R, Naeije R, Mols P, Lejeune P (1984) Deleterious effect of nifedipine on pulmonary gas exchange in chronic obstructive pulmonary disease. Am Rev Respir Dis 130:612–616
35. Bratel T, Hedenstierna G, Nyquist O, Ripe E (1990) The use of a vasodilator, felodipine, as an adjuvant to long-term oxygen treatment in COPD patients. Eur Respir J 3:46–54
36. Reyes A, Barberà JA, Roca J, Wagner PD, Rodriguez-Roisin R (1990) Intravenous aminophylline does not cause further ventilation-perfusion mismatch during exacerbation of chronic obstructive pulmonary disease (abstract). Eur Resp J 3 (suppl 10): 117S
37. Mélot C, Naeije R, Rothschild, Mertens P, Mols P, Hallemans R (1983) Improvement in ventilation-perfusion matching by almitrine in COPD. Chest 83:528–533
38. Castaing Y, Manier G, Guénard H (1986) Improvement in ventilation-perfusion relationships by almitrine in patients with chronic obstructive pulmonary disease during mechanical ventilation. Am Rev Respir Dis 134:910–916
39. Ferrer A, Viegas C, Montserrat JM, Roca J, Wagner PD, Rodriguez-Roisin R (1991) Gas exchange response to bronchodilators in chronic obstructive pulmonary disease (abstract). Am Rev Respir Dis (in press)
40. Ballester E, Reyes A, Roca J, Guitart R, Wagner PD, Rodriguez-Roisin R (1989) Ventilation-perfusion mismatching in acute severe asthma: effects of salbutamol and 100% oxygen. Thorax 44:258–267
41. Wong CS, Pavord ID, Williams J, Britton JR, Tattersfield AE (1990) Bronchodilator, cardiovascular, and hypokaliemic effects of fenoterol, salbutamol, and terbutaline in asthma. Lancet 336:1396–1399
42. Annat G, Viale JP, Dereymez CP, Bouffard YM, Delafosse BX, Motin JP (1990) Oxygen cost of breathing and diaphragmatic pressure-time index. Measurement in patients with COPD during weaning with pressure support ventilation. Chest 98:411–414
43. Caldwell PRB, Echeverri U, Kilcoyne MM, Fritts HW Jr (1970) Observations on a model of proliferative lung disease: II. Description of pulmonary gas exchange and comparison of Fick and dye cardiac outputs. J Clin Invest 49:1311–1315
44. Light RB (1988) Intrapulmonary oxygen consumption in experimental pneumococcal pneumonia. J Appl Physiol 64:2490–2495
45. Hubmayr RD, Loosbrock LM, Gillespie DJ, Rodarte JR (1988) Oxygen uptake during weaning from mechanical ventilation. Chest 94:1148–1155

Control of Ventilation and Response to Loading

J. Milic-Emili

Introduction

There are several reasons for studying the respiratory responses to loads:

1. to elucidate basic physiology,
2. to improve understanding and treatment of disturbances in patients with respiratory diseases, and
3. to assist in the design and use of breathing equipment for medical or other purposes.

Several reviews on respiratory responses to loading are available [1–3]. In this chapter, no attempt is made to cover the vast literature available on respiratory loading. Instead, a synthesis of old and new observations will be provided.

Classification of Loads

The classification of loads must take into account the nature of the load *(what),* the respiratory phase during which it is applied *(when),* and the site of application *(where).* Thus loads can be external (i.e. applied to the airway opening or body surface) or internal (i.e. within respiratory system). Loads can be inspiratory, expiratory, or continuous if applied to both phases of the respiratory cycle. They can be elastic, flow resistive, or inertial depending on whether they are related to volume, flow, or acceleration. Furthermore they can be classified as linear or nonlinear. Addition of any of these loads results in increased mechanical impedance of the respiratory system; therefore they should be regarded as true mechanical loads. An example of external nonlinear resistive load is represented by the endotracheal tubes (Fig. 1).

Pressure applied to the respiratory system either at the airway opening or at the body surface is often referred to as mechanical loading, although it does not necessarily lead to increased respiratory mechanical impedance. For example, with application of moderate values of continuous positive pressure to the airway opening, the total respiratory system compliance may remain unchanged, whereas flow resistance may decrease because of an increased lung volume. This implies a decreased mechanical load; however, the burden on the inspiratory muscles should increase because of changes in their operating length due to increased lung volume and thus decreased effectiveness of their contraction [4, 5]. Accordingly, application of constant pressure is better defined as continuous pressure biasing [5]. Similarly inspiratory and expiratory threshold loads are not easy to classify. These loads

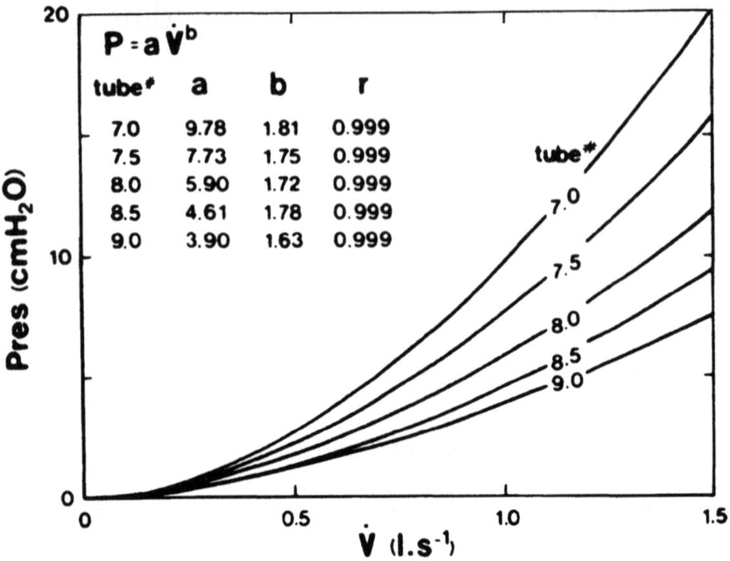

Fig. 1. Relationships between resistive pressure (Pres) and airflow ($\dot{V}$) for endotracheal tubes (and connectors) of standard length but different internal diameter (ranging from 7 to 9 mm). The pressure-flow relationships fit power functions of the form Pres = $a\dot{V}^b$, a and b are constants. (From [4] with permission)

prevent flow at the beginning of inspiration or expiration until a threshold pressure is exceeded [6]. In this connection, it should be noted that intrinsic PEEP is an internal inspiratory threshold load [7, 8].

Shifting from upright to supine position is an example of continuous internal pressure biasing in which the changes in pressure are mainly caused by abdominal hydrostatic forces. Because in the resting tidal volume range this postural shift is usually associated with decreased compliance and increased flow resistance of the respiratory system, this could also be regarded as a form of continuous internal flow-resistive loading and elastic unloading. Clearly, there are both conceptual and semantic difficulties in defining the respiratory loads, particularly the internal ones. Therefore, it seems necessary to always clearly define the *what, where,* and *when.*

Classification of Responses

Responses can be classified as *intrinsic* (nonneural) or *extrinsic* (neural). A nonneural response implies that during loading the intensity and timing of the neural drive remain unchanged. Intrinsic responses are influenced by the passive mechanical properties of the respiratory system when the respiratory muscles are relaxed and ventilation is sustained by artificial means and also by the properties of active contracting muscles during spontaneous breathing. The shape and distribution of the neural drive to the various respiratory muscles can profoundly modulate such responses [1–3].

Neural responses are those in which the intensity of the neural drive to the various respiratory muscles and/or its timing change. Neural responses include those in which the central drive changes and those in which it does not. This distinction is clear in the case of conscious or chemical responses versus spinal reflexes but not when reflex loops include higher centers. Active chemical responses are those in which the chemical composition of arterial blood and/or cerebrospinal fluid (CSF) are changed in a direction that increases the central drive. Active nonchemical responses may occur in the absence of chemical changes and may even be associated with decreased chemical drive.

In this context, it seems useful to scrutinize terms such as "load-compensating mechanisms and responses". The literature often refers to tidal volume (VT) or minute ventilation ($\dot{V}E$) load-compensatory mechanisms and responses. These are legitimate terms. In the last analysis, however, a given response is truly compensatory only if it defends alveolar ventilation and helps to maintain the normal chemical composition of arterial blood and CSF. A response that preserves minute ventilation is not necessarily compensatory in terms of arterial blood gas and CSF composition. This can readily be appreciated from the classic equation.

$$PaCO_2 = \frac{\dot{V}CO_2 K}{\dot{V}E(1 - VD/VT)} \tag{1}$$

where $PaCO_2$ is arterial CO_2 tension, $\dot{V}CO_2$ is metabolic CO_2 production, and VD is physiologic dead space. In terms of $PaCO_2$, load compensation clearly involves more than maintenance of $\dot{V}E$: the effects of loads on $\dot{V}CO_2$, VD, and VT must also be considered.

Intrinsic Mechanisms and Responses

Intrinsic (nonneural) responses to elastic and flow-resistive loads depend mainly on the magnitude of the volume-elastic and flow-resistive impedances of the respiratory systems relative to that of the imposed load: the larger the impedance of the respiratory system relative to the imposed one, the smaller the resulting decrement in VT and VE [3]. A high internal impedance, although costly in terms of energy expenditure, may be regarded as a mechanism by which added mechanical loads are compensated. When the muscles are relaxed, the impedance of the respiratory system is represented by the volume-elastic and flow-resistive impedances offered by the passive properties of the airways, lung, and chest wall. When muscles contract agonistically, their active force-length and force-velocity properties add to the internal impedance. The force-length properties add to the volume-elastic impedance (elastance, E) and force-velocity properties add to the flow-resistive impedance (flow resistance, R) [4, 8, 9]. Thus the intrinsic properties of the contracting muscles are load compensating in that they increase the internal impedance and render the respiratory system less susceptible to external influences. In addition, during active breathing there is distortion of the respiratory system that should also increase the elastance [4, 8] [10 and 11 for detailed accounts of passive and active impedances of the respiratory system].

The intrinsic responses to pressure biasing are of a different nature. The most common form of pressure biasing consists of changing body posture. Such natural biasing and various unnatural forms of pressure breathing (e.g. application of PEEP) shift the lung volume around which breathing takes place, i.e. the so-called midposition. These shifts result in changes in the operating characteristics of the respiratory system. Although ordinarily pressure biasing does not cause substantial changes in the overall respiratory mechanical impedance, this may increase substantially if the changes in midposition are large. Indeed the internal volume-elastic impedance of the respiratory system rises abruptly towards the upper and lower extremes of the vital capacity [12], and the flow-resistive impedance rises substantially at low lung volume [13].

Of greater significance are the changes in operating length of the respiratory muscles that are associated with shifts in midposition. Shifts in the inspiratory direction (e.g. those that accompany postural shifts from recumbency to upright or application of positive pressure at airway opening) cause a shortening of the inspiratory muscles and a lengthening of the expiratory muscles. In addition, there are concomitant changes in the geometry of the respiratory muscles that may change the effectiveness of the respiratory muscles as pressure generators (e.g. Laplaces's law) [4, 9, 14]. Indeed, at fixed neural drive the pressure developed by the inspiratory muscles decreases with increasing lung volume. The opposite is true for the expiratory muscles. The significance of these effects can be appreciated by comparing the intensity of diaphragmatic discharge observed during resting ventilation in upright and supine positions. In normal humans, the shift in midposition is about 15% of the vital capacity while the intensity of diaphragmatic discharge is about 5 times greater standing upright than in supine position (Fig. 2) [15]. It should be noted that during the experiments in Fig. 2 there were no significant differences in

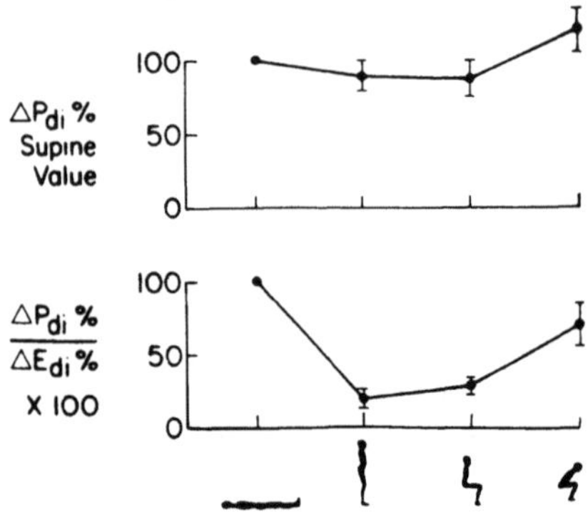

Fig. 2. Postural changes in the amplitude of integrated electrical activity of the diaphragm (ΔEdi) and transdiaphragmatic pressure (ΔPdi) during resting breathing. Mean data for 8 normal subjects obtained while standing and sitting erect and leaning forward, expressed as percent of supine values. The ratio ΔPdi%/ΔEdi% is an index of the effectiveness of the diaphragm as a pressure generator. (From [15] with permission)

VT and between body positions. These results underline the importance of operational length and geometry in determining the mechanical output of the principal inspiratory muscle, the diaphragm. They also emphasize the fact that, from the standpoint of stability of ventilation in response to postural changes, the neural mechanisms are paramount.

Neural Mechanisms and Responses

Neural mechanisms include automatic responses that can be regarded as reflex in nature and less automatic responses that are behavioral in nature. Two aspects of such responses must be distinguished: intensity and timing.

Intensity

The intensity of the motor command (neural drive) to the respiratory muscles is reflected by the rate of rise of the intensity of electrical discharge in the muscles themselves or in the motor nerves supplying them (electromyogram, EMG or electroneurogram, ENG recorded as moving time average) [16, 17]. The shape of the phrenic ENG and diaphragmatic EMG waves varies considerably among different species and also within the same species (Fig. 3) [10]. This has important implications not only in terms of ventilatory output but also in terms of the respiratory responses to loading [7, 11]. Appropriate shaping of the neural drive will render the respiratory system more stable in the face of a given load. This important aspect deserves future investigation.

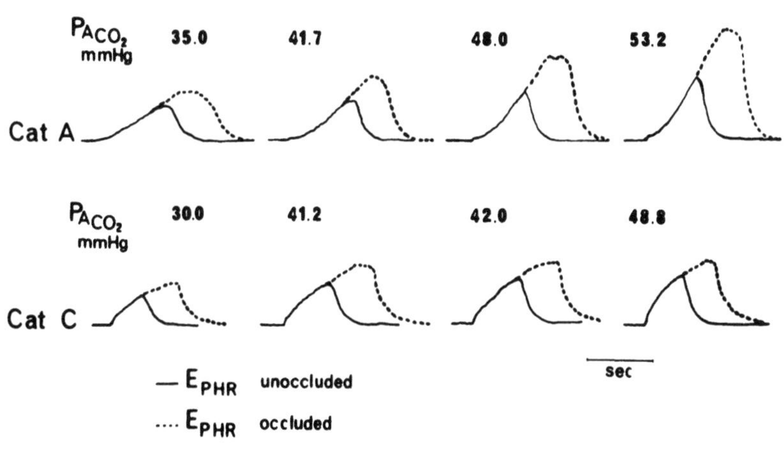

Fig. 3. Integrated phrenic activity (E_{PHR}) of breaths occluded at end-expiration and preceding unoccluded breaths in 2 cats anesthetized with pentobarbital sodium (35 mg/kg) at different levels of alveolar partial pressure of CO_2 ($PACO_2$). Phrenic activity was integrated by a "leaky integrator" with a time constant of 100 ms. Removal of volume-related vagal feedback by airway occlusion prolongs activity but initial E_{PHR} trajectory is not altered. (From [16] with permission).

The intensity of respiratory neural drive depends on chemoreceptor influences (Fig. 3): changes in blood and CSF gas composition provide a potentially powerful mechanism for load compensation. However, blood gases generally remain unchanged in conscious humans during loaded breathing, except when the external loads are very large [18]. Similarly, in patients with markedly altered mechanical properties of the respiratory system (increased flow resistance and decreased compliance), the arterial O_2 and CO_2 tensions are often within the normal range [19]. This implies nonchemical modulation of intensity in response to loading.

Muscle spindle and tendon organ reflexes provide potential load-compensatory mechanisms through intensity modulation. Although such reflexes may play an important role in the conscious state [20] their effectiveness in anesthetized preparations appears to be limited [2, 3]. Similarly the chemoreceptor responsiveness is generally depressed by anesthesia [21, 22]. Thus in the anesthetized state mechanical load compensation relies more heavily on timing responses.

Timing

The inspiratory (TI) and expiratory (TE) durations depend mainly on the interaction of the central inspiratory activity and reflex influences with the inspiratory off-switch and on-switch mechanisms. This topic is reviewed extensively elsewhere [23].

Three timing responses are of particular interest in terms of loading; each is related to volume and is vagally mediated. Clark and von Euler [24] were the first to note that the duration of inspiration can be importantly influenced by the rate at which lung volume increases: the lower the rate, the longer the inspiratory duration (Fig. 3). Furthermore they noted that in the same breath, TE was proportional to TI; thus the ratio of inspiratory or expiratory duration to total cycle duration (TT) tended to be preserved. Because the application of inspiratory mechanical loads causes decreased inspiratory flow, such inspiratory volume-related vagal reflex provides a potential mechanism for defending VT (but not necessarily $\dot{V}E$; see next section).

The expiratory duration is also influenced by the rate of lung emptying (among other factors) [25, 26]. Thus addition of flow-resistive loads during expiration will tend to retard lung emptying and prolong expiratory duration. This response is also mediated through a vagal reflex.

The effect of pressure biasing is characterized by marked changes in expiratory duration that are also vagally mediated, whereas inspiratory duration changes less [27–30].

The implications of the timing responses on the ventilatory output during loaded breathing can be appreciated by examining the ventilation equations.

Ventilation Equations

The classic equation defines VE as the product of VT and respiratory frequency (f)

$$\dot{V}E = VTf \tag{2}$$

Based on the analysis of the breathing cycle as the result of a driving and a timing mechanism, the following equation has been proposed [31, 32]

$$\dot{V}E = (VT/TI)(TI/TT) \tag{3}$$

where VT/TI is the mean inspiratory flow, and TI/TT is the "inspiratory duty cycle".

The advantage of equation (3) is that ventilation is partitioned into two components: one (TI/TT) reflects timing and the other (VT/TI) is related to neuromuscular inspiratory drive. More specifically, VT/TI depends on the intensity of the neural inspiratory drive and on the operating characteristics of the respiratory system (active impedance and operating length of inspiratory muscles). Equation (3) is useful in analysis of the effects of loading on ventilation. For example, the prolongation of TI, such as elicited by an added flow resistance or elastance, will defend VT but not necessarily VT/TI. Furthermore, if the load causes a proportional increase of inspiratory and expiratory durations, TI/TT will be unchanged. According to Equation (3), in this case the changes in timing induced by the loads will not defend ventilation. Note that most past reports have focused mainly on VT compensation and not on defense of either VE or alveolar ventilation.

To appreciate the contribution of nonneural load-compensatory mechanisms, model analysis has provided useful insight [2, 3].

Responses to Mechanical Loading

The responses to mechanical loading in awake humans and animals have been reviewed extensively [1-3]. This section is limited to general considerations.

During anesthesia the passive elastance and flow resistance of the respiratory system are, at least in humans, greater than in the awake state [31]. This implies less effective intrinsic load compensation in the awake state (Fig. 4). On the other hand, results from Agostoni et al. [29] and Axen and Haas [33] suggest that in many awake subjects there can be an increase of inspiratory motoneuron output during the first elastically or resistively loaded breath. In some instances the tidal volume of the first loaded breath is actually increased. In awake subjects the respiratory frequency commonly increases immediately after elastic loading [32-34] but tends to decrease with added flow resistances [33]. Thus, in awake subjects both intensity and timing of the neural drive can change substantially during the first loaded breath. These changes are characterized by marked intersubject variability. However, the ventilation during the first loaded breath is generally reduced [33, 34].

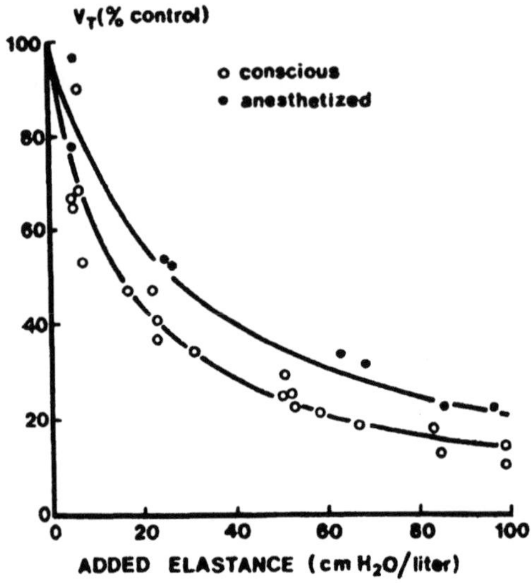

Fig. 4. Relationship between tidal volume (V_T) of the first loaded breath (expressed as percentage of the control value) and added elastance in a normal subject while conscious and anesthetized. (From [34] with permission)

During sustained respiratory loading, the differences in response between awake and anesthetized states are also very marked. In awake subjects:

a) ventilation tends to return more briskly towards control values than during anesthesia [34], and
b) under steady-state conditions there is generally little change of alveolar gas composition even in the face of substantial added elastic and flow-resistive loads [18, 32]. This implies that nonchemical neural load-compensatory mechanisms are more effective during wakefulness.

In awake state, the responses to loading can be modified by anticipation and previous experience and may also depend on individual personality traits. Sears [35] suggested that as soon as any interference to ventilation is detected, voluntary control supersedes automatic regulation and an appropriate new pattern of breathing is established. This new pattern then becomes automatic. Consequently, anticipation and experience should alter the responses to ventilatory load. Behavioral factors may explain the marked interindividual and intraindividual variability of responses to loading in the awake state [33]. Mechanical loading during anesthesia invariably leads to increased $PaCO_2$ and decreased PaO_2. In the conscious state, this occurs only when large loads are added. Similarly, in awake patients with markedly altered mechanical properties of the respiratory system (increased flow resistance and/or elastance), PaO_2 and $PaCO_2$ are very often within the normal range [19]. Because VT/TI is either normal or increased in patients [19], this implies increased intensity of neuromuscular inspiratory drive via as yet poorly understood nonchemical mechanisms.

In conscious subjects, sustained external elastic loading generally leads to increased respiratory frequency [32, 34] whereas flow-resistive loads cause decreased frequency [18]. By contrast, in anesthetized subjects the changes in respiratory frequency are small or absent and independent of the type of external loading [34].

The response of awake normal individuals appears to be useful in terms of minimization of the mechanical work of breathing [36, 37]. Note that in awake patients, a decreased frequency of breathing is seldom seen even in the face of markedly increased internal flow resistance [19]. This implies that internal respiratory loading is not analogous to external loading.

Responses to Pressure Biasing

The differences in response to pressure biasing between the anesthetized and the conscious state are as marked as the differences in responses to mechanical loading. In conscious humans, apnea is generally absent after the application of positive-pressure biasing [34]. This usually results in an immediate increase of inspiratory muscle activity [20, 38], which Mead [5] called the *operational length compensating (OLC) response*. The recent observation that quadriplegic patients show a prompt and powerful increase in diaphragmatic excitation when their midvolume is shifted in the inspiratory direction [38] suggests that the nature of the OLC response may be partly reflexive. However, in normal individuals a large part of the response must be cortical, as suggested by the wide variability in responses between and within subjects [20]. In normal conscious subjects, positive-pressure biasing generally elicits expiratory muscle activity (Fig. 5) [6, 39]. This has been termed the *operational length restoring (OLR) response* [5]. It may reflect a vagally mediated reflex, but the interindividual and intraindividual variability of the response suggests cortical involvement. As for mechanical loading, the short-term response to pressure biasing can be altered by previous instruction to the subject. Thus, if sub-

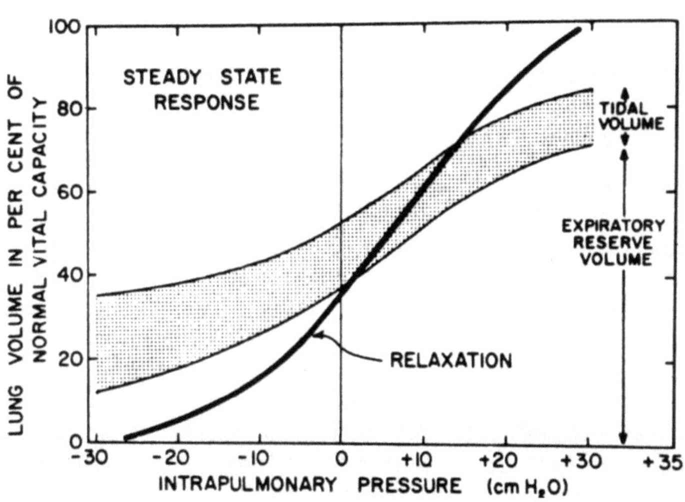

Fig. 5. Steady-state effects of continuous pressure biasing on tidal volume and inspiratory and expiratory reserve volumes. Average results of 10 seated conscious subjects. Note that, under steady-state conditions, end-expiratory volume deviates from the relaxation curve of total respiratory system (*solid line*), reflecting activity of expiratory muscles. (Adapted from [40])

jects are asked to relax, expiratory muscle activity may be absent and the end-expiratory volume lies on the static relaxation curve of the respiratory system [39].

Tolerance to pressure biasing and to mechanical loads

An important physiological limitation in positive-pressure biasing is the circulatory embarrassment caused by the elevation of intrathoracic pressure, which disturbs the normal gradient in venous pressure from the periphery to the heart. Excessive positive pressures lead eventually to syncope. The majority of subjects can tolerate positive pressures of about 20–30 cmH_2O; however, those accustomed to this maneuver can tolerate breathing up to about 60 cmH_2O [41]. Higher pressures lead rapidly to syncope and may also cause lung rupture.

An important physiological limit to negative-pressure breathing is probably pulmonary engorgement resulting from increased central blood volume. Most subjects can tolerate negative pressures of about −30 cmH_2O for prolonged periods [42]. A full account of the factors limiting the tolerance to positive- and negative-pressure breathing can be found elsewhere [41].

The foremost physiological limitation to mechanical and pressure biasing is respiratory muscle fatigue [42].

Conclusions

The respiratory system has a remarkable capacity to maintain ventilation within relatively narrow limits despite considerable changes in mechanical loading and pressure biasing. This ventilatory stability is provided by three main mechanisms:

1. the chemoreceptor-respiratory center control system,
2. nervous reflexes originating from pulmonary receptors and chest wall proprioceptors, and
3. mechanisms intrinsic to the ventilatory pump.

The last include the intrinsic properties of the respiratory muscles (force-length and force-velocity relationships), their mechanical arrangement and geometry, and the mechanical properties of the various structures comprising the ventilatory apparatus. In the conscious state, behavioral factors become prominent and the responses may be modified by a variety of factors (e.g. experience, instruction to subject, and individual personality traits). Although many of the factors that provide ventilatory stability in the face of pressure biasing and mechanical loading of breathing have been identified, little is known about their roles under the various conditions of daily life. Indeed, it should be stressed that conscious responses,which are characterized by marked interindividual and intraindividual variability, are very poorly understood.

References

1. Cherniack NS, Altose MD (1981) Respiratory responses to ventilatory loading. In: Hornbein TF (ed) Lung biology in health and disease. Regulation of breathing, vol. 17, pt. II, Dekker, New York, pp 905–964
2. Cherniack NS, Milic-Emili J (1985) Mechanical aspects of loaded breathing. In: Roussos C, Macklem PT (eds) The Thorax – Part B, Marcel Dekker Inc, New York, pp 751–786
3. Milic-Emili J, Zin WA (1986) Breathing responses to imposed mechanical loads. In: Cherniack NS, Widdicombe JG (eds) Handbook of physiology – the respiratory system II, Waverly Press Inc, Baltimore, pp 751–769
4. Pengelly LD, Alderson AM, Milic-Emili J (1971) Mechanics of the diaphragm. J Appl Physiol 30:797–805
5. Mead J (1979) Responses to loaded breathing. Bull Physio-Pathol Respir 15 (Suppl):61–71
6. Campbell EJM, Dickinson CJ, Dinnick OP, Howell BL (1961) The immediate effects of threshold loads on the breathing of men and dogs. Clin Sci 21:309–320
7. Gottfried SB, Rossi A, Higgs BD, et al. (1985) Noninvasive determination of respiratory mechanics during mechanical ventilation for acute respiratory failure. Am Rev Respir Dis 131:414–420
8. Goldman MD, Grassino A, Mead J, Sears TA (1978) Mechanics of the human diaphragm during voluntary contraction: dynamics. J Appl Physiol 44:840–848
9. Grassino A, Goldman MD, Mead J, Sears TA (1978) Mechanics of the human diaphragm during voluntary contraction: statics. J Appl Physiol 44:829–839
10. Milic-Emili J, Zin WA (1986) Relationship between neuromuscular respiratory drive and ventilatory output. In: Macklem PT, Mead J (eds) Handbook of physiology. Section 3, vol. III, mechanics of breathing, chapter 35, Am Physiol Soc Bethesda, pp 631–646
11. Younes M, Riddle W (1981) A model for the relation between respiratory neural and mechanical outputs. I.Theory. J Appl Physiol 51:963–978
12. Agostoni E, Mead J (1964) Statics of the respiratory system. In: Fenn WO, Rahn H (eds) Handbook of physiology. respiration, sect. 3, vol. I, Am Physiol Soc, Washington, DC, pp 387–409
13. Dubois AB (1964) Resistance to breathing. In: Fenn WO, Rahn H (eds) Handbook of physiology. respiration, sect. 3, vol. I, chapt. 16, Am Physiol Soc pp 451–462
14. Kim MJ, Druz WS, Danon J, Machnach W, Sharp JT (1976) Mechanics of the canine diaphragm. J Appl Physiol 41:369–382
15. Druz WS, Sharp JT (1982) Electrical and mechanical activity of the diaphragm accompanying body position in severe obstructive pulmonary disease. Am Rev Respir Dis 125:275–280
16. Siafakas NM, Chang HK, Bonora M, Gautier H, Milic-Emili J, Duron B (1981) Time course of phrenic activity and respiratory pressures during airway occlusion in cats. J Appl Physiol 51:99–108
17. Euler C von, Martilla I, Remmers JE, Trippenbach T (1976) Effects of lesions in the parabracial nucleus on the mechanisms for central and reflex termination of inspiration in the cat. Acta Physiol Scand 96:324–337
18. Zechman F, Hall FG, Hull WE (1957) Effects of graded resistance to tracheal air flow in man. J Appl Physiol 10:356–362
19. Milic-Emili J (1981) Recent advances in clinical assessment of control of breathing. Lung 160:1–17
20. Banzett R, Strohl K, Geffory B, Mead J (1981) Effect of transrespiratory pressure on PET_{CO2}–Pa_{CO2} and ventilatory reflexes in humans. J Appl Physiol 51:660–664
21. Gauthier H (1976) Pattern of breathing during hypoxia or hypercapnia of the awake or anesthetized cat. Respir Physiol 27:193–206
22. Hickey RF, Severinghaus JW (1981) Regulation of breathing: drug effects. In: Hornbein TF (ed) Lung biology in health and disease. regulation of breathing, vol. 17, pt. II, Dekker, New York, pp 1251–1312
23. Younes M, Remmers JE (1981) Control of tidal volume and respiratory frequency. In: Hornbein TF (ed) Lung biology in health and disease. regulation of breathing, vol. 17, pt. I, Dekker, New York, pp 621–671

24. Clark FJ, Euler C von (1972) On the regulation of depth and rate of breathing. J Physiol London 222:267–295
25. Gauthier H, Remmers JE, Bartlett D Jr (1973) Control of duration of expiration. Respir Physiol 18:205–221
26. Knox CK (1973) Characteristics of inflation and deflation reflexes during expiration in the cat. J Neurophysiol 36:284–295
27. Bishop B, Bachofen H (1972) Vagal control of ventilation and respiratory muscles during elevated pressures in the cat. J Appl Physiol 32:103–112
28. D'Angelo E, Agostoni E (1975) Tonic vagal influences on inspiratory duration. Respir Physiol 24:287–302
29. D'Angelo E, Agostoni E (1975) Immediate response to expiratory threshold load. Respir Physiol 25:269–284
30. Grunstein MM, Wyszogrodski I, Milic-Emili J (1975) Regulation of frequency and depth of breathing during expiratory threshold loading in cats. J Appl Physiol 38:869–874
31. Derenne JP, Couture J, Iscoe S, Whitelaw WA, Milic-Emili J (1976) Occlusion pressures in men rebreathing CO_2 under methoxyflurance anesthesia. J Appl Physiol 40:805–814
32. Milic-Emili J, Grunstein MM (1976) Drive and timing components of ventilation. Chest 70 (Suppl): 131–133
33. Axen K, Sperber Haas S (1979) Range of first-breath ventilatory responses to added mechanical loads in naive men. J Appl Physiol 46:743–751
34. Margaria CE, Iscoe S, Pengelly LD, Couture J, Don H, Milic-Emili J (1971) Immediate ventilatory response to elastic loads and positive pressure in man. Respir Physiol 18:347–369
35. Sears TA (1971) Breathing: a sensory-motor act. In: Sci Basis Med Annu Rev, chapt. 7, pp 129–147
36. Mead J (1960) Control of respiratory frequency. J Appl Physiol 15:325–336
37. Otis AB, Fenn WO, Rahn H (1950) Mechanics of breathing in man. J Appl Physiol 2:592–607
38. Banzett RB, Inbar GF, Brown R, Goldman M, Rossier A, Mead J (1981) Diaphragm electrical activity during negative lower torso pressure in quadriplegic men. J Appl Physiol 51:654–659
39. Green M, Mead J, Sears TA (1978) Muscle activity during chest wall restriction and positive pressure breathing in man. Respir Physiol 35:283–300
40. Rahn H, Otis AB, Chadwick LE, Fenn WO (1946) The pressure-volume diagram of the thorax and lung. Am J Physiol 146:161–178
41. Ernsting E (1965) The physiology of pressure breathing: In: Gilles JA (ed) The textbook of aviation physiology, Pergamon, Oxford, U.K.
42. Roussos C (1982) The failing ventilatory pump. Lung 160:59–84
43. Rahn H, Otis AB, Chadwick LE, Fenn WO (1946) The pressure-volume diagram of the thorax and lung. Am J Physiol 146:161–178

Diagnosing the Adequacy of Neural Stimulation

J. W. Fitting

Introduction

Ventilatory failure may result from a wide range of disorders of the respiratory system, from the respiratory centers to the alveoli. In a limited number of circumstances, ventilatory failure is solely due to an insufficient neural stimulation from the respiratory centers to the respiratory muscles. Such a failing ventilatory drive occurs for instance in drug overdose, anesthesia, or primary alveolar hypoventilation. The majority of cases of ventilatory failure, however, results from disorders of the airways, the lungs, and the chest wall. Still, the question may arise as to whether the ventilatory drive is adequate to cope with these situations of increased load. This chapter will review the parameters and methods available to the clinician for assessing the adequacy of neural stimulation in ventilatory failure.

The various steps of the process of breathing are described in Fig. 1. After integration of peripheral and cortical afferent, the rhythmic activation of the brain stem respiratory centers is transferred via alpha-motoneurons to the different respiratory muscles. The latter are activated, shorten, and apply tension to the various structures of the respiratory system. As a result, the chest wall and the lungs expand and generate inspiratory airflow.

Under experimental conditions, several parameters reflecting ventilatory drive may be measured. The closest signal to the respiratory centers is the electrical activity of the alpha-motoneurons which can be measured as the phrenic electroneurogram (ENG) [1, 2]. The next signal is the electrical activation of the respiratory muscles which can be measured as the electromyogram (EMG) of the diaphragm, or intercostal and accessory muscles [1, 3–5]. Respiratory muscle shortening can be measured by sonomicrometry in anesthetized or awake animals [6, 7]. During a dynamic contraction, a muscle consumes oxygen and generates tension in proportion with its EMG activity [8]. The oxygen cost of breathing can be measured as the difference in oxygen uptake between spontaneous and mechanical ventilation. The tension applied to the lungs can be measured as pleural pressure during unimpeded breathing, or as mouth or tracheal pressure during sustained [1, 2] or brief [9] airway occlusion. Finally, the neural output is transformed into movements of air that can be characterized as inspiratory flow and duration, tidal volume (VT), respiratory rate, or minute ventilation (VE).

Some of these parameters are limited to animal experiments, like phrenic ENG and respiratory muscle shortening. Others may be measured in humans but do not always reflect the respiratory neural output reliably. In the presence of acute ventilatory failure, what parameters can be used by the clinician to assess the respiratory

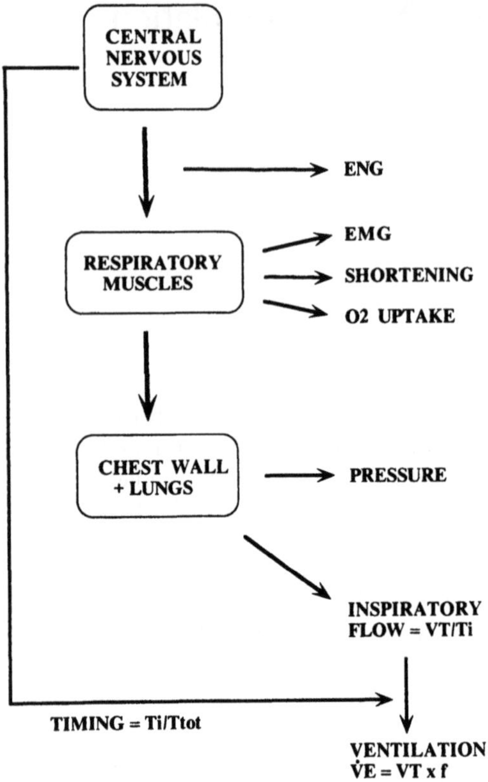

Fig. 1. Schema illustrating the process transforming neural output into ventilation and the various parameters used to test respiratory drive. *VT:* tidal volume. *Ti:* inspiratory time. *Ttot:* total breath time. *V̇E:* minute ventilation. *f:* breathing frequency

drive? They will be presented here, going from the periphery toward the respiratory centers.

Ventilatory Parameters

In the absence of neuromuscular, chest wall, and lung disorder, VE accurately reflects respiratory drive and has been extensively used to quantify the responsiveness to hypercapnia or hypoxia [10, 11]. VE is usually described as the product of VT times frequency (f): $\dot{V}E = VT \times f$. Milic-Emili and Grunstein [12] proposed another way to analyze VE which is more directly related to respiratory center output:

$$\dot{V}E = \frac{VT}{TT} \cdot \frac{TI}{Ttot}$$

where TI is inspiratory time, and Ttot is total breath time. The expression VT/TI is mean inspiratory flow which has been shown to track chemical drive [13] and velocity of shortening of the diaphragm [14]. Thus, VT/TI reflects the intensity of neural drive. The expressions TI and TI/Ttot indicate the timing of neural drive which is the other important determinant of VT.

This analysis of breathing pattern has led to a better understanding of control of breathing in disease. Thus, both normocapnic and hypercapnic patients with chronic obstructive pulmonary disease (COPD) breathe with a higher VT/TI than normal subjects [15]. However, hypercapnic patients are characterized by a shorter TI which results in a smaller VT and a higher breathing frequency. This altered timing and reduced VT may in itself explain the development of CO_2 retention, according to the following equation:

$$PaCO_2 = \frac{k \cdot \dot{V}CO_2}{\dot{V}E(1 - VD/VT)}$$

where $PaCO_2$ is arterial partial pressure of carbon dioxide, k is a constant, $\dot{V}CO_2$ is carbon dioxide production, and VD is physiological dead space.

The usefulness of mean inspiratory flow (VT/TI) is limited because it reflects neural drive only in the absence of neuromuscular, chest wall, and lung disease, i.e. only in a minority of cases of ventilatory failure. This parameter underestimates the intensity of neural drive in the presence of altered mechanics of the respiratory system, or of weakness of respiratory muscles [16].

However, the timing component of breathing pattern should be considered. Rapid shallow breathing is a common manifestation in several diseases, including COPD [15, 17] and neuromuscular disorders [18], and may lead to hypercapnia via an increased VD/VT ratio. Thus, the development of tachypnea may be considered as a potentially dangerous adaptation of respiratory controlling mechanisms to situations of increased load.

Airway Occlusion Pressure

The forces applied by the various inspiratory muscles to the lungs can be globally assessed by airway pressure during an occlusion. If the airways of anesthetized cats are occluded for 15–20 breaths, a progressive increase in inspiratory effort is observed. During such an occlusion, peak negative airway pressure and peak phrenic integrated ENG increase in parallel, showing a close linear correlation as displayed in Fig. 2 [1]. Similarly, peak airway occlusion pressure increases in parallel with phrenic ENG activity during CO_2 rebreathing tests [2]. Thus, peak airway occlusion pressure represents a valid index of the respiratory neural output. A clinical counterpart has been proposed by Marini et al. [19], consisting in occluding the endotracheal tube of mechanically ventilated patients for 20 sec in order to better assess inspiratory muscle strength. As the ventilatory drive increases during the occlusion, this maneuver actually tests respiratory neural output and inspiratory muscle strength together.

A sustained airway occlusion cannot be used to assess respiratory drive during spontaneous breathing because conscious subjects quickly react by increasing their effort or by holding their breath. To obviate this problem, it has been proposed to measure mouth pressure 0.1 sec or 0.15 sec after the onset of inspiratory effort against an occlusion, the so-called P0.1 or P0.15 [9, 21, 22]. By that time, the subject is still unaware of the occlusion, the reaction time to an occlusion being

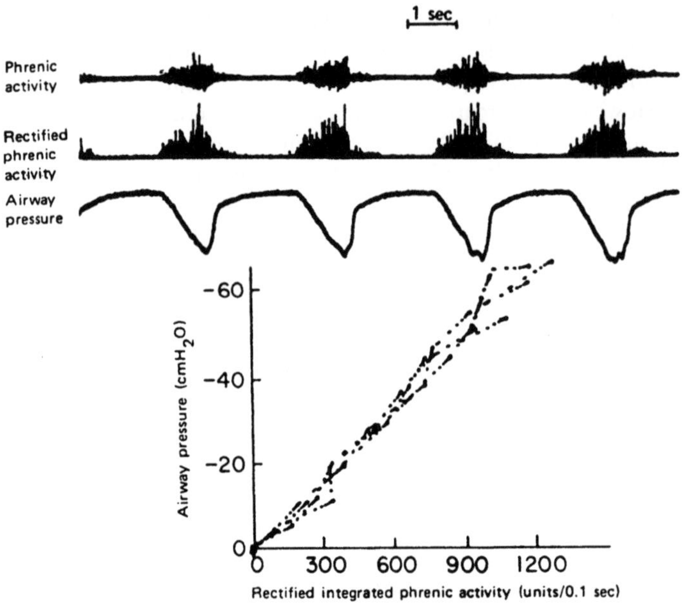

Fig. 2. Relationship between airway pressure and phrenic nerve activity during four consecutive occluded breaths in an anesthetized cat. Airway occlusion pressure increases linearly with phrenic electroneurogram activity. (From [1] with permission)

0.2–0.3 sec. Thus, mouth occlusion pressure represents an index of the respiratory neural output which is not artefactually modified by its own measurement.

It was originally assumed that the occlusion ensured an isometric contraction of inspiratory muscles and thereby eliminated pressure losses due to force-length and force-velocity relationships. Direct measurements of changes in diaphragm length by sonomicrometry in animals proved this assumption to be wrong. Indeed, diaphragm shortening after 0.1 sec was identical in occluded and unoccluded breaths during CO_2 rebreathing tests [20]. However, the amount of muscle shortening is probably insufficient to result in an important pressure loss.

Mouth occlusion pressure increases linearly with diaphragmatic EMG activity during CO_2 rebreathing in conscious humans [5, 23]. This noninvasive measurement can therefore be used to assess respiratory neural output. Several caveats must however be noticed. First, because P0.1 is the result of both neural and muscular output it can theoretically be modified by an impaired muscle performance. Although P0.1 is clearly less affected than VE during partial curarization, it can be expected to underestimate central neural drive in case of severe muscle weakness [16]. Second, P0.1 may sometimes be generated by the relaxation of abdominal muscles in early inspiration and may therefore bear no relationship with diaphragmatic activation. This is particularly likely to occur during stimulated breathing in the sitting position [24].

The interpretation of mouth occlusion pressure poses special problems in case of COPD. First, P0.1 measured at the mouth underestimates P0.1 measured in the esophagus or in the trachea [25, 26]. During an occlusion, the transmission of alveolar pressure to the mouth is function of a time constant which is the product of airway resistance and upper airway compliance. This product is normally small but increases sufficiently in COPD to explain the discrepancies between mouth and esophageal or tracheal occlusion pressure [26]. Second, hyperinflation is associated with a shorter and flatter diaphragm which reduces its tension output for a given activation and its pressure output for a given muscle tension. This represents another cause of underestimation of respiratory neural drive by P0.1. Third, because of incomplete lung emptying in COPD, a residual positive alveolar pressure frequently exists at the end of expiration, that has been termed intrinsic PEEP or auto-PEEP [27, 28]. This positive pressure must first be overcome by inspiratory effort before mouth or tracheal pressure starts to decrease. As a consequence, mouth or tracheal P0.1 may represent the pressure change occurring between 0.1 and 0.2 sec rather than that of the first 0.1 sec of inspiratory effort [26].

Mouth occlusion pressure has been used to assess respiratory neural output in chronic and acute ventilatory failure. Sorli et al. [15] found an increased P0.1 during resting breathing in patients with stable COPD, both with and without CO_2 retention. On average, P0.1 was 2.5 cm H_2O in normocapnic patients, 3.2 cm H_2O in hypercapnic patients, and 1.0 cm H_2O in normal subjects [15]. The ventilatory drive was found even higher in COPD patients with acute respiratory failure (ARF). Aubier et al. [17] reported an average P0.1 of 8.3 cm H_2O during ARF, decreasing to 3.9 cm H_2O with recovery, compared with 1.7 cm H_2O in normal subjects. This increase in respiratory drive is all the more important that it is underestimated by mouth occlusion pressure in severe COPD.

Tracheal occlusion pressure can be measured for assessing central neural output during weaning trials from mechanical ventilation. Patients at risk of weaning failure because of an insufficient respiratory drive may be recognized by an inadequately low P0.1 [29]. However, difficult weaning appears to be most often associated with an increased respiratory drive. Thus, in 20 patients Herrera et al. [30] reported weaning to be unsuccessful in 89% of cases with P0.1 >4.2 cm H_2O and successful in 78% of cases with P0.1 <4.2 cm H_2O. Similarly, in 12 patients Sassoon et al. [31] reported five weaning failures, all with P0.1 >6 cm H_2O, and seven successes, all with P0.1 <6 cm H_2O.

The weaning difficulties encountered with high airway occlusion pressure are probably related to respiratory muscle fatigue. Murciano et al. [32] measured tracheal occlusion pressure during short periods of spontaneous breathing in 16 COPD patients receiving mechanical ventilation for ARF. From the first to the last day of mechanical ventilation, the mean P0.1 decreased from 7.4 to 4 cm H_2O in the group successfully weaned, whereas it remained 6.4 cm H_2O in the group needing early reintubation. On the first day, the high/low ratio of diaphragmatic EMG consistently fell during the course of spontaneous breathing, indicating fatiguing contractions in both groups of patients. This EMG pattern of incipient fatigue was found at each session in the group with persistently high P0.1. In contrast, it disappeared when P0.1 decreased in the group with favorable weaning outcome. In this context, high occlusion pressures indicate that the respiratory muscles receive adequate neural stimulation to cope with increased loads but that they may contract beyond the threshold of fatigue [33].

A hypercapnic challenge has been proposed by Montgomery et al. [34] for predicting weaning outcome. Studying 14 trials in 11 patients considered marginal for weaning, these authors found that P0.1 on a T-piece trial was similarly increased in those patients who succeeded and in those who failed to wean. Each patient was submitted to a hypercapnic challenge, induced by inhaling a 3% CO_2 and 40% O_2 mixture for five minutes, which raised end-tidal PCO_2 by 10 mm Hg. The relative increase in P0.1 during the hypercapnic test was consistently higher in those patients who could be weaned. Thus, P0.1 increased always more than 40% in the group with successful weaning and always less than 30% in the group with weaning failure [34].

In summary, it appears from several studies that patients with difficult weaning most often breathe with an increased ventilatory drive, which may sometimes lead to respiratory muscle fatigue [30–32, 34, 35]. Conflicting data exist about the predictive value of absolute P0.1 in this circumstance (Table 1). Testing the patient's neuromuscular output reserve by a hypercapnic challenge may offer a better prediction of weaning outcome.

Work of Breathing

The work of breathing is computed from the pressure-volume diagram of the lung and chest wall, using esophageal pressure for pleural pressure [36]. The calculation of the work of breathing is usually performed to assess the load faced by the respiratory muscles rather than the ventilatory drive. However, it represents an indirect way to estimate respiratory neural output when ventilatory response cannot be used because of altered mechanics of the lung or chest wall. Indeed, important fluctuations in pleural pressure will be measured if the neural drive is high in the presence of an increased load. However, this method is seldomly used to test central neural drive because it is indirect and it requires an esophageal balloon.

Table 1. Prediction of weaning outcome from mechanical ventilation according to airway occlusion pressure

Reference	Diseases	P0.1 (cm H_2O)		Predictive
		Success	Failure	
Herrera [30]	Various	<4.2	>4.2	Yes
Sassoon [31]	COPD	<6.0	>6.0	Yes
Murciano [32]	COPD	4.0 ± 0.05	6.4 ± 0.03	Yes
Montgomery [34]	Various	3.7 ± 0.7	5.7 ± 1.4	No
Pourriat [35]	COPD	6.2 ± 0.6	8.2 ± 1.0	No

P0.1: Airway occlusion pressure after 0.1 sec of inspiration; *COPD:* Chronic Obstructive Pulmonary Disease.
Values are means ±SE.

Oxygen Cost of Breathing

Skeletal muscle contraction involves electrical activation, energy expenditure, and production of force and displacement. During submaximal dynamic contractions, the oxygen consumption ($\dot{V}O_2$) increases linearly with the force exerted and with the integrated EMG activity [8]. Thus, measurement of $\dot{V}O_2$ allows another indirect assessment of neural stimulation directed to a group of muscles.

The $\dot{V}O_2$ of the respiratory muscles can be estimated by indirect calorimetry in patients receiving mechanical ventilation. To this end, it is necessary to calculate the oxygen cost of breathing (OCB) which is the difference of total $\dot{V}O_2$ between total ventilatory support and spontaneous breathing. Numerous studies have reported the OCB during weaning trials from mechanical ventilation. The results are heterogeneous and difficult to compare because of differences in patients, methods of measurement, and of calculations. However, the OCB is generally 10–20% of total $\dot{V}O_2$ during mechanical ventilation, with occasionally much higher values [37–43]. Because the OCB of normal subjects is less than 5% [44], these results suggest that respiratory neural output is most often increased at the time of weaning from mechanical ventilation, as otherwise indicated by studies on airway occlusion pressure.

The interpretation of the OCB as an index of central neural drive requires some caution. First, the respiratory muscles may not be the sole contributors to the OCB. Some increase in $\dot{V}O_2$ is probably attributable to the increase in catecholamine levels observed during weaning [45]. Second, indirect calorimetry requires steady state conditions which are not always possible during discontinuation of ventilatory support. Thus, minute ventilation is likely to drop in the patient with an inadequately low respiratory drive, thereby preventing measurements in steady state.

Electromyogram

The activation of a muscle fiber takes place through a repeated depolarization-repolarization process propagating from the neuromuscular junction. Single fiber EMG recordings by means of microelectrodes provide information on the firing rate of a given motor unit. Global EMG recordings by means of surface electrodes are composed of oscillations of multiple frequencies and reflect both firing rates and recruitment of underlying motor units.

The EMG of the diaphragm can be recorded via skin or mucosal surface electrodes. The costal segment of the diaphragm is recorded by electrodes positioned in the 5th, 6th, and 7th intercostal spaces near the chondrocostal junctions. During stimulated ventilation, however, these electrodes will pick up cross-talk from adjacent expiratory muscles, i.e. the internal intercostal and the abdominal muscles. The crural segment of the diaphragm is recorded without interference by an esophageal electrode whose extremity is stabilized against the cardia of the stomach by an inflated balloon [46].

Electromyographic monitoring of scalene and sternocleidomastoid activity may be of interest because these muscles are invariably recruited in case of respiratory distress. Surface electrodes can be used to this end, but they will pick up the electrical activity of the platysma as well. As illustrated by Fig. 3, this superficial muscle may be strongly activated in the presence of an increased ventilatory load [47]. When limited to inspiration, the activation of the platysma probably reflects the global recruitment of accessory neck muscles. The use of implanted fine wire electrodes provides a specific recording of scalene or sternocleidomastoid activity, but requires greater expertise than surface electrodes [47].

An EMG study of the respiratory muscles first provides a simple qualitative assessment: is a given muscle activated or not? If no activity is found, the question arises of a failing central drive or of a neural lesion, for instance of the phrenic nerve.

The EMG may also provide a quantitative assessment of respiratory drive. Indeed, simultaneous recordings have shown that diaphragmatic EMG activity changes in parallel with phrenic nerve activity [48]. Different methods have been used to quantify diaphragmatic EMG activity. Electronic integration provides total electrical activity per breath but shows only poor correlation with $PaCO_2$ during rebreathing tests [5, 49]. Another common method consists in rectifying the raw signal, and smoothing it through a resistance-capacitance circuit or a higher order filter. The resulting signal is the moving time average and represents the average level of activity over the preceding 100 or 200 ms [5, 50]. Although not corresponding to an electronic integration, the moving time average of EMG is frequently referred to as "integrated EMG". The shape of diaphragmatic moving time average EMG is triangular, resembling that of the spirogram (Fig. 4). Both peak activity and rate of rise (slope) adequately reflect chemical drive [5, 49]. As shown by Fig. 5, both peak and slope of moving time average EMG increase linearly with $PaCO_2$ during tests of progressive hypercapnia [51].

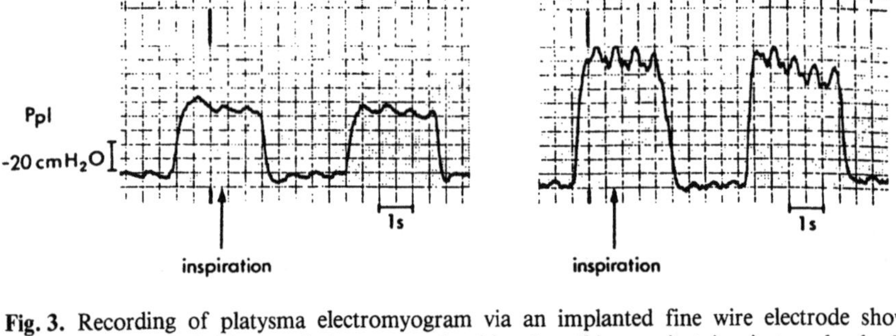

Fig. 3. Recording of platysma electromyogram via an implanted fine wire electrode showing strong activation of this muscle in a normal subject breathing against inspiratory loads. Left: inspiration with diaphragmatic emphasis; right: inspiration with rib cage muscle emphasis. (From [47] with permission)

Because diaphragmatic EMG recording is affected by such factors as electrode position, presence of esophageal air or mucus, and individual variations, a single absolute voltage is meaningless. Two methods of calibration have been proposed to allow intrasubject and intersubject comparisons. The peak EMG activity may be normalized to the peak activity obtained during an active inspiration at total lung capacity (TLC), which is reproducible in a given person [52]. When the respiratory neural output is assessed during stimulated breathing, the EMG response may be expressed as percent change from baseline activity [49].

Respiratory muscle EMG activity has the advantage of remaining a reliable indicator of neural drive in case of force failure, i.e. when there is dissociation between the electrical activation and the mechanical output, as with fatigue. This point is illustrated in Fig. 6 showing records of transdiaphragmatic pressure (Pdi), diaphragmatic electromyogram (Edi), and phrenic electroneurogram (Ephr) in an animal model of diaphragmatic fatigue induced by cardiogenic shock [53]. In this example, P0.1 is not shown but can be inferred from the rate of rise of Pdi. After 60 min of shock, there was an increase in Ephr, Edi, and Pdi (and consequently P0.1) attesting an enhanced respiratory drive. After 140 min of shock, there was further augmentation of Ephr and Edi, whereas in contrast Pdi declined as a result of diaphragmatic fatigue. At this time, P0.1 would no longer reflect neural drive. It should be noted that in this example peak activity of Ephr and Edi increased with a prolongation of inspiratory effort (and a reduced respiratory rate), but that the rate of rise of Ephr and Edi remained constant from 60 to 140 min of shock [53].

Thus, the quantified activity of respiratory muscle EMG offers the most direct index of central neural drive in humans. However, the relative complexity of signal recording and processing has until now prevented its general utilization in clinical settings.

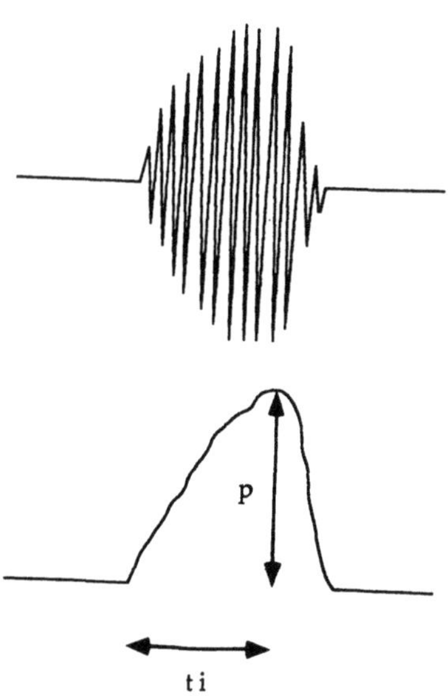

Fig. 4. Schematic representation of an electromyographic recording of the diaphragm. Top: raw EMG, which is adequate for detecting the presence or absence of muscle activation. *Bottom:* moving time average of EMG (often referred to as "integrated EMG"), which is adequate for quantifying the degree of muscle activation; *p:* peak EMG activity; *p/ti:* rate of rise (slope) of EMG activity

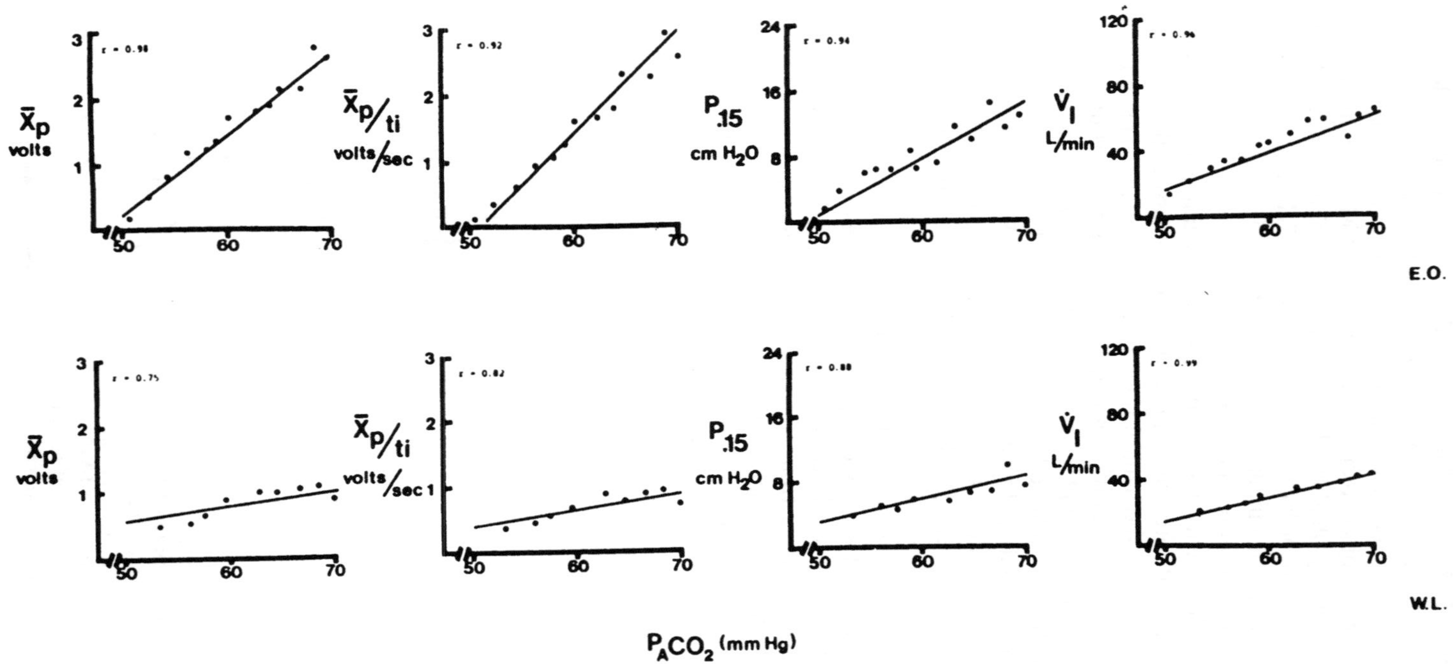

Fig. 5. Relationship between respiratory output variables and increasing alveolar PCO_2 ($PaCO_2$) during CO_2 rebreathing in two normal subjects. $\overline{Xp}$: peak of moving time average diaphragmatic EMG; $\overline{Xp}/ti$: slope of moving time average diaphragmatic EMG; *P* 0.15: mouth occlusion pressure at 0.15 sec., $\dot{V}I$: minute ventilation. The responses to CO_2 are linear. (From [52] with permission)

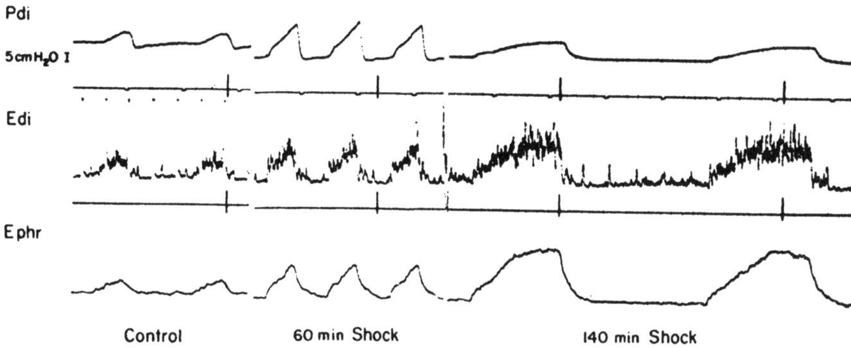

Fig. 6. Records of transdiaphragmatic pressure (Pdi), moving time average of diaphragmatic electromyogram (Edi) and of phrenic electroneurogram (Ephr) in a dog during cardiogenic shock. Airway occlusion pressure (P0.1) is not shown, but would change in proportion with the rate of rise of Pdi. After 60 min of shock, an enhanced neural drive is detected by an increase in Pdi, Edi, and Ephr. After 140 min of shock, Pdi declines as a result of diaphragmatic fatigue whereas Edi and Ephr increase further. At this point, P0.1 would no longer be a reliable index of neural stimulation. (From [53] with permission)

References

1. Eldridge FL (1975) Relationship between respiratory nerve and muscle activity and muscle force output. J Appl Physiol 39:567–574
2. Evanich MJ, Lopata M, Lourenco RV (1976) Phrenic nerve activity and occlusion pressure changes during CO_2 rebreathing in cats. J Appl Physiol 41:536–543
3. Agostoni E, Sant'Ambrogio G, Del Portillo Carrasco H (1960) Electromyography of the diaphragm in man and transdiaphragmatic pressure. J Appl Physiol 15:1093–1097
4. Petit JM, Milic-Emili J, Delhez L (1960) Role of the diaphragm in breathing in conscious normal man: an electromyographic study. J Appl Physiol 15:1101–1106
5. Lopata M, Evanich MJ, Lourenco RV (1977) Quantification of diaphragmatic EMG response to CO_2 rebreathing in humans. J Appl Physiol 43:262–270
6. Newman S, Road J, Bellemare F, Clozel JP, Lavigne CM, Grassino A (1984) Respiratory muscle length measured by sonomicrometry. J Appl Physiol 56:753–764
7. Easton PA, Fitting JW, Arnoux R, Guerraty A, Grassino AE (1989) Recovery of diaphragm function after laparotomy and chronic sonomicrometer implantation. J Appl Physiol 66:613–621
8. Bigland-Ritchie B, Woods JJ (1974) Integrated EMG and oxygen uptake during dynamic contractions of human muscles. J Appl Physiol 36:475–479
9. Whitelaw WA, Derenne JP, Milic-Emili J (1975) Occlusion pressure as a measure of respiratory center output in conscious man. Respir Physiol 23:181–199
10. Read DJC (1967) A clinical method for assessing the ventilatory response to carbon dioxide. Australasian Ann Med 16:20–32
11. Weil JV, Bryne-Quinn E, Sodal IE, et al. (1970) Hypoxic ventilatory drive in normal man. J Clin Invest 49:1061–1072
12. Milic-Emili J, Grunstein MM (1976) Drive and timing components of ventilation. Chest 70 (Suppl): 131–133
13. Newsom Davis J, Stagg D (1975) Interrelationships of the volume and time components of individual breaths in resting man. J Physiol (London) 245:481–495
14. Fitting JW, Easton PA, Grassino AE (1986) Velocity of shortening of inspiratory muscles and inspiratory flow. J Appl Physiol 60:670–677
15. Sorli J, Grassino A, Lorange G, Milic-Emili J (1978) Control of breathing in patients with chronic obstructive pulmonary disease. Clin Sci Mol Med 54:295–304

16. Holle RHO, Schoene RB, Pavlin EJ (1984) Effect of respiratory muscle weakness of P0.1 induced by partial curarization. J Appl Physiol 57:1150–1157
17. Aubier M, Murciano D, Fournier M, Milic-Emili J, Pariente R, Derenne JP (1980) Central respiratory drive in acute respiratory failure of patients with chronic obstructive pulmonary disease. Am Rev Respir Dis 122:191–199
18. Bégin R, Bureau MA, Lupien L, Bernier JP, Lemieux B (1982) Pathogenesis of respiratory insufficiency in myotonic dystrophy. Am Rev Respir Dis 125:312–318
19. Marini JJ, Smith TC, Lamb V (1986) Estimation of inspiratory muscle strength in mechanically ventilated patients: The measurement of maximal inspiratory pressure. J Crit Care 1:32–38
20. Easton PA, Fitting JW, Grassino AE (1987) Costal and crural diaphragm in early inspiration: free breathing and occlusion. J Appl Physiol 63:1622–1628
21. Shekleton M, Lopata M, Evanich MJ, Lourenco RV (1976) Effect of elastic loading on mouth occlusion pressure during CO_2 rebreathing in man. Am Rev Respir Dis 114:341–346
22. Lopata M, La Fata J, Evanich M, Lourenco RV (1977) Effects of flow-resistive loading on mouth occlusion pressure during CO_2 rebreathing. Am Rev Respir Dis 115:73–81
23. Lopata M, Evanich MJ, Lourenco RV (1977) Relationship between mouth occlusion pressure and electrical activity of the diaphragm: effects of flow-resistive loading. Am Rev Respir Dis 116:449–455
24. Grassino AE, Derenne JP, Almirall J, Milic-Emili J, Whitelaw W (1981) Configuration of the chest wall and occlusion pressures in awake humans. J Appl Physiol 50:134–142
25. Marazzini L, Cavestri R, Gori D, Gatti L, Longhini E (1978) Difference between mouth and esophageal occlusion pressure during CO_2 rebreathing in chronic obstructive pulmonary disease. Am Rev Respir Dis 118:1027–1033
26. Murciano D, Aubier M, Bussi S, Derenne JP, Pariente R, Milic-Emili J (1982) Comparison of esophageal, tracheal, and mouth occlusion pressure in patients with chronic obstructive pulmonary disease. Am Rev Respir Dis 126:837–841
27. Pepe PE, Marini JJ (1982) Occult positive end-expiratory pressure in mechanically ventilated patients with airflow obstruction. Am Rev Respir Dis 126:166–170
28. Rossi A, Gottfried SB, Zocchi L, et al. (1985) Measurement of static compliance of the total respiratory system in patients with acute respiratory failure during mechanical ventilation: The effect of intrinsic positive end-expiratory pressure. Am Rev Respir Dis 131:672–677
29. Montgomery AB, Stager MA, Schoene RB (1985) Marked suppression of ventilation while awake following massive ingestion of atenolol. Chest 86:920–921
30. Herrera M, Blasco J, Venegas J, Barba R, Doblas A, Marquez E (1985) Mouth occlusion pressure (P0.1) in acute respiratory failure. Intensive Care Med 11:134–139
31. Sassoon CSH, Te TT, Mahutte CK, Light RW (1987) Airway occlusion pressure. An important indicator for successful weaning in patients with chronic obstructive pulmonary disease. Am Rev Respir Dis 135:107–113
32. Murciano D, Boczkowski J, Lecocguic Y, Milic-Emili J, Pariente R, Aubier M (1988) Tracheal occlusion pressure: A simple index to monitor respiratory muscle fatigue during acute respiratory failure in patients with chronic obstructive pulmonary disease. Ann Intern Med 108:800–805
33. Bellemare F, Grassino A (1982) Effect of pressure and timing of contraction on human diaphragm fatigue. J Appl Physiol 53:1190–1195
34. Montgomery AB, Holle RHO, Neagley SR, Pierson DJ, Schoene RB (1987) Prediction of successful ventilator weaning using airway occlusion pressure and hypercapnic challenge. Chest 91:496–499
35. Pourriat JL, Lamberto C, Hoang PH, Fournier JL, Vasseur B (1986) Diaphragmatic fatigue and breathing pattern during weaning from mechânical ventilation in COPD patients. Chest 90:703–707
36. Agostoni E, Campbell EJM, Freedman S (1970) Energetics. In: Campbell EJM, Agostoni E, Newsom Davis J (eds) The respiratory muscles. London, Lloyd-Luke, pp 115–137
37. Field S, Kelly SM, Macklem PT (1982) The oxygen cost of breathing in patients with cardiorespiratory disease. Am Rev Respir Dis 126:9–13
38. Kemper M, Weissman C, Askanazi J, Hyman AI, Kinney JM (1987) Metabolic and respiratory changes during weaning from mechanical ventilation. Chest 92:979–983

39. Viale JP, Annat GJ, Bouffard YM, Delafosse BX, Bertrand OM, Motin JP (1988) Oxygen cost of breathing in postoperative patients. Pressure support ventilation vs continuous positive airway pressure. Chest 93:506–509
40. Hubmayr RD, Loosbrock LM, Gillespie DJ, Rodarte JR (1988) Oxygen uptake during weaning from mechanical ventilation. Chest 94:1148–1155
41. McDonald NJ, Lavelle P, Gallacher WN, Harpin RP (1988) Use of the oxygen cost of breathing as an index of weaning ability from mechanical ventilation. Intensive Care Med 14:50–54
42. Lewis WD, Chwals W, Benotti PN, et al. (1988) Bedside assessment of the work of breathing. Crit Care Med 16:117–122
43. Shikora SA, Bistrian BR, Borlase BC, Blackburn GL, Stone MD, Benotti PN (1990) Work of breathing: Reliable predictor of weaning and extubation. Crit Care Med 18:157–162
44. Otis AB (1954) The work of breathing. Physiol Rev 34:449–458
45. Kennedy SK, Weintraub RM, Skillman JJ (1977) Cardiorespiratory and sympatho-adrenal responses during weaning from controlled ventilation. Surgery 82:233–240
46. Grassino AE, Whitelaw WA, Milic-Emili J (1976) Influence of lung volume and electrode position on electromyography of the diaphragm. J Appl Physiol 40:971–975
47. Fitting JW, Bradley TD, Easton PA, Lincoln MJ, Goldman MD, Grassino A (1988) Dissociation between diaphragmatic and rib cage muscle fatigue. J Appl Physiol 64:959–965
48. Lourenco RV, Cherniack NS, Malm JR, Fishman AP (1966) Nervous output from the respiratory center during obstructed breathing. J Appl Physiol 21:527–533
49. Lopata M, Evanich MJ, Lourenco RV (1976) The electromyogram of the diaphragm in the investigation of human regulation of ventilation. Chest 70 (Suppl):162–165
50. Evanich MJ, Lopata M, Lourenco RV (1976) Analytical methods for the study of electrical activity in respiratory nerves and muscles. Chest 70 (Suppl):158–162
51. Lopata M, Zubillaga G, Evanich MJ, Lourenco RV (1978) Diaphragmatic EMG response to isocapnic hypoxia and hyperoxic hypercapnia in humans. J Lab Clin Med 91:698–709
52. Grassino A, Goldman M, Mead J (1974) Influence of chest wall configuration on the static and dynamic characteristics of the contracting diaphragm. In: Pengelly LD, Rebuck AS, Campbell EJM (eds) Loaded breathing. Don Mills, Ontario, Longman Canada, pp 64–72
53. Aubier M, Trippenbach T, Roussos C (1981) Respiratory muscle fatigue during cardiogenic shock. J Appl Physiol 51:499–508

Role of Extradiaphragmatic Musculature in Breathing

M. Decramer

Introduction

There is conclusive evidence now that quiet breathing and breathing under all possible circumstances require a coordinated contraction of different respiratory muscles to be accomplished [1–3]. The muscles regularly being activated during respiratory acts include: diaphragm, parasternal intercostals, scalenes, triangularis sterni, transversus abdominis, sternocleidomastoids, external intercostals and levatores costae. Although many studies on electromyogram (EMG) activity of these muscles are present, only scanty data are available on the mechanical outcome of contraction of individual respiratory muscles. Such data, however, are absolutely required to fully understand the act of breathing. This comprehension is of potential interest to patients with pulmonary disease or patients admitted to intensive care units. Indeed, pulmonary diseases were shown to be associated with important changes in respiratory muscle interaction [4, 5] which may affect both symptomatology and pathophysiology of these diseases. Moreover, therapeutic strategies aimed at altering respiratory muscle interaction may be tried, and may be successful in the treatment of the latter diseases. The purpose of the present review is to discuss respiratory muscle interaction with special emphasis on the mechanical outcome of muscle contraction and the contribution of the extradiaphragmatic musculature, and on alterations in respiratory muscle interaction induced by various circumstances associated to lung diseases.

Respiratory Muscle Interaction

Role of the Diaphragm

Diaphragmatic contraction undoubtedly has an important contribution to respiratory muscle interaction in all circumstances. The diaphragm consists of two muscles, the costal and crural parts (Fig. 1), each having their own motor innervation [4, 5], their own embryological origin [5], and possibly also their own fiber type [6–8]. Diaphragmatic action can be analyzed into three distinct components. First, diaphragmatic contraction is associated with fiber shortening and hence, with diaphragmatic descent [9–11] thereby increasing the craniocaudal diameters of the rib cage and accommodating the increase in lung volume into the lower rib cage and the abdominal wall [9]. Moreover, diaphragmatic contraction also increases lower rib cage dimensions, by two distinct mechanisms. First, the rise in abdominal

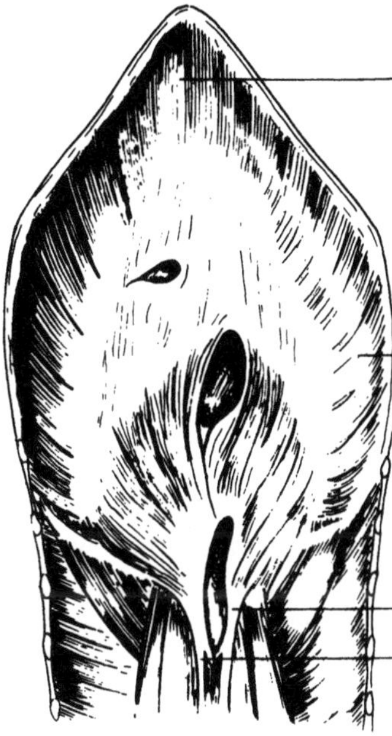

Fig. 1. Schematic diagram of the functional anatomy of the canine diaphragm

pressure caused by diaphragmatic contraction acts on the lower rib cage through the part of the diaphragm which is immediately apposed to the lower rib cage, the zone of apposition [9]. This is the appositional component of diaphragmatic action. Second, the costal diaphragm also has insertions into the lower rib cage by

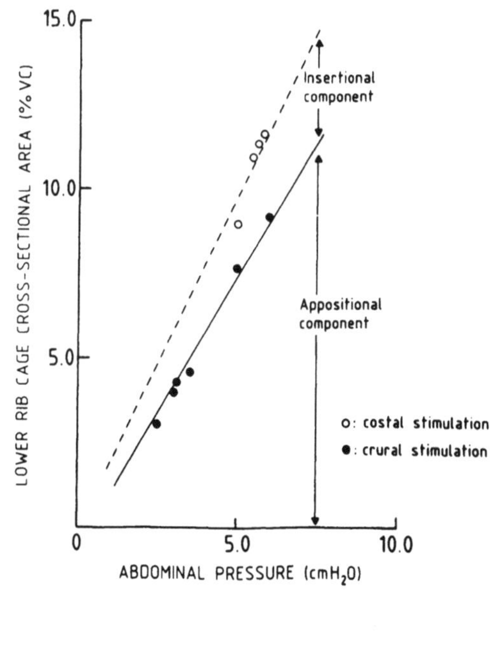

Fig. 2. Relationship between lower rib cage dimensions (cross-sectional area) and pressure acting on the lower rib cage (abdominal pressure), during separate stimulation of the costal (open circles) and crural parts of the diaphragm (closed circles), in one representative experiment. Data points represent plateau increases obtained during stimulation. Lines represent regression lines. Lower rib cage cross-sectional area is expressed as a percentage of the excursion during a vital capacity maneuver. Pressure is expressed in cm H_2O

virtue of which it increases lower rib cage dimensions during contraction. This is the insertional component of diaphragmatic contraction [9].

We attempted to estimate the relative significance of these actions in an animal model [12]. Indeed, since the crural part of the diaphragm has no insertions into the lower rib cage, crural stimulation will increase lower rib cage dimensions only because of an appositional component. By way of contrast, costal diaphragmatic action on the lower rib cage has both an insertional and an appositional component. As a consequence, the relationship between lower rib cage dimensions and abdominal pressure during separate costal and crural stimulation, allows to separate the appositional and insertional component. Figure 2 shows the results of a representative experiment. The appositional component was invariably far greater than the insertional component.

Moreover, in the same series of experiments, we studied the mechanical interdependence of the upper and lower canine rib cage. During phrenic nerve stimulation, the upper rib cage invariably deflated, the lower rib cage inflated, and virtually no mechanical interdependence between these two parts of the rib cage was present. Similarly, the human rib cage appeared to be a very distortable structure as well, although the mechanical interdependence between upper and lower rib cage was more significant than for the canine rib cage [13]. Since during quiet breathing in both dogs and humans upper rib cage expansion is clearly present, it must be obtained through contraction of the extradiaphragmatic musculature which thus contributes mechanically to the act of breathing.

Role of the Intercostal Muscles

The functional anatomy of the intercostal muscles is schematically shown in Fig. 3. The interosseus portion of the intercostal musculature consists of an outermost layer, the external intercostal, and an innermost layer the internal intercostal which have fiber orientations 90° perpendicular to one another. Inbetween the cartilage-

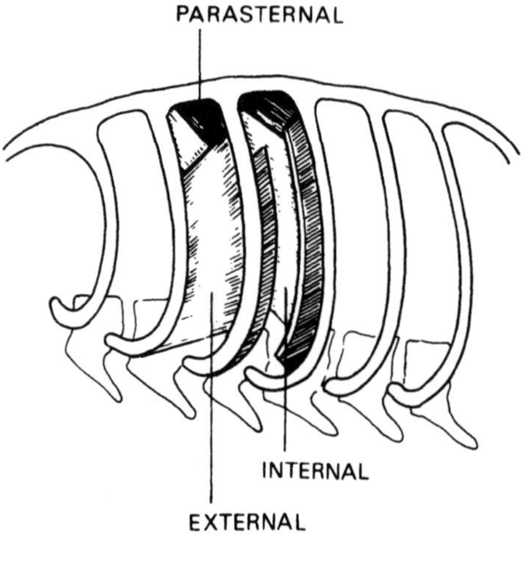

Fig. 3. Schematic diagram of the functional anatomy of the canine intercostal muscles

nous portions of the rib only one layer of intercostal muscle is present. It has the same fiber orientation as the internal intercostal and is called the parasternal intercostal. This muscle constitutes the most important respiratory part of the intercostal musculature [14–16]. We have attempted to estimate its mechanical contribution to inspiration in two consecutive series of experiments in dogs [17].

First, we developed a technique to measure changes in intramusculare pressure in the parasternal intercostals during respiratory maneuvers [17]. We showed that, during bilateral stimulation of the parasternal intercostals, an excellent correlation was present between the force exerted on the rib and the increase in intramuscular pressure. Figure 4 shows the experimental setup in this experiment. Figure 5 demonstrates the relationship between force and intramuscular pressure in a typical experiment. The slope of the relationship between force and intramuscular pressure appeared to be determined by the mass of the parasternal intercostal, and hence, by the body weight of the animal. Moreover, during active contraction of the parasternal intercostal in respiratory maneuvers, increases in intramuscular pressure were invariably found, and a correlation between the latter and the inspiratory fall in pleural pressure was present. This relationship is shown in Fig. 6. During passive inflation, when the parasternals were passively shortened, intramuscular pressure tended to decrease. By way of contrast, during passive deflation, when the parasternals were passively lengthened, intramuscular pressure invariably increased. As a consequence, during respiratory maneuvers, intramuscular pressure increased whenever the tension in the muscle increased either actively or passively, while it decreased whenever the tension in the muscle decreased. Hence, intramuscular pressure allows to measure the force developed during parasternal intercostal contraction correctly.

Second, we used the force developed during contraction as measured by the change in intramuscular pressure to estimate the parasternals' contribution to rib motion. We determined the relationship between intramuscular pressure and force as in the forementioned experiment. In addition, we determined the relationship between intramuscular pressure and rib motion measured with a linear displacement transducer, during bilateral stimulation of the parasternal intercostals. Final-

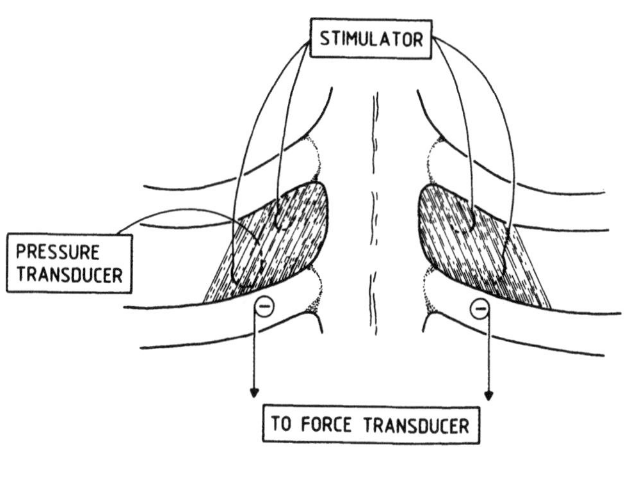

Fig. 4. Experimental setup during stimulation of the parasternal intercostals (From [17] with permission)

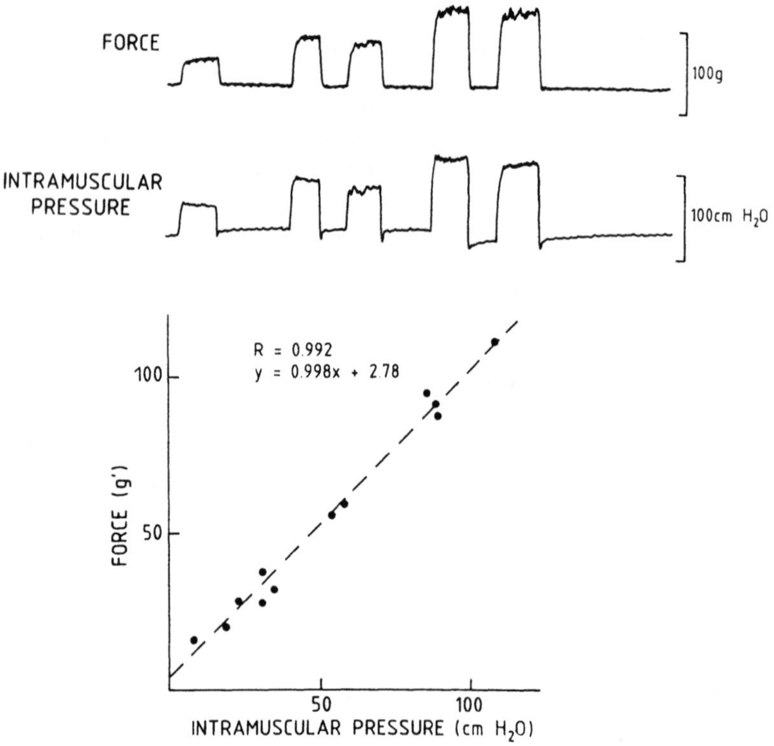

Fig. 5. Results of a typical experiment. *Upper panel,* tracing of force acting on the rib and intramuscular pressure during bilateral stimulation of the parasternal intercostals. *Lower panel,* relationship between force acting on the rib and intramuscular pressure during a typical experiment. Data points represent plateaus obtained during stimulation, dashed line represents regression line (From [17] with permission)

ly, intramuscular pressure and rib displacement were studied during a variety of respiratory maneuvers, thus allowing to estimate the parasternals' contribution to rib motion during these maneuvers. A representative experiment is summarized in Fig. 7. On the average, about 50–60% of the rib elevation was due to parasternal intercostal contraction during quiet breathing. The forementioned reasoning implicitly assumes that the relationship between a force exerted on the rib, and rib displacement is similar during bilateral stimulation of the parasternal intercostal in one intercostal interspace and during quiet breathing. This assumption strictly means that almost no mechanical interaction between different parasternal intercostals and different interspaces is present. This e.g. would be the case if the parasternals attach to the sternum at one end, and to the rib at the other end. Such a mechanical model is an oversimplification. Since, however, inspiratory shortening is vastly reduced after selective denervation [18, 19], the assumption appears to be reasonable and the mechanical interaction between parasternal intercostals in the different interspaces appears to be limited.

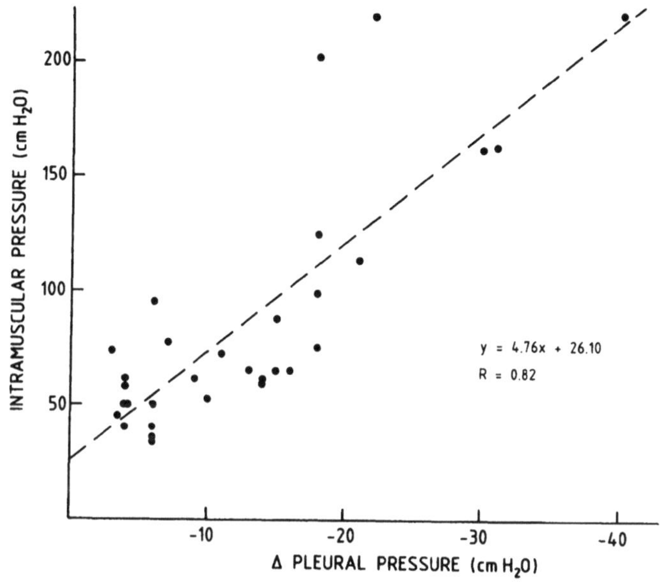

Fig. 6. Relationship between intramuscular pressure and swing in pleural pressure in eight animals, during quiet breathing, resistive loading and occluded inspiration. Dashed line is regression line. Pressures are expressed in cm H_2O. (From [17] with permission)

There is little doubt that the parasternal intercostals contribute importantly to inspiration in man as well. The muscles are always electrically active during inspiration in man [14]. Their mechanical contribution to inspiration is evidently more difficult to assess than in anesthetized dogs. Nevertheless, the close similarity of the anatomical arrangements, the high degree of distortability of the rib cage, and the upper rib cage expansion normally seen during inspiration, all suggest that similar concepts apply to humans.

Moreover, several lines of evidence suggest that in pulmonary disease with hyperinflation, the contribution of the parasternal intercostals vastly increases [20–22]. Hyperinflation is expected to be very severe in patients with chronic obstructive pulmonary disease (COPD) [23], and is probably even more pronounced in such patients admitted to intensive care units. The extent to which an increased contibution of the intercostal and accessory muscles in these patients may be associated with an increased sensation of dyspnea remains to be determined [24]. In any event, the increased contribution of the parasternal intercostals to inspiration with hyperinflation is likely to be related to the fact that the shortening of these muscles with hyperinflation is less pronounced than diaphragmatic shortening and hence, the mechanical disadvantage induced in the diaphragm is considerably more pronounced than in the parasternal intercostals to which hyperinflation may even be beneficial [20, 21].

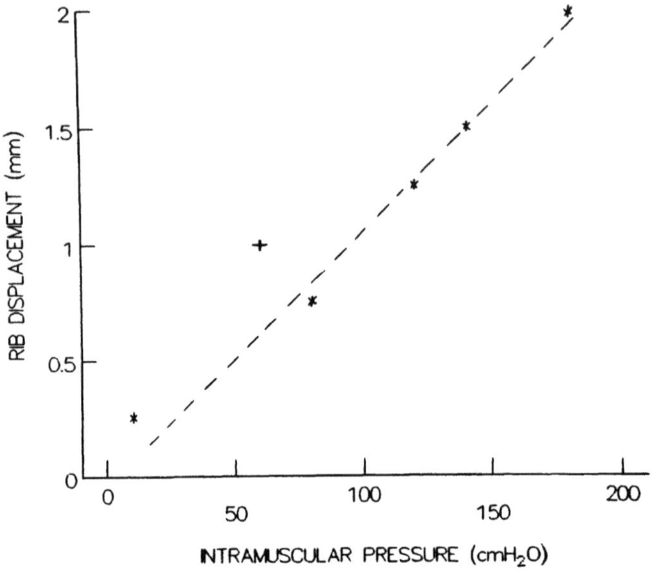

Fig. 7. Relationship between rib displacement (mm) and intramuscular pressure (cm H_2O) during bilateral stimulation of the parasternal intercostal (*, dashed line) and during quiet inspiration (+). The distance between the abscissa and the regression line represents the contribution of the parasternal intercostals to rib elevation, the distance between the regression line and + represents the contribution of other muscles

Role of the Scalenes

The scalenes are invariably active during inspiration in normal humans breathing quietly in the upright position [3]. Such activity is absent in anesthetized and awake dogs, and consequently animal models studying the mechanical outcome of scalene activity are more difficult to develop. Although it is difficult to quantify the mechanical contribution of the scalenes, data on tetraplegic subjects indicate that these muscles contribute mechanically to inspiration in humans [1].

Role of the Sternocleidomastoids and Other Accessory Muscles of Inspiration

These muscles are not active during quiet breathing in normal humans and are, therefore, termed accessory muscles of inspiration. The sternocleidomastoids are active in patients with high tetraplegia and profoundly hypertrophy in these patients, since they are innervated by the eleventh cranial nerve. They also are active during loaded inspiration, during inspiration in COPD-patients, and in patients with acute respiratory failure (ARF) [25]. Their mechanical contribution to inspiration remains to be determined.

Other potential inspiratory muscles include the pectoralis major, the shoulder girdle muscles and the levatores costae. Activity in the latter muscles was demonstrated during quiet breathing in dogs [26] and in cats [27]. In phrenicotomized animals, these muscles were contributing substantially to rib elevation, although even under these circumstances the parasternals still contributed the major part of the rib elevating action [26].

Role of the Expiratory Muscles

In humans during quiet expiration, expiratory muscle activity is usually absent in the supine position. In the upright position the abdominal muscles are tonically active in most subjects. The activity is tonic and greatest in the dependent regions of the abdomen [28–31] and may assist diaphragmatic function by preventing excessive diaphragmatic shortening during tilting from supine to upright position [32]. The abdominal muscle with the most important respiratory function is likely to be the transversus abdominis, which is often recruited during quiet inspiration in lightly anesthetized and awake dogs [33, 34]. This muscle does not contribute to quiet inspiration in humans, but is recruited during expiration below functional residual capacity (FRC), during laughing, coughing and speech [35]. In these maneuvers, the transversus abdominis is more easily recruited than the abdominal external oblique or the rectus abdominis.

The most important rib cage expiratory muscle is likely to be the triangularis sterni, which runs at the inner surface of the sternum between the caudal aspect and the lower ribs. The muscle is invariably active in supine anesthetized dogs during quiet breathing [36, 37] and contributes mechanically to inspiration by its relaxation. The muscle is not active during quiet expiration in humans [38], but is recruited during expiration below FRC, during speech, laughing and coughing.

Expiratory muscles may contribute up to 60% of tidal volume (VT) in upright dogs [39]. They thus constitute an important potential that may be recruited under certain circumstances. Such circumstances in humans include exercise [40]. To what extent expiratory muscles contribute to breathing in patients with ARF remains to be established, but clinical observation of these patients suggests that abdominal muscle contraction is frequently present.

Alterations in Respiratory Muscle Interaction

Several circumstances may exert a profound effect on respiratory muscle interaction and may profoundly alter the pattern of thoracoabdominal motion. These include: exercise, anesthesia, COPD, non-cardiogenic pulmonary edema, hyperinflation ... In most circumstances, the contribution of the extradiaphragmatic musculature to breathing vastly increases. In the last years, we studied two interventions, relevant to intensive care medicine, which were found to alter respiratory muscle interaction profoundly: hyperinflation and intravenous administration of aminophylline.

Hyperinflation

Hyperinflation is a common function abnormality accompanying diseases associated with air flow obstruction and acute respiratory pathology. Hyperinflation may be extremely severe in these patients with a FRC equalling or even exceeding predicted total lung capacity (TLC) [23]. In two series of experiments on a total of 21 supine anesthetized dogs, the effects of hyperinflation on inspiratory muscle mechanics were studied by applying large amounts of CPAP to make the animal breathe near its TLC. We found that hyperinflation profoundly reduced diaphragmatic mechanical effectiveness, as was evident from reduced abdominal motion, frequently even clear abdominal paradox, reductions in inspiratory rises in gastric pressure, frequently even inspiratory falls in gastric pressure, and reductions in diaphragmatic shortening while diaphragmatic EMG increased.

By way of contrast, rib cage expansion was much better preserved during breathing near TLC, while parasternal intercostal EMG tended to decrease. This suggested that the mechanical effectiveness of the parasternal intercostals was much better preserved with hyperinflation than diaphragmatic effectiveness. The latter hypothesis was confirmed by direct muscle stimulation experiments which demonstrated relatively unchanged swings in intramuscular pressure and force exerted on the rib, when the parasternals were stimulated at FRC and TLC [21]. Similar changes in the pattern of thoracoabdominal motion were observed in patients with hyperinflation [22]. An example of the effect of hyperinflation on the pattern of thoracoabdominal motion is shown in Fig. 8. It is clear that phrenicotomy profoundly affects the pattern of thoracoabdominal motion at FRC, while it almost does not affect it near TLC, which directly demonstrates the mechanical ineffectiveness of the diaphragm near TLC. It should be emphasized, however, that the

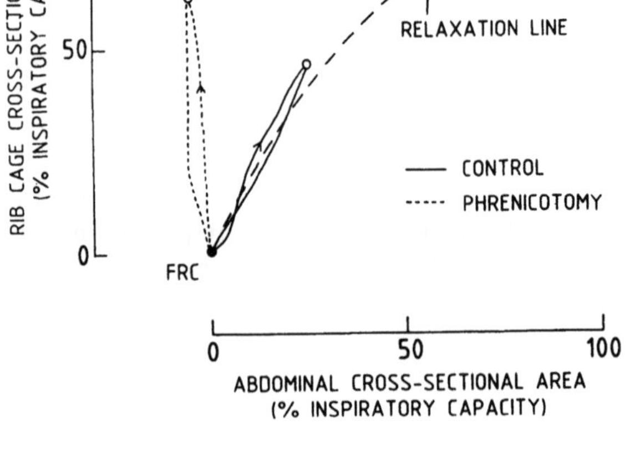

Fig. 8. Diagram relating rib cage cross-sectional area to abdominal cross-sectional area (Konno-Mead diagram). Dashed line is relaxation line. Loop represents animal breathing quietly at FRC and near TLC, before (solid line) and after bilateral phrenicotomy (dotted line). Cross-sectional areas are expressed as a percentage of the excursion during an inspiratory capacity maneuver. (From [20] with permission)

greater relative expansion of the rib cage near TLC, certainly in patients, does not necessarily indicate an increased contribution of the parasternal intercostals but could also be caused by an increased contribution of other inspiratory rib cage muscles, which were not explicitly studied in our experiments. Studies on the effects of hyperinflation on the other rib cage muscles, therefore, seem warranted.

Aminophylline

The effects of intravenous administration of progressively increasing doses of aminophylline (5, 10, 20, 40, 80 mg/kg), on respiratory muscle interaction were studied in 14 supine anesthetized dogs [41]. We observed that after aminophylline administration quiet inspiration became almost invariably biphasic, or if biphasic, inspiration was already present before to a certain extent, the magnitude of the first phase was clearly enhanced. A representative experiment is shown in Fig. 9. Biphasic inspiration was defined as an inspiration showing two distinct phases.

First, the onset of inspiration was characterized by a sudden increase in rib cage cross-sectional area often associated to a decrease in abdominal dimensions. Dur-

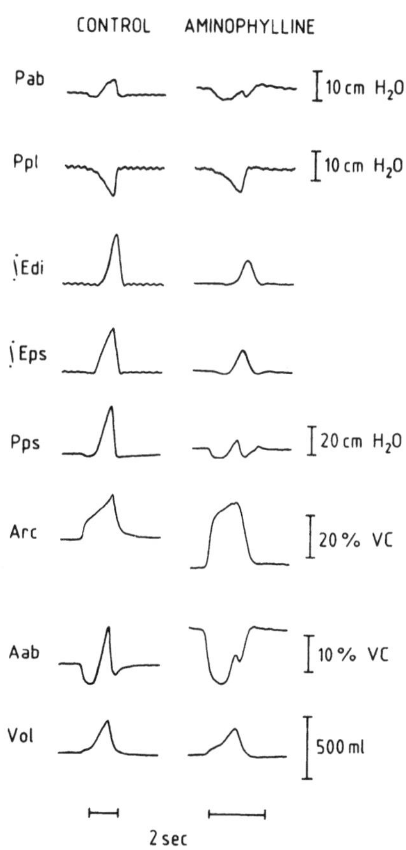

Fig. 9. Effects of aminophylline (80 mg/kg) on respiratory muscle interaction in one representative experiment. Abdominal pressure (Pab), pleural pressure (Ppl), integrated diaphragm EMG (E_{di}), integrated parasternal intercostal EMG (E_{ps}), parasternal intramuscular (Pps), rib cage cross-sectional area (Arc), abdominal cross-sectional area (Aab) and lung volume are shown. Pressures are expressed in cm H_2O, cross-sectional areas as a percentage of the excursion during a vital capacity maneuver and lung volume in ml. Note that after administration of aminophylline abdominal pressure decreases during inspiration, diaphragmatic and parasternal EMG decrease, and the sudden increase in Arc and the initial dip in Aab at the onset of inspiration are markedly enhanced, signalling enhanced recruitment of expiratory muscles

ing this initial part of inspiration, the parasternals and the diaphragm were electrically silent, confirming that it was achieved by relaxation of expiratory muscles. Further inspiration occurred predominantly through expansion of the abdomen. On the average, $40 \pm 27\%$ of the rib cage expansion was due to expiratory muscle relaxation at a dose of 80 mg/kg vs $20 \pm 22\%$ under control conditions ($p < 0.05$).

In this study, expiratory muscle recruitment was further confirmed by a clear increase in triangularis sterni EMG ($319 \pm 300\%$ control at a dose of 80 mg/kg), a tendency of transversus abdominus EMG to increase, and by significant increases in end-expiratory abdominal and pleural pressure. This study thus clearly demonstrated that in supine anesthetized dogs aminophylline administration promoted recruitment of expiratory muscles. More work is needed to clarify the extent to which the observed changes in respiratory muscle interaction might affect diaphragm length and to what extent changes in diaphragm length might be involved in the changes in diaphragmatic contractility induced by aminophylline, observed by others [42, 43]. Whatever the effects of expiratory muscle recruitment on diaphragm length and diaphragmatic contractility might be, it is, if it were to be present in patients with respiratory failure, expected to significantly alter the sensation of dyspnea. Indeed, to the extent that the latter sensation is expected to be related to the force developed by a given inspiratory muscle during inspiration, recruitment of expiratory muscles and hence, partitioning of the work of breathing between inspiratory and expiratory muscles is expected to reduce the force developed by each inspiratory muscle and consequently, to reduce the sensation of dyspnea. The significance of the latter mechanism in relation to other mechanisms by which aminophylline might reduce the sensation of dyspnea still remains to be assessed [44].

Acknowledgments. The author thanks Dr. Eric Derom and Dr. Han Jiang-Na for the stimulating discussions we had on this subject. He further thanks the "Fonds voor Geneeskundig Wetenschappelijk Onderzoek", "National Lottery - Belgium" and "Nationale Vereniging tot Steun aan de Gehandicapten" for their financial support. The expert secretarial assistance of Ms. Hilde Santermans is gratefully acknowledged.

References

1. De Troyer A, Estenne M (1988) Functional anatomy of the respiratory muscles. In: Belman MS (ed) Respiratory muscles: function in health and disease. Clin Chest Med 9:175–193
2. Decramer M (1987) How does the vital pump work. Bull Europ Physiopath Resp (editorial) 23:199–202
3. De Troyer A, Estenne M (1984) Coordination between rib cage muscles and diaphragm during quiet breathing in humans. J Appl Physiol 57:899–906
4. De Troyer A, Sampson M, Sigrist S, Macklem PT (1981) The diaphragm: two muscles. Science 213:237–238
5. De Troyer A, Sampson M, Sigrist S, Macklem PT (1982) Action of costal and crural parts of the diaphragm on the rib cage in dogs. J Appl Physiol 53:30–39
6. Riley DA, Berger AJ (1979) A regional histochemical and electromyographic analysis of cat respiratory diaphragm. Exp Neurol 66:636–649

7. Sieck GC, Ray RR, Powell P, Bianco C, Edgerton VR, Harper RM (1983) Muscle fiber type distribution and architecture of the cat diaphragm. J Appl Physiol 55:1386–1392
8. Reid MB, Ericson GC, Feldman HA, Johnson RL Jr (1987) Fiber types and fiber diameters in the canine respiratory muscles. J Appl Physiol 62:1705–1712
9. Mead J, Loring SH (1982) Analysis of volume displacement and length changes of the diaphragm during breathing. J Appl Physiol 53:750–755
10. Loring SH, Mead J (1982) Action of the diaphragm on the rib cage inferred from a force-balance analysis. J Appl Physiol 53:756–760
11. Decramer M, Jiang TX, Reid MB, Kelly S, Macklem PT, Demedts M (1986) Relationship between diaphragm length and abdominal dimensions. J Appl Physiol 61:1815–1820
12. Jiang TX, Demedts M, Decramer M (1988) Mechanical coupling of upper and lower canine rib cages and its functional significance. J Appl Physiol 64:620–626
13. Ward M, Ward J, Bellemare F, Macklem PT (1988) Distortability of the human rib cage. The Physiologist (abstract) 31:A222.
14. De Troyer A, Sampson M (1982) Activation of the parasternal intercostals during breathing efforts in human subjects. J Appl Physiol 52:524–529
15. Decramer M, De Troyer A (1984) Respiratory changes in parasternal intercostal length. J Appl Physiol 57:1254–1260
16. Decramer M, Kelly S, De Troyer A (1986) Respiratory and postural changes in intercostal muscle length in supine dogs. J Appl Physiol 60:1686–1691
17. Leenaerts P, Decramer M (1990) Respiratory changes in parasternal intercostal intramuscular presure. J Appl Physiol 68:868–875
18. De Troyer A, Farkas GA (1989) Passive shortening of canine parasternal intercostals during breathing. J Appl Physiol 66:1414–1420
19. De Troyer A, Farkas GA (1989) Mechanical arrangement of the parasternal intercostals in the different interspaces. J Appl Physiol 66:1421–1429
20. Decramer M, Jiang TX, Demedts M (1987) Effects of hyperinflation on inspiratory muscle use. J Appl Physiol 63:1493–1498
21. Jiang TX, Deschepper K, Demedts M, Decramer M (1989) Effects of acute hyperinflation on the mechanical effectiveness of the parasternal intercostals. Am Rev Respir Dis 139:522–528
22. Gilmartin JJ, Gibson GJ (1984) Abnormalities of chest wall motion in patients with chronic airflow obstruction. Thorax 39:264–271
23. Decramer M (1989) Effects of hyperinflation on respiratory muscles. Eur Respir J (editorial) 2:299–302
24. Ward M, Eidelman D, Stubbing DG, Bellemare F, Macklem PT (1988) Respiratory sensation and pattern of respiratory muscle activation during diaphragm fatigue. J Appl Physiol 65:2181–2189
25. Efthimiou J, Fleming J, Spiro SG (1987) Sternocleidomastoid muscle function and fatigue in breathless patients with severe respiratory disease. Am Rev Respir Dis 136:1099–1105
26. De Troyer A, Farkas GA (1989) Inspiratory function of the levator costae and external intercostal muscle in the dog. J Appl Physiol 67:2614–2621
27. Hilaire GG, Nichols JG, Sears TA (1983) Central and proprioceptive influences on the activity of the levator costae motorneurons in the cat. J Physiol London 342:527–548
28. De Troyer A (1983) Mechanical role of the abdominal muscles in relation to posture. Respir Physiol 53:341–353
29. Floyd WF, Silver PHS (1950) Electromyographic study of patterns of activity of the anterior abdominal wall muscles in man. J Anat 84:132–145
30. Loring SH, Mead J (1982) Abdominal muscle use during quiet breathing and hyperpnea in uninformed subjects. J Appl Physiol 52:700–704
31. Strohl KP, Mead J, Banzett RB, Loring SH, Kosch PC (1981) Regional differences in abdominal muscle activity during various maneuvers in humans. J Appl Physiol 51:1471–1476
32. Strohl KP, Mead J, Banzett RB, Lehr J, Loring SH, O'Cain C (1984) Effect of posture on upper and lower rib cage motion and tidal volume during diaphragm pacing. Am Rev Respir Dis 130:320–321

33. Gilmartin JJ, Ninane V, De Troyer A (1987) Abdominal muscle use during breathing in the anesthetized dog. Respir Physiol 70:159–171
34. De Troyer A, Gilmartin JJ, Ninane V (1989) Abdominal muscle use during breathing in unanesthetized dogs. J Appl Physiol 66:20–27
35. De Troyer A, Estenne M, Ninane V, Vangansbeke D, Gorini M (1990) Tranversus abdominis muscle function in humans. J Appl Physiol 68:1010–1016
36. De Troyer A, Ninane V (1986) Triangularis sterni: a primary muscle of breathing in the dog. J Appl Physiol 60:14–21
37. Ninane V, Decramer M, De Troyer A (1986) Coupling between triangularis sterni and parasternal during breathing in dogs. J Appl Physiol 61:539–544
38. De Troyer A, Ninane V, Gilmartin JJ, Lemerre C, Estenne M (1987) Triangularis sterni muscle use in supine humans. J Appl Physiol 62:919–925
39. Farkas GA, Estenne M, De Troyer A (1989) Expiratory muscle contribution to tidal volume in head-up dogs. J Appl Physiol 67:1438–1442
40. Grimby G, Goldman M, Mead J (1976) Respiratory muscle action inferred from rib cage and abdominal V-P partitioning. J Appl Physiol 41:739–751
41. Decramer M, Deschepper K, Jiang TX, Derom E (1991) Effects of aminophylline on respiratory muscle interaction. Am Rev Respir Dis (in press)
42. Sigrist S, Thomas D, Howell S, Roussos CS (1982) The effect of aminophylline on inspiratory muscle contractility. Am Rev Respir Dis 126:46–50
43. Murciano D, Aubier M, Lecocguic Y, Pariente R (1984) Effects of theophylline on diaphragmatic strength and fatigue in patients with chronic obstructive pulmonary disease. N Eng J Med 311:349–353
44. Murciano D, Auclair MH, Pariente R, Aubier M (1989) A randomized, controlled trial of theophylline in patients with severe chronic obstructive pulmonary disease. N Eng J Med 320:1521–1525

Respiratory Failure: Dynamics of Breathing and Coordination

B.M. Hagan and R.D. Hubmayr

Introduction

Fatigue of the respiratory muscles is thought to play an important role in the pathophysiology of CO_2 retention and respiratory pump failure [1]. Fatigue is a condition in which there is a loss in the capacity for developing force or velocity of a muscle resulting from muscle activity under load and which is reversible by rest [2]. A fatiguing load alters the timing and coordination of respiratory muscle use. The pathophysiological basis of respiratory muscle dynamics and coordination in experimental fatigue syndromes and in the context of respiratory pump failure in patients is the subject of this chapter.

Mechanical Determinants of Respiratory Muscle Fatigue

Respiratory muscle fatigue occurs whenever the load on the respiratory muscles exceeds a threshold that varies in proportion to their strength. Several investigators have tested and confirmed this hypothesis by studying ventilatory load responses in normal volunteers under controlled experimental conditions [1, 3–8]. In these studies, the respiratory pump was loaded with an external resistance while subjects were instructed to generate a predetermined airway or transdiaphragmatic target pressure (Pdi) during each breath. The inability to continue this task for prolonged periods of time was considered evidence for muscle fatigue. The validity of this assumption has been subsequently confirmed with the twitch occlusion technique [9].

Figure 1 shows the determinants of extrinsic load-induced diaphragm fatigue as they have emerged from above experiments [3, 4]. The quantity Pdi/Pdimax on the abscissa is the target pressure or inspiratory load expressed as a fraction of the maximal force, or more specifically, the pressure generating capacity of the diaphragm. The quantity Ti/Ttot, or duty cycle, on the ordinate is the inspiratory time expressed as a fraction of the total breath duration. Any combination of variables that defines a point to the right and upwards of the shaded area identifies a load as non-sustainable or fatiguing, while a point to the left and down implies that the load will not induce fatigue and can be sustained "indefinitely". According to Fig. 1., any load that is large relative to the maximal strength of the diaphragm, and which has to be sustained over a large portion of the respiratory cycle, is fatiguing. Because of the hyperbolic interface between the fatigue and non-fatigue zones (shaded area), fatiguing loads can be distinguished from non-fatiguing loads

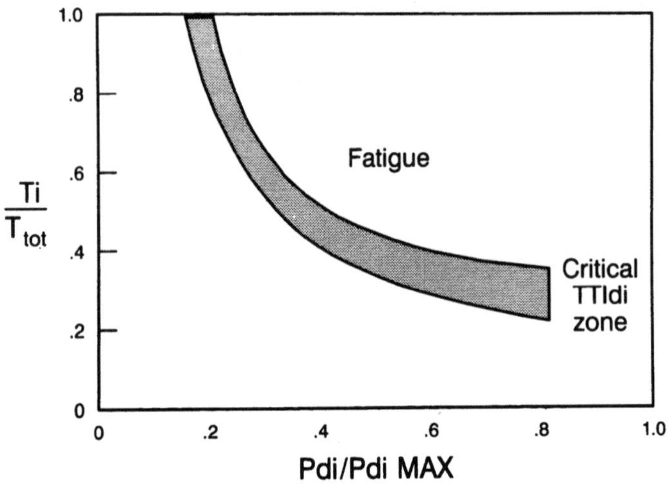

Fig. 1. Determinants of the tension time index of the diaphragm (TTIdi) and its predictive value in experimental diaphragm fatigue. (Adapted from [4] with permission). See text for further explanation

on the basis of a single variable, which is the product of Pdi/Pdimax and Ti/Ttot. This product is known as the tension time index of the diaphragm (TTIdi). According to Fig. 1, whenever TTIdi is greater than 0.15, performance failure of the respiratory pump is predicted [3].

Despite its strong scientific underpinning, TTIdi has not proven useful in the clinical diagnosis of impending respiratory pump failure. One possible reason for this is the complex interaction between intrinsic load and the system's load response. In contrast to laboratory based experiments during which known, invariant load (i.e. Pdi target) can be imposed to study ventilatory responses, patients with diseases of the respiratory system are not constrained to generate a unique Pdi. Presumably, the respiratory pump's response to a load is designed to minimize the required force or power output of the respiratory muscles [8, 10, 11]. The compensatory response of the respiratory pump to loading, thus modifies the effective load on the respiratory muscles. A response that is out of proportion to the magnitude or type of mechanical load implies intrinsic respiratory muscle disease, impending muscle fatigue, or impending pump failure [12]. This is distinct from overt failure, which is associated with hypoventilation and hypercarbia. What constitutes an appropriate load response requires a basic understanding of respiratory muscle dynamics and coordination. Defining impending pump failure on the basis of an abnormal load response is void of any mechanistic assumptions. Nevertheless, such an operational definition may be useful to the clinician, who must decide when to intervene and unload the respiratory pump with mechanical ventilation (MV).

The Mechanical Interactions Between Respiratory Muscles and Thorax: Basic Concepts

Changes in intrinsic load affect both rate and magnitude of the pressure the respiratory muscles exert on the respiratory system [13–16]. These variables can be inferred from time based recordings of volume, flow, or airway occlusion pressure. A limiting assumption is that all inspiratory muscles are represented by a single contractile element, which shortens against elastic, resistive, or inertive loads. The load is assumed proportional to simple mechanical constants such as elastance (Ers), flow resistance (Rrs), and inertance (Irs) of the relaxed respiratory system, while the properties of the contractile element are usually derived from classic models of muscle mechanics. These are embodied in the length/tension and force/velocity relationships of skeletal muscles. It is commonly assumed that the initial length of the contractile element is a function of lung volume and that muscle shortening and shortening velocity are proportional to tidal volume and inspiratory flow [14].

Figure 2 depicts the mechanical interactions between the respiratory apparatus and the inspiratory muscles in schematic form. For the moment, energy dissipation will be ignored, i.e. the respiratory apparatus will be represented by a spring, and the properties of the muscle element by isometric length/tension curves. Muscle length (L) is expressed as percent of optimal length (Lo) and is shown on the abscissa. Tension, expressed as a percent of maximal tension (To), is shown on the ordinate. The solid lines are isometric length/tension curves of a muscle between Lo and 40% Lo. The uppermost curve represents the performance envelope of the muscle, i.e. its length/tension relationship during maximal activation. The curves below represent varying levels of lesser activation. The line, which intercepts the length axis at Lo represents the length/tension relationship of a linear elastic ele-

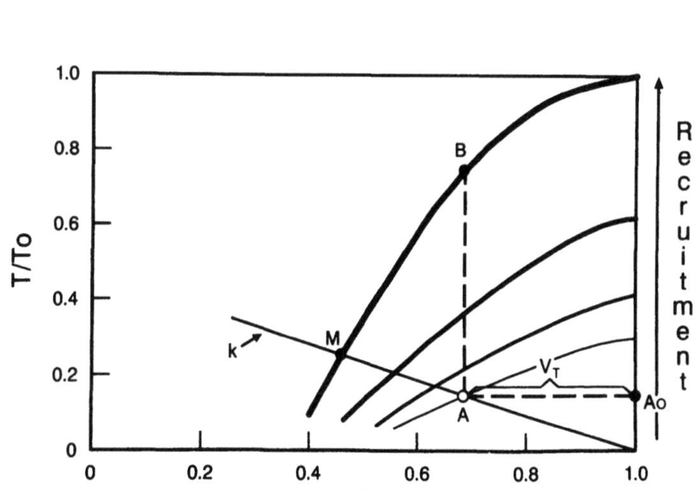

Fig. 2. Schematic representation of the mechanical interactions between the inspiratory muscles and the thorax. Abbreviations: *L/Lo:* length of the contractile element as a fraction of optimal length; *T/To:* tension of the contractile element as a fraction of maximal tension; *k:* spring constant of the elastic element; *VT:* tidal volume. See text for further explanation

ment. It can be thought of as a spring which is arranged in series with the muscle and is under no tension at Lo. The slope of the spring curve (k) defines the stiffness of the elastic element. The combined length of the elastic element and the muscle is assumed constant. When the muscle shortens from Lo by an amount equal to ΔL, the spring is being stretched by $-\Delta L$.

The intersections of each muscle curve with the length/tension curve of the spring element define unique solutions for

1. the length of the elastic element (lung volume),
2. its length change from a state of zero tension (tidal volume, VT),
3. the elastic recoil of the spring (Pel,rs)
4. the active length of the muscle at end-inspiration (L′/Lo),
5. its fractional shortening (ΔL/Lo),
6. muscle tension or its pressure equivalent (Pmus, which must be in equilibrium with Pel,rs), and
7. the pressure reserve of the muscle (Pmus/Pmusmax).

The slope of the spring curve and the relative shapes of the muscle curves define the level of muscle activation (drive) that is necessary to raise lung volume by an amount equal to VT. The intercept of the spring curve with the maximal length/tension curve of the muscle (point M) defines the maximal length of the elastic element (analogous to total lung capacity, TLC). Extension of the spring element by a lesser amount (e.g. from Ao to A) requires less muscle activation. Point B represents the maximal tension that can be generated at a length corresponding to point A. The tension at point A relative to that at point B, thus reflects the force reserve of the muscle at end-inspiration.

Many clinical measurements of respiratory muscle function have their foundation in this model. They include the pressure the respiratory muscles must generate (Pmus) to displace the thorax [13, 17], the inspiratory airway occlusion pressure P0.1 [18], the pressure/volume work and the power output of the inspiratory muscles. The relationship between Pmus and the mechanical properties of the respiratory system is defined by the equation of motion

$$\mathrm{Pmus} = (\mathrm{Pel,rs_i} + \mathrm{Ers}) \cdot (\mathrm{VT} + \mathrm{Rrs}) \cdot (\dot{V} + d\dot{V}/dt) \cdot \mathrm{Irs} \qquad (1)$$

whereby $\mathrm{Pel,rs_i}$ is the elastic recoil pressure of the respiratory system at the beginning of inspiration (analogous to intrinsic PEEP, $\mathrm{PEEP_i}$), VT is the tidal volume, $\dot{V}$ the mean inspiratory flow, and $d\dot{V}/dt$ the change in inspiratory flow with respect to time. During quiet breathing, the component of Pmus attributable to inertance is small and is usually ignored. For a breath initiated from relaxation volume, $\mathrm{Pel,rs_i}$ is 0, but this term must not be ignored in patients with airflow obstruction and dynamic hyperinflation [19, 20].

The ability of inspiratory muscles to exert pressure on the respiratory system declines with increasing volume [21]. This is illustrated in Fig. 3A, in which the airway occlusion pressure during maximal inspiratory and expiratory efforts (PImax, PEmax) has been plotted against lung volume (expressed as % vital capacity, VC). Also shown is the pressure/volume curve of the relaxed respiratory system

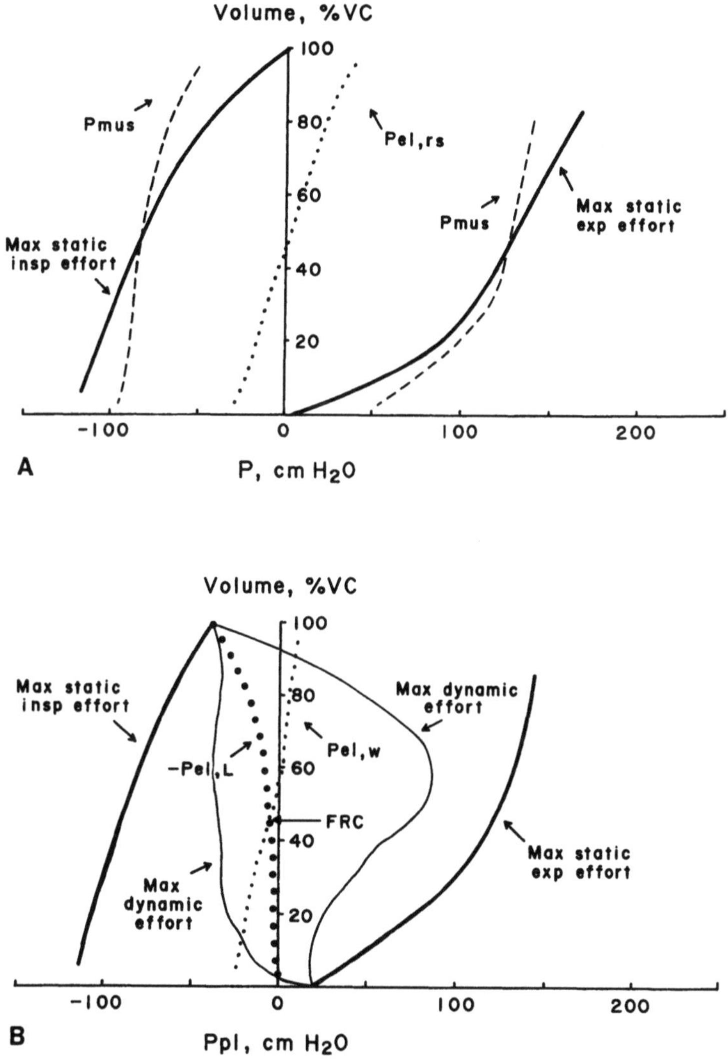

Fig. 3A, B. Respiratory pressures in a normal subject during maximal static (**A**) and dynamic (**B**) efforts. (From [25] with permission) See text for further explanation

(Pel,rs/V curve, dotted line). PImax and PEmax reflect the sum of two pressures that act on the respiratory system: Pmus and Pel,rs. Pmus can, therefore, be calculated at each volume from Pmax and Pel,rs and is represented by the thin broken lines. As represented by point M in Fig. 2, PImus and Pel,rs are equal and opposite near TLC (100% VC), indicating that all of PImus is required to counterbalance Pel,rs at that volume. The decline in PImus with volume can be attributed to a fall in the force generating capacity of the respiratory muscles at lengths less than optimal length [21, 22]. An alternative explanation, for which there is some experimental evidence [23, 24], is a volume dependent change in the mechanical efficiency of the inspiratory muscles as pressure generators.

Since breathing is a dynamic event, the pressure reserve of the inspiratory muscles may be considerably smaller than is assumed in Fig. 2 and 3A. According to Equation (1), any increase in $\dot{V}$ requires additional pressure, the magnitude of which depends on Rrs [25]. Secondly, the ability of skeletal muscles to generate pressure declines as their rate of shortening increases [26, 27]. This is illustrated in Fig. 3B, which contrasts the pleural pressure (Ppl) volume relationships during maximal static efforts (airway occluded) to those during maximal dynamic efforts (in the presence of flow). The Pel,rs/V curve of Fig. 3A has been replaced by its components, i.e. the lung curve (−Pel,L/V curve, heavy dotted line) and the chest wall curve (Pel,W/V curve, thin dotted line). During a breath hold with the glottis open, Pel,L, the elastic recoil pressure of the lungs, is counterbalanced by the actions of the inspiratory muscles (−Pel,L). The difference between −Pel,L and Ppl during a maximal static inspiratory effort is a measure of the pressure reserve of the inspiratory muscles. This reserve is available to produce inspiratory flow. During a maximal dynamic inspiratory effort (thin solid line) the reserve becomes 0 as all of Pmus is required to counterbalance Pel,L and to generate the pressure that is required to overcome the inspiratory flow resistance. The separation between the static and dynamic inspiratory pressure/volume curves reflects the force loss of the inspiratory muscles caused by the effects of shortening. The separation between the maximal dynamic Ppl/V curve and the lung curve, on the other hand, reflects the added pressure needed to overcome the viscous resistance of airways and lung parenchyma. Considering Fig. 1, a fall in inspiratory pressure reserve to 0 implies that the load on the muscles is equal to their maximal force generating capacity and cannot be sustained. These concepts have been used to explain exercise limitation on the basis of inspiratory muscle function [28].

The airway occlusion pressure 100 msec after the beginning of a breath (P0.1) also has its basis in this simple model of muscle interactions with the respiratory system [18]. In a sense, P0.1 is the change in Pmus over the initial 100 msec of a breath and is influenced by respiratory drive. To assume that P0.1 uniquely reflects the level of inspiratory motor recruitment requires a critical appraisal of the model's assumptions and their validity in disease.

These assumptions include

1. the rate of activation of inspiratory muscles over the initial 100 msec of a breath is the same whether the airway is patent or occluded;
2. inspiratory muscles contract isometrically during airway occlusion;
3. there is a unitary relationship between respiratory pressures and muscle force;
4. the contractile properties of inspiratory muscles and their initial lengths are constant;
5. the activity of expiratory muscles remains constant during the measurement; and
6. changes in intrathoracic pressure are instantaneously transmitted to the airway.

Since there are no conditions under which all these assumptions are satisfied, the measurement of P0.1 may be viewed as too simplistic [29]. Yet some consider it useful in the assessment of respiratory muscle function and drive in patients with respiratory failure [30, 31].

The Determinants of Tidal Volume and Respiratory Rate: Mechanical Perspective

Normal individuals maintain a given alveolar ventilation by adjusting the rate of breathing so that the average force generated by the respiratory muscles is minimized [11]. Minimizing force and muscle tension also minimizes blood flow requirements to respiratory muscles [32]. Experimental fatigue of the respiratory muscles produces a fall in VT and an increase in respiratory rate [6]. From an energetic perspective, such a change in breathing pattern might be maladaptive. It has been speculated, therefore, that respiratory control mechanisms down-regulate the use of fatigued muscles in order to minimize the perception of effort. In normal individuals, the perception of inspiratory effort varies in proportion to Pmus and the maximal pressure generating capacity of the inspiratory muscles [33]. During experimental fatigue, the perception of inspiratory effort at a given Pmus is heightened [34]. Thus, changes in effort perception together with a reduction in inspiratory muscle strength may account for the rapid shallow breathing which has been observed in experimental and clinical fatigue syndromes [6, 35–39].

Recall from Fig. 1 and 2 that adopting a strategy of rapid shallow breathing may lower the probability that a load will be fatiguing. A reduction in VT usually requires less Pmus to be generated per breath and is thus associated with a lower TTIdi provided Ti/Ttot remains the same. Ti/Ttot is similar in normals and in patients with different diseases of the respiratory system [40]. Furthermore, changes in Ti/Ttot are relatively small when ventilatory demand increases [41]. This means that during intrinsic loading the ordinate of Fig. 1 collapses to a narrow band ($0.3 \geq Ti/Ttot \leq 0.45$) and that fatigue is primarily determined by Pmus and the maximal pressure generating capacity of the inspiratory muscles [1, 5].

Rapid shallow breathing is a general manifestation of respiratory load compensation, but it is not a specific sign of respiratory muscle fatigue [42]. Figure 4A depicts the effects of elastic loading on muscle mechanics using the model presented in Fig. 2. A new spring curve with a slope $k' = 2k$ has been added to reflect an increase in the elastic load on the muscle element. The contractile properties of the muscle element have not been altered. Given the shape of the maximal length/tension curve of the muscle, the maximal length of the elastic element (point M′) is now reduced. In addition, a greater level of muscle activity (drive) is required to keep VT constant, i.e. to stretch the spring element to a length corresponding to point A in the original example (point A′ on the new spring curve). Such a breathing strategy, however, would require that a greater percentage of maximal tension be generated during each breath (tension at point A′ relative to that at point B). Preserving VT would increase the probability that the load will be fatiguing and would raise the subject's awareness of respiratory effort. If respiratory activity

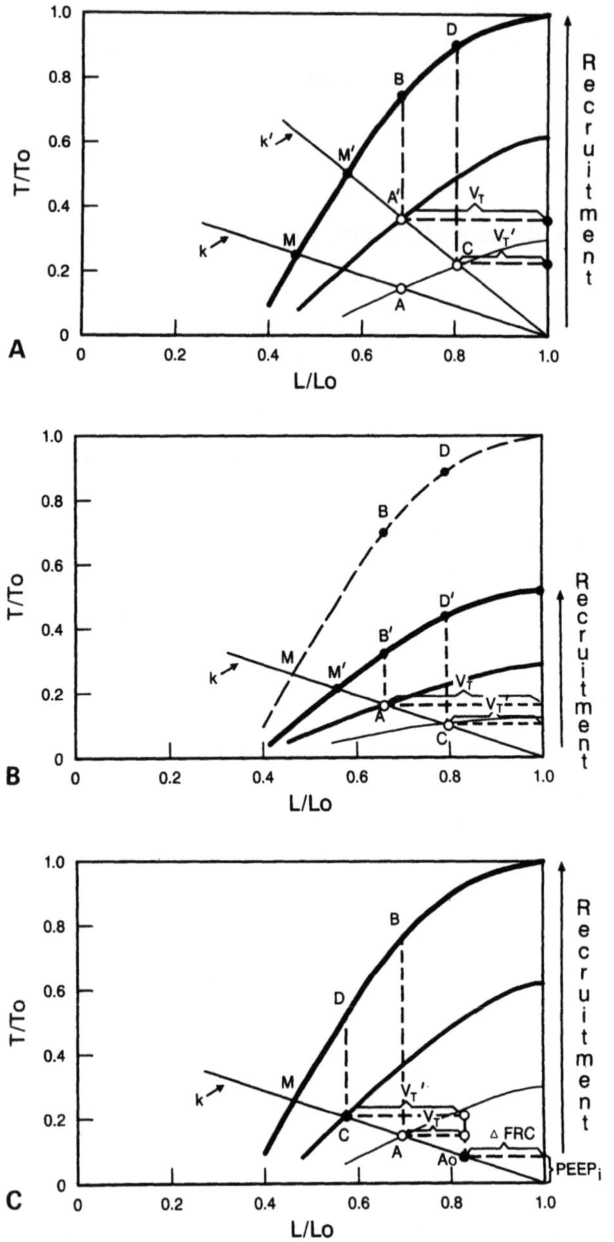

Fig. 4A–C. Schematic of the interactions between inspiratory muscles and thorax during elastic loading (**A**), in the presence of muscle weakness (**B**), and during dynamic hyperinflation (**C**). See text for discussion

(drive) did not increase in response to the added load, the length of the spring element at "end inspiration" would decline from A′ to C. Such a strategy would lead to a fall in tidal shortening commensurate with a reduction in VT to VT′, and would allow the system to operate with a greater force reserve (A′/B ≫ C/D). Because of the shape of the length tension curves, the muscle tension (Pmus) at point

C would still be greater than before loading (point A), thereby minimizing the anticipated fall in VT. This mechanism, which has been referred to as intrinsic load compensation, determines in part the VT response of individuals during the first loaded breath [14, 43]. The steady state ventilatory responses to elastic loading are determined by an interplay between intrinsic load compensation and changes in muscle recruitment (drive). The strategy represented by point A′ (complete preservation of VT) has not been observed experimentally [42]. A fall in VT influences proprioceptive afferent nerve traffic to the respiratory controller and would result in an increase in arterial CO_2 tension ($PaCO_2$) unless met by an increase in respiratory rate.

The same principles can be applied to analyze the effects of muscle weakness or fatigue on the dynamics of breathing (Fig. 5B). Instead of increasing the elastic load as was done in Fig. 5A, assume that the contractile properties of the muscle have changed. This is reflected in a downward shift of each muscle curve compared with Fig. 2 and 4A. To extend the spring element to point A requires a considerable increase in fractional muscle tension ($A/B' \gg A/B$) and would have to be met with an increase in respiratory drive. A reduction in tidal shortening to VT′ (point C) would lower Pmus, raise the force reserve in the new operating range ($A/B' \gg C/D'$), and possibly reduce the effective load below a fatigue threshold.

Rapid shallow breathing can lead to dynamic hyperinflation, particularly in the presence of expiratory airflow limitation [19, 20]. The consequences of having to initiate a breath from a lung volume other than static equilibrium volume (SEV) can also be examined in the context of this simple model (Fig. 4C). SEV is represented by the intercept of the elastic element curve with the length axis, where spring tension and Pmus ar 0 and the muscle length is assumed equal to Lo. Initiating a breath from a volume above SEV, e.g. from point Ao, means that the spring element is under some initial tension ($Pel,rs_i = PEEP_i \gg 0$), that Pmus must be generated first to counterbalance the passive tension in the spring before it can be stretched further to point A, and that tidal shortening is reduced in proportion to the increase in SEV (ΔFRC). It can be appreciated that hyperinflation limits the options for dynamic load compensation, especially in the presence of airways obstruction and impaired inspiratory muscle function. Alveolar ventilation cannot be restored by increasing VT to VT′ because of the consequences on the inspiratory force reserve. The use of expiratory muscles to maintain an end-expired lung volume near SEV (drive point Ao to the right) is ineffective because of expiratory flow limitation. Further reductions in end-inspired volumes would impose additional rate demands, which are likely to cause mor hyperinflation.

Although the concepts embodied in Fig. 5 provide a useful initial appraisal of the interactions between respiratory muscles and thorax, there are a number of additional factors which have not been considered. As alluded to in the example of Fig. 3B, motion is associated with dissipation of energy within the contractile machinery [7, 8, 25–27]. While visco-elastic energy losses of the respiratory system can be approximated using the equation of motion (Eq. 1), it is much harder to model the effects of motion on the required level of muscle recruitment. When a muscle shortens, the shape of its length-tension curve is not unique. It is determined by the number and type of active motor units (recruitment) and varies with motor unit firing rates (rate coding) and the phase relationships among active units (synchron-

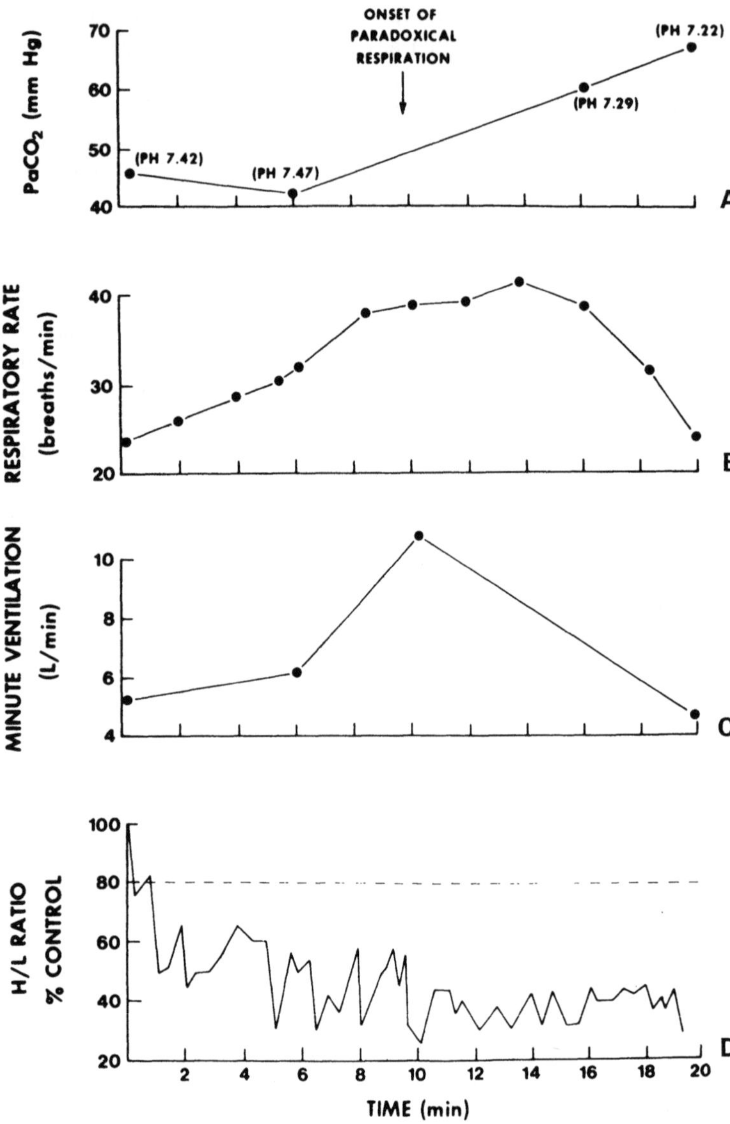

Fig. 5. Changes in $PaCO_2$, respiratory rate, minute ventilation, and the power spectrum of the diaphragm EMG expressed as high-to-low ratio in a patient during weaning from MV (From [38] with permission)

ization) [44]. Furthermore, during submaximal activation, the peak force produced by a muscle is not determined only by its final active length, but also by its initial length, shortening velocity, and the absolute amount of shortening [26, 27]. These factors are undoubtedly also important in modifying the rate and VT responses of the respiratory pump in fatigue.

Breathing Pattern and Respiratory Muscle Fatigue: Neurobiologic Perspective

The motor unit firing rate of limb muscles declines when a fatiguing task is performed [45]. This occurs in conjunction with a shift of the muscle's force frequency curve to the left. A leftward shift implies that force generation (relative to the maximal force) is better preserved at low stimulation frequencies. The changes in shape of the force frequency curve of fatigued muscles reflect a slowing of the muscle's rate of relaxation. The fall in spontaneous motor unit discharge rates takes advantage of these changes. It is suspected, but not proven, that similar events occur in the phrenic nerve and diaphragm during breathing against a fatiguing load. What has been demonstrated is that during experimental fatigue, the relaxation rate of the diaphragm is prolonged [46] and that the power spectrum of the diaphragm EMG is altered [38, 47]. Gallagher et al [6] demonstrated that breathing patterns during recovery from experimental respiratory muscle fatigue were similar in individuals with and without impaired diaphragm strength as long as the power spectrum of the diaphragm EMG remained abnormal.

Respiratory muscle fatigue is a process that involves both afferent and efferent limbs of respiratory motor control. Afferent information to the respiratory centers is derived not only from vagal pathways, but also from mechano-receptors of the chest wall. The diaphragm has virtually no muscle spindles but contains type III and type IV fibers, which modulate phrenic nerve activity [48]. The new tendon organs of the diaphragm are thought to mediate the inhibition of phrenic nerve traffic during passive muscle stretch [48, 49]. It has been shown that afferent activity from mechano-receptors of intercostal muscles plays a role in shaping the overall motor output of respiratory centers and may be involved in the mediation of the tachypnea so characteristic of the fatigue syndrome [50]. The main effect of intercostal afferent stimulation appears to be an inhibition of phrenic nerve activity [48, 49, 51, 52], although studies are complicated because of the complex deformations of the rib cage and associated musculature. It has been postulated that the primary determinants of f and VT under resting conditions are not vagally mediated, but are derived from intercostal afferents [53] which provide information on the shape and stress distributions of the rib cage. This information may allow the respiratory centers to impose a breathing strategy which minimizes the overall stress on the rib cage musculature. On the other hand, there is evidence that vagotomy profoundly alters the breathing patterns and alveolar ventilation in anesthetized dogs with experimental respiratory muscle fatigue [54]. It is unclear whether type III and type IV fibers are of importance in mediating the changes in muscle activation patterns during loaded breathing. By their functions in other tissues, it is assumed that they serve as nociceptors and may convey to the central nervous system information on the metabolic state of the respiratory muscles, and thereby induce changes in breathing strategy, although this has not been demonstrated.

The assumption of rapid shallow breathing in fatigue is obviously not the consequence of a simple change in a single input variable, but requires the integration of many signals. It has been demonstrated that load compensation varies with the state of consciousness and the naivete of the subject. Prolongation of inspiratory time in the face of an inspiratory resistive load is greatly diminished during sleep and anesthesia [55, 56]. Prior exposure to a load has also been shown to affect the response to the load. Naive subjects exposed to continuous positive airway pressure (CPAP) will attempt to defend lung volume by recruitment of expiratory muscles and prolongation of expiratory time. In contrast, experienced subjects breathing with CPAP allow lung volume to increase and compensate for any mechanical disadvantage of the inspiratory muscles by increasing diaphragm motor output [57].

Dynamics and Muscle Coordination in Respiratory Failure: Clinical Observations

A description of the physiologic expressions of impending respiratory muscle fatigue can be obtained from studies of patients during weaning from MV. Fig. 5 shows the time course of $PaCO_2$, respiratory rate, minute ventilation ($\dot{V}E$), and the power spectrum of the diaphragm EMG in a patient with weaning-induced overt respiratory failure [38]. The power spectrum of the diaphragm EMG was expressed as a ratio of the signal contents at high and low frequencies (H/L ratio). On the basis of a decreased H/L ratio, the authors concluded that peripheral diaphragm fatigue was responsible for weaning failure. Although the sensitivity and specificity of the H/L ratio as predictor of muscle fatigue have been questioned [58, 59], the observed trends in breathing pattern and chest wall motion as overt gas exchange failure evolved are in line with many other reports [35–39, 60]. Initially, the respiratory rate increases out of proportion to the fall in VT, explaining the rise in $\dot{V}E$. At that stage, arterial CO_2 is still normal although tachypnea and a change in the pattern of chest wall motion (paradoxic breathing) indicate a heightened respiratory motor output.

Since weaning from MV is a clinical response test to intrinsic loading, it seems prudent to ask whether one can distinguish between sustainable and nonsustainable loads on the basis of breathing pattern and chest wall motion. Available data suggest that tachypnea is an important sign of respiratory load compensation but not a specific predictor of weaning outcome [37]. This is in keeping with the rationale presented in Fig. 4. Therefore, one must consider additional degrees of freedom with which the respiratory pump can cope.

These include

1. a redistribution of motor output among different groups of respiratory muscles, and
2. acceptance of a lower alveolar ventilation to minimize the respiratory muscles' force requirements.

Respiratory Muscle Coordination

Chest wall shape and displacement. The respiratory pump is driven by many different muscles which need not be recruited in unison. Their interplay and different mechanical actions on the thorax can be inferred from the displacements and deformation of rib cage and abdomen and from the changes in pressure within these compartments [61–65]. Given the complex mechanical properties of the chest wall, thus far it has not been possible to satisfactorily relate chest wall shape to the topographical distribution of stresses. Furthermore, it remains to be seen if known stress distributions can be singularly attributed to individual respiratory muscles or muscle groups.

In 1967, Konno and Mead [63] described the movements of the respiratory system by plotting the relative displacements of rib cage and abdomen through time (Fig. 6). During normal quiet breathing, the rib cage and abdomen are displaced along their relaxation characteristics, that is, they describe the configuration of the chest wall when it is undistorted by respiratory muscle forces (Fig. 6, left panel). Initially, this observation was inferred to mean that the mechanical events during breathing were relatively simple, with the diaphragm acting as the only significant inspiratory muscle. Subsequently, it has been shown that the mechanical interactions between the diaphragm and rib cage are quite complex [61, 65], and that breathing requires the coordinated use of the diaphragm and of muscle groups with primary actions on the rib cage [66–68].

During a normal inspiration, the diaphragm shortens and moves caudally like a piston, thereby lowering intrathoracic pressure. Despite the fall in Ppl, the rib cage expands more or less as a unit, because the diaphragm inflates the lower rib cage, and because other respiratory muscles (foremost the parasternal intercostals and scaleni) provide restoring forces which prevent or minimize distortions of the rib cage [68]. The force exerted by the diaphragm on the lower rib cage has two distinct components: an insertional component and abdominal pressure. At volumes below TLC, the muscle fibers of the diaphragm are apposed to the lower rib cage and are oriented in a cranio-caudal direction. Because the diaphragm uses the abdominal contents as a fulcrum, its fibers lift the lower ribs on which they insert. Furthermore, the zone of apposition allows abdominal pressure to be transmitted to the lower rib cage and thereby helps to inflate it [69].

The Konno-Mead analysis has been used to study chest wall motion during intrinsic and extrinsic loading of the respiratory system in health and disease [36, 40,

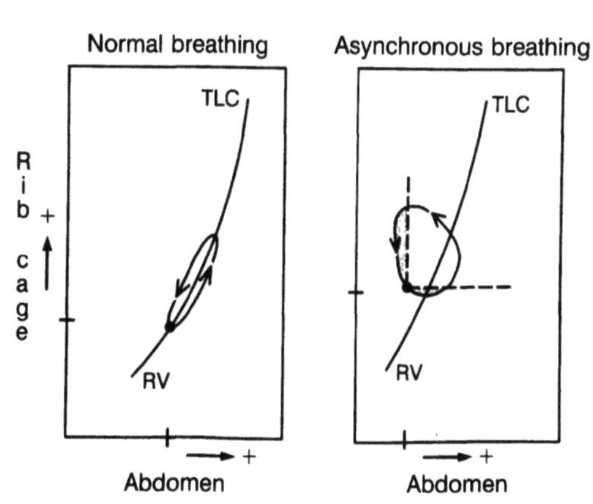

Fig. 6. Schematic of a Konno-Mead diagram during normal quiet breathing *(left panel)* and during asynchronous breathing *(right panel)*. The line between TLC and residual volume (RV) illustrates the relative dimensions of rib cage and abdomen during quasi-static relaxation maneuvers between the volume extremes. The relative dimensions during breathing are shown by the broken lines. Upward arrows on the breathing loops identify inspiration, downward arrows expiration. The shaded areas during asynchronous breathing quantify portions of the loop during which rib cage or abdominal dimension are smaller than at end-expiration

62, 70]. In particular, the analysis has been useful in describing varying degrees of asynchrony between the motions of rib cage and abdomen (Fig. 6, right panel). Several indices have been proposed to quantify the degree of asynchrony. One approach has been to measure the phase angle, Θ, between rib cage and abdominal signals [21]. Others have focused on the area encompassed by the Konno-Mead plot, which is a measure of the differences (hysteresis) among chest wall shapes during inspiration and expiration. Degrees of thoraco-abdominal paradox have been quantified by measuring the area fraction of the loop, which lies outside a 90° window anchored at FRC. A few general conclusions can be derived from such studies.

Asynchrony and distortions of the chest wall during breathing are common

1. in patients with airways obstruction [62, 71],
2. in the presence of neuromuscular diseases [72], and
3. during weaning from MV [35, 36].

The goal to link certain displacement patterns unequivocally leading to fatigue of a muscle or muscle group, however, remains elusive. This is not surprising given the inherent assumptions of the Konno-Mead approach and considering the multiplicity of factors which determine thoraco-abdominal shape.

A departure of thoraco-abdominal shape from its relaxed configuration implies a distortion of the chest wall by muscular forces relative to some minimum energy state. The Konno-Mead diagram characterizes these distortions, provided rib cage and abdomen behave as single, independent units. Distortions within rib cage and abdomen add additional degrees of freedom, complicating the interpretation of chest wall surface measurements. Although it has been implied that breathing near "the relaxation line" is advantageous for energetic reasons, there is no evidence that the normal respiratory system is designed or constrained to maintain a unique relationship between lung volume and chest wall shape during breathing. Departures from the relaxation line and widening of the hysteresis loop between inspiration and expiration are commonly seen in normal individuals during voluntary hyperventilation and during exercise [57]. From a purely mechanical perspective, there could be trade offs between using muscles to prevent distortions within the rib cage compartment and to preserve thoraco-abdominal shape near the relaxation configuration. In diseases like COPD, structural adaptations of the chest wall and hyperinflation affect the mechanical efficiency of respiratory muscle groups relative to each other [71].

Therefore, asynchrony, distortions, and hysteresis of the chest wall loop may reflect

1. the altered mechanical actions of the diaphragm on the hyperinflated chest [73],
2. the effects of muscular forces during active expiration,
3. changes in diaphragm recruitment relative to inspiratory rib cage and accessory muscles, or
4. a true change in the intrinsic contractile properties of the diaphragm (peripheral fatigue).

The determinants of relative recruitments of diaphragm, rib cage inspiratory muscles, and abdominal muscles are incompletely understood and most hypotheses concerning the coordinated use of these muscle groups have been teleologic in nature. For example, it has been postulated that the abdominal muscles are recruited during inspiration in an attempt to optimize the pressure generating capacity of the diaphragm in the presence of hyperinflation. The diaphragm is considered to be the most important inspiratory muscle in man. A change in its contribution to overall Pmus alters the relative displacements of rib cage and abdomen and affects the pressure swings within thorax and abdomen. As has been illustrated in Fig. 5, thoraco-abdominal paradox is a common clinical manifestation of respiratory distress and reflects a decreased downward displacement of the diaphragm during inspiration. Possible causes of thoraco-abdominal paradox include

1. an increased relative recruitment of inspiratory muscles with primary actions on the rib cage, and
2. the activation of abdominal muscles during inspiration.

In principle, neither mechanism requires that contractile failure of the diaphragm is present. Indeed, there is mounting evidence that thoraco-abdominal paradox is a strategy used for load compensation which is abandoned as soon as the load is removed [70].

Tobin et al. [36] systematically evaluated chest wall motion in patients during weaning from MV. Patients who failed weaning had more asynchronous chest wall movements than those who succeeded. However, there was a great deal of overlap between groups, and none of the asynchrony parameters had sufficient predictive value to aid in clinical decision making. There was greater breath-to-breath variability of chest wall displacement patterns in the failure group. This was reflected by a greater standard deviation about the fraction of VT which was attributable to rib cage expansion (ΔVRC/VT). Individual ΔVRC/VT values were not clustered around two means as would be the case for true "respiratory alternans". Respiratory alternans describes an oscillation in chest wall displacement patterns between two distinct states, classically between rib cage and abdominal breathing [1]. Such a strategy has been thought to provide alternating "rest" to different sets of respiratory muscles, i.e. diaphragm and inspiratory rib cage muscles. Regardless of the uncertainties in underlying mechanisms and strict definitions, respiratory alternans or breath-to-breath variability in chest wall motion appears to be one of the most specific predictors of impending respiratory failure [74].

Regional respiratory pressures. The relative contribution of the various respiratory muscles during breathing determines, in part, the distribution of pressure swings within thorax and abdomen. The difference between abdominal and pleural pressure swings (ΔPab and ΔPpl, respectively) is often used to infer the contribution of the diaphragm during breathing ($\Delta Pab - \Delta Ppl = \Delta Pdi$). During quiet breathing in erect normal man, the ratio of ΔPdi/ΔPpl is ≤ -1, averaging -1.95 ± 0.86 [75]. As the contribution of the rib cage and accessory inspiratory muscles to Pmus increases, ΔPpl/ΔPdi approaches zero. In the presence of diaphragm paralysis or extreme weakness, ΔPab becomes negative (falls during inspiration), raising ΔPab/ΔPdi above 0. This is usually associated with asynchronous chest wall movements and thoraco-abdominal paradox. One of the advantages of measuring regional respiratory pressures and Pdi is in the assessment of inspiratory muscle function in patients who are unable to perform maximal respiratory maneuvers [76]. Unfortunately, measurements of ΔPdi are exquisitely sensitive to changes in lung volume [21, 77], respiratory system geometry [23, 24], and abdominal impedance [78], and are affected by the pressure contribution by other inspiratory muscles to overall Pmus [79]. It is, therefore, not possible to clearly define the intrinsic contractile properties of the diaphragm in a spontaneously breathing patient on the basis of regional pressure measurements. In keeping with these limitations, the monitoring of ΔPdi has not proven useful in the early diagnosis of respiratory pump failure during weaning [60].

Demonstrating a reversible change in the contractile properties of respiratory muscles in a clinical setting would facilitate the interpretation of specific load response patterns. It would also strengthen the relevance of experimental studies during which peripheral muscle fatigue has been induced by extrinsic loads. Figure 7A shows a recording of gastric pressure (Pga), flow ($\dot{V}$), and esophageal pressure (Pes) in a ventilator dependent patient at the end of a 1-hour weaning trial that had to be aborted because of dyspnea. At that time, the respiratory rate had risen to 44 breaths/min. The shape of the expiratory flow wave tracing, with its convexity towards the time axis, demonstrates the presence of airways obstruction. Palpation of the abdomen revealed active expiration which probably accounts for the increase in Pes to +10 cm H_2O at end-expiration. The inspiratory swings in Pes were relatively large (20 cm H_2O) and accompanied by a fall in Pga as abdominal muscle activity decayed early during each breath. Fig. 7B shows the result of two twitch occlusion tests, one performed before weaning (left panel) and one 5 min after the

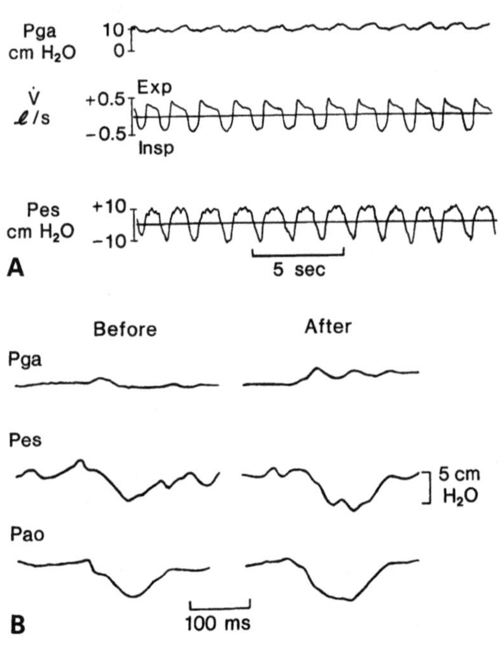

Fig. 7A, B. Measurements of gastric pressure (Pga), flow ($\dot{V}$), and esophageal pressure (Pes) in a patient at the end of a symptom-limited weaning trial (**A**). Measurements of Pga, Pes, and airway occlusion pressure (Pao) during bilateral twitch stimulations of the phrenic nerves before and after weaning in the same patient (**B**). See text for discussion

symptom-limited weaning trial (right panel). Even after prolonged respiratory muscle rest before weaning, intrathoracic (ΔPes and ΔPao) and abdominal pressure swings (ΔPga) during supramaximal twitch stimulation of the phrenic nerves were significantly reduced. Normal volunteers generate a twitch Pdi ≥ 20 cm H_2O near SEV [77] as opposed to the 6 cm H_2O in this patient, who suffered from profound diaphragm weakness. After weaning, there was no further reduction in twitch Pdi, suggesting that weaning had not induced peripheral diaphragm fatigue. These observations are consistent with the hypothesis that respiratory distress and compromise need not reflect contractile failure of the respiratory muscles themselves (peripheral fatigue) but may involve load perception and integrative responses on a central level. The example also points out that weakness and fatigue may share common load responses in terms of respiratory dynamics and muscle coordination.

Effects of Breathing Pattern on CO_2 Elimination

$\dot{V}E$ combined with the mechanical impedance of the respiratory system determines the power output of the respiratory muscles and, thus, their load. The relationships between fatigue-induced changes in breathing patterns and their effects on pulmonary gas exchange are not straightforward. A fall in VT must result in an increase in the dead space (VD) to VT ratio (VD/VT) compromising pulmonary CO_2 elimination ($\dot{V}CO_2$). To minimize the increase in arterial CO_2 tension ($PaCO_2$) and body CO_2 stores, respiratory rate must increase. From an energetic perspective, it would be preferable to accept alveolar hypoventilation as a means of reducing the mechanical load on the inspiratory muscles and modifying VT and rate responses accordingly. If that were indeed the case, O_2 and CO_2 would change and exert their own independent effects on breathing pattern and respiratory motor output. Cause and effect between rapid shallow breathing and hypercarbia would thus be obscure.

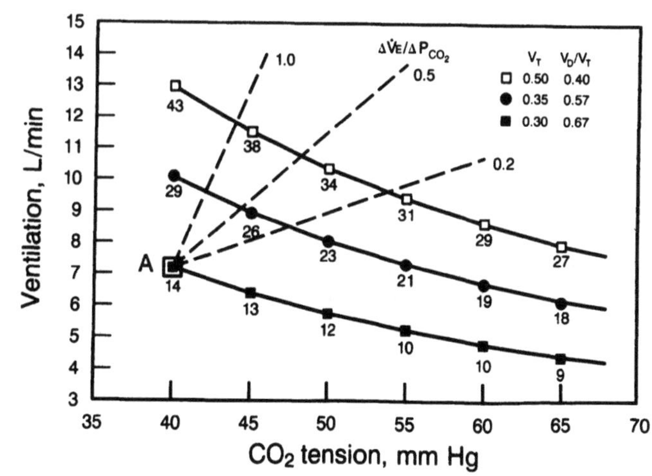

Fig. 8. Schematic illustration of the interdependency between breathing pattern, dead space (VD), alveolar ventilation, arterial CO_2 tension, and the ventilatory response to CO_2. See text for further explanation

The relationships between $\dot{V}E$ and $PaCO_2$ can be represented by metabolic hyperbolae as has been illustrated in Fig. 8. Assume for the purpose of simplicity that CO_2 production and its elimination by the lungs are equal ($\dot{V}CO_2$ = 0.2 l/min) and do not change as a function of VT or rate. The three hyperbolae in Fig. 8 represent VE to VT isopleths (VD/VT = 0.4, 0.57, and 0.67, respectively) and illustrate all possible combinations of $\dot{V}E$ and $PaCO_2$ at a given VD/VT. VD itself is assumed constant (VD = 0.2 l/breath), a value consistent with moderately severe intrinsic lung disease. Since VD is constant each VD/VT isopleth is also a VT isopleth (VT = 0.50, 0.35, and 0.30, respectively). Respiratory rate changes with $\dot{V}E$ along each isopleth as indicated numerically. Let point A represent some baseline state during which a subject breathes with a VT of 0.5 l and a rate of 14 breaths/min maintaining a $PaCO_2$ of 40 mm Hg. As VT decreases in response to an insult (or load), the relationships between $PaCO_2$ and $\dot{V}E$ shift to a different isopleth. For example, a fall in VT from 0.5 l to 0.35 l would result in a change in VD/VT from 0.4 to 0.57 and would be accompanied by CO_2 retention unless respiratory rate increased to 29 bpm. A fall in VT to 0.3 l would mandate a disproportionate rate increase to 43 bpm in order to preserve isocapnea. In principle, the relationship between $PaCO_2$ and $\dot{V}E$ describes the CO_2 responsiveness of the respiratory pump. Three hypothetical response curves with slopes between 1.0 l/min/mm Hg and 0.2 l/min/mm Hg are shown as broken lines. In theory, a blunted chemo-responsiveness ($\Delta\dot{V}E/\Delta PaCO_2$ = 0.2 l/min) would allow the subject to reduce VT to 0.3 l unaccompanied by an inordinate increase in rate, albeit at the expense of hypercarbia.

The slope of the ventilatory response curve to CO_2 is not a load independent expression of intrinsic respiratory drive [80]. Alveolar ventilation may, therefore, decline when the respiratory muscles are faced with an otherwise fatiguing load. What is not clear is how large an increase in $PaCO_2$ can be tolerated without foregoing the possibility of reaching a new steady state. Fig. 8 illustrates how the gas exchange function of the lung, expressed here by a single parameter (VD), sets limits to the mechanical load compensation that can occur on a muscle level. The agency through which these limits may be expressed is the CO_2 responsiveness of the respiratory pump.

At high respiratory rates the cost associated with dynamic dissipation of muscle pressure may exceed the benefit derived from minimizing the elastic pressure. Yamashiro et al [10, 41] have shown that minimization of total respiratory work (as opposed to Pmus as % maximal Pmus) is achieved asymptomatically as the level of ventilation rises during exercise. Fig. 8 also underscores the constraints imposed by CO_2 homeostasis on patients with expiratory flow limitation, who cannot increase respiratory rates into the 40 sec without suffering the consequences of additional hyperinflation. In addition, one must consider the added burden of rate compensation on CO_2 produced by the respiratory muscles, which would shift the metabolic hyperbolae even further towards higher $PaCO_2$ or $\dot{V}E$ values.

Dunn et al. [81] examined the effects of intrinsic loading on alveolar ventilation in ventilator dependent patients during weaning. The CO_2 responsiveness of the unloaded respiratory pump was measured with the recruitment threshold technique [82]. Measurements of respiratory motor output were made during MV and the settings adjusted until phasic inspiratory muscle activity was suppressed. The CO_2 recruitment threshold (CO_2RT) was defined as the lowest $PaCO_2$ at which the supplementation of CO_2 caused the reappearance of phasic motor activity. Since CO_2RT was determined during MV, it was interpreted as a measure of the CO_2 sensitivity of the unloaded respiratory pump. CO_2RT was then compared in each patient to the $PaCO_2$ during unassisted spontaneous breathing (CO_2SB). Seven of 10 patients who failed weaning because of dyspnea or sustained tachypnea (respiratory rate ≥ 30) retained CO_2SB compared with CO_2RT by more than 3 mm Hg. In contrast, the 5 patients who were weaned successfully maintained CO_2SB within 2 mm Hg of CO_2RT. Patients who failed weaning tended to be weaker. There was a considerable overlap in parameters reflective of mechanical load or inspiratory drive among the groups. These findings underscore the demands placed by the intrinsic load and the subsequent load response on CO_2 homeostasis. They also suggest that large elevations in $PaCO_2$ as they follow from the example in Fig. 8 (depressed CO_2 response curve) preclude the assumption of a new steady state.

References

1. Roussos C, Macklem PT (1982) The respiratory muscles. N Engl J Med 307:786–797
2. NHLBI workshop summary (1990) Respiratory muscle fatigue: Report of the respiratory muscle fatigue workshop group. Am Rev Respir Dis 142:474–480
3. Bellemare F, Grassino A (1982) Effect of pressure and timing of contraction on human diaphragmatic fatigue. J Appl Physiol 53:1190–1195
4. Bellemare F, Grassino A (1982) Evaluation of human diaphragm fatigue. J Appl Physiol 53:1196–1206
5. Roussos C, Macklem P (1977) Diaphragmatic fatigue in man. J Appl Physiol 43:189–197
6. Gallagher CG, Im Hof V, Younes M (1985) Effect of inspiratory muscle fatigue on breathing pattern. J Appl Physiol 59:1152–1158
7. McCool FD, McCann DR, Leith DE, Hoppin FG (1986) Pressure-flow effects on endurance of inspiratory muscles. J Appl Physiol 60:299–303
8. Jones GL, Killian KJ, Summers E, Jones NL (1985) Inspiratory muscle forces and endurance in maximum resistive loading. J Appl Physiol 58:1608–1615
9. Aubier M, Murciano D, Lecocguic Y, Viires N, Pariente R (1985) Bilateral phrenic stimulation: A simple technique to assess diaphragmatic fatigue in humans. J Appl Physiol 58:58–64
10. Yamashiro SM, Daubenspeck JA, Lauritsen TN, Grodins FS (1975) Total work of breathing optimization in CO_2 inhalation and exercise. J Appl Physiol 38:702–709
11. Mead J (1960) Control of respiratory frequency. J Appl Physiol 15:325–336
12. Rochester DF (1988) Does respiratory muscle rest relieve fatigue or incipient fatigue. Am Rev Respir Dis 138:516–517
13. Otis AB, Fenn WO, Rahn H (1950) Mechanics of breathing. J Appl Physiol 2:592–607
14. Younes M, Riddle W (1981) A model for the relation between respiratory neural and mechanical outputs. I. Theory. J Appl Physiol 51:979–989
15. Younes M, Riddle W, Polacheck J (1981) A model for the relation between respiratory neural and mechanical outputs. III. Experimental validation. J Appl Physiol 51:990–1001
16. Riddle W, Younes M (1981) A model for the relation between respiratory neural and mechanical outputs. II. Methods and evaluation of assumptions. J Appl Physiol 51:979–989
17. Campbell EJM (1958) The respiratory muscles and the mechanics of breathing. The Year Book Publishers, Chicago
18. Whitelaw WA, Derenne JP, Milic-Emili J (1975) Occlusion pressure as a measure of respiratory center output in conscious man. Respir Physiol 23:181–199
19. Pepe PE, Marini JJ (1982) Occult positive end-expiratory pressure in mechanically ventilated patients with airflow obstruction: The auto-PEEP effect. Am Rev Respir Dis 126:166–170

20. Milic-Emili J, Gottfried SB, Rossi A (1987) Dynamic hyperinflation: Intrinsic PEEP and its ramifications in patients with respiratory failure. In: Vincent JL (ed) Update in intensive care and emergency medicine: Update 1987, Vol 5. Springer, Berlin-Heidelberg-New York, pp 192–198
21. Agostoni E, Rahn H (1960) Abdominal and thoracic pressures at different lung volumes. J Appl Physiol 15:1087–1092
22. Grassino A, Goldman MD, Mead J, Sears TA (1978) Mechanics of the human diaphragm during voluntary contraction: Statics. J Appl Physiol 44:829–839
23. Marshall R (1962) Relationships between stimulus and work of breathing at different lung volumes. J Appl Physiol 17:917–921
24. Hubmayr RD, Sprung JJ, Nelson SB (1990) The determinants of transdiaphragmatic pressure in dogs. J Appl Physiol 69:1050–1056
25. Rodarte JR, Rehder K (1986) Dynamics of Respiration. In: Handbook of physiology, Section 3, Volume III, The respiratory system. Waverly Press, Baltimore, pp 131–144
26. Edman KAP (1981) Deactivation of the contractile system induced by shortening of striated muscle. In: The regulation of muscle contraction. Academic Press Inc., San Diego, pp 281–296
27. Edman KAP (1980) Depression of mechanical performance by active shortening during twitch and tetanus of vertebrate muscle fibers. Acta Physiol Scand 109:15–26
28. Bai TR, Rabinovitch BJ, Pardy RL (1984) Near maximal voluntary hyperpnea and ventilatory muscle function. J Appl Physiol 57:1742–1748
29. Marazzini L, Cavestri R, Gori D, Gatti L, Longhini E (1978) Difference between mouth and esophageal occlusion pressure during CO_2 rebreathing in chronic obstructive pulmonary disease. Am Rev Respir Dis 118:1027–1033
30. Sassoon CSH, Te TT, Mahutte CK, Light RW (1987) Airway occlusion pressure: An important indicator for successful weaning in patients with chronic obstructive pulmonary disease. Am Rev Respir Dis 135:107–113
31. Murciano D, Bockowski J, Lecocguic Y, Milic-Emili J, Pariente R, Aubier M (1988) Tracheal occlusion pressure: A simple index to monitor respiratory muscle fatigue during acute respiratory failure in patients with chronic obstructive pulmonary disease. Ann Int Med 108:800–805
32. Rochester DF, Bettini G (1976) Diaphragmatic blood flow and energy expenditure in the dog: Effects of inspiratory airflow resistance and hypercapnia. J Clin Invest 57:661–672
33. Killian KJ, Gandevia SC, Summers E, Campbell EJM (1984) Effect of increased lung volume on perception of breathlessness, effort, and tension. J Appl Physiol 57:686–691
34. Gandevia SC, Killian KJ, Campbell EJM (1981) The effect of respiratory muscle fatigue on respiratory sensations. Clin Sci 60:463–466
35. Ashutosh K, Gilbert R, Auchincloss JH, Peppi D (1975) Asynchronous breathing movements in patients with obstructive pulmonary disease. Chest 67:553–557
36. Tobin MJ, Guenther SM, Perez W et al (1987) Konno-Mead analysis of rib cage-abdominal motion during successful and unsuccessful trials of weaning from mechanical ventilation. Am Rev Respir Dis 135:1320–1328
37. Tobin MJ, Perez W, Guenther SM et al (1986) The pattern of breathing during successful and unsuccessful trials of weaning from mechanical ventilation. Am Rev Respir Dis 134:1111–1118
38. Cohen CA, Zagelbaum G, Gross D, Roussos CR, Macklem PT (1982) Clinical manifestations of inspiratory muscle fatigue. Am J Med 73:308–316
39. Gilbert R, Auchincloss JH, Peppi D, Ashutosh K (1974) The first few hours off a respirator. Chest 65:152–157
40. Tobin MJ, Chadha TS, Jenouri G, Birch SJ, Gazeroglu HB, Sackner MA (1983) Breathing Patterns. 2. Diseased Subjects. Chest 84:286–294
41. Yamashiro SM, Grodins FS (1973) Respiratory cycle optimization in exercise. J Appl Physiol 35:522–525
42. Younes M, Remmers J (1981) Control of tidal volume and respiratory frequency. In: Hornbein T (ed) Control of breathing. Vol 17 of series: Lenfant C (ed) Lung biology in health and disease. Marcel Dekker, New York, Part 1, pp 617–667

43. Campbell EJM, Dinnick OP, Howell JBL (1961) The immediate effects of elastic loads on breathing of man. J Physiol London 156:260–273
44. Burke RE, Edgerton VR (1975) Motor unit properties and selective involvement in movement. Exercise Sport Sci 3:31–81
45. Bigland-Ritchie B, Johansson R, Lippold OCJ, Woods JJ (1983) Contractile speed and EMG changes during fatigue of sustained maximal voluntary contractions. J Neurophysiol 50:313–324
46. Esau SA, Bellemare F, Grassino A, Permutt S, Roussos C, Pardy RL (1983) Changes in relaxation rate with diaphragmatic fatigue in humans. J Appl Physiol 54:1353–1360
47. Gross D, Grassino A, Ross WRD, Macklem PT (1979) Electromyogram pattern of diaphragmatic fatigue. J Appl Physiol 46:1–7
48. Cheeseman M, Revelette WR (1990) Phrenic afferent contribution to reflexes elicited by changes in diaphragm length. J Appl Physiol 69:640–647
49. Speck DF, Revelette WR (1987) Attenuation of phrenic motor discharge by phrenic nerve afferents. J Appl Physiol 62:941–945
50. Roussos C (1984) Ventilatory muscle fatigue governs breathing frequency. Bull Eur Physiopathol Respir 20:445–451
51. Hernandez YM, Lindsay BG, Shannon R (1989) Intercostal and abdominal muscle afferent influence on caudal medullary expiratory neurons that drive abdominal muscles. Exp Brain Res 78:219–222
52. Shannon R, Lindsey BG (1987) Expiratory neurons in the region of the retrofacial nucleus: Inhibitory effects of intercostal tendon organs. Exp Neurol 97:730–734
53. von Euler C (1986) Brain stem mechanisms for generation and control of breathing pattern. In: Cherniak N, Widdicombe JG (ed) Handbook of physiology, vol 2. Control of breathing. American Physiological Society, Bethesda, pp 463–524
54. Adams JM, Farkas GA, Rochester DF (1988) Vagal afferents, diaphragm fatigue, and inspiratory resistance in anesthetized dogs. J Appl Physiol 64:2279–2286
55. Read DJ, Freedman S, Kafer ER (1974) Pressures developed by loaded inspiratory muscles in conscious and anesthetized man. J Appl Physiol 37:207–218
56. Weigland L, Zwillich CW, White DP (1988) Sleep and the ventilatory response to resistive loading in normal men. J Appl Physiol 64:1186–1195
57. Green M, Mead J, Sears TA (1974) Effects of loading on respiratory muscle control in man. In: Pengelly LD, Rebuck AS, Campbell EJM (eds) Loaded breathing. Churchill Livingstone, Edinburgh pp 73–80
58. Sieck GC, Mazar A, Belman M (1985) Changes in EMG spectra during hyperpneic loads. Respir Physiol 61:137–152
59. Bazzi AR, Korten JB, Haddad GG (1986) Increase in electromyogram low power in nonfatigued contracting skeletal muscle. J Appl Physiol 61:1012–1017
60. Swartz M, Marino P (1985) Diaphragmatic strength during weaning from mechanical ventilation. Chest 88:736–739
61. Mead J, Loring SH (1982) Analysis of volume displacement and length changes of the diaphragm during breathing. J Appl Physiol 53:750–755
62. Sharp JT, Goldberg NB, Druz WS, Fishman HC, Danon J (1977) Thoracoabdominal motion in chronic obstructive pulmonary disease. Am Rev Respir Dis 115:47–56
63. Konno K, Mead J (1968) Static volume-pressure characteristics of the rib cage and abdomen. J Appl Physiol 24:544–548
64. Agostoni E, Mognoni P (1966) Deformation of the chest wall during breathing efforts. J Appl Physiol 21:1827–1832
65. Loring SH, Mead J (1982) Action of the diaphragm on the rib cage inferred from a force-balance analysis. J Appl Physiol: Respirat Environ Exercise Physiol 53:756–760
66. De Troyer A, Estenne M (1988) Functional anatomy of the respiratory muscles. Clin Chest Med 9:175–193
67. De Troyer A, Sampson MG (1982) Activation of the parasternal intercostals during breathing efforts in human subjects. J Appl Physiol 52:524–529
68. De Troyer A, Estenne M (1984) Coordination between rib cage muscles and diaphragm during quiet breathing in humans. J Appl Physiol 57:899–906

69. Urmey WF, De Troyer A, Kelly KB, Loring SH (1988) Pleural pressure increases during inspiration in the zone of apposition of diaphragm to rib cage. J Appl Physiol 65:2207–2212
70. Tobin MJ, Perez W, Guenther SM, Lodato RF, Dantzker DR (1987) Does rib cage-abdominal paradox signify respiratory muscle fatigue? J Appl Physiol 63:851–860
71. Sharp JT, Van Lith P, Nuchprayoon CV, Briney R, Johnson FN (1968) The thorax in chronic obstructive lung disease. Am J Med 44:39–46
72. Mortola JP, Sant'Ambrogio G (1978) Motion of the rib cage and the abdomen in tetraplegic patients. Clin Sci 54:25–32
73. Hoover CF (1920) The diagnostic significance of inspiratory movements of the costal margins. Am J Med Sci 159:633–646
74. Krieger BP, Ershowsky P (1988) Noninvasive detection of respiratory failure in the intensive care unit. Chest 94:254–261
75. Lisboa C, Pare PD, Pertuze J et al (1986) Inspiratory muscle function in unilateral diaphragmatic paralysis. Am Rev Respir Dis 134:488–492
76. Hillman DR, Finucane KE (1988) Respiratory pressure partitioning during quiet inspiration in unilateral and bilateral diaphragmatic weakness. Am Rev Respir Dis 137:1401–1405
77. Hubmayr RD, Litchy WJ, Gay PC, Nelson SB (1989) Transdiaphragmatic twitch pressure: Effects of lung volume and chest wall shape. Am Rev Respir Dis 139:647–652
78. Smith J, Bellemare F (1987) Effect of lung volume on in vivo contraction characteristics of human diaphragm. J Appl Physiol 62:1893–1900
79. Hershenson MB, Kikuchi Y, Loring SH (1988) Relative strength of the chest wall muscles. J Appl Physiol 65:852–862
80. Dempsey JA (1976) CO_2 response: Stimulus definition and limitations. Chest 70:114–118
81. Dunn WF, Nelson SB, Hubmayr RD (1990) The determinants of arterial CO_2 tension during weaning from mechanical ventilation. Chest 97 (Suppl 3):68S–69S
82. Prechter GC, Nelson SB, Hubmayr RD (1990) The ventilatory recruitment threshold for carbon dioxide. Am Rev Respir Dis 141:758–764

Assessment of Respiratory Muscle Strength

W. P. Sexauer, G. J. Criner, and S. G. Kelsen

Introduction

The last decade has seen a considerable advance in our understanding of the motor control and mechanical action of the respiratory muscles and the effects of alterations in lung function, body metabolism (e.g. undernutrition) and blood chemistry (e.g. hypocalcemia) on respiratory muscle contractile function. This chapter will briefly review the determinants of respiratory muscle strength, the causes of respiratory muscle weakness and the techniques currently used to assess respiratory muscle strength in man.

Generally, respiratory muscle strength refers to the capacity to generate force or pressure at a given level of muscle activation. The greater the strength of a muscle, the greater its force output. Respiratory muscle weakness may be defined as a condition in which the capacity of a rested muscle to generate force or pressure is impaired [1]. Respiratory muscle weakness should be distinguished from muscle fatigue, which also impairs muscle force generation. Respiratory muscle fatigue has been defined as a condition resulting from muscle activity under load in which there is a loss in the capacity for developing force and/or velocity of a muscle, and which is reversible by rest [1]. Although the distinction between weakness and fatigue is important for understanding the pathophysiological basis for respiratory muscle dysfunction, in clinical practice a clear-cut separation is often difficult, and both processes may co-exist simultaneously. Indeed, it appears that respiratory muscle weakness predisposes to fatigue by requiring a higher percentage of maximum force for a given level of ventilation than when muscle strength is normal [2]. The present discussion will focus on currently available techniques for the assessment of respiratory muscle strength, realizing that in many instances a reduction in force output may be due wholly or partly to fatigue rather than muscle weakness.

Determinants of Respiratory Muscle Strength

The respiratory muscles are striated skeletal muscles and as such the force they develop depends upon:

1. muscle mass and fiber composition;
2. fiber length;
3. velocity of shortening; and
4. intensity of motor outflow.

Muscle Fiber Composition and Mass

Slow oxidative (Type I) muscle fibers are highly fatigue resistant and generate approximately 80 kN/m^2 cross sectional area [3]. Fast oxidative (Type II A) fibers are also highly fatigue resistant and generate approximately 100 kN/m^2 cross sectional area. Fast glycolytic fibers (Type II B), on the other hand, are highly susceptible to fatigue but generate approximately 130 kN/m^2 cross sectional area. Generally, slow oxidative fibers have the smallest cross sectional area while fast glycolytic fibers tend to have the largest [3]. The precise mix of fibers in any given respiratory muscle, therefore, determines not only its resistance to fatigue but also its force generating capacity. Although the fiber composition of the respiratory muscles in man have not been studied extensively, data are available for the human diaphragm. The diaphragm of adult human subjects appears to consist of approximately 50% slow oxidative fibers, 25% fast oxidative fibers, and 25% fast glycolytic fibers [4, 5]. It is clear, however, that there are considerable interindividual variations in diaphragm fiber composition which are likely to underlie differences in muscle strength as well as muscle endurance.

Muscle mass refers to the cross sectional area of the entire muscle and in turn depends both on the average muscle fiber diameter and fiber number. Diaphragm muscle mass appears to vary considerably between subjects, in part because of differences in body habitus and differences in the level of diaphragm activity. For example, diaphragm thickness and weight appear to be greater in heavy manual laborers than sedentary adults [6].

Length-Tension Relationship

All striated muscles (including the respiratory muscles) obey the length-tension relationship (Fig. 1). At any given level of muscle activation, changes in muscle fiber length alter active and passive tension. However, at some muscle fiber length, active tension is maximal. Changes in muscle fiber length above or below this optimal length (L_o) result in reductions in active tension. Respiratory muscle length depends largely upon lung volume and to a lesser extent on thoracoabdominal configuration [7–9]. Progressive increases in lung volume shorten the inspiratory muscles and lengthen the expiratory muscles [10].

The *in vivo* position of the respiratory muscles on their length-tension curve and hence their mechanical advantage at a given lung volume and thoracoabdominal configuration has not been defined in man. To date such an assessment has only been performed in canine respiratory muscles since determination of muscle mechanical advantage requires *in vivo* measurement of precontraction fiber length followed by performance of a length-tension determination of the same muscle segment *in vitro*. However, such experiments performed in the supine anesthetized dog have provided important information and indicate that the diaphragm and parasternal intercostal muscles are very close to L_o at lung volumes between functional residual capacity (FRC) and residual volume (RV) [11], while the sternocleidomastoid and scalene muscles appear to be situated at lengths shorter than L_o at FRC and approach L_o only in the upright position [12]. In contrast, some of the

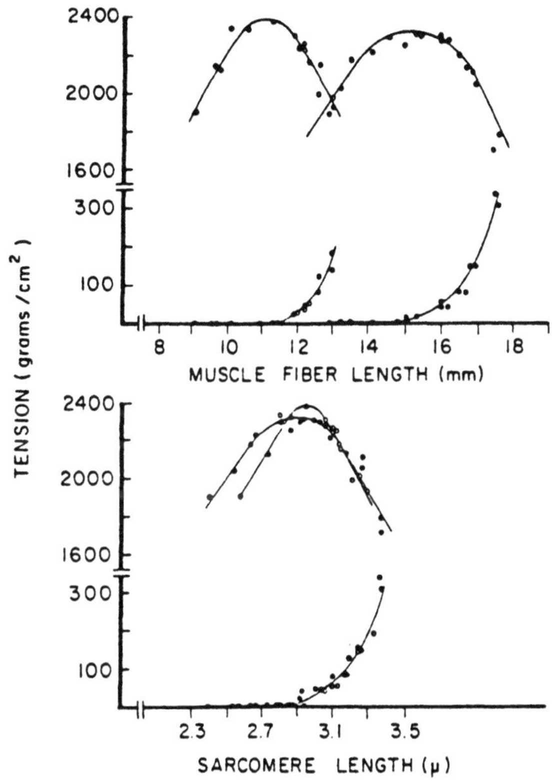

Fig. 1. Active *(upper trace each panel)* and passive, lower trace in each panel, length tension curves of muscle fiber bundles of the costal diaphragm. Data shown compare the results obtained for diaphragms from emphysematous *(open circles)* and normal *(solid circles)* hamsters. The top panel demonstrates the fiber length-tension relationship while the lower panel represents the sarcomere length-tension relationship. The apex of the active length-tension curves for both fiber length and sarcomere length represents the optimum length (L_O) for tension generation. Note in the top panel, the displacement of both the active and passive length-tension curves toward shorter fiber lengths in the emphysematous compared to the normal animals. Leftward movement of the length-tension curve tends to reestablish L_O at the shorter diaphragm fiber length present due to hyperinflation, and reduces the precontraction fiber length of all inspiratory muscles. Leftward displacement of the curve would tend to improve the tension generating ability of the diaphragm and, hence, reserve the mechanical disadvantage of tension generation imposed by hyperinflation. In contrast, the sarcomere length relationship is virtually identical in emphysema and normal. Therefore, shifts in the fiber length-tension curve in the emphysematous animal indicate that emphysema alters the relationship between fiber length and sarcomere length. Reductions in the number of sarcomeres arranged in series along the muscle fiber in the chronically hyperinflated emphysematous state explain this finding. (From [16] with permission)

expiratory muscles of the abdominal wall are at greater than L_o at FRC (e.g. rectus abdominus) and approach L_o as lung volume increases [13].

Changes in thoracoabdominal configuration may also alter the fiber length or configuration of the respiratory muscles independent of changes in lung volume. For example, Grassino et al. [8] found that transdiaphragmatic pressure (Pdi) at isolung volume and a given level of diaphragm electrical activity depended on thoracoabdominal configuration. Changes in abdominal volume had a threefold greater effect on Pdi than did similar changes in rib cage volume. At isolung volume, reductions in abdominal volume increased Pdi while reductions in rib cage volume decreased Pdi. These authors, however, did not measure diaphragm length or configuration at any given thoracoabdominal configuration.

In a later study, Loring et al. [9] assessed the effect of changes in lung volume and thoracoabdominal configuration on diaphragm length (measured indirectly by X-ray, ultrasound, and magnetometers) in normal subjects. Diaphragm length depended on both rib cage and abdominal displacement, but to unequal degrees. In agreement with the results of Grassino, Loring et al. found that a given volume displacement of the abdominal compartment changed diaphragm length on average twice as much as did an equal volume displacement of the rib cage.

Body posture also appears to be an important determinant of respiratory muscle mechanical advantage. Sharp et al. [14] studied the effect of posture on diaphragmatic function and accessory muscle electrical activity in a group of COPD patients. Subjects with severe hyperinflation (TLC 149% of predicted) demonstrated increased Pdi (without effecting diaphragm EMG) and reduced accessory muscle activity in the leaning forward and supine postures, compared to the standing or sitting postures. These authors suggested that in the leaning forward and supine postures the effect of gravity and/or abdominal compression enhanced diaphragm mechanical advantage. Postural change may also effect other respiratory muscles. For example, in the dog, Farkas and Rochester [12] have found that sternocleidomastoid and scalene muscle fiber length largely depends on the position of the head.

It is important to note however, that chronic alterations in lung volume and thoracoabdominal configuration may change muscle fiber structure and alter the position of the length-tension characteristic of the diaphragm. For example, in emphysematous hamster, chronic hyperinflation produces reductions in sarcomere number and a leftward displacement of the length-tension characteristic of the costal region of the diaphragm (Fig. 1) [15, 16]. These alterations in muscle fiber length-tension characteristic may help to restore the mechanical advantage of the diaphragm in chronically hyperinflated states [17].

Force-Velocity Relationship

The force developed by contracting skeletal muscle is inversely related to its velocity of shortening. The shape of the force-velocity relationship of skeletal muscle conforms to a rectangular hyperbola (Fig. 2). Isometric contractions generate greater levels of force than isotonic (shortening) contractions, and lengthening contractions generate the greatest force of all [18]. In man, strength of the respiratory muscles is usually assessed indirectly from changes in airway or esophageal pressure. Changes in pressure anywhere in the respiratory system require some degree of muscle shortening and changes in thoracic volume and/or configuration. Since muscle shortening reduces force output, the assessment of respiratory muscle force in man is usually performed utilizing techniques to minimize muscle shortening

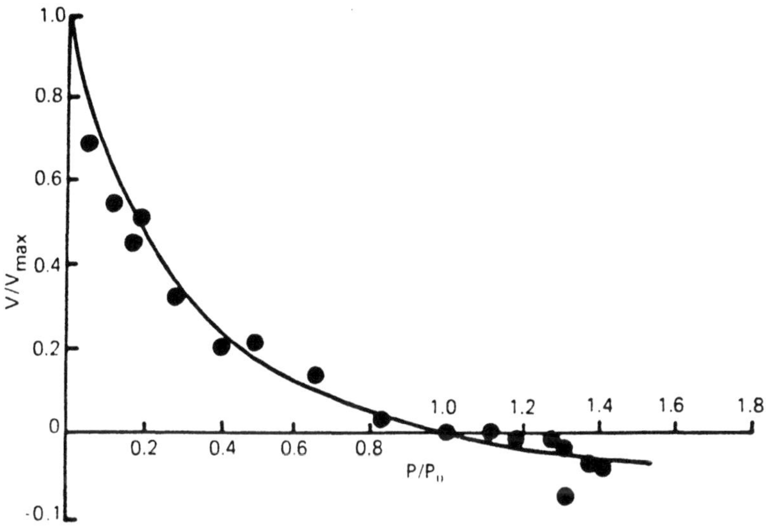

Fig. 2. Representative isotonic force-velocity relationship for skeletal muscle. Note that velocity decreases as external load (expressed as a percent of isometric force-P_O) increases. Note also that the greatest levels of force are generating during lengthening contractions (demonstrated as negative values of velocity). It is likely that lengthening contractions may develop under some circumstances when paradoxical movements of rib cage and abdomen occur. Performance of maximum diaphragm contractions during combined expulsive and Mueller maneuvers is one such circumstance. (From [88] with permission)

during contractions, such as airway occlusion and abdominal binding. The degree to which the respiratory muscles shorten in man when respiratory muscle strength is assessed is unclear and largely unstudied. However, Newman et al. [19], utilizing sonomicrometry to assess changes in diaphragm muscle length in the supine anesthetized dog, demonstrated marked diaphragmatic shortening during inspiratory efforts against an occluded airway. Of note, attempts to limit rib cage deflation or abdominal expansion and thereby minimize diaphragmatic shortening were not employed. These results suggest that diaphragm shortening may be considerable despite attempts to produce an isometric contraction by occluding the airway.

Motor Outflow

Force-frequency relationship. Application of depolarizing levels of current to an axon supplying a motor unit (or to a single fiber) initiates contraction and the development of active tension. Tension increases in a curvilinear fashion as a function of the axonal firing rate until a firing frequency is reached which is associated with maximal tension (force-frequency relationship) (Fig. 3). For the diaphragm, firing rates of 50–75 depolarizations per second are sufficient to develop a fully fused contraction and hence maximum force output [20]. The increase in tension as stimulation frequency rises is due to the progressive summation of individual contrac-

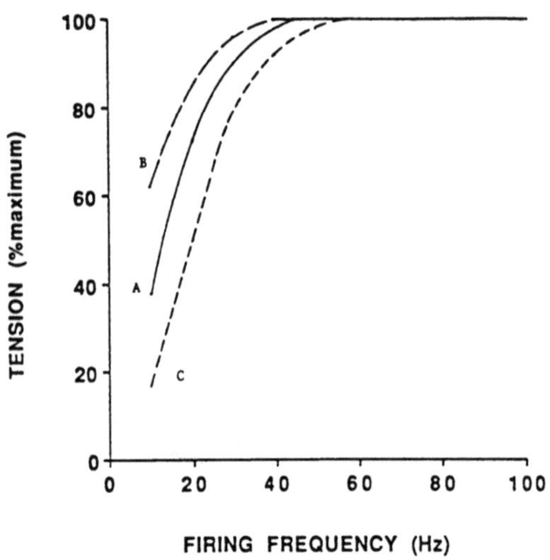

Fig. 3. Schematic representation of the force-frequency relationship of respiratory skeletal muscle. Note that tension increases as the frequency of axonal firing rises. At some level of firing frequency, tension reaches a maximum. In general, maximum tension is achieved when firing frequency exceeds 50 Hz (i.e. cycles per second). Curves B and C demonstrate the effects of changes in the percentages of fast and slow twitch fibers or the effects of temperature. Curve B is the condition in which the muscle is composed of a lower percentage of fast twitch fibers or when the temperature of the muscle is decreased. In contrast, curve C demonstrates the condition in which a greater percentage of the muscle is made up of fast twitch fibers or when muscle fiber temperature is increased

tions. The slower the rate of tension development and relaxation during a twitch of any given muscle, the greater the tendency for contractions to summate and the lower the stimulation frequency needed to achieve full summation. Therefore, reductions in muscle temperature which slow the rate of tension development and relaxation shift the curve to the left [21, 22]. In contrast, the greater the percentage of fast fibers in a given muscle, the greater the tendency of the force-frequency curve to shift to the right [22].

Motor unit recruitment. Force output of a contracting respiratory skeletal muscle is increased by recruitment of additional motor units which may have been quiescent when the muscle is inactive. During eupneic breathing, it is generally believed that only motor units comprised of slow oxidative fibers are active [23]. Increasing inspiratory muscle activity is associated with progressive recruitment of motor units comprised of fast oxidative and ultimately fast glycolytic motor units [23]. Of interest, motor unit size (i.e. the number of muscle fibers innervated by a single alpha motor neuron) is least for slow oxidative fibers, intermediate for fast oxidative fiber motor units, and greatest for fast glycolytic motor units [24]. Progressive increases in inspiratory drive or effort are, therefore, associated with recruitment of progressively larger motor units capable of generating more force per motor unit and per fiber in any given motor unit.

Causes of Respiratory Muscle Weakness

The disease processes that may impair respiratory muscle strength are numerous. Table 1 categorizes these processes [25–31]. A comprehensive discussion of each of these conditions is beyond the scope of this chapter. However, the respiratory mus-

Table 1. Respiratory muscle weakness

Category	Examples	Potential mechanisms	References
Neuromuscular			
Myopathic	Polymyositis	Muscle inflammation and necrosis	[25]
Demyelinating	Multiple sclerosis	Denervation atrophy	[25]
Myoneural synaptic dysfunction	Myasthenia gravis	Acetylcholine receptor antibodies; impaired muscle excitation	[25]
Malnutrition	Anorexia nervosa	Loss of contractile proteins	[26, 27]
Endocrine	Corticosteroid excess	Muscle fiber atrophy (Type II)	[28]
Metabolic	Hypercapnia	Altered intracellular pH (?); impaired excitation-contraction coupling	[29]
Mineral and electrolyte	Hypophosphatemia	Impaired excitation-contraction coupling	[30]
Post-surgical	Coronary artery Bypass surgery	Thermal or ischemic injury to phrenic nerves	[31]

cle dysfunction associated with chronic obstructive lung disease deserves special mention because of its complexity and frequency of occurrence.

The hyperinflation associated with chronic obstructive pulmonary disease (COPD) can impair inspiratory muscle strength via several mechanisms. Hyperinflation may foreshorten inspiratory muscle precontraction length and move muscle fibers to a less advantageous position on their length-tension curve [32]. Hyperinflation may also diminish the pressure generated by the inspiratory muscles at a given level of tension by complex effects on muscle fiber configuration and alignment with the rib cage. For example, depression and flattening of the normally highly curved dome of the diaphragm may realign the costal and crural muscle fibers such that the fibers contract in series rather than in parallel [33]. Forces generated by muscles mechanically arranged in series are equal to the greatest force generated by one muscle alone. In contrast, the force generated by muscles mechanically arranged in parallel represents the sum of the forces generated by the two muscles [34]. Realignment of costal and crural muscle fibers toward a series rather than a parallel arrangement diminishes the total diaphragmatic force. In the markedly flattened diaphragm, costal and crural muscle fibers may be rearranged perpendicularly rather than parallel to the chest wall (cephalo-caudal orientation). Contraction of these perpendicularly oriented fibers results in paradoxical inward movement of the lower rib cage (Hoover's sign) [32]. Hyperinflation also effectively reduces the inspiratory action of the costal and crural diaphragm on the lower rib cage by reducing the area of the zone of apposition of the costal diaphragm with the lower rib cage [34]. The zone of apposition of the costal diaphragm allows positive abdominal pressure generated during inspiration by contraction of the costal and crural diaphragm to produce an inspiratory action on the lower rib cage.

Respiratory muscle function in COPD may be impaired by mechanisms other than mechanical disadvantage. For example, in patients with COPD, wasting of the respiratory muscles is common, is related to the severity of airway obstruction, and is an independent factor contributing to an increased mortality [35, 36]. Reductions in muscle mass diminish the capacity of both the inspiratory and expiratory muscles to generate pressure [26]. In undernourished patients, the weight, thickness and surface area of the muscular region of the diaphragm appears to be diminished [6]. Atrophy of both fast and slow twitch muscle fibers of the diaphragm has been demonstrated in patients with COPD compared to normals, but whether this change is related to nutritional factors is unclear [4].

Finally, increases in $PaCO_2$ may reversibly diminish the tension generating ability of the diaphragm [29]. Even modest hypercapnia (e.g. arterial $PaCO_2$ 50–55 mm Hg) may depress transdiaphragmatic pressure at a given level of diaphragm muscle electrical activity during graded static voluntary inspiratory efforts in normal subjects [29]. It seems likely that similar effects are present in patients with COPD.

Methods of Assessing Respiratory Muscle Strength

History and Physical Examination

The signs and symptoms of respiratory muscle weakness are usually non-specific and of limited value in the assessment of respiratory muscle strength. Moreover, the clinical manifestations of respiratory muscle weakness depends on the specific muscle (or muscles) involved and their extent of dysfunction. Patients may be asymptomatic with mild weakness, but dyspnea on exertion becomes the predominant symptom as weakness becomes more severe. Patients with expiratory muscle weakness may have an impaired cough. Disturbed sleep and daytime hypersomnolence resulting from nocturnal alveolar hypoventilation may occur in subjects with diaphragm weakness [37]. As respiratory muscle weakness becomes more severe, CO_2 retention may ensue.

Respiratory muscle strength may be impaired by pathological processes that cause generalized skeletal muscle weakness. Atrophy or fasciculation of the respiratory muscles (intercostals, neck accessory muscles) may suggest such involvement. However, the degree of respiratory muscle involvement, if any, cannot be accurately inferred by simply assessing the degree of limb muscle involvement [38]. In fact, respiratory muscle dysfunction may occur in isolation. It is thus essential to specifically test for respiratory muscle weakness when signs or symptoms of pulmonary impairment occur in patients with neuromuscular disease.

In contrast to other causes of respiratory muscle weakness, patients with isolated severe diaphragm muscle weakness or paralysis may present with a characteristic clinical picture. They are often asymptomatic in the upright position but develop dyspnea when lying supine. In this position, there may be prominent paradoxical inward movement of the upper abdomen, resulting from passive movement of the diaphragm into the thorax as a result of the negative inspiratory pressure generated by the intercostal and neck accessory inspiratory muscles [39]. In the upright posture, such paradoxical movement is minimized by the effect of gravity on the abdominal contents. Abdominal paradox occurs when the transdiaphragmatic pressure is less than 30 cm H_2O and represents a crude measure of diaphragm strength [37].

Pulmonary Function Studies

When inspiratory muscle weakness is advanced, vital capacity falls because of a decrease in TLC. For example, isolated bilateral diaphragm paralysis results in a fall in the vital capacity (VC) and TLC with a normal RV [39, 40]. Even more useful in this setting is the measurement of VC in the upright and supine postures. Patients with bilateral diaphragm paralysis generally have a greater than 30% reduction in VC in moving from the seated to the supine position [40]. Normal subjects will have a reduction in VC of less than 30% [41]. The RV may increase when expiratory muscle function is impaired [42].

However, since lung and chest wall diseases may reduce VC in the absence of respiratory muscle weakness, the specificity of a reduction in VC is poor. Sensitivity is also poor since a reduction in VC will only occur with advanced respiratory muscle weakness.

Arterial blood gas abnormalities usually occur only with severe respiratory muscle weakness. Hypoxemia, usually mild, may occur as a result of microatelectasis and subsequent ventilation-perfusion mismatch. In addition, patients with significantly impaired muscle strength have impaired cough and retained secretions. Hypercapnia is also an insensitive measure of respiratory muscle strength. In a study of 53 patients with proximal myopathy, Braun et al. [42] found that $PaCO_2$ did not increase until respiratory muscle strength (as measured by maximal inspiratory and expiratory pressures) was less than 50% of predicted. These same authors found similar results in 30 patients with COPD [43].

In summary, spirometry and arterial blood gas analysis poorly reflect respiratory muscle strength and have a limited role in detecting and quantitating the severity of respiratory muscle weakness.

Radiology

In severe generalized inspiratory muscle weakness or bilateral diaphragm paralysis, inspiration is limited and the lung volume on a chest radiograph appears reduced. Unilateral hemidiaphragm paralysis produces an elevated diaphragm on the affected side. Neither radiographic appearance, however, is specific for respiratory muscle weakness.

Fluoroscopy is often employed in the assessment of diaphragmatic paralysis. In unilateral diaphragm paralysis, a positive "sniff test" (the patient makes a forceful sniff in the supine position) may demonstrate paradoxical upward movement of the affected hemidiaphragm [39]. This test may have a false positive rate as high as 6% in normal subjects [44]. The use of the sniff test to diagnose bilateral diaphragm paralysis is limited by compensatory contraction of the abdominal muscles. With abrupt cessation of abdominal muscle contraction during early inspiration, the abdominal contents descend, the abdominal wall moves outward and the diaphragm shows a net descent. In addition, the observational field of the diaphragm with fluoroscopy is limited to a band encompassing the diaphragmatic dome and adjacent ribs. If rib cage rostral movement exceeds diaphragm ascent, the diaphragm will appear to descend lower in the thorax and may falsely suggest diaphragm shortening [39].

Maximum Respiratory Pressures

Maximal static inspiratory and expiratory pressures, measured at the airway opening during a voluntary contraction against an occluded airway, are the simplest and most commonly performed tests of respiratory muscle strength. Although several variations on the basic technique have been described, the most widely used method is that of Black and Hyatt [45]. In this technique, pressure was measured utilizing an hand-held aneroid manometer with the patient seated with a mouthpiece in place and a nose clip on. During maneuvers, the patient pursed the lips inside a circular rubber mouthpiece to prevent perioral air leakage. A small orifice (2 mm in diameter, 15 mm in length) in the circuit served as an air leak to minimize the contribution of the facial muscles to airway pressure and to keep the glottis open. Maximal expiratory pressures (PE_{MAX}) were measured at or near TLC. Maximal inspiratory pressures (PI_{MAX}) were measured near residual volume after a maximal expiration. In each case, efforts were maintained for at least one second.

Black and Hyatt studied 120 adults, 60 males and 60 females, ranging in age from 20 to 86 years, and established "normal" values based on age and sex (Table 2). Table 2 also lists published values from other investigations for comparison [45–51].

As can be seen in Table 2, reported values for PE_{MAX} and PI_{MAX} in normal subjects vary widely. Potential reasons for this variation in results include important differences in technique that must be recognized. For example, there is a significant learning effect in the performance of these maneuvers. Patients usually require careful instruction and encouragement and performance of multiple attempts before meaningful results are obtained. Differences in results from different laboratories, therefore, may reflect the degree of instruction and repetition employed. For example, Rinqvist [46], using 10 or more trials per subject, obtained significantly higher values for PE_{MAX} and PI_{MAX} than did Leech [47], who reported the best value of only three trials. Other technique-related factors that may influence results include the type of mouthpiece used [52], and the development of fatigue during testing [53].

Lung volume effects. A major factor affecting PI_{MAX} and PE_{MAX} is lung volume. PE_{MAX} is greatest at TLC because the expiratory muscles are at greatest mechanical advantage and because the inward elastic recoil of the respiratory system is greatest. Likewise, PI_{MAX} is greatest at RV, where the inspiratory muscles are at greatest mechanical advantage and the outward elastic recoil of the respiratory system is maximum. Figure 4 illustrates the effect of lung volume on PI_{MAX} and PE_{MAX}. Only at FRC, where respiratory system recoil pressure measured at the airway opening is zero, are PI_{MAX} and PE_{MAX} solely a function of the pressure generated by the actively contracting respiratory muscles (Pmuscle). In practice, therefore, PI_{MAX} and PE_{MAX} are often measured at FRC [48]. Alternatively, Pmuscle may be measured from maximum static esophageal pressure (Pes) [54]. Unlike maximum airway pressure, maximum static Pes is not affected by lung recoil pressure or pressure artifacts from glottic closure or facial muscle contraction.

Changes in lung volume due to lung or chest wall pathology have important effects on maximal respiratory pressures. For instance, patients with COPD and hyperinflation have a larger FRC and RV than normals and therefore PI_{MAX} performed at RV or FRC are usually lower than values obtained in age and sex matched normal subjects [43]. Rochester and Braun [43] studied maximal respiratory pressures and their relation to lung volume and diaphragm length in 32 patients with COPD (mean $FEV_1 = 35\%$ predicted). PI_{MAX} was reduced in the group as a whole. Of interest, PE_{MAX} was reduced in one half of the patients. After correcting for hyperinflation, PI_{MAX} was in the normal range in patients with a normal PE_{MAX}, but still reduced in the patients with a low PE_{MAX}. Since reduc-

Table 2. Reported values for maximal static airway pressures in normal adults

Study	Sex	Number of subjects	Age range (years)	PI_{MAX} (cmH_2O)	PE_{MAX} (cm H_2O)	Coefficient of variation	References
Black and Hyatt 1969	Males	60	20–54	124 ± 22	233 ± 42	9%	[45]
	Females	60	20–54	87 ± 16	152 ± 27		
Rinqvist 1966	Males	100	18–83	130 ± 32	237 ± 46	6%	[46]
	Females	100	18–83	98 ± 25	165 ± 30		
Leech, et al. 1983	Males	325	17–35	114 ± 36	154 ± 82	Not given	[47]
	Females	480	15–35	71 ± 27	94 ± 33		
Rochester, Arora, 1983	Males	80	19–49	127 ± 28	216 ± 41	Not given	[48]
	Females	121	19–49	91 ± 25	138 ± 39		
Vincken, et al. 1987	Males	46	16–79	105 ± 25	140 ± 38	Not given	[49]
	Females	60	16–79	71 ± 23	89 ± 24		
Cooke, et al. 1964	Males	17	18–47	133 ± 39	237 ± 45	"Non-	[50]
	Females	9	18–32	100 ± 19	146 ± 34	significant"	
Wilson, et al. 1984	Males	48	19–65	106 ± 31	148 ± 34	PE_{MAX} = 7.1%	[51]
	Females	87	18–65	73 ± 22	93 ± 17	PI_{MAX} = 10.2%	

Values are mean ± standard deviation.

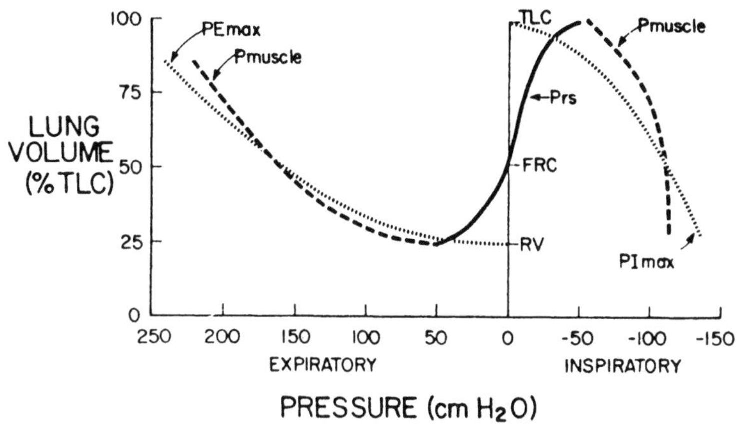

Fig. 4. The effect of lung volume on maximum static inspiratory (PI_{max}) and expiratory (PE_{max}, stippled line) pressures measured at the airway opening. Note that increasing lung volume reduces PI_{max} but increases PE_{max}. The pressure generated by the actively contracting muscle (P muscle, dashed line) however, represents the difference between PI_{max} (or PE_{max}) and respiratory system recoil pressure (Prs, solid line). Note that at FRC, where respiratory system recoil pressure is equal to 0, maximum static pressure at the airway opening is equal to Pmuscle. At all lung volumes other than FRC, recoil pressure contributes to PI_{max} and PE_{max}. (From [48] with permission)

tions in PE_{MAX} cannot be explained by hyperinflation, these authors suggested that reduction in PE_{MAX} in this subject population represented generalized muscle weakness. These results suggest that a reduction in PI_{MAX} in COPD patients may be due either to mechanical disadvantage or to a more generalized process causing skeletal muscle dysfunction, such as skeletal muscle atrophy.

Likewise, reduction in TLC due to restrictive lung disease may reduce PE_{MAX}. It is thus important to realize that in patients with pathologically altered lung volumes, all or part of a reduction in PI_{MAX} or PE_{MAX} may be due to mechanical disadvantage. The effects of varying body postures or alterations in thoracoabdominal configuration on maximal respiratory pressure have not been studied.

The effects of age and sex. The aging process may affect the respiratory musculature in several ways. Aging is associated with changes in respiratory system elastance [55] and lung volume [56], and hence may affect respiratory muscle load, recoil pressure, and muscle mechanical advantage. In addition, animal studies indicate that aging may directly affect respiratory muscle contractility. Zhang and Kelsen [57] studied the contractile properties of the costal diaphragm from young (mean age 4.9 months), middle aged (mean age 12.8 months), and elderly (mean age 18.8 months) adult Golden hamsters [57]. They found that maximal isometric tension at a given fiber length during electrically stimulated contractions *in vitro* was less in the elderly animals compared to the other two groups (Fig. 5). L_o was similar in all 3 groups. Of interest, there was no significant difference between the young and middle aged groups, suggesting that changes in muscle strength occur only at an advanced age.

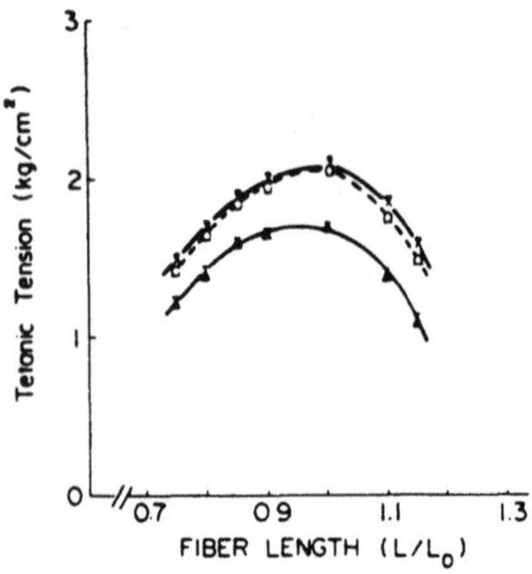

Fig. 5. The effects of aging on the maximum isometric force generating capacity of the costal region of the hamster diaphragm over a range of fiber lengths. Values shown are for 4 months (x), 12 months (open circles), and 18 months (solid triangles) old animals. Note that isometric tension generating ability is decreased at any given fiber length only in 18 month old animals. Therefore, reductions in tension generating ability do not appear to be progressive throughout life but appear to occur only in the extremely aged animals (i.e. 18 months). (From [57] with permission)

The effect of age on maximum respiratory pressures in humans has been studied by several investigators. Rinqvist [46] found that in 200 subjects, PI_{MAX} (measured at RV) decreased linearly with age in both males and females, and that PE_{MAX} (measured at TLC) decreased curvilinearly with age in male subjects. Vincken et al. [49], in a study of 106 normal subjects, also found that PI_{MAX} decreased linearly with age, whereas PE_{MAX} rose to a peak in middle age (age 35 in woman, 45 in men) before decreasing. Black and Hyatt [45] found a significant inverse relationship between PE_{MAX} and age in 25 males and females 55 years or older, and of PI_{MAX} in females. No relationship was found between PI_{MAX} or PE_{MAX} and age in subjects younger than 55 years of age.

In contrast to the above studies, McElvaney et al. [58] recently studied 104 normal subjects over the age of 55 (40 male, 64 female) and found no statistically significant relationship between PI_{MAX} or PE_{MAX} and age. However, graphic display of their data suggests a decrease in both PI_{MAX} and PE_{MAX} with advancing age for both sexes, especially for subjects over age 65. Like others, these authors found wide interindividual variation for both PE_{MAX} and PI_{MAX}. They speculated that a significant correlation between PI_{MAX} and PE_{MAX} may have been found if larger numbers of patients had been studied. An effect of age on PI_{MAX} and PE_{MAX} may also have been observed if results were compared to a younger population.

Tolep et al. [59] recently studied the effect of age on diaphragmatic function in normal young (mean age 24 years) and elderly (mean age 69 years) adult men as assessed by transdiaphragmatic pressure (Pdi). Maximum Pdi was assessed during a two-step explusive-Mueller maneuver (see below). Subjects were healthy nonsmokers with normal body weight and lung function. They found that maximum Pdi was significantly lower in the elderly (142 ± 10 cm H_2O) compared to the young subjects (176±9 cm H_2O), though there was considerable overlap between the two groups (Fig. 6).

The preponderance of evidence, therefore, suggests that age is an important determinant of maximal static pressures.

A universal finding in all studies of maximal respiratory pressures in normal subjects is that women have lower values for both PI_{MAX} and PE_{MAX} than men. For the studies listed in Table 2, PI_{MAX} in females ranged from 62–75% and PE_{MAX} ranged from 61–70% of values obtained in males. This female/male difference in strength resembles differences observed for measurements of limb skeletal muscle strength (e.g. hand grip) [60]. Although not studied directly, these differences may be related to differences in muscle mass between the sexes [49]. However, potential differences in respiratory muscle fiber type and/or number as explanations for differences in respiratory muscle strength in men and women remain unstudied. Although interindividual variability is large, the intraindividual variability in most studies has ranged from 6–9% [45, 46, 51]. This value for variability is similar to results of limb muscle strength testing [61]. Measurements of maximum static airway pressure are particularly useful, therefore, for assessing changes in respiratory muscle strength in a given subject over time.

Maximal inspiratory pressure (MIP) is commonly utilized as a measure of respiratory muscle strength in patients receiving mechanical ventilation. Bedside variations on the technique of Black and Hyatt have been advocated as a predictor of weaning success or failure [62]. A major problem with the use of MIP in mechanically ventilated patients is the frequent inability of these patients to generate a maximal effort either because of the underlying disease(s) or altered mental status.

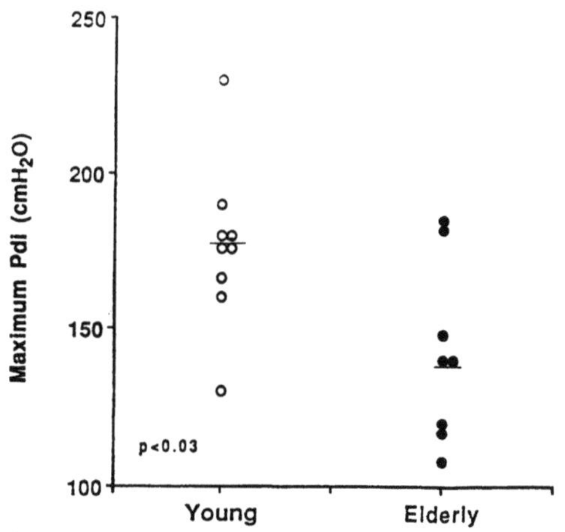

Fig. 6. Comparison of maximum static transdiaphragmatic pressure in young (<35 years of age) and elderly (greater than 65 years of age) normal adult males. Subjects performed maximum expulsive followed by Mueller maneuvers using visual feedback from a storage oscilloscope to generate maximum static transdiaphragmatic pressures. Symbols represent values obtained in individual subjects. As may be seen, for the group as a whole, maximum static pressure is significantly reduced in elderly as compared to younger subjects

Marini et al. [63] have described a standardized technique to improve the reproducibility of MIP measurements in mechanically ventilated patients. They compared MIP measurements obtained by 2 techniques:

1. total occlusion of the inspiratory and expiratory limbs of the breathing circuit for 20–25 sec; and
2. occlusion of the inspiratory limb of the circuit only with a unidirectional valve permitting exhalation to a lower lung volume.

In the latter technique, successive inspiratory efforts could be initiated from progressively lower lung volumes. Peak inspiratory pressure increased with successive breaths over time with both techniques. A maximum value was usually obtained after approximately 20 sec, or about 10 breaths (Fig. 7). Sustained occlusion of the inspiratory circuit for 20–25 sec may increase chemical drives to breathe (i.e. increased PCO_2 and decreased PO_2). These increases in respiratory drive stimulate increased respiratory motor output and hence progressively greater inspiratory efforts. MIP's obtained with method two (i.e. inspiratory occlusion and the use of a unidirectional exhalation valve) were on average 34% greater than those obtained using method one. Addition of the unidirectional exhalation valve may have augmented respiratory muscle mechanical advantage and/or respiratory drive by allowing reductions in lung volumes. Of note, the mental status of the patients, which ranged from alert to comatose, had no significant effect on MIP measurements in either method.

Multz et al. [64] measured MIPs on mechanically ventilated patients using the technique of Marini. Several different investigators performed the measurements

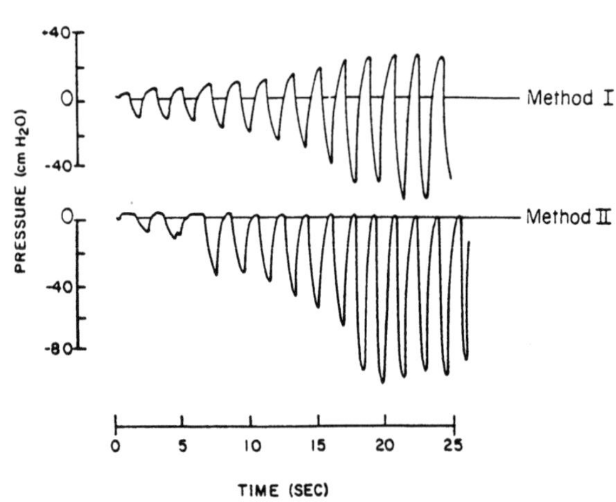

Fig. 7. Shows the change in peak inspiratory airway pressure (MIP) during maintained occlusion of the airway for 25 sec. In method I occlusion is performed during both inspiration and expiration while in method II the airway is occluded during inspiration only. In the latter method, lung volume can be reduced progressively during unobstructed expiration through an undirectional value. Note that peak inspiratory pressure increases progressively over time and reaches a maximum within 20–25 sec with both methods. Greater values of inspiratory pressure are obtained with method II. Progressively greater efforts with the two approaches appear to be explained by increasing chemical drives to breathe during airway occlusion. (From [63] with permission)

on a given patient over a period of one to seven days. They found that MIP measured by a single investigator during a single study had a coefficient of variation of approximately 12%, but was more widely variable when measured by different investigators on the same day (coefficient of variation = 32%). In addition, MIPs measured by the same investigator on different days varied widely without an obvious change in clinical status of the patient. These data suggest that technique related factors may contribute to the variability of measured MIP in mechanically ventilated patients and underscore the difficulty in assessing respiratory muscle strength in the severely ill, mechanically ventilated patient.

Despite the limitations discussed above, measurement of maximal static pressures at the airway opening remains the most widely applied bedside test of respiratory muscle strength. Furthermore, the method of Marini has distinct advantages since it yields higher MIP values compared to other methods, allows reduction in lung volume, and controls for the time of airway occlusion.

Transdiaphragmatic Pressure

While maximal static airway pressures are useful measures of global respiratory muscle strength, they do not assess the function of individual respiratory muscles. Since the diaphragm is the primary muscle of inspiration and may be susceptible to isolated injuries or disease processes (i.e. phrenic nerve paralysis due to cardiac surgery), specific testing of diaphragm strength is desirable. Assessment of diaphragm strength can be made by measuring abdominal (Pab) and esophageal (Pes) pressures via balloon tipped catheters placed in the stomach and mid-esophagus, respectively. Transdiaphragmatic pressure (Pdi) is then calculated as the algebraic substraction of Pes from Pab (Pdi = Pab − Pes).

The maneuvers utilized to elicit maximal transdiaphragmatic pressure (Pdi_{MAX}) have been the subject of extensive study. Early studies measured Pdi during maximal static inspiratory efforts against a closed airway (Mueller maneuver) at either FRC or RV. However, there is evidence that this maneuver may result in submaximal activation of the diaphragm, with the degree of activation varying widely from subject to subject [65]. During a Mueller maneuver, most subjects generate a large negative Pes, but a small and variable Pab. A few subjects even generate a negative Pab [42, 66, 67], possibly due to passive movement of the diaphragm into the thorax. Alternatively, if the increase in abdominal volume due to expansion of the lower rib cage is greater than the reduction in abdominal volume due to diaphragmatic descent, Pab may be negative. Intraindividual coefficients of variation as high as 40% have been attained when measuring Pdi_{MAX} during a Mueller maneuver [62].

Laporta and Grassino [68] compared 5 different maneuvers for measuring Pdi_{MAX} to determine the optimal technique for producing maximal and reproducible values in 35 subjects (10 normals, 12 COPD, 13 restrictive lung disease). The maneuvers employed were:

1. Mueller maneuver with a mouthpiece;
2. Mueller maneuver without a mouthpiece;

3. an expulsive maneuver with an open glottis during which abdominal pressure is increased maximally by the combined contraction of the diaphragm and abdominal muscles;
4. a two-step maneuver in which the subject first performs an explusive maneuver and superimposes a Mueller maneuver; and finally
5. a feedback maneuver in which the two-step maneuver is performed using visual feedback of Pes and Pab on an oscilloscope to maximize Pdi by simultaneously achieving maximal positive abdominal and negative esophageal pressures.

Pdi_{MAX} was greatest during the feedback maneuver (maneuver number 5) as compared to the other four maneuvers. This was the case despite the fact that greater values for Pab or Pes occurred during the expulsive and Mueller maneuvers, respectively. These authors found that the feedback maneuver was easily mastered (with an average of 5 trials required in normal subjects) and more reproducible ($\leq 10\%$ variation) than any of the other maneuvers.

The explanation as to why the highest values for Pdi_{MAX} were obtained during the feedback maneuver is the subject of some debate. Laporta and Grassino speculated that this combined maneuver with feedback resulted in greater activation of the diaphragm than either the Mueller or explusive maneuver alone. This appears to be supported by the data of Hershenson et al. [65] who found that bilateral phrenic nerve stimulation at one Hz (twitch) elicited a transient increase in Pdi when superimposed on Pdi during a Mueller maneuver. However, the twitch induced little or no increase in Pdi when superimposed during a combined expulsive and Mueller maneuver. These results suggest that the diaphragm was submaximally activated during the Mueller maneuver alone but maximally activated during the combined expulsive and Mueller maneuvers. Another reason suggested for the increased Pdi during the feedback maneuver is that changes occur in diaphragm geometry that may be more favorable to force generation [8]. A third possible explanation was proposed by Hillman et al. [69] who found evidence that diaphragm fiber lengthening occurs during the expulsive maneuver which may yield greater tension than during isometric contraction alone, independent of a change in muscle activation. Using fluoroscopy, these investigators demonstrated diaphragmatic ascent into the thorax during a maximal expulsive maneuver and extrinsic abdominal compression as well as changes in thoracoabdominal configuration that would be consistent with diaphragm lengthening.

Major disadvantages of transdiaphragmatic pressure as a measure of diaphragm strength are its relative invasiveness and requirement for specialized equipment. Operators performing the test require expertise in catheter placement, patient instruction, and interpretation of results. There is also some question regarding the ability of subjects to maximally activate the diaphragm during voluntary static efforts (see below).

Phrenic Nerve Stimulation

A crucial factor in the measurement of diaphragm strength is the ability to consistently attain maximal activation of the diaphragm during a voluntary effort. Electrophrenic stimulation is a method that has been recently utilized to consistently activate the diaphragm. Phrenic nerve stimulation as a means of providing artificial respiration in patients has been known since the 1950's [70], but the application of this technique to assess diaphragm contractile function has occurred only in the last decade. Besides assessing diaphragm strength, this technique offers the added advantage of assessing phrenic nerve conduction and the possibility of phrenic nerve injury in patients with diaphragm weakness of unknown cause [71].

The phrenic nerves are stimulated in the neck near the posterior border of the sternocleidomastoid muscle at the level of the cricoid cartilage, where the phrenic nerves are most superficial. Stimulations may be performed either transcutaneously with surface electrodes [66] or percutaneously with needle [72] or wire [73] electrodes. Transcutaneous stimulation has the advantage of being non-invasive, but may be more painful than needle electrodes because of the higher voltages necessary to overcome skin resistance. Stimulation with needle electrodes may be less painful, but poses the potential hazards of phrenic nerve or vascular injuries.

Phrenic stimulation is usually performed with the patient in either the seated or supine position in a relaxed state. Stimulations are performed at FRC with the airway occluded. Abdominal binding or casting is sometimes used to limit diaphragmatic shortening. Electrodes to record the diaphragm muscle action potential (DMAP) may be placed bilaterally in the anterior sixth, seventh, or eighth intercostal spaces or in the esophagus. Transdiaphragmatic pressures are measured as previously described.

Regardless of the electrodes used, stimulation of the phrenic nerves must be demonstrated to be supramaximal with regard to voltage and current. Supramaximal conditions are ensured by increasing the stimulus intensity until maximal DMAP or Pdi is achieved. DMAP is then checked periodically throughout the study to ensure that constancy is maintained. Voltage or current levels up to 1.5 times the amount needed to obtain maximal Pdi are employed to ensure supramaximal conditions.

The use of tetanizing stimulation frequency (i.e. 75 HZ) to assess maximal Pdi has been attempted by several investigators [20, 74], but has generally been abandoned because tetanic stimulations are painful and commonly activate surrounding neck and arm muscles and dislodge the stimulating electrode. In addition, contraction of neck muscles may effect Pdi by creating a more negative Pes and hence limiting diaphragm shortening.

The most commonly used technique of electrophrenic stimulation now employs a frequency of one pulse per second (i.e. 1 Hz) to measure Pdi during a single, unfused twitch contraction (i.e. Pdi_{TWITCH}). Table 3 lists values obtained by several investigators for peak transdiaphragmatic pressure by bilateral electrophrenic stimulation in healthy adults. The usefulness of Pdi_{TWITCH} as a measure of diaphragm strength is dependent upon the demonstration that all diaphragm muscle fibers are fully activated (see above).

Phrenic nerve stimulation may be performed either unilaterally or bilaterally. When an identical supramaximal stimulus is administered separately to the right and left phrenic nerves, the values for Pdi_{TWITCH} obtained from the left side are usually greater than from the right, and the algebraic sum of the values obtained from the separate simulation of the two sides is less than the value obtained during bilateral simultaneous twitch stimulation [75, 76]. This is felt to occur because unilateral phrenic nerve stimulation results in shortening of the stimulated hemidia-

Table 3. Reported values for bilateral twitch Pdi in seated normal adults at end-expiratory lung volume

Study	Number of subjects	Age range (years)	Pdi Peak (cm H_2O)	Range
Bellemare et al., 1984 [77]	9	23–55	48 ± 13 SD abd bound closed glottis	(34–70)
Aubier et al., 1985 [72]	6M	27–35	34 ± 4 SE ext. airway occlusion	(22–50)
Bellemare et al., 1986 [74]	6 (5M:1F)	23–34	42 ± 10 SD abd bound closed glottis	—
			33 ± 10 SD	—
Hubmayr et al., 1989 [73]	6M	28–48	31 ± 3 SE	(19–36)
Mier et al., 1989 [76]	20 (10M:10F)	24–73	21 ± 5 SD closed glottis	(9–33)
Similowski et al., 1989 [79]	6 (5M:1F)	24–38	33 ± 10 SD ext. airway occlusion	(23–50)

M = male; F = female

phragm and passive lengthening of the contralateral non-stimulated hemidiaphragm. The reason for the disparity between right and left Pdi_{TWITCH} is unknown. It has been speculated, however, that differences in compliance of the two hemithoraxes due to the presence of the heart on the left side affect muscle shortening and hence Pdi_{TWITCH} [71].

Pdi_{TWITCH} has been used to assess maximal static Pdi indirectly via the twitch-occlusion technique (Fig. 8) [77, 78]. In this method, single twitches are superimposed on progressively stronger voluntary diaphragm contractions. As voluntary effort and Pdi increase, the increment in Pdi produced during the twitch (twitch deflection superimposed on the Pdi) decreases. When no twitch Pdi deflection is descernible, it is assumed that the diaphragm is maximally activated, and thus the voluntary Pdi at that point represents Pdi_{MAX}. Bellemare and Bigland-Ritchie [77] and Gandevia and McKenzie [78] proposed a method for estimating Pdi_{MAX} during submaximal voluntary efforts from the inverse linear relationship between the amplitude of the superimposed twitch and the Pdi during voluntary effort. The extrapolation of the line to zero superimposed twitch Pdi has been taken as maximum static Pdi. Bellemare and Bigland-Ritchie [77] found that this relationship may not be linear at high levels of voluntary effort, but this has not been confirmed on a large number of subjects.

There is some controversy as to whether all diaphragm muscle fibers can be maximally activated during the different maneuvers employed to assess diaphragm strength. Gandevia and McKenzie [78] found maximal activation of the diaphragm (as assessed by twitch occlusion) during both a Mueller and expulsive maneuver. Hershenson et al. [65], however, found evidence that the diaphragm was submaximally activated during the Mueller maneuver, whereas maximal activation was

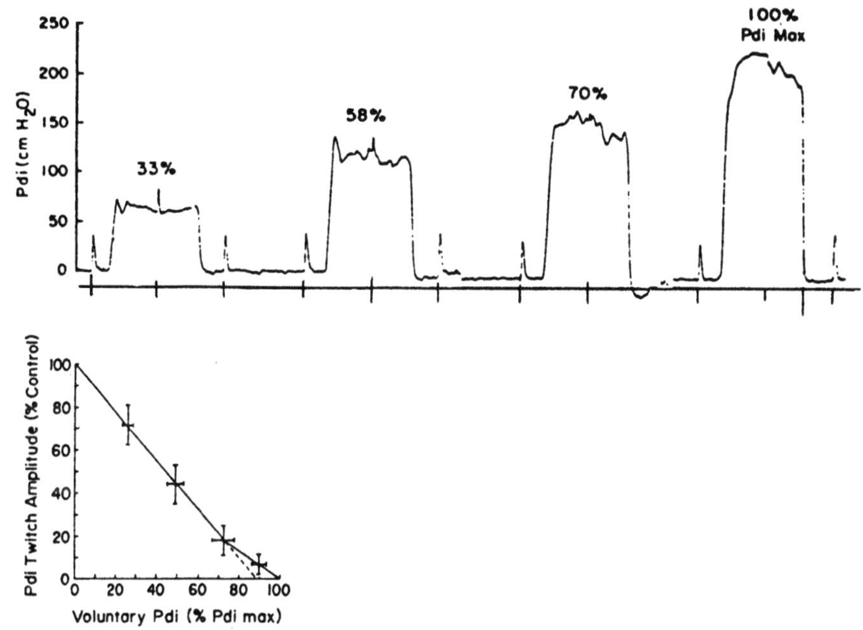

Fig. 8. Effect of increasing (voluntarily generated) transdiaphragmatic pressure on the amplitude of superimposed twitch contractions. Twitches during expiratory breath hold are the largest spike deflections. As may be seen, transdiaphragmatic pressure increases from 33% to 100% of maximum, the magnitude of the superimposed twitch diminishes steadily and, in fact, is absent at 100% Pdi. The lower panel demonstrates the relationship between the magnitude of the voluntary Pdi and the magnitude of the superimposed twitch. Control values represent the twitch amplitude during expiration. As may be seen the relationship is inversely linear. The use of the twitch occlusion technique, therefore, during a range of submaximal diaphragm contractions can be used to calculate maximum static transdiaphragmatic pressure by extrapolation of the relationship to 0 superimposed twitch. This approach holds promise as a method of assessing the diaphragm strength without requiring full activation of the muscle. (From [77] with permission)

found only during the explusive and combined expulsive-Mueller maneuver. To date, the discrepancy between these two investigators remains unresolved.

Recently, a technique using magnetic stimulation of the phrenic nerves has been described [79]. In this technique, the phrenic nerves are stimulated using a magnetic coil encased in a 9 cm diameter plate, with the center of the plate placed on the neck posteriorly over the spinous process of C7. An electrical current applied to this coil creates a pulsed magnetic field in a plane parallel to the coil, which in turn produces secondary electrical (stimulating) currents in the phrenic nerves. The position of the coil and the intensity of the stimulus can be varied to maximize phrenic nerve stimulation and minimize activation of surrounding muscles and nerves. Magnetic stimulation produced Pdi_{TWITCH} and Pdi_{TWITCH}/Pdi_{MAX} ratios (Pdi_{MAX} was performed by a combined expulsive-Mueller maneuver) comparable to those previously obtained with needle or surface electrodes. This technique offers the advantages of being painless, non-invasive, and without known adverse effects. The disadvantage of this technique is that the stimulus cannot be localized solely to the phrenic nerve, but involves the brachial plexus and hence surrounding muscles including the sternocleidomastoid, deltoid, trapezius, and rhomboids.

Few studies have directly assessed twitch Pdi in patients with suspected diaphragm weakness. Mier et al. [71] measured bilateral twitch Pdi in the supine posture in 20 normal subjects and 15 patients with diaphragm weakness due to a variety of disorders. In addition, they measured maximal Pdi during a forceful sniff (Pdi_{SNIFF}) in the seated position. Pdi_{SNIFF} was used as an index of Pdi_{MAX} because of its relative ease of performance and reproducibility, even though higher values for transdiaphragmatic pressure can be obtained by other maneuvers [63]. Pdi_{TWITCH} in the controls ranged from 9 to 33 cm H_2O and from 3 to 27 cm H_2O in 10 patients. Six out of the 10 patients had Pdi_{TWITCH} values that fell within the range of the control group. All control subjects had a normal Pdi_{SNIFF} value and all patients demonstrated a reduced Pdi_{SNIFF}. Although the patients tended to demonstrate a lower Pdi_{TWITCH} than the controls (15 vs 21 cm H_2O), there was no significant difference in Pdi_{TWITCH} between the two groups. These authors concluded that Pdi_{TWITCH} is relatively insensitive for diagnosing diaphragm weakness given the wide overlap in Pdi_{TWITCH} values in patient and control groups. The Pdi_{TWITCH} was found to be clearly out of the normal range only when weakness was severe.

There is also evidence that phrenic nerve stimulation, in some instances, may be useful in detecting and differentiating upper from lower phrenic motor neuron lesions [80, 81]. Mier-Jedrzejowicz and Green [81] demonstrated a reduced Pdi_{MAX} during 3 separate maneuvers (maximal sniff, Mueller maneuver, and an inspiration to TLC) in 3 patients with cerebellar atrophy. All three subjects had normal values for Pdi_{TWITCH} and normal phrenic nerve conduction times. The reduced Pdi_{MAX} was not felt to be volitional in any patient. The authors concluded that because the lower motor phrenic neurons and diaphragm muscle itself behaved normally during phrenic stimulation, diaphragm dysfunction was caused by an upper motor neuron abnormality – most likely cerebellar ataxia. That these findings can also be applied to other causes of upper motor neuron disease (i.e. stroke) has not been shown. These results emphasize the point that diaphragm dysfunction cannot be excluded by normal values for Pdi_{TWITCH}.

Maximal Sniff and Other Maneuvers

In an attempt to overcome variable effort performance during voluntary maximal static contractions against an occluded airway, alternative maneuvers have been investigated. Of these, the maximal sniff maneuver has been the most extensively studied. In this technique, subjects perform a vigorous sniff against an unoccluded airway. During such an effort, the nose acts as a Starling resistor or flow limiting segment [82], thereby generating intrathoracic pressures approaching those obtained during inspiratory efforts against an occluded airway (see below). Proponents argue that this maneuver approaches a more "natural" respiratory effort than other types of maneuvers used to measure maximal airway pressure, and thus should be more easily mastered and reproducibly performed.

The maximal sniff maneuver has been applied to the evaluation of diaphragm muscle strength. Miller et al. [83] compared transdiaphragmatic pressure during a maximal sniff (Pdi_{SNIFF}) and during a Mueller maneuver ($Pdi_{MUELLER}$) in 64 normal subjects. They found that Pdi_{SNIFF} yielded a higher mean value (137 vs 90 cm H_2O) and narrower range (82–204 vs 16–164 cm H_2O) than did $Pdi_{MUELLER}$. In addition, they found Pdi_{SNIFF} to be easily learned and more reproducible than $Pdi_{MUELLER}$ (coefficient of variation of 7% vs 13% for $Pdi_{MUELLER}$). Of note, however, the values for Pdi_{SNIFF} and $Pdi_{MUELLER}$ obtained by these authors were substantially lower than those reported by Laporta and Grassino [68] for the combined feedback maneuver.

The maximal sniff technique has also been applied to the study of global inspiratory muscle strength. Laroche et al. [84] measured pleural pressure with an esophageal catheter in 61 subjects with suspected respiratory muscle weakness. Esophageal and transdiaphragmatic pressures were measured during a maximal sniff (Pes_{SNIFF}, Pdi_{SNIFF}) and a Mueller maneuver (PI_{MAX}, $Pdi_{MUELLER}$). In 36 of 61 subjects, normal values for PI_{MAX} and Pes_{SNIFF} were obtained and subjects were believed to have normal respiratory muscle strength. Pdi_{SNIFF} was normal or moderately reduced in these same subjects. In 13 subjects, a low PI_{MAX} correlated with a similar reduction in Pes_{SNIFF} and Pdi_{SNIFF}. However, 11 subjects had a low PI_{MAX} but a normal Pes_{SNIFF}. These subjects also had normal or moderately reduced Pdi_{SNIFF} values. The authors concluded that Pes_{SNIFF} is a more useful test of inspiratory muscle strength than PI_{MAX} because Pes_{SNIFF} correlated more closely to Pdi_{SNIFF} than did PI_{MAX}.

However, this study has several flaws which limits the interpretation of their results. First, this study had no proper controls. In addition, no information is given describing whether Pes_{SNIFF} and Pdi_{SNIFF} were measured on simultaneous breaths and whether the discrepancy in Pes_{SNIFF} and PI_{MAX} compared to Pdi_{SNIFF} may be due to variations in breathing efforts or changes in the pattern of rib cage and abdominal expansion. Finally, the maneuver for measuring transdiaphragmatic pressure that has been shown to produce the highest and most reproducible values (the combined feedback maneuver of Laporta and Grassino) was not employed as the standard of reference.

To avoid the need for placement of esophageal balloons for measurement of Pes_{SNIFF}, Koulouris et al. [85] recently correlated mouth (Pmo) and nasopharyngeal (Pnp) pressures with Pes_{SNIFF} in 10 normal subjects and 12 patients with muscle weakness. Pressures were measured simultaneously in the esophagus, nasopharynx, and mouth during a maximal sniff. They found that Pnp and Pmo correlate closely with Pes in both normals and patients with respiratory muscle weakness. These authors concluded that Pnp and Pmo may provide a less invasive method of measuring maximal respiratory pressures during a sniff maneuver than Pes. However, this technique has not been studied in subjects with obstructive airways disease, in whom delay in equilibration of pressures between the thorax and the upper airway may cause Pmo or Pnp to underestimate Pes.

Values for Pdi, Pes, and Pab obtained by the maximal sniff maneuver appear to be similar to or slightly lower than values obtained during static maneuvers. Although the airway is not occluded, increases in thoracic volume are likely to be small due to the brief duration of inspiration and the high airflow resistance across the nose. However, prospective studies are needed to compare these maneuvers to the combined feedback maneuver of Laporta and Grassino to determine the reproducibility and efficacy of the maximum sniff maneuver as a reflection of respiratory muscle strength.

Measurement of positive esophageal pressures during a forceful cough (Pes_{COUGH}) has been proposed as a measure of expiratory muscle strength. Pes_{COUGH} has been shown to decrease in parallel with PE_{MAX} when expiratory muscle weakness is induced by progressive curarization, during which Pes_{COUGH} was approximately 82% of PE_{MAX} at any level of weakness [86]. This technique has been used in the evaluation of cough performance after thoracotomy [87].

Conclusions

The assessment of inspiratory and expiratory muscle strength from maximum static inspiratory and expiratory pressures has generated a great deal of clinically useful information. It is now clear that factors such as breathing technique, the learning factor, lung volume, patient motivation, age and sex have an important effect on measurements of respiratory muscle strength. In addition, common clinical problems such as undernutrition, electrolyte disturbances, hypoxemia, and hypercapnia can all depress measurements of respiratory muscle strength.

The dependence of maximum static inspiratory and expiratory pressure on behavioral factors (motivation and learning) has led to attempts to develop newer techniques which allow respiratory muscle strength to be assessed in a more standard fashion. Recently, a number of studies have demonstrated that electrical stimulation of the phrenic nerves is a safe and effective way to assess the contractile performance of the diaphragm without subject cooperation. These newer techniques offer the prospect that inspiratory muscle function can be examined with a greater level of sophistication and consistency than was previously possible. Phrenic nerve stimulation may be useful in determining the degree of activation of the diaphragm during voluntary efforts and indirectly in determining Pdi_{MAX} by using the twitch occlusion method of electrophrenic diaphragm stimulation. The technique of cervical electromagnetic stimulation has considerable promise as a non invasive modality which may allow diaphragm function to be assessed repeatedly in the same subject. In addition, the ability to examine the twitch pressure waveform during electrically stimulated contractions offers the possibility that the intracellular processes which affect muscle contractility may be assessed with greater detail.

References

1. Aubier M, Banzett RB, Bellemare F, et al (1990) Respiratory muscle fatigue: report of the respiratory muscle fatigue workshop group. Am Rev Respir Dis 142:474–480
2. Rochester DF (1986) Respiratory effects of respiratory muscle weakness and atrophy. Am Rev Resp Dis 134(5):1083–1086
3. Eddinger TJ, Moss RL (1987) Mechanical properties of skinned single fibers of identified types from rat diaphragm. Am J Physiol 253:C210–C218
4. Sanchez J, Derenne JP, Debesse B, Riquet M, Monod H (1982) Typology of the respiratory muscles in normal men and in patients with moderate chronic respiratory diseases. Eur Physiopath Resp 18:901–914

5. Lieberman DA, Faulkner JA, Craig AB, Maxwell LC (1973) Performance and histochemical composition of guinea pig and human diaphragm. J Appl Physiol 34(2):233–237
6. Arora NS, Rochester DF (1982) Effect of body weight and muscularity on human diaphragm muscle mass, thickness, and area. J Appl Physiol 52(1):64–70
7. Smith J, Bellemare F (1987) Effects of lung volume on in vivo contraction characteristics of human diaphragm. J Appl Physiol 62(5):1893–1900
8. Grassino A, Goldman MD, Mead J, Sears TA (1978) Mechanics of the human diaphragm during voluntary contraction: statics. J Appl Physiol 44(6):829–839
9. Loring SH, Mead J, Griscom NT (1985) Dependence of diaphragmatic length on lung volume and thoracoabdominal configuration. J Appl Physiol 59(6):1961–1970
10. Rahn H, Otis AB, Chadwick LE, Fenn WO (1946) The pressure-volume diagram of the thorax and lung. Am J Physiol 146(6):161–178
11. Farkas GA, Decramer M, Rochester DF, De Troyer A (1985) Contractile properties of intercostal muscles and their functional significance. J Appl Physiol 59(2):528–535
12. Farkas GA, Rochester DF (1986) Contractile characteristics and operating lengths of canine neck inspiratory muscles. J Appl Physiol 61(1):220–226
13. Farkas GA, Rochester DF (1988) Characteristics and functional significance of canine abdominal muscles. J Appl Physiol 65(6):2427–2433
14. Sharp JT, Drutz WS, Moisan T, Foster J, Machnach W (1980) Postural relief of dyspnea in severe chronic obstructive pulmonary disease. Am Rev Respir Dis 122:201–211
15. Farkas GA, Roussos C (1982) Adaptability of the hamster diaphragm to exercise and/or emphysema. J Appl Physiol 53(5):1263–1272
16. Supinski GS, Kelsen SG (1982) Effect of elastase-induced emphysema on the force-generating ability of the diaphragm. J Clin Invest 70:978–988
17. Oliven A, Supinski GS, Kelsen SG (1986) Functional adaptation of diaphragm to chronic hyperinflation in emphysematous hamsters. J Appl Physiol 60(1):225–231
18. Joyce GC, Rack PMH, Westbury DR (1969) The mechanical properties of cat soleus muscle during controlled lengthening and shortening movements. J Appl Physiol 204:461–474
19. Newman S, Road J, Bellemare F, Clozel JP, Lavigne CM, Grassino A (1984) Respiratory muscle length measured by sonomicrometry. J Appl Physiol 56(3):753–764
20. Aubier M, Farkas G, De Troyer A, Mozes R, Roussos C (1981) Detection of diaphragmatic fatigue in man by phrenic stimulation. J Appl Physiol 50(3):538–544
21. Prezant DJ, Richner B, Valentine DE, et al (1990) Temperature dependence of rat diaphragm muscle contractility and fatigue. J Appl Physiol 69(5):1740–1745
22. Segal SS, Faulkner JA (1985) Temperature-dependent physiological stability of rat skeletal muscle in vitro. Am J Physiol 248:C265–C270
23. Sieck GC, Fournier M (1989) Diaphragm motor unit recruitment during ventilatory and nonventilatory behaviors. J Appl Physiol 66(6):2539–2545
24. Fournier M, Sieck GC (1988) Mechanical properties of muscle units in the cat diaphragm. J Neurophysiol 59(3):1055–1066
25. Kaminski MJ, Young RR (1985) Neuromuscular and neurological disorders affecting respiration. In Roussos C, Macklem PT (eds) The Thorax (Part B). Marcel Dekker, New York, pp. 1023–1087
26. Arora NS, Rochester DF (1982) Respiratory muscle strength and maximal voluntary ventilation in undernourished patients. Am Rev Respir Dis 126:5–8
27. Lewis MI, Belman MJ (1988) Nutrition and the respiratory muscles. Clin Chest Med 9(2):337–348
28. Viires N, Pavlovic D, Pariente R, Aubier M (1990) Effects of steroids on diaphragmatic function in rats. Am Rev Respir Dis 142:34–38
29. Juan G, Calverley P, Talamo C, Schnader J, Roussos C (1984) Effect of carbon dioxide on diaphragmatic function in human beings. N Engl J Med 310:874–879
30. Aubier M, Murciano D, Lecocguic Y, et al (1985) Effect of hypophosphatemia on diaphragmatic contractility in patients with acute respiratory failure. N Engl J Med 313:420–424
31. Estenne M, Yernault JL, De Smet JM, et al (1985) Phrenic and diaphragm function after coronary artery bypass grafting. Thorax 40:293–299
32. Sharp JT (1986) The respiratory muscles in chronic obstructive pulmonary disease. Am Rev Respir Dis, Annual Meeting Highlights pp. 1089–1090

33. Macklem PT (1984) Hyperinflation. Am Rev Respir Dis 129 (Editorial): 1–2
34. Macklem PT, Macklem DM, De Troyer A (1983) A model of inspiratory muscle mechanics. J Appl Physiol 55:547–557
35. Hunter AB, Cavoy MA, Larsh HW (1981) The nutritional status of patients with chronic obstructive pulmonary disease. Am Rev Resp Dis 124:376–381
36. Wilson DO, Rogers RM, Wright EC, Anthonisen NR (1989) Body weight in chronic obstructive pulmonary disease: The National Institutes of Health intermittent positive pressure breathing trial. Am Rev Resp Dis 139:1435–1438
37. Mier-Jedrzejowicz A, Brophy C, Moxham J, Green M (1988) Assessment of diaphragm weakness. Am Rev Resp Dis 137:877–883
38. Mier-Jedrzejowicz AK, Brophy C, Green M (1988) Respiratory muscle function in myasthenia gravis. Am Rev Respir Dis 138:867–873
39. Loh L, Goldman M, Newsom Davis J (1977) The assessment of diaphragm function. Medicine 56(2):165–169
40. Laroche CM, Carroll N, Moxham J, Green M (1988) Clinical significance of severe isolated diaphragm weakness. Am Rev Respir Dis 138:862–866
41. Allen SM, Hunt B, Green M (1985) Fall in vital capacity with posture. Br J Dis Chest 79:267–271
42. Braun N, Arora NS, Rochester DF (1983) Respiratory muscle and pulmonary function in polymyositis and other proximal myopathies. Thorax 38:616–623
43. Rochester DF, Braun N (1985) Determinants of maximal inspiratory pressure in chronic obstructive pulmonary disease. Am Rev Respir Dis 132:42–47
44. Alexander C (1966) Diaphragm movements and the diagnosis of diaphragmatic paralysis. Clin Radiol 17:79–83
45. Black LF, Hyatt RE (1969) Maximal respiratory pressures: Normal values and relationship to age and sex. Am Rev Respir Dis 99:696–702
46. Rinqvist T (1966) The ventilatory capacity in healthy adults: An analysis of causal factors with special reference to the respiratory forces. Scand J Clin Lab Invest 18(Suppl 88):1–111
47. Leech JA, Ghezzo H, Stevens D, Becklake MR (1983) Respiratory pressures and function in young adults. Am Rev Respir Dis 128:17–23
48. Rochester DF, Arora NS (1983) Respiratory muscle failure. Med Clin North Am 67(3):573–598
49. Vincken W, Ghezzo H, Cosio MG (1987) Maximal static respiratory pressures in adults: normal values and their relationship to determinants of respiratory function. Bull Eur Physiopathol Respir 23:435–439
50. Cooke CD, Mead J, Orzalesi MM (1964) Static volume-pressure characteristics of the respiratory system during maximal efforts. J Appl Physiol 95(5):1016–1022
51. Wilson DO, Cooke NT, Edwards RHT, Spiro SG (1984) Predicted normal values for maximal respiratory pressures in caucasian adults and children. Thorax 39:535–538
52. Koulouris N, Mulvey DA, Laroche CM, Green M, Moxham J (1988) Comparison of two different mouthpieces for the masurement of PImax and PEmax in normal and weak subjects. Eur Respir J 1:863–867
53. Rochester DF (1988) Tests of respiratory muscle function. Clin Chest Med 9(2):249–261
54. De Troyer A, Yernault JC (1980) Inspiratory muscle force in normal subjects and patients with interstitial lung disease. Thorax 35:92–100
55. Turner JM, Mead J, Wohl ME (1968) Elasticity of human lungs in relation to age. J Appl Physiol 25(6):664–671
56. Leith DE, Mead J (1967) Mechanisms determining residual volume of the lungs in normal subjects. J Appl Physiol 23(2):221–227
57. Zhang Y, Kelsen SG (1990) Effects of aging on diaphragm contractile function in Golden hamsters. Am Rev Resp Dis 142:1396–1401
58. McElvaney G, Blackie S, Morrison NJ, Wilcox PG, Fairbarn MS, Pardy RL (1989) Maximal static respiratory pressures in the normal elderly. Am Rev Respir Dis 139:277–281
59. Tolep K, Kelsen SG, Muza SR, Criner G (1991) Transdiaphragmatic pressure generation in healthy elderly subjects. Am Rev Resp Dis 143(2 Part 2):A366
60. Wilmore JH (1974) Alterations in strength, body composition and anthropometric measurements consequent to a 10-week weight training program. Med Sci in Sports 6(2):133–138

61. Tornvall G (1963) Assessment of physical capabilities: With special reference to the evaluation of maximal voluntary isometric muscle strength and maximal working capacity: An experimental study on civilian and military subject groups. Acta Physiol Scand (Suppl 201) pp. 19–55
62. Sahn SA, Lakshminarayan S, Petty TL (1976) Weaning from mechanical ventilation. JAMA 235:2208–2212
63. Marini JJ, Smith TC, Lamb V (1986) Estimation of inspiratory muscle strength in mechanically ventilated patients: the measurement of maximal inspiratory pressure. J Crit Care 1(1):32–38
64. Multz AS, Aldrich TK, Prezant DJ, Karpel JP, Hendler JM (1990) Maximal inspiratory pressure is not a reliable test of inspiratory muscle strength in mechanically ventilated patients. Am Rev Respir Dis 142:529–532
65. Hershenson MB, Kikuchi Y, Loring SH (1988) Relative strengths of the chest wall muscles. J Appl Physiol 65(2):852–862
66. Macklem PT, Gross D, Grassino A, Roussos C (1978) Partitioning of the inspiratory pressure swings between diaphragm and intercostal/accessory muscles. J Appl Physiol: Respir Environ Exercise Physiol 44(2):200–208
67. De Troyer A, Estenne M (1981) Limitations of measurement of transdiaphragmatic pressure in detecting diaphragmatic weakness. Thorax 36:169–174
68. Laporta D, Grassino A (1985) Assessment of transdiaphragmatic pressure in humans. J Appl Physiol 58(5):1469–1476
69. Hillman DR, Markos J, Finucane KE (1990) Effect of abdominal compression on maximum transdiaphragmatic pressure. J Appl Physiol 68(6):2296–2304
70. Sarnoff SJ, Sarnoff LC, Whittenberger JL (1951) Electrophrenic respiration VII – The motor point of the phrenic nerve in relation to external stimulation. Surg Gynaecol Obstet 93:190–196
71. Mier H, Brophy C, Moxham J, Green M (1987) Phrenic nerve stimulation in normal subjects and in patients with diaphragmatic weakness. Thorax 42:885–888
72. Aubier M, Murciano D, Lecocguic Y, Viires N, Pariente R (1985) Bilateral phrenic stimulation: a simple technique to assess diaphragmatic fatigue in humans. J Appl Physiol 58(1):58–64
73. Hubmayr RD, Litchy WJ, Gay PC, Nelson SB (1989) Transdiaphragmatic twitch pressure: Effects of lung volume and chest wall shape. Am Rev Respir Dis 139:647–652
74. Bellemare F, Bigland-Ritchie B, Woods JJ (1986) Contractile properties of the human diaphragm in vivo. J Appl Physiol 61(3):1153–1161
75. McKenzie DK, Gandevia SC (1985) Phrenic nerve conduction times and twitch pressures of the human diaphragm. J Appl Physiol 58(5):1496–1504
76. Mier A, Brophy C, Moxham J, Green M (1989) Twitch pressures in the assessment of diaphragm weakness. Thorax 44:990–996
77. Bellemare F, Bigland-Ritchie B (1984) Assessment of human diaphragm strength and activation using phrenic nerve stimulation. Resp Physiol 58:263–277
78. Gandevia SC, McKenzie DK (1985) Activation of the human diaphragm during maximal static efforts. J Physiol 367:45–56
79. Similowski T, Fleury B, Launois S, Cathala HP, Bouche P, Derenne JP (1989) Cervical magnetic stimulation: a new painless method for bilateral phrenic nerve stimulation in conscious humans. J Appl Physiol 67(4):1311–1318
80. Mier A, Brophy C, Havard CW, Green M (1988) Severe diaphragm weakness in spinocerebellar degeneration. Thorax 43:78–79
81. Mier-Jedrzejowicz A, Green M (1988) Respiratory muscle weakness associated with cerebellar atrophy. Am Rev Respir Dis 137:673–677
82. Bridger GP, Proctor DF (1970) Maximum nasal inpiratory flow and nasal resistance. Ann Otol Rhinol Laryngol 79:481–488
83. Miller JM, Moxham J, Green M (1985) The maximal sniff in the assessment of diaphragm function in man. Clin Sci 69:91–96
84. Laroche CM, Mier AK, Moxham J, Green M (1988) The value of sniff esophageal pressures in the assessment of global inspiratory muscle strength. Am Rev Respir Dis 138:598–603

85. Koulouris N, Mulvey DA, Laroche, CM, Sawicka EH, Green M, Moxham J (1989) The measurement of inspiratory muscle strength by sniff esophageal, nasopharyngeal, and mouth pressures. Am Rev Respir Dis 139:641–646
86. Arora NS, Gal TJ (1981) Cough dynamics during progressive expiratory muscle weakness in healthy curarized subjects. J Appl Physiol 51(2):494–498
87. Byrd RB, Burns JR (1975) Cough dynamics in the post-thoracotomy state. Chest 67(6):654–657
88. Curtin NA, Davies RE (1972) Chemical and mechanical changes during stretching of activated frog skeletal muscle. Cold Spring Harbor Symposia on Quantitative Biology 37:619–626

Ventilatory Muscle Fatigue and Failure

C. Roussos and S. Lakynthinos

Introduction

The importance of respiratory, chiefly inspiratory, muscle fatigue has become well recognized in the last decade. If inspiratory muscles fail, so does ventilation. Neuromuscular fatigue had previously been defined as the inhability to maintain the required or expected force or power output, which follows a sustained muscular contraction and is reversible by rest. In this regard, fatigue of the inspiratory muscles had been defined as the inability to continue to generate sufficient pressure for an adequate alveolar ventilation. Recently, the definition of muscle fatigue has been revised; it is defined as a condition in which there is a loss in the capacity for developing force and/or velocity of a muscle, resulting from muscle activity under load and which is reversible by rest [1]. According to this definition, fatigue may be present at a time considerably preceding the point in time at which a muscle is unable to continue to perform a particular task (exhaustion or task failure). In applying this concept to the inspiratory muscles, one concludes that they may be fatigued before there is hypercapnia (task failure) due to inadequate alveolar ventilation. Furthermore, it is now clear that during fatigue from dynamic contractions the maximum force and velocity of shortening often change independently, whereas previous definition implied that force and power output necessarily change in parallel. Fatigue should be distinguished from muscle weakness, which is defined as a condition in which the capacity of a rested muscle to generate force is decreased [1], although the presence of such muscle weakness may predispose to muscle fatigue.

The site and mechanism of fatigue have remained a subject of controversy over the last century. Theoretically, the site of fatigue may be located at any link in the long chain of events involved in muscular contraction leading from the brain to the contractile machinery (brain, spinal cord, nerve, neuromuscular junction, muscle cell membrane, transverse tubular system, calcium release, actin-myosin activation, and cross-bridge formation). We distinguish between failure to generate force because of a reduced central motor output (central fatigue), and failure to generate force because of fatigue at the neuromuscular junction, or within the muscle machinery (peripheral fatigue). Then the question, first formulated in the early part of this century [2, 3] arises: do the respiration controllers become too tired to drive the muscles to maintain adequate ventilation when the respiratory system is presented with a fatiguing load, or do the muscles become unable to generate the required force despite an adequate neural drive? These investigators, who where the first to study respiratory muscle fatigue, deduced that both types of fatigue, central and peripheral, may exist. Recently, there has been an increasing bulk of evidence that about one-half of the force decline during diaphragmatic fatigue can be attributed to reduced central motor drive and the remainder to peripheral muscle contractile failure [1, 4]. However, whether such a depression of the central nervous system (CNS) is due to primary central failure or to an adaptation of the CNS to the changes in the contracting muscle reflecting a protective mechanism, remains unclear.

Pathophysiology of Respiratory Muscle Fatigue

During a voluntary contraction, a chain of events is triggered starting with an electical signal originating in the motor cortex and terminating with the energy-dependent interaction of actin and myosin in the muscle fiber.

These events can be divided into three categories:

1. The process of delivering sufficient electrical activation from the CNS to the muscle;
2. the metabolic and enzymatic process providing energy for the contractile mechanism; and
3. the excitation-contraction coupling process that link these two.

Hence, since the generation of a voluntary contraction involves the whole pathway from the brain to the muscles, the various potential sites of failure can be divided into three broad categories:

1. those which lie within the CNS (central fatigue);
2. those concerned with nerve transmission from the CNS to muscle (transmission fatigue); and
3. those within the individual muscle fibers (contractile fatigue) (Table 1).

Table 1. Diagnostic features of diaphragmatic fatigue. (From [120] with permission)

Type of fatigue	Voluntary effort		Phrenic nerve stimulation		Direct muscle stimulation (animal)
	EMG Response	Pdi Response	EMG Response	Pdi Response	
Central Transmission	Decreased	Decreased	Normal	Normal	Normal
	Decreased	Decreased	Decreased	Decreased	Normal
Contractile	Normal	Decreased	Normal	Decreased	Decreased

Abbreviations: *EMG* = electromyogram; *Pdi* = transdiaphragmatic pressure

Central Fatigue

Central fatigue is considered present when a maximal voluntary contraction generates less force than does maximal electrical stimulation [5, 6]. In fact, if maximal electrical stimulation superimposed on a maximal voluntary contraction can potentiate the force generated by a muscle, a component of central fatigue is said to exist. The procedure applied for the diaphragm consists of the twich occlusion test, which it is argued may separate central from peripheral fatigue [1, 4, 7]. Some studies show that the force generated with maximal electrical stimulation may exceed that of voluntary contraction [4, 5]. However, lack of motivation during voluntary contraction or methodological difficults during stimulation may account for some of the discrepancies observed. In contrast, Merton [6] previously found no differences in the forces generated by voluntary or by electrically stimulated contraction. Furthermore, Merton et al. [8] found no decline in the muscle mass action potential evoked by periodic stimulation of the motor cortex in humans during fatiguing maximal voluntary contraction. This observation reveals that electrical propagation is not limited at any site in the motor pathway between cortex and muscle and strongly suggests that central fatigue is not responsible for loss of force. However, central fatigue must not be confused with progressive decrease in the firing rate during maximum contraction, during which superimposed supramaximal electric tetanic stimulation does not increase muscle force [9].

Several investigators have clearly shown that the central firing rate decreases during fatiguing muscle contraction [10, 11]. Experimentally, the gradual loss of force following prolonged maximum voluntary contraction can be accurately mimicked with electrical stimulation if the stimulation frequency can be accurately reproduced. Conversely, if high stimulation frequencies are maintained too long, force loss is more rapid. Thus, it is possible that the decrease in firing frequency represents an adaptive protecting mechanism to the alteration of muscle contractile characteristics, preventing an undue reduction of intrinsic muscle fiber strength [1, 10].

It is well known that fatigue is characterized not only by loss of force, but also by slowing of the muscle contractile speed. In addition, it is established that for any muscle of motor unit the minimum excitation frequency required to generate force, and tetanic fusion is proportional to its contractile speed. Thus, if during fatigue the degree of contractile slowing matches the decline in motoneuron firing rate, the latter does not result in any additional reduction in muscle force. Such an adaptation would be rather beneficial. In fact, it would avoid failure of impulse propagation associated with high-frequency fatigue as well as the complete depletion of vital chemicals within the muscle cell, which might otherwise occur if high frequency excitation was maintained. Of course, an interesting question is how such an adaptation is brought on. It seems likely that activation of muscle afferents by some fatigue-induced change within the muscle inhibits motoneuron activity by reducing its firing rates. In this regard, Hannerz and Grimby [12] have presented evidence that motor neurons receive a tonic inhibitory drive from peripheral sources and that during a maximum voluntary contraction the motor neuron discharge rate increases if muscle afferents are partially blocked. Such an alteration in the firing rate of the diaphragm during fatigue is not known. However, it has been shown that afferent information via large (type I and II) and small (type III and IV) fibers affects the central respiratory controller's discharge in terms of firing rate, firing time and frequency of breathing [12]; the latter is observed in states of diaphragmatic fatigue in both animal and humans [13, 14]. It is tempting therefore to hypothesize that, as the contractile properties and the diphragmatic chemistry change during fatigue, chest wall or respiratory muscle afferents via the phrenic nerve may affect the output of respiratory centers in terms of firing rate or timing (frequency of breathing, duty cycle).

The strong interaction between the respiratory muscles and the CNS is well known. The interrelationship between respiratory muscle energy expenditure and its central control was first suggested by Otis [15], who concluded that for a given alveolar ventilation and mechanical properties of the respiratory system, there is an optimal frequency at which minimal work is performed. Similarly, Mead [16] pointed out that the optimal frequency during spontaneous breathing is more closely associated with the minimum average force. In this regard, someone can propose that fatigue is not mainly just a failure of physiologic function, but rather a protective mechanism for survival when the torax is under excessive stress. Therefore, as speculated above, a regulatory mechanism must exist within the CNS to coordinate the motor neuron discharge to the changes in the contractile speed of the motor unit they supply, and/or alteration in the muscle chemistry.

An alternative hypothesis is that, when fatigue ensues, the CNS alters either its firing output or its rhythmicity, which can be called "central fatigue". The work of Bellemare et al. [4, 17] supports the fact that a central component of diaphragmatic fatigue exists. It may be responsible for about 50% on the force decline [1, 4]. However, whether such a "central fatigue" is due to primary central failure and not to an adaptation of the CNS needs further investigation.

In summary, as fatigue ensues, central discharge firing rate decreases and contractile slowing increases, either as primary central failure (central fatigue) or an adaptation to the altered chemistry and/or contractile characteristics of the muscles, which may prevent their self-destruction by excessive activation. These changes in motoneuron activity is postulated to be mediated by chest wall or respiratory muscle afferents.

Transmission Fatigue

During artificial stimulation of a motor neuron, especially at high frequencies, muscle force declines rapidly in association with the decline in action-potential amplitude. This response, known as "high frequency fatigue", is attributed to failure of impulse propagation across the neuromuscular junction and/or over the muscle surface membrane. This failure may occur postsynaptically (from a decrease in end-plate excitability) or presynaptically (probably in fine terminal filaments of the motor nerve or, less frequently, from depletion of synaptic transmitter substance) [18, 19].

The development of this type of failure during voluntary contraction is questionable. First, evoked muscle compound action potential (M-wave) amplitudes are generally found to remain unimpaired. Second, no unique relation between muscle force and electromyographic (EMG) activity has been observed [1]. Evidence that neuromuscular transmission and cell membrane excitation are adequate has been found in experiments in dogs in cardiogenic and septic shock (Fig. 1 and 2) [13, 20]. As the diaphragm became fatigued, the relationship between integrated phrenic nerve activity (Ephr) and diaphragmatic EMG activity remained unaltered. In

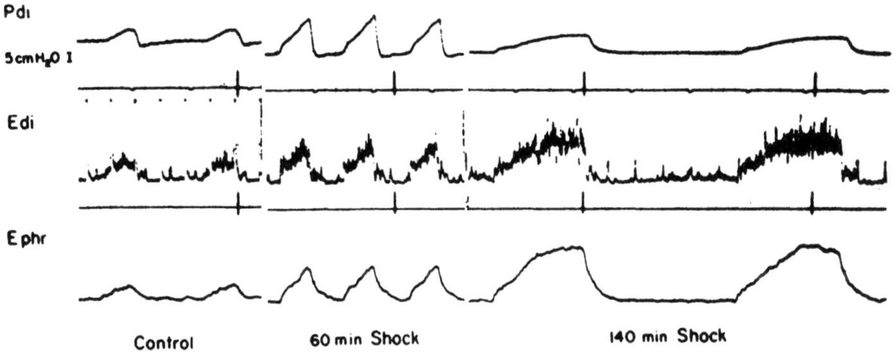

Fig. 1. Tracings from a dog in cardiogenic shock show typical evolution of transdiaphragmatic pressure (Pdi), integrated electrical activity of the diaphragm (Edi), and integrated electrical activity of the phrenic nerve (Ephr). The left panel represents a control. The middle panel shows a reading made 60 min after onset of cardiogenic shock. The right panel shows a reading made 140 min after onset of cardiogenic shock and just before the death from respiratory arrest. While Edi and Ephr continue to increase, Pdi decreases (fatigue). The decrease in size of electrocardiographic artifact on Edi trace is a consequence of injection of saline into pericardium. (From [13] with permission)

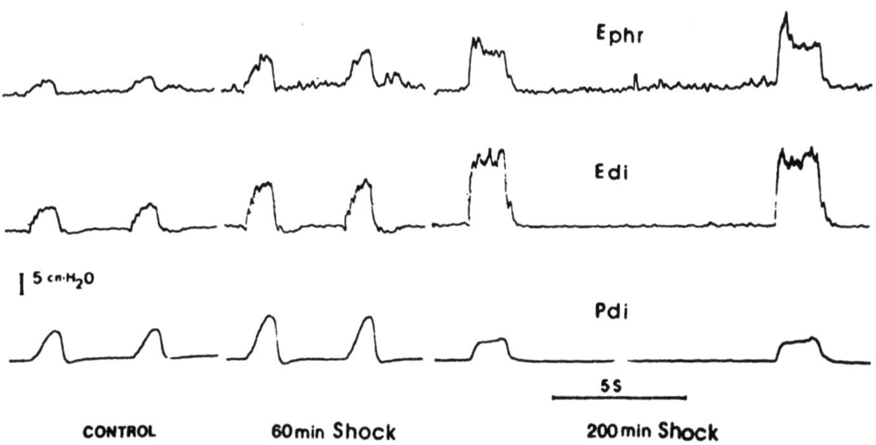

Fig. 2. Representative tracings of dog during endotoxic shock showing changes in integrated phrenic neurogram (Ephr), integrated diaphragmatic electromyogram (Edi), and transdiaphragmatic pressure (Pdi). Left, during control; middle, 60 min after onset of endotoxic shock; right, 200 min after onset of endotoxic shock and prior to death of animal. While Ephr and Edi continue to increase, Pdi decreases due to peripheral fatigue (impaired excitation-contraction coupling). (From [20] with permission)

other words, when the diaphragm started failing as a force generator, and greater stimulation was needed for an increment of transdiaphragmatic pressure, the relationship between Ephr and EMG was similar to that observed during the control period and to the earlier stage of the fatigue. However, these experiments may not be specific in testing this question; for example, changes in the wave form of action potential through the run may have compensated for discrepancies between Ephr and EMG [9]. Teleologically, transmission block could be beneficial in some instances. As suggested by some authors [21–23], if failure occurs at the neuromuscular junction or in the excitation of the cell membrane, it may protect the muscle against excessive depletion of its ATP stores, which would lead to rigor mortis. If high-frequency fatigue is due to failure of the neuromuscular junction, it may be speculated that such a failure can exist in the diaphragm of man. In fact, it has been clearly shown that normal subjects breathing against inspiratory loads develop high-frequency fatigue [24], which may reflect neuromuscular junction failure.

Contractile Fatigue

Most studies conclude that the major factors underlying neuromuscular fatigue occur within the muscle fibers and mainly result from depletion of muscle energy stores or pH changes from lactic acid accumulation [1]. The substances directly involved in transformation of chemical energy into mechanical work in skeletal muscle are ATP, ADP, inorganic phosphate (Pi), hydrogen ions (H^+), magnesium ions (Mg^{2+}) and phosphocreatine (Pc). ATP leaves the mitochondria and diffuses in the contractile machinery of the cell, where ATPase enzymes hydrolyze one of the pyrophosphate bonds, liberating large quantities of energy in the process,

$$\mathrm{ATP} + \mathrm{H_2O} \xrightarrow[\text{ATPases}]{} \mathrm{ADP} + \mathrm{Pi} + \mathrm{H}^+ + \text{Energy}$$

High levels of exercise or hypoxia result in the accumulation of ADP, Pi and lactate, as well as decreases in Pc and pH. The decrease in Pc and the concomitant increase in Pi provide a convenient index of cellular energy state: the Pc/Pi ratio [25]. In the past, measures of this ratio could be obtained only by destructive tissue biopsy procedures. This has changed with the introduction of 31-phosphorus magnetic resonance spectroscopy (^{31}P-MRS), a technique that makes it possible to sequentially monitor changes in Pc, Pi and ATP in the muscle during hypoxia, exercise or fatigue in an accurate and non-invasive manner [25]. Using this technique, Dawson et al. [26] showed that during fatigue, Pc breaks down progressively, and creatine, ADP, and H^+ levels rise, while ATP, the direct source of energy, is reduced only by 25%. The latter finding is consistent with the results obtained in normal subjects performing dynamic exercise until exhaustion [27]. They found that at high work loads, when Pc was practically depleted, ATP decreased to 40% of its control value. Why then does the muscle become unable to generate force in the presence of adequate sources of ATP? To answer this, we must consider the above mentioned hydrolysis of ATP. As the muscles fatigue, the concentration of all by-products increases considerably, and therefore this reaction is delayed. This leads to the hypothesis, so far untested in the diaphragm, that the decline in muscle force is not due to the depletion of ATP but to the reduced rate of ATP breakdown because of product accumulation.

The increase in energy demands in the working skeletal muscles, including the respiratory muscles, is provided mainly by the conbustion of fat, blood glucose, and glycogen of the muscle. During submaximal prolonged heavy exercise, exhaustion coincides with the depletion of muscle glycogen, whereas exercise capacity is enhanced when the storage of muscle glycogen is increased [28]. Similar observations have been made in the diaphragm of dogs with a low cardiac output [29]. However, why glycogen depletion coincides with fatigue is not clear. During prolonged intermittent heavy exercise that depends on aerobic metabolism, the rate of utilization of fatty acids and glucose is high; although these substances circulate in large amounts in the bloodstream, they cannot provide sufficient energy to the muscle to meet the demands. Hence, muscle glycogen must be used to supplement the blood-borne fuels, and fatigue will occur when it is depleted.

A great deal of attention has been focused on the role that lactic acid plays in the development of fatigue. That is the result of a form correlation between lactic acid accumulation in the muscle and contractile force [26, 30]. Similarly, blood lactate elevation has been found in subjects breathing through high inspiratory loads to exhaustion [31], but there is no direct evidence that the lactic acid produced by the respiratory muscles is the culprit in diaphragmatic fatigue. Furthermore, animals in cardiogenic shock develop substantially less lactic acidosis if they are mechanically ventilated than if they are breathing spontaneously [29], indicating that the respiratory muscles produce great amounts of lactic acid if they are working under fatiguing conditions.

The effect of lactic acid on force generation is believed to be mediated by lowering the pH, which is a well-established reason of decrease in skeletal muscle force. At low pH, Ca^{2+} is sequestered in the sarcoplasmic reticulum [32] and a larger amount of Ca^{2+} is needed to produce a given tension [33]. In addition, hydrogen ions exert a direct negative effect on the contractile process itself [34].

Metzger and Fitts [35], using glass microelectrodes, found decreases in intracellular pH from 7.03 to 6.33 with stimulation in a rat diaphragm preparation as it developed high and low frequency fatigue. They concluded that intracellular acidosis was associated with muscle fatigue, probably produced by the inhibition of phosphofructokinase, a key enzyme in the control of glycolysis. However, to date, it is not entirely clear if intracellular acidosis is the cause and not a manifestation of diaphragmatic fatigue [25]. It seems that intracellular acidosis may have a more important effect during the recovery period than during active contraction [36]. It also appears that extracellular acidosis plays a key role during recovery from fatigue [37] since lactate efflux from cells ceases when the extracellular pH falls to 6.8. Furthermore, Fitzgerald et al. [38], using ^{31}P-MRS to study the effects of metabolic and compensated metabolic acidosis on an *in vitro* rat diaphragm preparation, proved that the decrease in diaphragmatic force during acidosis is not the result of a loss of high energy phosphates, Pi or ATP, but the consequence of acidosis *per se*.

To summarize, glycogen depletion, lactic acid accumulation, acidosis of every kind, inability to utilize blood-borne substances and decrease in the rate of ATP hydrolysis are merged to explain loss of force, but the exact interplay of all these factors is not yet identified in either the diaphragm or the other skeletal muscles.

Impaired excitation-contraction coupling. All processes that link the electrical activation of the muscle fiber and the various metabolic and enzymatic processes providing energy to the contractile machinery are called excitation-contraction coupling processes. Impaired excitation-contraction coupling is thought to be responsible when the loss of force is not accompanied by a parallel decline in the electrical activity [6]. This type of fatigue is characterized by a selective loss of force at low frequencies of stimulation (low frequency fatigue) despite maintenance of the force generated by high frequencies of stimulation, indicating that the contractile proteins continue to generate force. This type of fatigue is not related to depletion of ATP or Pc and is characteristically long-lasting, taking several hours to recover. The mechanism of this type of fatigue is not well known. It may occur because of a reduced supply of Ca^{2+} or a change in the affinity of the troponin binding site for Ca^{2+}. These defects would reduce the twitch and hence would reduce the force developed at low stimulation. In contrast, at higher stimulation frequencies, a relatively normal force can be generated when the interior of the fiber is saturated with Ca^{2+} [39, 40]. Other possibilities include a structural damage [41] or an alteration in the compliance of the series-elastic component of the muscle [42].

Impaired excitation-contraction coupling occurs in the diaphragm of the dog during cardiogenic shock [13]; despite a threefold increase of the integrated EMG, Pdi decreased (Fig. 1). In addition, low-frequency fatigue, and by inference impaired excitation-contraction coupling, has been found in the diaphragm and sternocleidomastoid of normal subjects after they breathed against very high inspiratory resistance (Fig. 3) [24, 43].

Integrated View of Respiratory Muscle Fatigue

Fatigue is likely to be the result of a dynamic process in which compensatory mechanisms are overwhelmed in a closed loop system consisting of central motor drive, peripheral impulse propagation, excitation/contraction coupling, depletion of energy substrates and/or metabolite accumulation and feedback-modulating reflexes [1]. The site of fatigue may be placed at any level from the CNS to the contractile machinery depending on the experimental setting. For an individual muscle, a close relationship exists between excitation and energy metabolism [26]. It has been shown that a protective mechanism may exist at the site of the action potential or beyond, so that, when there is a depletion of fuel, failure of the activation system occurs, and in extreme fatigue, prevents the muscle form destroying itself, which would happen if the ATP level fell to zero. A decrease in excitation may result from failure of the neuromuscular junction [18, 21–23], or it may stem from a reduced rate of firing by the CNS [11], or both. In the respiratory system, in addition to the reduction in firing frequency, the CNS may respond by altering the frequency and the duty cycle [13]. Although it has not yet been proved, such an alteration in the responses of central controllers could be brought about by afferents from the fatiguing inspiratory muscles and the chest wall. During fatigue, the

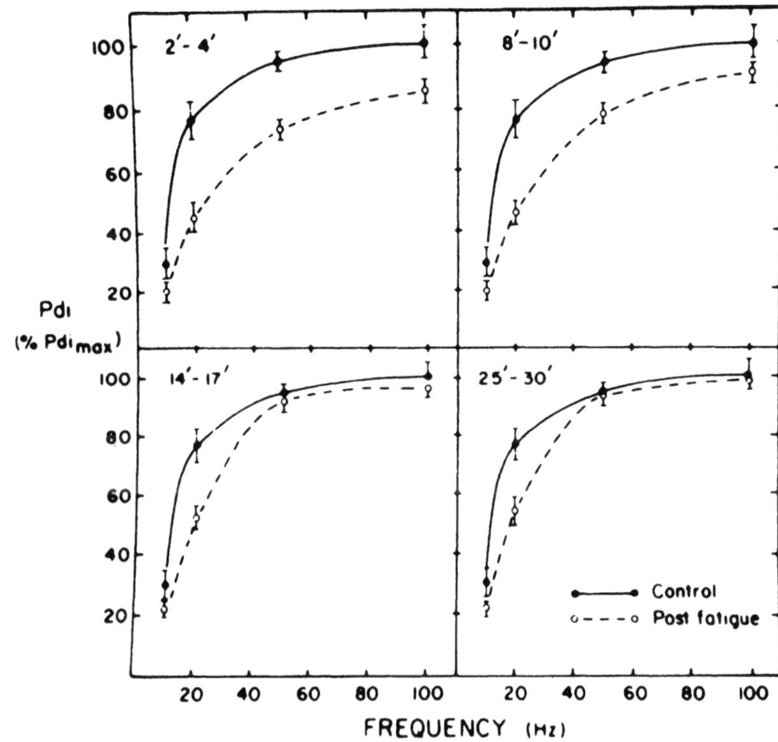

Fig. 3. Progression of changes in pressure-frequency curves of diaphragm of four subjects up to 30 min after fatigue. Solid lines, average of three curves before fatigue (control); dotted lines, average of three curves at different times during recovery from fatigue; bars ± 1 SE. Transdiaphragmatic pressure (Pdi) is expressed as percent of Pdi generated with supramaximal phrenic nerve stimulation at frequency of 100 Hz (% Pdi, max); 30 min after fatigue, Pdi generated at high frequencies of stimulation (50 Hz) approaches control values, whereas low frequencies of stimulation cannot generate prefatigue Pdi values. (From [24] with permission)

normal inhibitory influence from Golgi tendon organs presumably declines with the loss of force, but concomitant fatigue of intrafusal fibers might reduce the excitatory response of muscle spindles. Furthermore, free nerve endings within the muscle might inhibit motoneuron activity in response to muscle stretch and fatigue. As it has shown, afferent information via large (type I and II) and small (type III and IV) fibers affects the central respiratory controllers in terms of firing rate, firing time and frequency of breathing [12].

Diagnosis of Respiratory Muscle Fatigue

It is obvious in the definition of fatigue that its detection requires techniques that estimate force, particularly if these relate to the degree of muscle excitation. More specifically, the force should be related to the intensity and frequency of stimulation, the fiber length and the velocity of shortening. If this is achieved, contractility can be estimated. The bedside clinical diagnosis of fatigue, however, is hampered by the inability to measure the baseline before fatigue [1]. It may be possible only to infer fatigue retrospectively by its reversibility after a period of rest.

Currently, there are the following tests to detect respiratory muscle fatigue:

1. tests that measure the pressures generated by the respiratory muscles (maximal inspiratory mouth pressure (P_{Imax}) and transdiaphragmatic pressure with respect to inspiratory time and respiratory rate (pressure-time index and Pdi_{max});
2. tests that measure diaphragmatic or other inspiratory muscle electrical activity (power spectral analysis and integrated electrical activity (Edi), or some combination of electrical activity and pressure development (Edi/Pdi));
3. tests that aim to assess the capacity of the diaphragm to generate pressure independent from central control mechanisms (bilateral phrenic nerve twich stimulation and pressure-frequency (Pdi/frequency) curves), and finally
4. tests that measure the increase in Pdi when a twitch is superimposed on the naturally activated diaphragm to detect the relative degree of motor unit recruitment through central pathways (twitch occlusion tests).

The measurement of force-frequency curves is a useful and specific technique for detecting peripheral fatigue. Measurement of the force-frequency curve of the diaphragm is made possible by stimulating the phrenic nerve and recording transdiaphragmatic pressure [44, 45]. The curve can easily be documented for the sternocleidomastoid muscle by stimulation of the muscle with surface electrodes [43]. Loss of force at low-frequency stimulation indicates impairment of excitation-contraction coupling (Fig. 3). Loss of force at high frequency stimulation indicates impairment of the neuromuscular junction or of membrane excitation. There are however several sources of errors in the use of such curves. It is not possible to supramaximally stimulate the phrenic nerve transcutaneously. Thus, when comparing curves, it is important to evaluate that the nerve received exactly the same stimulation. Furthermore, the contraction must be isometric, or the degree and velocity of shortening as well as the initial fiber length and geometry of the diaphragm must be identical. Provided these variables are properly controlled, the change in the force-frequency curve gives information about the underlying mechanism of the peripheral fatigue, as previously mentioned. When one cannot be certain that the nerve received the same stimulation, curves measured at different times can still be usefully analyzed by comparing the ratio of pressure developed at a given frequency with that obtained at 100 Hz; this gives information on the shape of the curve. The ratio is high in high-frequency fatigue and low in low-frequency fatigue [46].

The force developed for a given degree of excitation can also be estimated by relating Pdi to the integrated electrical activity of the diaphragm (Edi) during a Muller maneuver against a closed airway. A reduction in the Pdi/Edi ratio at constant length and geometry is a good index of muscle fatigue. Care must be taken to ensure that the contraction is isometric (i.e. no displacement occurs of either ribcage or abdomen) and that electrode placement and electrical impedance are identical.

Among the tests that measure the pressures generated by the respiratory muscles, the detection of progressive decrease of Pimax during an inspiratory task at a defined lung volume may easily provide some information regarding fatigue. However, under such conditions, there is always the possibility that inadequate effort may give false results.

As fatigue develops, the time that a muscle takes to relax is known to be prolonged. The assessment of decay of the relaxation rate of the diaphragm during fatigue has been found to correlate significantly with the rate of decay of H/L (EMG) [47]. The test can be performed easily and non-invasively by using sniffs as a means of generating maximal voluntary diaphragmatic contractions [48].

Twitch Occlusion Test

This is the only test among those used to detect respiratory muscle fatigue that may separate central from peripheral fatigue. Using bilateral phrenic nerve stimulation and Pdi changes, both the maximal strength of the diaphragm and its relative degree of activation by the CNS under any breathing conditions are assessed [7]. It has been shown that the amplitude of Pdi twitches superimposed on graded voluntary contractions declines linearly as the voluntary Pdi increases (twitch occlusion). In fact, during maximal voluntary contractions (Pdi_{max}) no superimposed twitches could be detected. Thus, in the absence of fatigue, the CNS is capable of recruiting all diaphragm motor units to respond with maximum tetanic force [7]. By this method originally introduced by Merton [6], the decline in intrinsic muscle strength is measured from changes in the contractile response to electrical stimulation delivered to the relaxed muscle between voluntary contractions. Changes in the degree to which the muscle is (or can be) activated by the CNS are assessed by comparing these values to the extra force that can be elicited when twitches are superimposed on the voluntary contractions. For this purpose, it is important to be certain that the intensity of the stimulus remains unchanged by, for example, monitoring the amplitude of the evoked M-wave, which also tests the integrity of neuromuscular transmission. This test had been enthusiastically endorsed by the NHLBI workshop [1]. It was recommended that this test be evaluated and compared with the other ones in order to determine the value and utility of each, and thus to describe their specificity and sensitivity. This technique is particularly appropriate for clinical studies since it is relatively painless, easy to apply, and can be used on muscles where the motor nerve is not readily accessible. Moreover, maximal muscle strength can be indirectly and accurately assessed under conditions where the patient is unable, or unwilling to make a truly maximal effort.

One drawback when using this technique to investigate fatigue of the diaphragm is that consistent supramaximal bilateral tetanic stimulation of the phrenic nerves has so far proved unreliable [1]. Thus, changes in intrinsic muscle strength can so far only be assessed from changes in the twitch responses elicited from the relaxed muscle. These responses may be subject to fluctuations, e.g. substantial degrees of twitch potentiation or “low frequency fatigue”, not seen when tetanic stimulation is applied. Despite the drawbacks, it is felt that information obtained from bilateral transcutaneous supramaximal phrenic nerve twitch stimulation has the best potential of becoming a diagnostic test of respiratory muscle fatigue [1].

Recently, in order to minimize the invasivity of the balloon-catheter technique to measure twitch transdiaphragmatic pressure, which limits its clinical use, the measurement of mouth pressure twitch against an occluded airway has been developed [49]. Although it can potentially be used as a twitch occlusion test, more rigorous evaluation needs to be done before it can be recommended for general use [1].

EMG Spectral Shift

Analysis of the frequency components of EMG delineates its power spectrum; with fatigue, this spectrum shifts to lower frequencies. This approach has been used for many years in other skeletal muscles [50] and the last decade in the respiratory muscles [51]; however, the underlying cellular mechanisms remain unknown. Among the theories which attempt to explain this shift, the most popular remains the slowing of conduction velocity [52]; the spectral shift observed during fatigue could be explained by a progressive slowing of conduction velocity, which would in turn prolong the fiber action-potential wave form. Mortimer et al. [53] suggested that slowing of conduction velocity may result from the accumulation of metabolites, such as lactic acid. The accumulation of lactate is unlikely in itself to explain the EMG changes because patients with myophosphorylase deficiency who do not produce lactic acid have the same change in EMG power spectrum during fatigue [54]. However, the finding of other authors [55, 56] indicate they were unable to find any relation between conduction velocity and changes in the power spectrum during both fatiguing and non-fatiguing muscle contractions. They concluded that factors other than changes in the wave form of individual muscle fiber action potentials must contribute to the observed shift in the total EMG frequency components.

The relationship between power-spectral shift and fatigue is empirical. It occurs in the diaphragm before failure to develop adequate force, and thus is a useful objective measure to predict and precede the onset of fatigue (Fig. 4). With the new definition of respiratory muscle fatigue [1] which dictates that fatigue may be present at a time considerably preceding the point in time at which a muscle is unable to continue to perform a particular task, it is possible that the power spectral shift tracks the development of fatigue with considerable accuracy [57]. However, a single measurement of the power spectrum is insufficient, and a change must be observed in order to predict fatigue. In addition to the fact that the electrical activity of inspiratory muscles is influenced by changes in the spatial relationships between the recording electrodes and the muscle, power spectrum changes can result from conditions other than muscle fatigue. Thus, there is evidence casting doubt upon the sensitivity and specificity of this technique [1].

Further work is needed to elucidate the pathogenesis of the changes in the EMG power spectrum [46]. Such studies should help to understand the mechanism and site of fatigue. What is clear so far is that one cannot equate EMG indexes of fatigue to contractile fatigue. Under certain experimental conditions, changes in EMG power spectrum are associated with high-frequency fatigue, whereas EMG power spectrum is normal in low-frequency fatigue [58]. Thus, the power-spectral shift might signal fatigue due to reduced central firing frequency, neuromuscular

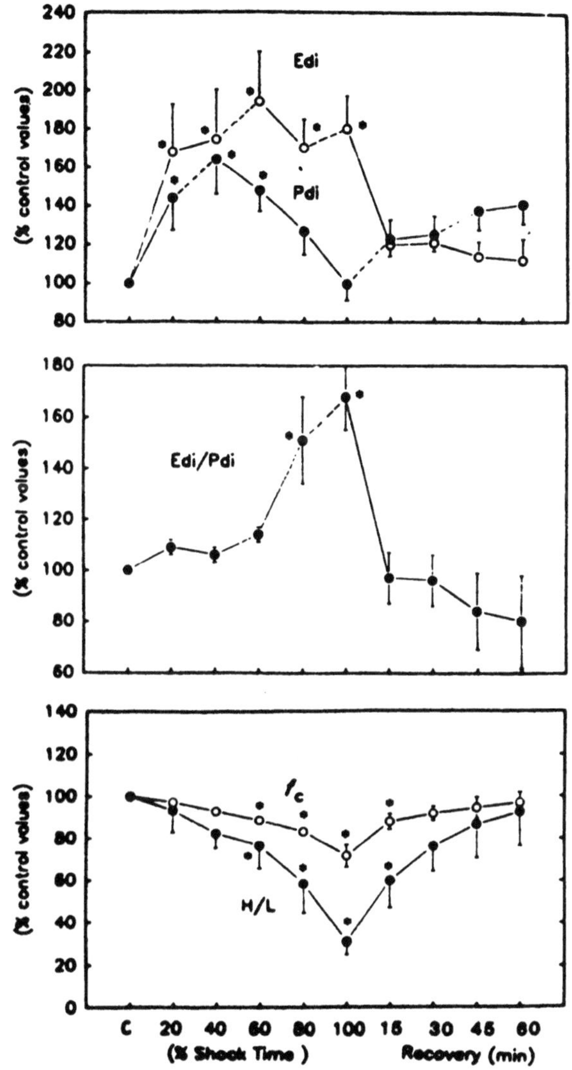

Fig. 4. Changes in the peak values of integrated spontaneous EMG activity of diaphragm (Edi) and corresponding spontaneous transdiaphragmatic pressure (Pdi; *top*), ratio of Edi to Pdi (Edi/Pdi, *middle*), and centroid frequency (fc), and ratio of high and low frequencies of diaphragmatic EMG (H/L, *bottom*), during shock induced by a balloon inflation in the inferior vena cava in a canine model and recovery. Means ± SE. $P<0.05$ compared with control values. Although Edi/Pdi rose at 80 and 100% of shock time only, both fc and H/L decline immediately and progressively after decline in arterial pressure. (From [121] with permission)

junction failure, failure in the excitation of sarcolemma, or failure in the synchronization that occurs during fatigue. Conversely, the shift may be insensitive to failure in excitation-contraction coupling or in the contractile machinery [46].

Clinical Detection of Fatigue

An interesting and important feature of the fatiguing inspiratory muscles is the alternation in the contribution of each group of muscles (diaphragm or intercostal/accessory) to the breathing task [14, 59, 60]. When a normal subject breathes against a fatiguing load, during which he attempts to maintain a constant mouth pressure, 3 stages of breathing have been observed from the point of view of breathing pattern and ability to maintain the required task (Fig. 5). At the beginning, the timing of breathing and the mouth pressure remain constant. This period is called the stage of "infinite possibilities"; that is, the subject has no indication that the task is of limited duration and, hence, the run might be from very short to very long. The last period, mainly the terminal 4–5 breaths, the stage of "exhaustion", is when the subject can no longer sustain the breathing task and stops the effort. Between these two periods is the third period, the stage of "alternative strategies". During this period, whenever the breathing task eventually leads to exhaustion because it is above the critical level, the subject uses all possible strategies to maintain the target pressure or work to preserve ventilation. During this stage, although mouth pressure remains constant, the pleural, or gastric, and transdiaphragmatic pressure vary almost in an alternating fashion. These changes may be interpreted as the result of recruitment and derecruitment between the diaphragm and intercostal/accessory muscles. This alternation can also be explained as a strategy of partial resting of one group of muscles while the other group is doing most of the work.

The three stages of breathing have also been observed in patients breathing against a load that might lead to fatigue, as in patients who cannot be weaned from the ventilator [14]. These patients had also demonstrated respiratory muscle fatigue, as detected by EMG measurements (Fig. 6). Very early, after discontinuation of mechanical assistance, there is an increase in frequency of breathing (tachypnea), while the muscles can still generate adequate ventilation. Bradypnea ensues. In many of these patients, paradoxic chest wall respiration results from either inward motion of the abdominal wall (abdominal paradox) or alternating breathing (respiratory alternans), and invariably coincides with a decrease in inspiratory muscle pressure because of fatigue. Finally, if artificial ventilation is not instituted, bradypnea follows and central apnea ensues (Fig. 7). The clinician can observe abdominal paradox and/or alternating breathing by simple inspection and/or by palpation of the chest wall and detect respiratory muscle fatigue.

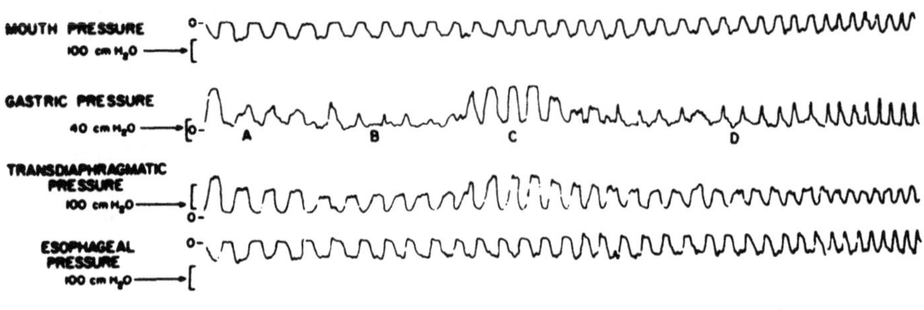

Fig. 5. Tracings of an experimental run in a man breathing against an inspiratory resistive load. With each breath, subject generated 75% of maximum mouth pressure. All pressures, except transdiaphragmatic pressure, were measured relative to atmospheric pressure. Only gastric and transdiaphragmatic pressure varied; mouth and esophageal pressures remained constant throughout the run. Gastric pressures increased during periods A and C and declined during periods B and D, indicating alternation of inspiratory muscle recruitment. (From [60] with permission)

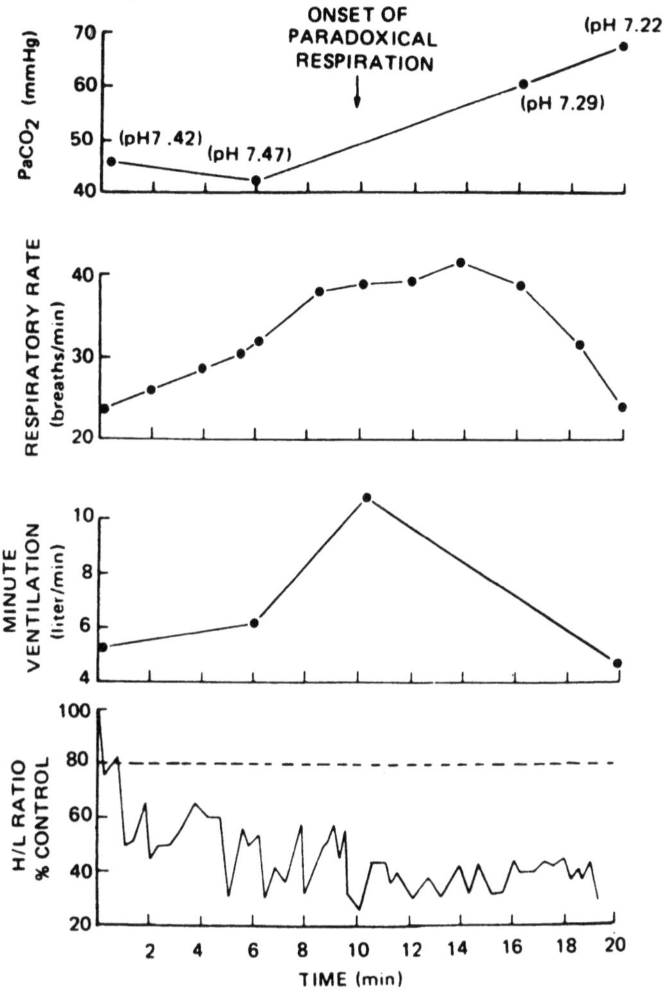

Fig. 6. Sequence of changes in $PaCO_2$, respiratory rate, minute ventilation, and high/low (H/L) ratio of the diaphragm in a patient during a 20-min attempt at discontinuation of mechanical assistance. The initial change was the fall in high/low ratio ventilated (indicating fatigue), followed by a progressive increase in respiratory rate. The $PaCO_2$ fell initially, and the patient became alkalemic. Paradoxical abdominal displacements were not noted untill after there had been a substantial increase in respiratory rate and minute ventilation. Hypercapnia and respiratory acidosis did not develop until after abdominal paradox and alternation between rib cage and abdominal breaths were noted. Just before the artificial ventilation was reinstituted, there was a sharp fall in respiratory frequency and minute ventilation. (From [14] with permission)

Management of Respiratory Muscle Fatigue

Experimental muscle develops when the demands on the respiratory pump are excessive in relation to pump capacity. However, it is not yet clear whether in the clinical setting of ventilatory failure overt peripheral muscle fatigue develops or

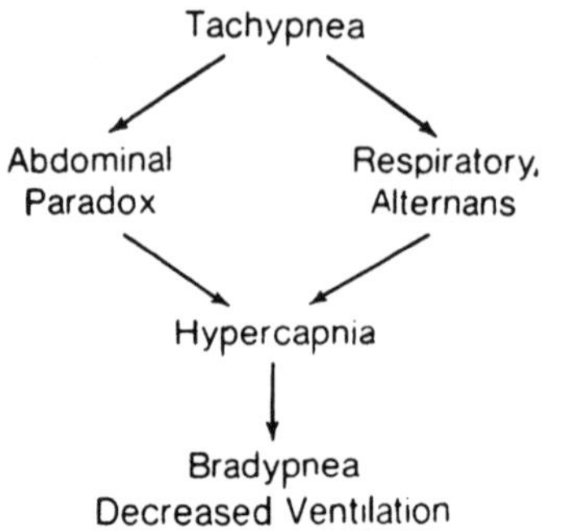

Fig. 7. Schematic representation of the clinical signs of respiratory muscle fatigue, in sequence from top to bottom.

whether an adaptive feedback reduction of central drive avoids such fatigue, albeit at the cost of hypoventilation [1]. The three components of the system (demand, capacity, and drive) are closely linked, and for the patient proceeding to ventilatory failure, a small alteration in one variable may crucially determine outcome. It is rational, therefore, to direct therapeutic efforts at minimizing demand, maximizing capacity, and optimizing respiratory drive.

Decreasing the Demands of the Respiratory Muscles

If the work of breathing or pressure-time index increases and exceeds a critical value, the energy requirement will also increase, and fatigue may develop. This may explain the inability or normal subjects to maintain high levels of ventilation for long periods [61–63] or to sustain normal ventilation when the work of breathing is excessive. Therefore, in patients with increased work of breathing, fatigue may be avoided by therapy if it reduces the load applied on the ventilatory pump below the fatiguing threshold. In the clinical situation, this is most often achieved by treatment directed at reducing airway resistance and increasing pulmonary compliance.

Muscle strength is an important factor when considering muscle energy demands; thus pressure should be normalized by expressing it as a fraction of Pmax at the same fiber length. The greater the work required to sustain adequate ventilation, the greater the value of P/Pmax, and the greater the energy demand. Thus, at constant pressure the energy demand will increase as Pmax decreases [46]. This is of considerable physiological significance since Pmax is a function of fiber length; thus for the respiratory muscles it is determined, in part, by lung volume. Hyperinflation strongly predisposes to fatigue, not only by increasing the driving pressure but also by decreasing Pmax [60, 64]. Furthermore, if the efficiency of the respiratory muscles decreases, which occurs with an increase in airway resistance, the O_2 cost of breathing and energy demands increase for the same external power [65], further predisposing to fatigue. Airway obstruction frequently leads to dynamic hyperinflation, further decreasing the efficiency of the respiratory muscles because of the shortening on the fiber length and obliging the muscles to perform an isometric contraction in the beginning of inspiration in order to overcome auto-PEEP.

Increasing the Capacity of the Respiratory Muscles

Rational therapy of respiratory muscle fatigue includes training, nutritional repletion, rest and muscle pharmacotherapy. These measures prevent fatigue by increasing the capacity of the respiratory muscles. Furthermore, as weak muscles are susceptible to fatigue, treatable or avoidable causes of weakness must not be ignored; these include hypercapnia [66, 67], acidosis [68, 69] hypocalcemia [70], hypokalemia and hypophosphatemia [71], as well as thyroid, alcohol, steroid, drug-induced and infammatory myopathies [1].

Pharmacological agents. Only recently has attention been focused on the effects that various pharmacological agents may have on improving the contractility and endurance of the respiratory muscles. Respiratory muscle function can be modulated pharmacologically by acting at the level of either the excitation-contraction coupling process, or the energy supply to the muscles. Drugs acting at the level of excitation-contraction coupling are xanthines [44, 72, 73] and digitalis [74, 75], while those acting by increasing the energy supply are isoproterenol [76] and dopamine [77]. Studies in animals [72], isolated preparations [73, 78], normal subjects [44] and patients [79, 80], have shown that theophylline has a positive inotropic effect on respiratory muscles, enhancing their contractility at therapeutic dose level. Hence, theophylline restored the ability of the fatigued diaphragm to generate adequate forces increasing its endurance. Its effects appear to be greater in the fatigued than in the fresh state. The mechanism of action is not yet clear, but recent studies indicate that theophylline may facilitate the influx of Ca^{2+} through the slow channels, and perhaps activate a Ca^{2+} induced Ca^{2+} release from the sarcoplasmic reticulum [81].

Training. Specific training of the respiratory muscles, like other skeletal muscles, can enhance their strength and endurance, the latter being most relevant to patients with chronic ventilatory loads or weaning difficulties. Ventilatory muscle strength has been increased by 55% in subjects performing repeated maximum static inspiratory and expiratory pressure maneuvers [63]. By increasing inspiratory muscle strength, the pressure developed per breath expressed as a fraction of the maximum, will diminish, thus reducing the vulnerability to fatigue.

An increase in the endurance of respiratory muscle performance has been achieved in both healthy individuals [63, 82] and patients with a variety of conditions, i.e. chronic airflow limitation [83, 84], cystic fibrosis [85], and quadriplegia [51]. In quadriplegic patients [51] improvement of inspiratory muscle strength and endurance has been achieved by imposing resistive loads during inspiration for several periods each day for 6–8 weeks. Strength progressively increased over an 8-week period and endurance improved over a 12-week period. Leith and Bradley [63] have reported that normal subjects who spent 30–45 min/day for 5 week hyperventilating under normocapnic conditions were able to increase the sustainable maximum voluntary ventilation (MVV) by 14%. A 5-week period was required for MVV to return to control values after cessation of the training. However, it is well known that training produces improvements in the task being trained for, with ver benefit to other tasks. Further, such programs may also have a sub-cebo effect [1].

The cellular adaptations that the respiratory muscles undergo during training are in all likelihood similar to those found in other skeletal muscles. Keens et al. [85] found an increase in the oxidative capacity of the diaphragm and intercostals when he chronically increased the ventilatory load in rats. Furthermore, the diaphragm responded with an increase in the proportion of muscle fibers with the myofibrillar ATPase-staining characteristics of slow-twich fibers [86]. Similarly, Farkas and Roussos [87, 88] found that emphysematous hamsters increased the oxidative capacity of the inspiratory muscles while the endurance of the diaphragm increased. The diaphragm subjected to chronic hyperinflation became shorter, so its length-tension curve was shifted to the left. This adaptation was achieved by reducing the number of sarcomeres and allowing the diaphragm to operate optimally at a shorter length (Fig. 8) [87].

The literature on respiratory muscle training leaves many clinically important questions unanswered; for example, which patients are likely to benefit from training, how much training in terms of intensity and duration produces maximal results, which training devices are most effective, and how much long-term training is required to avoid de-training. Furthermore, although training of respiratory muscles with significant reserve capacity may improve performance, training of muscles, already being driven at the limit of their capacity may produce myopathic changes, well recognized in overtrained athletes, recovery from which can be prolonged [1].

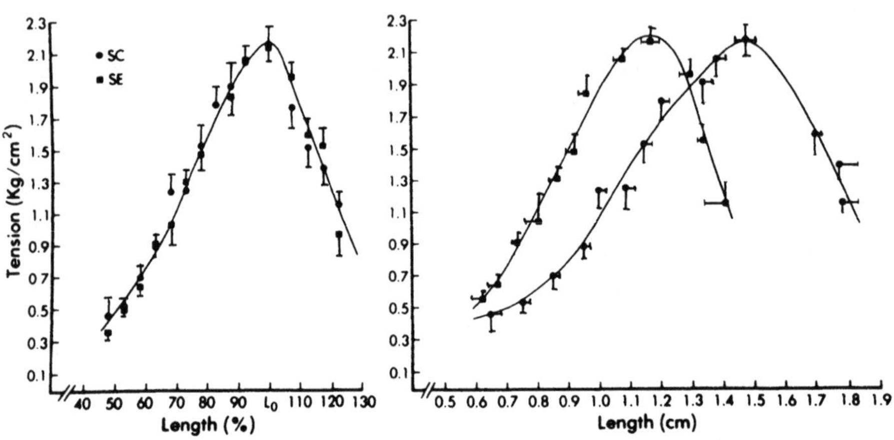

Fig. 8. Active length tension curves obtained from diaphragm strips of sedentary control (SC) and sedentary emphysematous (SE) animals. *Left:* tension expressed as kilograms per cross-sectional area of muscle. Both groups achieve same Pmax. *Right:* fiber length expressed in absolute terms. Active length tension curve of SE group is significantly shifted to the left; Pmax is generated at a shorter length in this group. (From [122] with permission)

Nutritional repletion. Malnutrition is an extremely important complicating factor in critically ill patients requiring mechanical ventilation as well as in patients with a variety of chronic lung disease [89]. It has been shown that it is associated with impaired respiratory muscle structure and function in humans [90, 91]. Nutritional repletion can improve the strength and endurance of the ventilatory pump [1, 92].

Rest. A logical approach to restore the contractility and endurance of a muscle from fatigue would be to put the muscle at rest. Available data clearly demonstrate long-term benefit to patients with chronic chest wall disorders and neuromuscular disease from the non-invasive use of assisted ventilation, usually nocturnal, using both positive and negative pressure-ventilators [93–97]. Similarly, several studies have shown a significant improvement in patients with severe stable COPD and CO_2 retention, in terms of decreasing CO_2 and increasing the strength of the respiratory muscles, using mainly negative pressure ventilating devices [98–101]. The recent development of non-invasive positive pressure ventilation via a face or nose mask in acute exacerbations of COPD [102–104], makes it possible to apply this technique to stable COPD patients. Although such mechanical ventilation rests the respiratory muscles, the mechanism whereby respiratory function, ventilatory failure and symptoms are improved is not yet clear. The hypothesis that the improvement in these patients is a result of respiratory muscle rest reversing muscle fatigue remains speculative [1].

Respiratory Muscle Fatigue and Ventilatory Failure

Ventilatory failure resulting in CO_2 retention implies alveolar hypoventilation for a given level of CO_2 production ($\dot{V}CO_2$). The respiratory equation relates the arterial carbon dioxide tension ($PaCO_2$) to alveolar ventilation ($\dot{V}A$):

$$PaCO_2 = K\frac{\dot{V}CO_2}{\dot{V}A}$$

where K demotes the constant of proportionallity. Since $\dot{V}A = \dot{V}E\text{-}VD$, where $\dot{V}E$ denotes minute ventilation and $\dot{V}D$ dead space ventilation, the respiratory equation may be expressed as follows:

$$PaCO_2 = K\frac{\dot{V}CO_2}{\dot{V}E - \dot{V}D} = K\frac{\dot{V}CO_2}{\dot{V}E(1 - \dot{V}D/\dot{V}E)}$$

$$= K\frac{\dot{V}CO_2}{\dot{V}E(1 - fVD/fVT)} = K\frac{\dot{V}CO_2}{\dot{V}E(1 - VD/VT)}$$

$$= K\frac{\dot{V}CO_2}{VT \cdot f(1 - VD/VT)}$$

where f is frequency.

This equation states that $PACO_2$ will rise if carbon dioxide production increases without increasing alveolar ventilation, or when, for a given $\dot{V}CO_2$, alveolar ventilation decreases by virtue of a rise in the ratio of VD/VT (either by increasing VD or decreasing VT at a constant total ventilation ($\dot{V}E$ or VTf), or when minute ventilation decreases at constant VD/VT, or both). An important point that may be deduced from this equation also is that, at constant $\dot{V}E$, CO_2 may rise by increasing the frequency, with a concurrent fall in tidal volume and hence increase in VD/VT. $\dot{V}E$ in the above equation may further be separated to its two components, namely inspiratory flow and duty cycle:

$$\dot{V}E = VT \cdot f = VT \cdot \frac{1}{TT} = \frac{VT}{TI} \cdot \frac{TI}{TT}$$

Thus, a reduction in mean inspiratory flow (VT/TI), duty cycle (TI/TT) or both, will cause retension of carbon dioxide. In these equations, it becomes apparent that $PaCO_2$ may rise due either to inability of the muscles to generate pressure and, in turn, inspiratory flow (VT/TI), or to alterations in the pattern of breathing (f, TI/TT), or even to reduced neural output. As fatigue ensues, the last two mechanisms of CO_2 retention might be implicated either as an adaptation to the altered characteristics of the respiratory muscles via a feedback loop, or as central fatigue.

Fatigue as Cause of Respiratory Failure

In a number of conditions, as in cardiogenic (Fig. 1) and septic shock (Fig. 2) in dogs or in patients during the weaning period from ventilators (Fig. 6), respiratory muscle fatigue is recognized as a cause of respiratory failure, whereas in other conditions, it is very likely that patients hypoventilate due to fatigue. Because hypercapnia occurs either acutely, as in cardiogenic shock with pulmonary edema or chronically as in COPD, it follows that, if fatigue plays a role in the CO_2 retention, it may occur either acutely or chronically (Table 2).

Fatigue and, in turn, hypercapnia of acute onset are usually due to a combination of increased mechanical loading of the lung, a reduced muscle strength, decreased efficiency, and reduced energy supplies to the inspiratory muscles. The mechanisms responsible for CO_2 retention are both decreasing VE and increasing VD/VT. The sequence of events in this condition has been postulated to be as follows: if the energy supply is inadequate for the demand, the patients with weak and/or loaded respiratory muscles must avoid other factors that predispose to fatigue, e.g. hyperinflation [105]. Big tidal breaths force the muscles to shorten more than small tidal breathing. Thus, by reducing TI and keeping everything else constant, the respiratory muscles operate at an optimal length, and yet will not substantially affect its geometry while the energy demand per breath (expressed by the pressure-time index-P.TI) decreases, and theoretically, muscle fatigue is postponed. Such a pattern of breathing will reduce TT and VE, VD/VT will increase and, therefore, PCO_2 must increase. This reduction in TI, however, is usually compen-

Table 2. Clinical conditions in which fatigue may be a cause of ventilatory failure. (From [105] with permission)

Hypercapnia of acute onset
Lung diseases
Asthma
Acute on chronic respiratory failure
Chest wall diseases
Prematurity
Atrophy secondary to artificial ventilation
Neuromuscular disorders
Lung and chest wall disease
Cardiogenic shock
Noncardiogenic pulmonary edema
Respiratory distress syndrome of infants
Hypercapnia of insidious onset
Lung diseases
Bronchitis
Emphysema
Bronchiectasis
Chest wall diseases
Kyphoscoliosis
Thoracoplasty
Pleural thickening
Extreme obesity
Neuromuscular disorders
Lung and chest wall diseases
Scleroderma
Polymyositis
Systemic lupus

sated at least at the beginning by increasing frequency so that VE is maintained or increased allowing adequate alveolar ventilation (Fig. 6). Such a frequency of breathing however is no longer optimal [106] and for the same alveolar ventilation, the energy demand will increase. Thus, although the non-optimal frequency seems to be a better option than prolonging TI, it too might finally lead to muscle fatigue. This period during which the subject uses all possible strategies to maintain the ventilation represents the stage of "alternative strategies" (Fig. 5 and 7) as may be deduced from the review in the section of clinical detection of fatigue. Later, in the stage of "exhaustion", pressure will decrease, and as a result, VT and VE will decrease while VD/VT further increases. The reduction in pressure will obviously decrease the P.TI and the energy demands per breath, but VA will be further reduced and $PaCO_2$ will rise. Later, just before death from respiratory arrest [13], TI increases again and respiratory frequency gradually decreases. In fact, as the muscles are unable to displace the thorax to develop high or even adequate flows, they can afford longer periods of excitation (TI) without largely deviating from optimal length and geometry. But to reduce the energy demands per minute, that is to avoid increases in TI/TT, the frequency of breathing decreases. Finally, at extreme fatigue, the CNS reduces the output signals per breath, further reducing P and VT and eventually leading to respiratory arrest.

Patients with chronic hypercapnia usually develop CO_2 retention insidiously. They may have to breathe against increased loads imposed either by the lung (as in COPD), the chest wall (as in kyphoscoliosis and extreme obesity), or both (as in scleroderma). The mechanism by which these patients develop CO_2 retention insidiously is unknown. We can hypothesize, however, that as the disease progresses, the critical level of power output is exceeded in order to maintain normal alveolar ventilation. Thus, it is possible that the muscles become fatigued chronically or, alternatively the CNS controllers may set a lower level of ventilation reducing the power output below the critical value. This hypothesis is consistent with the findings of Sorli et al. [107] who showed that in COPD patients with CO_2 retention, the inspiratory time was reduced with a concomitant decrease in VT while VT/TI, TI/TT, VE, and central drive were not different from those in patients with COPD who did not retain carbon dioxide (Table 3). In addition, the CO_2 retainers had a lower FEV_1, higher effective impedance, higher weight and higher FRC and FRC/TLC, compared to non-CO_2 retainers. In this regard, it is reasonable to speculate that CO_2 retainers prefer to terminate TI early, avoiding substantial deviation from the optimal muscle length and perhaps substantial geometrical alteration of the diaphragm and intercostal muscles, as well as minimizing the energy demands per breath (by the decrease of P.TI), than to take a large VT (long TI). This reduction in VT results in an increase in VD/VT, which in turn, as the respiratory equation predicts, will raise $PaCO_2$. Although afferent stimuli arising from the chest wall, stretch or irritant or J-receptors must be responsible for this reduction in TI, the possibility of direct alterations in the rhythm of the respiratory centers due to chronic CO_2 retention and hypoxia [108] must not be ignored. COPD patients with CO_2 retention may have to develop pressures at the end of inspiration which approach or exceed the critical inspiratory pressures, thus leading the inspiratory muscle to fatigue. To approach this question, Roussos (unpublished work) studied 12 patients with COPD (6 CO_2 retainers, $PCO_2 > 45$ mm Hg) and grouped his results with those of Bellemare and Grassino [109]. He found that patients with CO_2 retention developed a Pdi which was 25–30% of Pdimax while the peak tidal Pdi in patients with no CO_2 retention was 10% of Pdimax. Both groups of patients, particularly the CO_2 retainers, were hyperinflated, but the CO_2 retainers had a higher

Table 3. Mean values (±SD) of FEV_1 (% Predicted) and of pulmonary gas exchange data in 15 stable COPD patients breathing room air at rest. (From [107] with permission)

	FEV_1 (% predicted)	$PaCO_2$ (mm Hg)	$\dot{V}E$ (liters/min)	VT (liters)	VD[a] (liters)	$\dot{V}CO_2$ (liters/min)
Group A (n=8)	38±16	38±3.6	10.6±1.8	0.71±0.09	0.32±0.07	0.26±0.03
Group B (n=7)	22± 5	50±8.7	9.4±1.0	0.56±0.07	0.32±0.05	0.28±0.05
Group A vs group B	$p<0.05$	$p<0.005$	NS	$p<0.01$	NS	NS

[a] VD includes equipment dead space of 70 ml

frequency, while TI/TT was not different in both groups. In normal subjects, the critical pleural pressure (i.e. the pressure developed per inspiration, which precipitates fatigue to 25–30% at the maximum) occurs at FRC plus ½ IC. By this guideline, CO_2 retainers may be placed at or above the critical zone of fatigue, while the non-CO_2 retainers remain in the non-fatiguing zone. In addition, it is known that undernutrition is a problem involved in some COPD patients and it might play a role in CO_2 retention. In fact, body weight less than 85% of the predicted value occurs in approximately 20% of patients with COPD, and it is accompanied by a reduction in the diaphragm muscle mass [110] and by a reduction in the thickness of the sternocleidomastoid muscle [111]. These changes may be partly responsible for the reduction in Pimax observed in these patients. Furthermore, it is important to note that patients whose Pimax is less than −50 mm Hg have chronic CO_2 retention [112]. Thus the combination, in some patients, of increased work of breathing due to disease, decrease in mechanical efficiency due to hyperinflation and/or airway resistance, and muscle weakness due to hyperinflation and/or atrophy and undernutrition, may predispose the respiratory muscles to fatigue and CO_2 retention. In this regard, it is tempting to speculate either that the CO_2 retainers are in a chronic state of fatigue or that the CNS sets a pattern of breathing in an attempt to avoid exhaustion. These authors favor the latter and we speculate that afferents from the small fibers (type III and IV) stimulated by the heavy work (ergoreceptors, type III) or by noxious substances like lactic acid (nociceptors, type IV) modify the CNS output. The mechanism is not known, but the production of endogenous opioids may play an important role. In this regard, the results of Edelman et al. [113–119] are interesting. They have shown that in both patients and animals breathing against a heavy load, or under conditions of brain hypoxia, endogenous opioids alter the central controllers significantly while naloxone prevents or reverses this effect.

References

1. NHLBI Workshop (1990) Respiratory muscle fatigue: report of the respiratory muscle fatigue workshop group. Am Rev Respir Dis 142:474–480
2. Davies HW, Haldane JS, Priestly JG (1919) The response to respiratory resistance. J Physiol London 53:60–69
3. Davies HW, Brown GR, Bringer CAL (1925) The respiratory response to carbon dioxide. J Exp Med 41:37–52
4. Bellemare F, Bigland-Ritchie B (1987) Central components of diaphragmatic fatigue assessed by phrenic nerve stimulation. J Appl Physiol 62 (3):1307–1316
5. Bigland-Ritchie B, Jones DA, Hosking GP, Edwards RHT (1978) Central and peripheral fatigue in sustained maximal voluntary contractions of human quadriceps muscle. Clin Sci Mol Med 54:609–614
6. Merton PA (1954) Voluntary strength and fatigue. J Physiol London 13:553–564
7. Bellemare F, Bigland-Ritchie B (1984) Assessment of human diaphragm strength and activation using phrenic nerve stimulation. Respir Physiol 58:263–277
8. Merton PA, Hill DK, Morton HB (1981) Indirect and direct stimulation of fatigued human muscle. In: Porter R, Whelan J (eds) Human Muscle Fatigue: Physiological mechanisms, Pitman Medical, London (Ciba Found Symp 82) pp 120–126
9. Roussos C (1990) Respiratory muscle fatigue and ventilatory failure. Chest 97 (Suppl 3): 89–96

10. Bigland-Ritchie B, Johannsson R, Lippold OCL, Woods JJ (1983) Contractile speed and EMG changes during fatigue of sustained maximal voluntary contractions. J Neurophysiol 50:313–324
11. Grimby L, Hannerz J, Hedman B (1981) Fatigue and voluntary discharge properties of single motor units in man. J Physiol London 316:543–554
12. Jammes Y, Buchler B, Delpierre S, Rasidakis A, Grimand C, Roussos C (1986) Phrenic afferents and their role in inspiratory control. J Appl Physiol 60:854–860
13. Aubier M, Trippenbach T, Roussos C (1981) Respiratory muscle fatigue during cardiogenic shock. J Appl Physiol 51:449–508
14. Cohen C, Zagelbaum G, Gross D, Roussos C, Macklem PT (1982) Clinical manifestations of inspiratory muscle fatigue. Am J Med 73:308–316
15. Otis AB (1954) The work of breathing. Physiol Rev 34:449–458
16. Mead J (1960) Control of respiratory frequency. J Appl Physiol 15:325–336
17. Bigland-Ritchie B, Bellemare F, Woods JJ (1981) Central and Peripheral fatigue in intermittent submaximal contractions. In: Porter R, Whelan J (eds) Human muscle fatigue: physiological mechanisms, Pitman Medical, London (Ciba Found Symp 82)
18. Krnjevic K, Miledi R (1958) Failure of neuromuscular propagation in rats. J Physiol London 140:440–461
19. Krnjevic K, Miledi R (1959) Presynaptic failure of neuromuscular propagation in rats. J Physiol London 288:285–300
20. Hussain S, Simkus G, Roussos C (1985) Respiratory muscle fatigue: a cause of ventilatory failure in septic shock. J Appl Physiol 58:2033–2040
21. Nassar-Gentina V, Passoneau JV, Vergard JL, Rapoport SI (1978) Metabolic correlates of fatigue and of recovery from fatigue in single frog muscle fibers. J Gen Physiol 72:593–606
22. Kugelberg E, Lindergren B (1979) Transmission and contraction fatigue of rat motor units in relation to succimate dehydrogenase activity of motor unit fibers. J Physiol London 288:285–300
23. Wilkie D (1981) Shortage of chemical fuel as a cause of fatigue. In: Porter R, Whelan J (eds) Human muscle fatigue: physiological mechanisms, Pitman Medical, London (Ciba Found Symp 82) pp 102–114
24. Aubier M, Farkas G, De Troyer A, Mozes R, Roussos C (1981) Detection of diaphragmatic fatigue in man by phrenic stimulation. J Appl Physiol 50:538–544
25. Gutierrez G, Palizas F, Marini CE (1990) Cellular energy metabolism. Recent advances in the study of the diaphragm with magnetic resonance spectroscopy. Chest 97:975–982
26. Dawson MJ, Gardian DG, Wilkie DR (1978) Muscular fatigue investigated by phosphorous nuclear magnetic resonance. Nature London 274:863–866
27. Hultman E, Bergstrom J, Mc Lennan-Anderson (1967) Breakdown and resynthesis of phosphoryl-creatine and adenosine triphosphate in connection with muscular work in man. Scand J Clin Lab Invest 19:56–66
28. Bergstrom J, Hermansen L, Hultman E, Saltin B (1967) Diet, muscle glycogen and physical performance. Acta Physiol Scand 71:140–150
29. Aubier M, Viires N, Syllie G, Mozes R, Roussos C (1982) Respiratory muscle contribution to lastic acidosis in low cardiac output. Am Rev Respir Dis 126:648–652
30. Fitts RH, Holloszy JO (1976) Lactate and contractile force in frog muscle during development of fatigue and recovery. Am J Physiol 231:430–433
31. Jardim J, Farkas G, Prefaut C, Thomas D, Macklem PT, Roussos C (1981) The failing inspiratory muscles under normoxic and hypoxic conditions. Am Rev Respir Dis 124:274–279
32. Nakamura Y, Schwartz A (1970) Possible control of intracellular calcium metabolism by (H^+): sarcoplasmic reticulum of skeletal and cardiac muscle. Biophys Res Commun 41:830–839
33. Robertson S, Kerrick W (1976) The effect of pH on submaximal and maximal Ca^{2+} activated tension in skinned frog skeletal fibers. Biophys J (Abstract) 16:73A
34. Fabiato A, Fabiato F (1978) Effects of pH on the myofilaments and the sarcoplasmic reticulum of skinned cell from cardiac and skeletal muscles. J Physiol London 53:233–255

35. Metzger JM, Fitts RH (1987) Role of intracellular pH in muscle fatigue. J Appl Physiol 62:1392–1397
36. Mainwood GW, Remaud JM (1985) The effect of acid-base balance on fatigue of skeletal muscle. Can J Physiol Pharmacol 63:403–416
37. Mainwood GW, Alward M (1982) Evidence for an extracellular mechanism for the action of H+ on recovery of muscles following fatigue. Can J Physiol Pharmacol 60:1720–1724
38. Fitzgerald RS, Howell S, Pike MM, Jacobus WE (1988) NMR study of rat diaphragm exposed to metabolic and compensated metabolic acidosis. J Appl Physiol 65:2278–2284
39. Edwards RHT, Hill DK, Jones DA, Merton PA (1977) Fatigue of long duration in human skeletal muscle after exercise. J Physiol London 272:769–778
40. Edwards RHT, Young A, Hosking CP, Jones DA (1977) Human skeletal muscle function: description of texts and normal values. Clin Sci Mol Med 52:283-290
41. Edwards RHT, Mills KR, Newham DJ (1981) Greater low frequency fatigue produced by eccentric than concentric muscle contraction. J Physiol London 317:17
42. Vigreux B, Cnockaert JC, Pertuzon E (1980) Effects of fatigue on the series elastic component of human muscle. Eur J Appl Physiol 45:11–17
43. Moxham J, Wiles CM, Newham D, Edwards RHI (1980) Sternomastoid muscle function and fatigue in man. Clin Sci Mol Med 59:463–468
44. Aubier M, De Troyer A, Sampson M, Macklem PT, Roussos C (1981) Aminophylline improved diaphragmatic contractility. N Engl J Med 305:249–252
45. Moxham J, Morris AJR, Spiro SG, Edwards RHT, Green M (1981) Contractile properties and fatigue of the diaphragm in man. Thorax 36:164–168
46. Roussos C, Macklem PT (1986) Inspiratory muscle fatigue. In: Fishman AP, Macklem PT, Mead J, Geiger SR (eds) Handbook of Physiology. The Respiratory system: Mechanics of Breathing, part 2, American Physiological Society, Bethesda, pp 511–527
47. Esau SA, Bellemare F, Grassino A, Permutt S, Roussos C, Pardy RL (1983) Changes in relaxation rate with diaphragmatic fatigue in humans. J Appl Physiol 54:1353–1360
48. Esau SA, Bye PTP, Pardy RL (1983) Changes in rate of relaxation of sniffs with diaphragmatic fatigue in humans. J Appl Physiol 55:731–735
49. Similowski T, Gauthier AP, Yan S, Macklem PT, Bellemare F (1990) Mouth pressure twich during phrenic stimulation in COPD patients. Eur Respir J (suppl 10) Abstract:195s
50. Lindstrom L, Kadefors R, Petersen I (1977) An electromyographic index for localized muscle fatigue. J Appl Physiol 43:750–754
51. Gross D, Grassino A, Ross WRD, Macklem PT (1979) Electromyogram pattern of diaphragmatic fatigue. J Appl Physiol 46:1–7
52. Lindstrom L, Magnusson R, Petersen I (1970) Muscular fatigue and action potential conduction velocity changes studies with frequency analysis of EMG signal. Electromyography 10:341–355
53. Mortimer JT, Magnusson R, Petersen I (1970) Conduction velocity in ischemic muscle: effect on EMG frequency spectrum. Am J Physiol 219:1324–1329
54. Wiles CM, Jones DA, Edwards RHT (1981) Fatigue in human metabolic myopathy. In: Porter R, Whelan J (eds) Human Muscle Fatigue: Physiological mechanisms, Pitman Medical, London (Ciba Found Symp 82) pp 264–282
55. Bigland-Ritchie B, Donovan EF, Roussos C (1981) Conduction velocity and EMG power spectrum changes in fatigue of sustained maximal efforts. J Appl Physiol 51:1300–1305
56. Roussos C (1979) Respiratory muscle fatigue in the hypercapnic patient. Bull Eur Physiopathol Respir 15:117–126
57. Macklem PT (1990) The importance of defining respiratory muscle fatigue. Am Rev Respir Dis 142:274
58. Moxham J, Edwards PHT, Aubier M et al (1982) Changes in EMG power spectrum (high-to-low ratio) with force fatigue in humans. J Appl Physiol 53:1094–1099
59. Lopes JM, Muller NL, Bryan MH, Bryan AC (1981) Synergistic behavior of inspiratory muscles after diaphragmatic fatigue in the newborn. J Appl Physiol 51:547–551
60. Roussos C, Fixley M, Gross D, Macklem PT (1979) Fatigue of inspiratory muscles and their synergic behavior. J Appl Physiol 46:897–904
61. Zocche GP, Fritts HW Jr, Cournand A (1960) Fraction of maximum breathing capacity available for prolonged hyperventilation. J Appl Physiol 15:1073–1074

62. Tenney SM, Reese RE (1968) The ability to sustain great breathing efforts. Respir Physiol 5:187–201
63. Leith DE, Bradley M (1976) Ventilatory muscle strength and endurance training. J Appl Physiol 41:508–516
64. Farkas F, Roussos C (1984) Acute diaphragmatic shortening; in vitro mechanics and fatigue. Am Rev Respir Dis 130:434–438
65. Mc Gregor M, Becklake MR (1961) The relationship of oxygen cost of breathing to respiratory mechanical work and respiratory force. J Clin Invest 40:971–980
66. Juan G, Calverley P, Talamo C, Schnader J, Roussos C (1984) Effect of carbon dioxide on diaphragmatic function in human beings. N Engl J Med 310:874–879
67. Schnader JY, Juan G, Howell S, Fitzgerald R, Roussos C (1985) Alterial CO_2 partial pressure affects diaphragmatic function. J Appl Physiol 58:823–829
68. Fitzgerald RS, Carfinkel F, Silbergeld E, Loscutoff S (1976) Factors in the interpretation of mouth occlusion pressure during measurements of chemosensitivity. Chest 70:145–149
69. Fitzgerald RS, Hauer MC, Bierkamper GG, Raff H (1983) Rat diaphragm response to unbuffered acidosis/alkalosis. Federation Proc (Abstract) 42:422
70. Aubier M, Viires N, Piquet J et al (1985) Effects of hypocalcemia on diaphragmatic strength generation. J Appl Physiol 58:2054–2061
71. Aubier M, Murciano D, Lecocguic Y et al (1985) Effect of hypophosphatemia on diaphragmatic contractility in patients with acute respiratory failure. N Engl J Med 313:420–423
72. Sigrist S, Thomas D, Howell S, Roussos C (1982) The effect of aminophilline on inspiratory muscle contractility. Am Rev Respir Dis 126:46–50
73. Jones DA, Howell S, Roussos C, Edwards RHT (1982) Low frequency fatigue in isolated skeletal muscles and the effects of methylxanthines. Clin Sci 63:161–167
74. Aubier M, Viires N, Murciano D, Seta JP, Pariente R (1986) Effects of digoxin on diaphragmatic strength generation. J Appl Physiol 61:1767–1774
75. Aubier M, Murciano D, Viires N et al (1987) Effects of digoxin on diaphragmatic strength generation in patients with chronic obstructive pulmonary disease during acute respiratory failure. Am Rev Respir Dis 135:544–548
76. Howell S, Roussos C (1984) Isoproterenol and aminophylline improve contractility of fatigued canine diaphragm. Am Rev Respir Dis 129:118–124
77. Aubier M, Murciano D, Menu Y, Boczkowski J, Mal H, Pariente R (1989) Dopamine effects on diaphragmatic strength during acute respiratory failure in chronic obstructive pulmonary disease. Ann Intern Med 110:107–123
78. Viires N, Aubier M, Murciano D, Marty C, Pariente R (1986) Effects of theophylline on isolated diaphragmatic fibers: a model for pharmacological studies on diaphragmatic contractility. Am Rev Respir Dis 133:1060–1064
79. Murciano D, Aubier M, Lecocguic Y, Pariente R (1984) Effects of theophylline on diaphragmatic strength and fatigue in patients with chronic obstructive pulmonary disease. N Engl J Med 311:349–353
80. Murciano D, Auclair MH, Pariente R, Aubier M (1989) A randomized controlled trial of theophylline in patients with severe chronic obstructive pulmonary disease. N Engl J Med 320:1521–1525
81. Aubier M, Murciano D, Viires N, Lecocguic Y, Pariente R (1983) Diaphragmatic contractility enhanced by aminophylline: role of extracellular calcium. J Appl Physiol 54:460–464
82. Bradley ME, Leith DE (1987) Ventilatory muscle training and the oxygen cost of sustained hyperpnea. J Appl Physiol 45:885–892
83. Bellemare F, Grassino A (1982) Evaluation of human diaphragm fatigue. J Appl Physiol 53:1196–1206
84. Pardy RI, Rivington RN, Despas PJ, Macklem PT (1981) The effects of inspiratory muscle training on exercise performance in chronic airflow limitation. Am Rev Respir Dis 123:426–433
85. Keens TG, Bryan AC, Levison H, Ianuzzo CD (1978) Developmental pattern of muscle fiber types in human ventilatory muscles. J Appl Physiol 44:909–913
86. Keens TG, Chen V, Patel P, O'Brien P, Levison H, Ianuzzo CD (1978) Cellular adaptations of the ventilatory muscles to a chronic increased respiratory load. J Appl Physiol 44:905–908

87. Farkas G, Roussos C (1988) Adaptability of the hamster diaphragm to excercise and/or emphysema. J Appl Physiol 53:1263–1272
88. Farkas G, Roussos C (1985) Histochemical and biochemical correlates of ventilatory muscle fatigue in emphysematous hamsters. J Clin Invest 74:1214–1220
89. Lewis MI, Belman MJ (1988) Nutrition and the respiratory muscles. Clin Chest Med 9 (2):337–348
90. Arora NS, Rochester DF (1982) Effect of body weight and muscularity on human diaphragm muscle mass, thickness, and area. J Appl Physiol 52:64–70
91. Arora NS, Rochester DF (1982) Respiratory muscle strength and maximal ventilation in undernourised patients. Am Rev Respir Dis 126:5–8
92. Armengaud MH, Rigaud D, Pariente R, Aubier M, Murciano D (1990) Effects of renutrition on respiratory and diaphragmatic function in patients with severe mental anorexia. Eur Respir J (suppl 10) (Abstract):196
93. Hoeppner VH, Cockcroft DW, Dosman JA, Cotton DJ (1984) Nighttime ventilation improves respiratory failure in secondary kyphoscoliosis. Am Rev Respir Dis 129:240–243
94. Garay SM, Turino GM, Godling RM (1981) Sustained reversal of chronic hypercapnia in patients with alveolar hypoventilation syndromes. Am J Med 70:269–274
95. Dunkin LJ (1983) Home ventilatory assistance. Anaesthesia 38:644–649
96. Marino W, Braun NMT (1982) Reversal of the clinical sequelae of respiratory muscle fatigue by intermittent mechanical ventilation. Am Rev Respir Dis 125:85
97. Bach JR, Alba A, Bohatiuk J, Saporito L, Lee M (1987) Mouth intermittent positive pressure ventilation in the management of postpolio respiratory insufficiency. Chest 91:859–864
98. Braun NMT, Marino WD (1984) Effect of daily intermittent rest of respiratory muscles in patients with severe chronic airflow limitation (CAL). Chest 85 (suppl 6):59s–60s
99. Cropp A, Dimarco AF (1987) Effects of intermittent negative pressure ventilation on respiratory muscle function in patients with severe chronic obstructive pulmonary disease. Am Rev Respir Dis 135:1056–1067
100. Gutierrez M, Boroiza T, Contreras G et al (1988) Weekly cuirass ventilation improves blood gases and inspiratory muscle strength in patients with chronic air-flow limitation and hypercarbia. Am Rev Respir Dis 138:617–623
101. Ambrosino N, Montagna T, Nava S et al (1990) Short term effect of intermittent negative pressure ventilation in COPD patients with respiratory failure. Eur Respir J 3:502–508
102. Bach JR, Alba A, Mosher R, Delaubier A (1987) Intermittent positive ventilation via nasal access in the management of respiratory insufficiency. Chest 92:168–170
103. Elliot MW, Steven MH, Phillips GD, Branthwaite MA (1990) Non-invasive mechanical ventilation for acute respiratory failure. Br Med J 300:358–360
104. Brochard L, Isabey D, Piquet J et al (1990) Reversal of acute exacerbations of chronic obstructive lung disease by inspiratory assistance with a face mask. N Eng J Med 323:1523–1530
105. Roussos C (1985) Ventilatory failure and respiratory muscles. In: Roussos C, Macklem PT (eds) The Thorax, Marcel Dekker, New York, pp 1253–1279
106. Roussos C (1985) Energetics. In: Roussos C, Macklem PT (eds) The Thorax, Marcel Dekker, New York, pp 437–492
107. Sorli J, Grassino A, Loragne G, Milic Emili J (1978) Control of breathing in patients with chronic obstructive lung disease. Clin Sci Mol Med 54:295–304
108. Remmers JE, Martilla I (1975) Action of intercostal muscle afferents on the respiratory rhythm of anesthetized cats. Resp Physiol 24:31–41
109. Bellemare F, Grassino A (1983) Force reserve of the diaphragm in patients with chronic obstructive pulmonary disease. J Appl Physiol 55:8–15
110. Arora NS, Rochester DF (1982) Effects of chronic obstructive pulmonary disease on diaphragm muscle dimensions. Am Rev Respir Dis (Abstract) 123 (part 2):176
111. Arora NS, Rochester DF (1982) Effect of chronic obstructive pulmonary disease on sternocleidomastoid muscle. Am Rev Respir Dis (Abstract) 125 (part 2):252
112. Rochester DF, Braun NMI, Arora NS (1979) Respiratory muscle strength in chronic obstructive lung disease. Am Rev Respir Dis 119 (part 2):151

113. Santiago TV, Remolina C, Scoles V, Edelman NH (1981) Endorphins and the control of breathing. N Engl J Med 304:1190–1195
114. Scardella AT, Parisi RA, Phair DK et al (1986) The role of endogenous opioids in the ventilatory response to acute flow-resistive loads. Am Rev Respir Dis 133:26–31
115. Neubauer JA, Posner MA, Santiago TV, Edelman NH (1987) Naloxone reduces ventilatory depression of brain hypoxia. J Appl Physiol 68:699–706
116. Petrozzino JJ, Scardella AT, Krawciw J, Edelman NH, Santiago TV (1990) Effect of naloxone on spectral shifts of the diaphragm EMG during respiratory loading. J Appl Physiol 68:1376–1385
117. Scardella AT, Petrozzino JJ, Mandel M, Edelman NH, Santiago TV (1990) Endogenous opioid effects on abdominal muscle activity during inspiratory loading. J Appl Physiol 69:1104–1109
118. Melton J, Neubauer J, Edelman H (1990) GABA antagonism reverses hypoxic respiratory depression in the cat. J Appl Physiol 69:1296–1301
119. Scardella AT, Santiago TV, Edelman NH (1989) Naloxone alters the early response to an inspiratory flow-resistive load. J Appl Physiol 67:1747–1753
120. Tobin MJ (1990) Respiratory monitoring during mechanical ventilation. In: Tobin MJ (ed) Mechanical Ventilation. WB Saunders Co., Philadelphia, p 691
121. Hussain S, Marcotte JE, Burnet H et al (1988) Relationship among EMG and contractile responses of the diaphragm elicited by hypotension. J Appl Physiol 65:649–656
122. Farkas G, Roussos C (1982) Adaptability of the hamster diaphragm to exercise and/or emphysema. J Appl Physiol 53:1263–1273

Training and the Respiratory Muscles

B. Celli

Introduction

Maintenance of ventilation depends upon the ability of the respiratory pump to move air in and out of the gas exchange portion of the system, the lung. The respiratory muscles constitute a vital link in the pump and it is their contraction, during portions of the breathing cycle, that will change the anatomic configuration of the thorax and displace its components so that air moves in and out [1–3]. This chapter will review the effect of training on respiratory muscles, without loosing sight of their special relationship with the other components of the pump, the respiratory centers, the conducting nerves and the ribcage and abdomen. All these links must function in an orchestrated manner to guarantee effective ventilation at a low energy cost. The review will devote most of its content to chronic airflow obstruction (CAO) since this is the condition that afflicts most of the patients in whom training is considered and where most of the data has been obtained. Many of the concepts are nevertheless applicable to patients with other pulmonary (restrictive interstitial disease, lung cancer and lung transplant) and non-pulmonary (chest wall disorders, neuromuscular diseases, pre and post-operative treatment) conditions. A review is made of the little data that has been obtained from patients undergoing weaning with the hope that we can stimulate more research in this vital area.

Anatomical and Mechanical Considerations

The diaphragm is the best studied respiratory muscle [2]. Normally, it is thought to exert its inflating action on the ribcage by three mechanisms:

1. by using the abdomen as a fulcrum against which it leans exerting an expanding action on the ribcage,
2. by the vertical and downward orientation of its fibers and the curvature of its shape, and
3. the transmission of the increase in abdominal pressure during contraction to the ribcage through its zone of apposition [2–5]

It is thought that with the hyperinflation of CAO as the fibers become more horizontal, the curvature of the diaphragm decreases and this decreases its capacity to generate pressures [6]. Recent evidence suggests that the diaphragm adapts to the chronic changes of CAO by shortening the optimal length of its fibers, so that each bundle generates its maximal tension for that new length [7, 8]. If this is correct, the decreased diaphragmatic pressure generating capacity is due to mechanical derangement or to contractile dysfunction and not to simple length tension changes. The external intercostals, the parasternal part of internal intercostal and scalene are essential muscles of respiration, which are active even during quiet breathing in normals [9]. Their functional importance increases with the hyperinflation of CAO, since they appear to undergo less marked shortening and are at less of a mechanical disadvantage than the diaphragm [10]. Other important muscles are called "accessory" inspiratory muscles because they are inactive during quiet breathing in normal subjects, but because of their anatomic arrangement, may be inspiratory in action under certain circumstances. The sternocleidomastoid, subclavian, pectoralis minor and major, serratus anterior, upper and lower trapezius and latissimus dorsi hold and extrathoracic anchoring point (shown for same of them in Figs. 1 and 2) and a ribcage insertion, if they are fixed on their extrathoracic anchoring point, they may exert a pulling force on the ribcage [11]. Except for the sternocleidomastoid and pectoralis, the respiratory function of these muscles has not been fully studied. They are probably inactive during quiet breathing in normal subjects, but may be called to partake in ventilation during strenuous circumstances. This may explain the common observation that normal subjects will

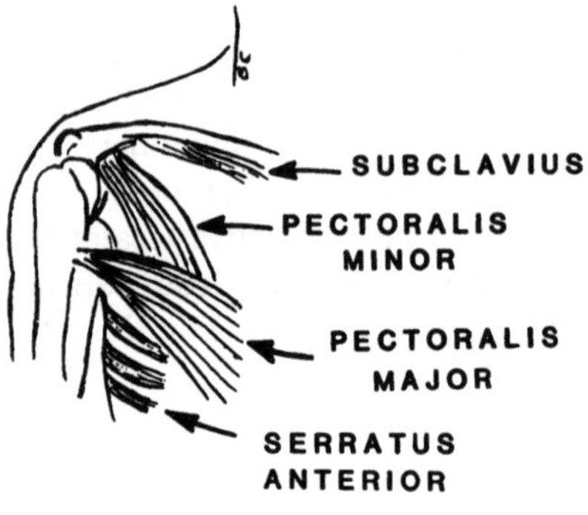

Fig. 1. Anterior shoulder girdle muscles that may partake in respiration when anchored extrathoracically

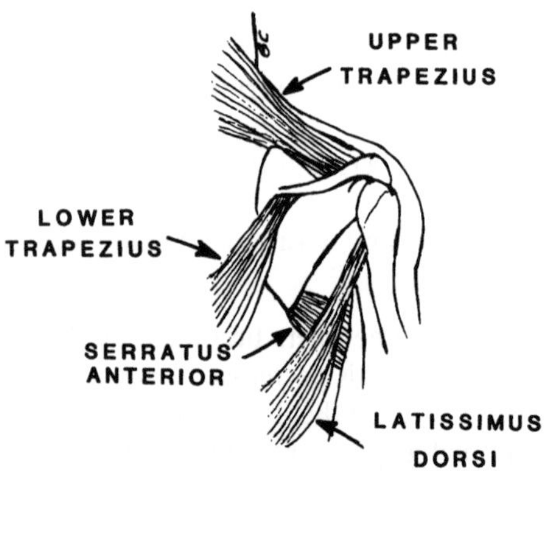

Fig. 2. Posterior shoulder girdle muscles that may partake in respiration when anchored extrathoracically

brace their arms after fatiguing exercise. Three recent studies confirm this observation. Banzett et al. [12] showed that normal volunteers could sustain a higher ventilatory target if their arms were braced on a table than if they were unsupported at the sides, Maestro et al. [13] showed that normal volunteers would have similar work loads when cycling with the arms elevated vs supported on the ergometer handle. We have shown that unsupported arm exercise may be more limiting than leg exercise and have hypothesized that this is due to derecruitment of these muscles from its ventilatory contribution during unsupported arm activity [14]. As we shall discuss later, these muscles become most important in patients with poorly functioning diaphragm and the understanding of their functions opens a therapeutic avenue through techniques different from generalized ventilatory muscle training.

The abdominal muscles are considered muscles of expiration. In as much as they oppose diaphragmatic contraction by helping generate abdominal pressure, they are also inspiratory. It is also thought that by contracting during expiration, they tend to decrease end-expiratory lung volume, a position in which the chest wall stores elastic energy that assists in the subsequent inspiratory effort [15]. We have recently shown that, with worsening of airflow obstruction, there is progressive recruitment of the abdominal muscles of exhalation [16]. It is unclear why patients with the most severe CAO would choose a breathing strategy that tends to close even more, already compromised airways. The best explantation is that by recruiting accessory muscles during inspiration and the abdominal muscles during expiration, the patients may shift work, away from an overworked and inefficient diaphragm. We have observed this to be the case during pursed lip breathing, whereby using this strategy, the patients are capable of breathing larger tidal volumes (VT) at similar transdiaphragmatic pressures.

Composition, Metabolism, Blood Flow and Coordination of the Respiratory Muscles

The diaphragm and other respiratory muscles are composed of striated muscle fibers. The fibers can be of 3 types: Type I or slow twitch oxidative (SO) have well developed oxidative enzyme systems and are fatigue-resistant. Type II-A or fast twitch oxidative glycolytic (FOG) have well developed oxidative and glycolytic enzyme system. They are more resistant to fatigue than the fast twitch glycolytic fibers but not as much as Type I-SO fibers. Finally, some fibers possess a well developed glycolytic enzyme system and have a fast twitch response to a stimulus. They constitute the fast twitch glycolytic fibers (FG) or Type II-B, and are more suited for fast, powerful activities not requiring endurance. The actual composition of most of the accessory muscles remain unknown. The human diaphragm contains approximately 55% Type I or II-A (fatigue-resistant) fibers, perhaps reflecting the enduring work it has to perform through an individual's life [17]. During quiet breathing in normals only a fraction the fibers (presumably most Type I fibers) are used. With progressive efforts (loads) more fibers are recruited so that training involves the loading of muscles so that the fibers may hypertrophy (strength), or change its composition to one that is more fatigue resistant (endurance).

Very important in training is the state of blood flow and energy supply since it is believed that imbalances in energy supply and demand result in fatigue. Most of what is known concerns the diaphragm. Like the heart, diaphragmatic perfusion occurs preferentially during relaxation and decreases during contraction, even though the diaphragm is supplied by a well developed system that is arranged to minimize the decrease in blood flow during inspiration. Two factors determine the contracting compromise of the diaphragm during breathing. The duration of contraction or duty cycle, which can be expressed as the ratio of inspiratory time to total cycle time (TI/Ttot) and the load which can be inferred by relating the pressure needed to perform the ventilatory effort, as a function of the maximal pressure that the muscle can generate. The latter relationship have been defined as Pdi/Pdi_{max} for the diaphragm or PI/Pi_{max} for the sum of the inspiratory pressure measured at the mouth. The product of both ratios has been termed tension time index (TTi) and in the case of the diaphragm, has been shown to relate to electromyographic and other signals of muscle fatigue [18]. It follows that training should also be aimed at changing the above mentioned factors: decrease PI, increase Pi_{max} or decrease contraction time. If successful, this sould result in improved muscle function and fatigue resistance. On the other hand, the possibility exists that excessive overload (of already loaded muscles) may lead to more dysfunction and perhaps overt fatigue. Finally, if overt fatigue were present, the best therapeutic avenue is rest, so that the muscle may recover.

Neural Control, Coordination

The diaphragm and the other respiratory muscles are innervated by a wide array of motor neurons that range from cranial nerve 11 (C–11) to lumbar roots L2–L3. The respiratory cycle is regulated by a complex series of centrally organized neurons. This complex arrangement maintains rhythmic breathing that goes usually unnoticed, but can be voluntarily overridden by cortical connection. Since we only use primarily the diaphragm, the scalene and some intercostals to quiet breath, the system is capable to function without problems. Some of the respiratory muscles serve other purposes. Upper torso and shoulder girdle muscles partake in positioning of the upper chest and upper extremity, while the diaphragm and muscles of the abdomen partake in the generation of sound (speech, singing), cough, defecation and parturition. It has been postulated that the autonomic and voluntary ventilatory pathways are different. Along the same line, studies in humans and animals show that the respiratory and tonic functions of these muscles are driven from different central nervous areas and integrated at the spinal level [19, 20]. In patients in whom some of these muscles are partaking in respiration to be able to perform non-ventilatory work, they must maintain a high degree of coordination. Either because of the load or because of competing central integration, muscle function may become dyscoordinated and result in dysfunction. We have shown this to occur in patients with CAO when asked to perform unsupported arm exercise. We studied a group of 12 patients with severe CAO (mean $\pm$ SD, FEV_1 of 0.68 ± 0.21 l) during unsupported arm exercise and compared the results with exercise performed in a leg cycle ergometer. Even though peak $\dot{V}O_2$, $\dot{V}E$ and heart rate were lower for arm exercise than leg ergometry, patients stopped arm exercise earlier. Arm, but not leg, exercise was associated with development of thoracoabdominal dyssynchrony, that was not due to diaphragmatic fatigue since maximal post exercise Pdi fell by the same degree in both exercises. We postulated that unsupported arm exercise leads to early fatigue of the muscles involved in arm positioning and that dyssynchrony between ribcage and diaphragm-abdomen may be caused by the competing output of the various driving centers that control rhythmic respiratory and tonic activities of the accessory ventilatory muscles and the diaphragm [14]. This dyssynchrony may be perceived as dyspnea. Its occurrence has been observed in normal subjects made to breath against resistive loads and in patients with CAO breathing during voluntary hyperventilation [21]. Thus, training should include considerations regarding the composition, the energy and blood supply, the pattern of contraction and the anatomic arrangement of the respiratory muscles.

From this review, it is clear that training may involve several different approaches and that perhaps simply associating it with strength or endurance training is too limiting and simplistic.

We shall now review the following concepts:

Respiratory muscle function and exercise conditioning
- Leg exercise
- Arm exercise
- Breathing coordination retraining

Respiratory muscle function: specific strength and endurance training.

Respiratory Muscle Function and Exercise Conditioning

Leg exercise conditioning. It is generally accepted that exercise conditioning diminishes dyspnea, improves exercise performance and improves quality of life. Table 1 shows two randomized studies in which control groups were included. There were no changes in strength of quadriceps, minute ventilation (VE) but there was a significant increase in 12 minute walking distance and peak oxygen uptake [22, 23]. These studies are important because they had a control group and the training only involved gradual inpatient and outpatient exercise. The study by Sinclair et al. [22] showed a significant increase in FVC, and it is only speculative whether this im-

Table 1. Controlled studies of patients with chronic airflow obstruction

Author	No. Patients	Duration	Course	Results
Cockroft et al. [23]	18 T	Daily	16 Weeks	↑12 MW. ↑VO_2
	16 C	—	—	No change
Sinclair and Ingram [22]	17 T	Daily	40 Weeks	↑FVC. ↑12 MW
	16 C	—	—	No change

T = Treated; *C* = Controls; *12 MW* = 12 minute walk test; *FVC* = Forced vital capacity; *VO_2* = Peak oxygen uptake

provement may have been due to improved respiratory muscle strength. Numerous studies have used the untreated patients as their own control. Most of them have shown increased exercise endurance, but the mechanism for the improvement remain debatable. Some have shown a drop in heart rate at similar work level, a hallmark of training effect, perhaps through a decrease in exercise lactate level [24, 25]. Other studies have not found changes in maximum oxygen uptake, decreases in heart rate or lactate at similar work rate. The study by Belman and Kendregan [26] is interesting since the patients had muscle biopsy specimens taken from the trained limbs. They found no decrease in heart rate for the same work load as represented by $\dot{V}O_2$, no change in the muscle biopsy enzyme content. Nevertheless, they observed improved exercise endurance, that they concluded, was not due to improved cardiovascular or local muscle performance. None of these studies evaluated respiratory muscle function but it is reasonable to assume no change, since in most of the studies in which it was measured, no changes were observed in FVC, a test that depends extent, on respiratory muscle strength.

Arm exercise. Much less information exists on the consequences of arm training on respiratory function even though many of the shoulder girdle muscles have a dual (respiratory and postural) function. Tangri and Wolf [27] used a pneumobelt to study 7 patients with COPD and showed that they developed an irregular and rapid pattern of breathing with unsupported arm activities (tying shoes, brushing teeth). After the exercise, they breathed deeper. We have documented dyssynchron-

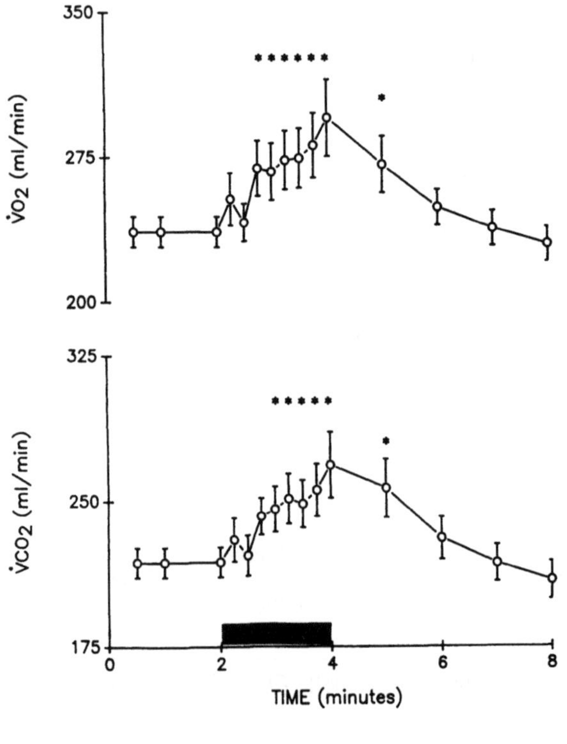

Fig. 3. The oxygen uptake ($\dot{V}O_2$) and carbon dioxide output ($\dot{V}CO_2$) increase in patients with chronic airflow obstruction when they elevate the arm to shoulder level (shaded area). Both values normalize after 1 min of arm down position

ous thoracoabdominal motions during arm exercise in patients with severe airflow obstruction, that is not due to diaphragmatic fatigue [14]. We have also evaluated ventilatory muscle function during simple arm elevation, arm exercise and before and after training. Martinez et al. [16] in our lab evaluated the metabolic and respiratory consequences of simple arm elevation to a 90° angle at shoulder level in patients with CAO. The results shown in Fig. 3 shows a significant increase in $\dot{V}O_2$, $\dot{V}CO^2$. There were similar increase in pulse and V_E. When ventilatory muscle recruitment was evaluated using continuous recording of end-oesophageal (Ppl) abdominal (Pg) and transdiaphragmatic (Pdi) pressures, there is a shift in the contribution to ventilation by the different muscle groups (Fig. 4). There is increased diaphragmatic and abdominal muscle use and lesser contribution by the inspiratory muscles of the ribcage. This shift is also present during unsupported arm exercise. We postulated that the reason for this shift is the recruitment of some of the muscles of the shoulder girdle to help position the arm with a decrease in their contribution to ventilation. There also is recruitment of abdominal and torso muscles to help maintain arm position. From this analysis, it follows that arm training, aimed at allowing the arms to perform more work, or to decrease the ventilatory requirement for the same work, could result in improved capacity to perform activities of daily living and perhaps in the inspiratory muscle function of those muscles of the shoulder girdle that have a dual function. This possibility has been raised by others. There are several studies that have utilized both arm and leg training and have shown that the addition of arm training results in improved performance and that

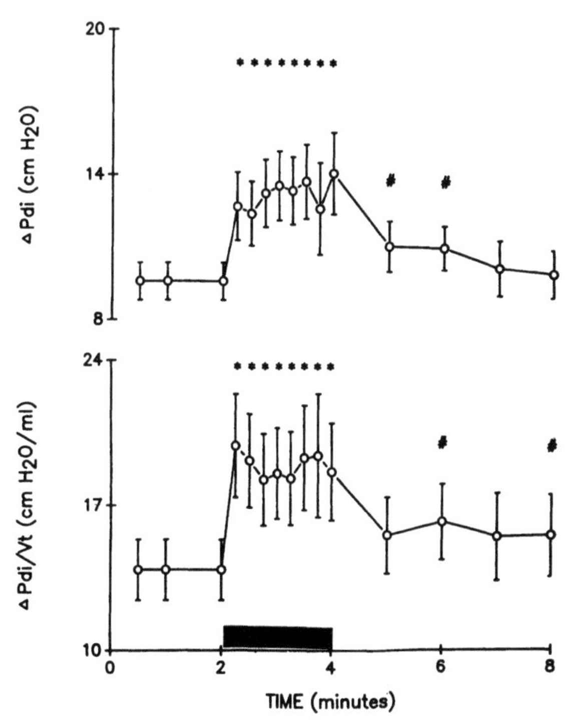

Fig. 4. The upper panel shows that the changes in transdiaphragmatic pressures (ΔPdi) increases significantly during arm elevation (shaded area) in patients with CAO. The lower panel indicate that the changes were not only due to increases in tidal volume (VT) since the ΔPdi/VT value increased significantly during arm elevation

for the most part the improved performance is task specific (Table 2). One of the studies included 6 patients who underwent upper limb exercises only and there were no differences in pulmonary functions, maximal inspiratory and expiratory pressures and respiratory muscle endurance [28]. In contrast, Keens et al [29] studied a group of cystic fibrosis patients with upper extremity exercise consisting of swimming and rowing and observed increases in maximum sustained ventilatory capacity that was similar in his group to the affect achieved by hyperventilatory isocapneic respiratory muscle training. In a very important study, Ries et al. [30] randomized patients to two forms of arm exercise, gravity resistance exercise (GR) which were low resistance high repetition in nature and prospective neuromuscular facilitation (PNF), which involved lower frequency, progressive resistance training. The control group received the educational component of the program and all patients underwent walking training. With upper extremity training, there was improvement in exercise tolerance with a decrease in the perception of effort for the task. The authors observed no improvement in respiratory muscle function as measured by

Table 2. Controlled studies of arm exercise in patients with chronic obstructive lung disease

Authors	# Patients	Duration	Course	Type	Results
Keens et al. [29]	7 Arms	1.5 hr qd	4 wks	Swimming/ Canoeing	↑VME (56%)
	4 VMT	15 min qd	4 wks	VMT	↑VME (52%)
	4 Control	—	—	VMT	↑VME (22%)
Belman and Kendregan [26]	8 Arms	20 min 4×Wk	6 wks	Arm ergometry	↑Arm cycle No ↑PFT
	7 Legs	20 min 4×Wk	6 wks	Cycle ergometry	↑Leg cycle No ↑PFT
Lake et al. [28]	6 Arms	1 hr 3×Wk	8 wks	Several types	No change PI_{max} VME
	6 Legs	1 hr 3×Wk	8 wks	Walking	No change PI_{max} VME
	7 Arms & Legs	1 hr 3×Wk	8 wks	Combined	No change PI_{max} VME
Ries et al. [30]	8 Gravity Resistance Arms	15 min qd	6 wks	Low resistance High repetition	↑Arm endurance ↓Dyspnea
	9 Neuro-muscular Facilitation Arms	15 min qd	6 wks	Weight lifts	↑Arm endurance ↓Dyspnea
	11 Controls	—	6 wks	Walk	No change
Epstein et al. [31]	13 Arm	30 min qd	8 wks	UAE	↓$\dot{V}O_2$ and $\dot{V}E$ for arm elevation No ↑PI_{max}
	10 VMT	30 min qd	8 wks	VMT	↑PI_{max} and VME

VMT = Ventilatory muscle training; *VME* = Ventilatory muscle endurance; *PFT* = Pulmonary function tests; PI_{max} = Maximal inspiratory pressure

the size of the orifice that the patients could tolerate a resistive breathing run. We have shown that 8 weeks of 3 times weekly unsupported arm exercise results in significant decreased in $\dot{V}E$, $\dot{V}O_2$ and $\dot{V}CO_2$ for simple arm elevation [31], with no changes in maximum transdiaphragmatic pressure and pulmonary functions. Our results shown in Fig. 5 indicate a significant drop in the ventilatory and metabolic cost of simple arm elevation and may help explain the improvement in endurance reported by most. We have recently completed a study of 24 patients randomly assigned to unsupported arm training or to ventilatory muscle training as the only forms of exercise. The patients in the arm training group manifested a significant lower rise in $\dot{V}O_2$ and $\dot{V}E$ with arm elevation that was not seen with the ventilatory muscle training group. There were no changes in PI_{max} or respiratory muscle endurance. More interestingly, the decrease in VE for arm elevation was due to a decrease in respiratory rate and work of breathing. In summary, arm exercise results in improved performance in arm acitivities and a drop in metabolic and ventilatory requirements for similar arm activities. Some studies indicate an improvement in respiratory muscle endurance, but more research is needed in this important area.

Coordination. If it is not the usual cardiovascular response that is responsible for the improved exercise performance seen after rehabilitation, then what are the possible reasons? As discussed in the introduction, the breathing apparatus is complex and more so, the neuromuscular array that make possible pressure generation during ventilation. In patients with COPD, as the diaphragm becomes impaired, more and more accessory muscles increase their contribution to ventilation even during quiet breathing. The system is further stressed during exercise and in many patients

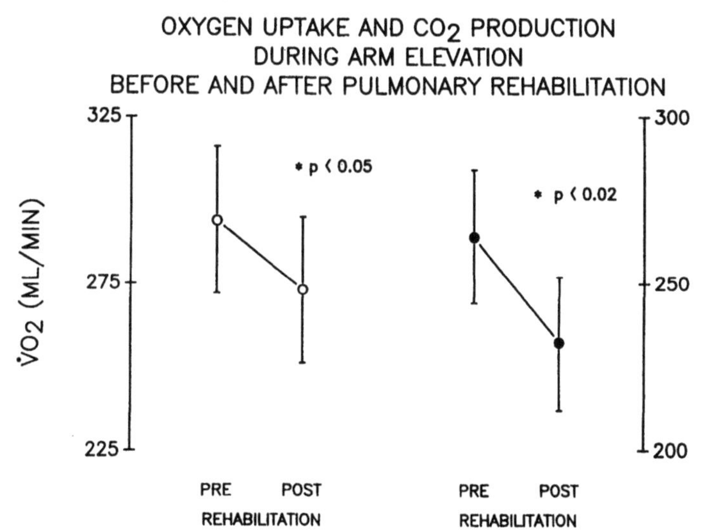

Fig. 5. Pulmonary rehabilitation did not improve forced expiratory volume in 1 sec (FEV_1), Functional residual capacity (FRC) and maximal transdiaphragmatic pressure (Pdi_{max}) in 14 patients with CAO

$\dot{V}E$ during peak exercise may exceed MVV. It is known that patients with COPD stop exercising because of dyspnea and recent evidence indicate that dyspnea relates better to respiratory muscle function than to airflow obstruction [16, 32–34]. It has been shown that dyspnea increases, as the ratio between the pressure needed to ventilate and the maximal pressure that the muscles can generate (Pdi/Pdi_{max}) decreases. It also increases with increases in the duration of the contraction (TI/Ttot) and respiratory frequency. Since these are also the factors that have been shown to be associated with EMG evidence of muscle fatigue, changes in any of them may help explain the observed increase or decrease in exercise performance after training. Finally, dyspnea may relate to recruitment of accessory ribcage and neck muscles, specially if their contraction is dyssynchronous with the diaphragm as shown in Fig. 6 [35]. With this in mind, it seems reasonable to postulate treatment goals that may result in improved respiratory muscle performance with systemic (legs, arms, etc.) or even specific (ventilatory muscle training) training. They are:

1. Reduction in inspiratory forces during breathing;
2. Increases in maximal inspiratory pressures;
3. Shortening of inspiratory time;
4. A decrease in respiratory frequency;
5. Better coordination among the different respiratory muscles.

It does not seem as if decreased load is a mechanism likely to occur since in most

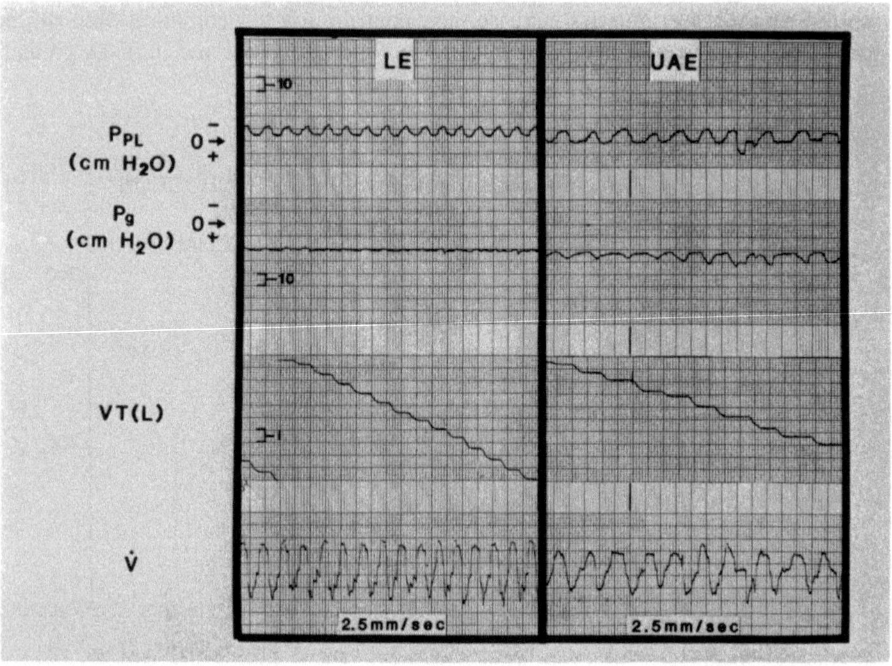

Fig. 6. Tracings of endoesophageal (Ppl), gastric (Pg), volume (VT and flow ($\dot{V}$) in a patient with CAO during leg (LE) and unsupported arm (UAE) exercise at the same volume. UAE resulted in increased diaphragm-abdomen contribution to pressure generation and there was development of irregular dyssynchronous thoraco-abdominal excursions

studies, systemic training does not change pulmonary functions. Similarly, results from a limited numbers of study where this has been measured, respiratory muscle strength, is not increased. Figure 7 shows the lack of change in either PFT's or Pdi_{max} after rehabilitation including leg and arm exercise in a group of 14 patients with CAO. We shall then review data that suggest that it may be through the last 2 mechanisms (decrease in respiratory frequency and/or better coordination of different respiratory muscles) that systemic training in COPD may result in improved exercise endurance and perhaps respiratory muscle function. Casciari et al. [36] studied 22 patients with COPD (FEV_1/FVC less than 0.50) before, during and after 9 weeks of rehabilitation that included exercise on a treadmill 3 times weekly. At the end of 6 weeks, 12 of the patients continued to exercise and served as controls. In contrast, the experimental group (10 patients) exercised and were trained with techniques aimed at improving breathing (breathing retraining). Although there were no changes in pulmonary functions, all patients improved their exercise per-

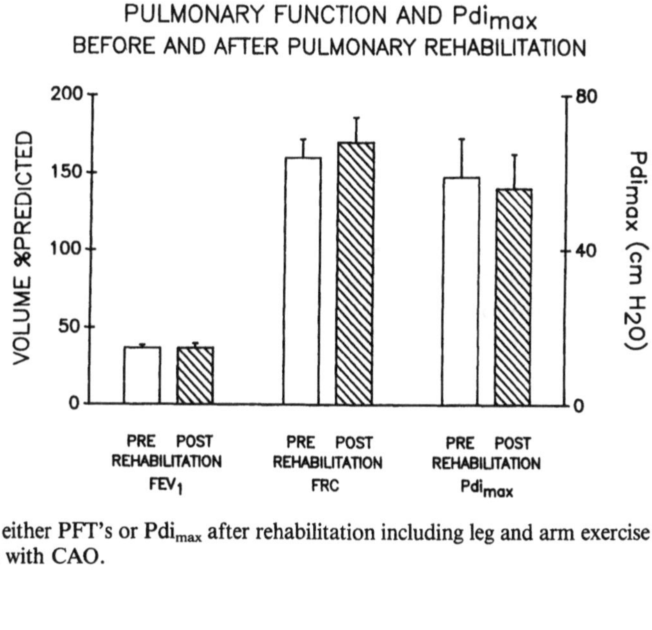

Fig. 7. Lack of change in either PFT's or Pdi_{max} after rehabilitation including leg and arm exercise in a group of 14 patients with CAO.

Table 3. Work of breathing, exercise endurance and maximal transdiaphragmatic pressure before and after pulmonary rehabilitation

	Endurance time (sec)	$F\delta$ Pesdt ($cmH_2O \cdot min^{-1}$)	Pdi_{max} (cmH_2O)
Pre-rehab	434	288	48
Post-rehab	512*	219*	52

* $p<0.05$

F δ Pesdt = Work of breathing as estimated by the pressure time index calculated from continuous recording of endesophageal pressure (Ppl); *Pdi_{max}* = Maximal transdiaphragmatic pressure

formance and their peak $\dot{V}O_2$. Of greater interest, the patients whose breathing was retrained, manifested a significantly larger increase in O_2 uptake and exercise endurance. Analysis of this results show an increase in VT and a drop in respiratory rate at rest and at end exercise. Cherniak [37] postulated that in patients with COPD, there is decreased efficiency of the respiratory muscles and that retraining may improve that efficiency. We [38] have recently studied some of these factors (Table 3). Work of breathing as determined by the pressure time integral of the excursions of the continuously recorded Ppl, was measured before and after rehabilitation in 16 patients with COPD. In there patients, there were no changes in pulmonary functions but there was a significant decrease in F δ Pesdt at the exercise isotime after rehabilitation. This drop was mostly due to a decrease in respiratory frequency. Finally, retraining in breathing techniques or pursed lip breathing that decrease breathing frequency, have been shown to result in increases in VT oxygen saturation and decreases in dyspnea.

Taken as a whole, there is limited but important evidence that systemic training improves some aspects of respiratory muscle function. It seems that most patients will return to an inefficient pattern of breathing if supervision is relaxed. The limited information available underscores the need for more systematic research where more aspects of respiratory muscle findings are better analyzed.

Respiratory Muscle Training

It has been 24 years since Leith and Bradley [39] first demonstrated that like their skeletal counterparts, the respiratory muscles of normal individuals could be specifically trained to improve their strength or their endurance. Subsequent to that observation multiple studies have shown that a training response will occur if there is enough stimulus. As discussed earlier, an increase in inspiratory muscle strength (and perhaps endurance) should result in improved respiratory muscle function by decreasing the PI/PI_{max}. Since reduced inspiratory muscle strength is evident in patients with COPD, considerable efforts have been made to define the role of respiratory muscles training in these patients.

Strength training. To achieve this goal a high intensity, low frequency stimulus is needed. Inspiratory muscles are trained by inspiratory maneuvers being performed against a closed glottis or shutter. Several studies have shown an increase in maximal inspiratory pressures when the respiratory muscles have been specifically trained for strength. Lecoq et al. [40] studied 9 patients (some of whom had COPD) and after 4 weeks showed a 50% increase in PI_{max}. Reid et al. [41] observed a 53% increase in 6 COPD patients after 5 weeks of training. Both groups noticed a smaller but significant increase in expiratory muscle pressure. The clinical importance of strength training for the respiratory muscles have not been explored and although theoretically important (decreasing PI/PI_{max}), it has not been shown to play a clinical role. It is nevertheless important to point out, that respiratory muscle strength has been shown to increase as a by product of the endurance training achieved with the use of resistive loads. It is then possible that some of the observed benefits reported after endurance training may relate to the increased strength.

Endurance training. This is achieved by low intensity, high frequency training programs. The programs that have been used are of 3 types: flow resistive loading, threshold loading and voluntary isocapneic hyperpnea.

In flow resistive training the load has consisted mainly of decreasing inspiratory breathing hole size. The load will increase provided that , VT and inspiratory time are held constant. Although most studies in patients with COPD have shown an improvement in the time that a given respiratory load can be maintained (ventilatory muscle endurance), the results have to be interpreted with caution since it has

Table 4. Controlled trials of ventilatory muscle resistive training in COPD

Author	# Pts.	Type	Frequency	Duration	Results
Pardy et al.	9	RB	BID	8 wks	↑E.T., ↑12 MW
[42]	8	PT	3×Wk	8 wks	No change
Larson et al.	10	RB	QD	8 wks	↑PI_{max}, ↑E.T.
[43]		30% PI_{max}	30 min		↑12 MW
	12	RB	QD	8 wks	No ↑ in PI,
		15% PI_{max}	30 min		End time or 12 MW
Harver et al.	10	RB	BID	8 wks	↑PI_{max},
[44]		6 level	15 min		↓Dyspnea
	9	RB	BID	8 wks	No change
		minimal	15 min		
Belman	8	RB	QD	6 wks	↑E.T.,
and Shadmehr			30 min		↑PI_{max}
[45]	9	RB	QD	6 wks	
		low intensity	(30 min)		
Chen et al.	7	RB	QD	4 wks	↑E.T.
[46]		(30 min)			
	6	Sham	QD	4 wks	No change
		(30 min)			
Bjerre et al.	14	RB	QD	6 wks	↑E.T.,
[47]		(45 min)			No ↑ exercise
	14	Sham	QD	6 wks	No change
		(45 min)			
Falk et al.	12	RB	QD	12 mo.	↑E.T.,
[48]		(45 min)			No ↑ exercise
	15	Sham	QD	12 mo.	No change
Noseda et al.	12	RB	QD	8 wks	↑E.T.
[49]		(30 min)			
	13	Breathing exercises	QD	8 wks	No change
Jones et al.	7	RB	QD	10 wks	↑Exercise end
[50]		(30 min)			
	6	Sham	QD	10 wks	↑Exercise end
	8	Exercise	QD	10 wks	↑Exercise end

RB = Resistive breathing; *PT* = Physical therapy; *ET* = Endurance time for loaded breathing; PI_{max} = Maximal inspiratory pressure; *BID* = Twice daily; *QD* = Once daily; *Exercise end* = Leg exercise endurance

been shown that endurance can be influenced and actually increased with changes in the pattern of breathing. Threshold loading has been employed and has been shown to result in some muscle training. This is done by assuring that at least the inspired pressure is high enough to ensure training, independent of inspiratory flow rate. Although breathing pattern is important (TI and respiratory rate) it is not as critically important. Many studies have not been controlled and it is very difficult to interpret the results as a product of the training. The controlled studies summarized in Table 4 have shown an increase in the endurance time that the ventilatory muscles could tolerate a known load [42–50], some of them have shown a significant increase in strength [43–45] and a decrease in dyspnea to inspiratory load [44]. In the studies where systemic exercise performance was evaluated, there was a minimal increase in walking distance [42, 43, 50]. It seems that the pressure required to achieve some training has to be at least 30% of maximal inspiratory pressure. From the data obtained, it is clear that VMT with resistive breathing, results in improved VM strength and endurance. It is not clear whether this effort results in decreased morbidity or mortality, or offers any clinical advantage that makes it worth the effort. In many of the studies, compliance was low with up to 50% of patients failing to complete the studies.

Ventilatory isocapnic hyperpnea is a training method by which patients maintain high levels of ventilation overtime (15 min, 2 or 3 times daily). The oxygen and carbon dioxide are kept constant in the breathing circuit. The results of an uncontrolled study showed that after 6 weeks of training, the patients with COPD not only increased their maximal sustained ventilatory capacity but also increased arm and leg exercise performance [51]. Two controlled studies also reported increases in MSVC in COPD in patients trained for 6 weeks, but their exercise endurance was not better than the improvement observed in the control group (Table 5) [52, 53].

It seems that respiratory muscle training results in increased strength and capacity of the muscles to endure a respiratory load. There is debate as to whether it also results in improved exercise performance or in performance of activities of daily living. From the respiratory muscle factors that may contribute to ventilatory limitation in COPD, it seems logical to predict that increases in strength and endurance should help respiratory muscle function but this is perhaps only important in the capacity of the patients to handle inspiratory loads, for example in acute exacerbations of their disease. It is less likely that ventilatory muscle training will greatly impact on systemic exercise performance.

Table 5. Controlled trials of ventilatory isocapneic hyperpnea in patients with COPD

Authors	# Patients	Type	Frequency	Duration	Results
Ries and	5	VIH	45 min	6 wks	↑MSVC. ↑Exercise
Moser [52]	7	Walking	45 min	6 wks	↑Exercise
Levine et al.	15	VIH	15 min	6 wks	↑MSVC. ↑Exercise
[53]	17	IPPB	15 min	6 wks	↑ADL
					↑ADL. ↑Exercise

VIH = Ventilatory isocapneic hyperpnea; *MSVC* = Maximal sustainable ventilatory capacity; *ADL* = Activities of daily living; *IPPB* = Intermittent positive pressure breathing

Ventilatory Muscle Training in the Patient in the Intensive Care

Very little objective data exists that allows a valid conclusion for this important question. It is apparent that as soon as a patient is left to breathe on his own (as during any form of weaning), his respiratory muscles are being retrained. Unconsciously, we have been using this methodology when we place patients on T-piece or low synchronized intermittent mandatory ventilation (SIMV), but we have not analyzed results in terms of this being a training method. More often, we think of training in terms of the addition of an external load above and beyond spontaneous respiration. There is very little experience in patients who have or are recovering from ventilatory failure. Belman reported improvement in two patients [54]. In a larger but still uncontrolled study, Aldrich et al. [55] recruited 30 patients with stable chronic respiratory failure for at least 3 weeks who failed repeated weaning attempts. Patients with active infections or unstable cardiovascular, renal or endocrine problems were not included. The authors also excluded patients with gross malnutrition (albumin <2.5 g/dl) and/or neuromuscular disease. The patients were intermittently trained by having them breath through one inspiratory resistor while the patients spontaneously breathed or were supported 2 to 8 breaths per minute with SIMV. In these patients, PImax improved from -37 ± 15 to -46 ± 15 cm H_2O while vital capacity increased from 561 ± 325 to 901 ± 480 ml. Of the 30 patients, 12 were weaned after 46 days of training (40% success). Because it is uncontrolled and used a very selective group of patients, these findings may not apply to most patients recovering from respiratory failure, and the success rate is not much different from those reported in weaning facilities that have not used VMT [56]. In spite of these encouraging reports, before ventilatory muscle training can be recommended as a form of treatment for patients with respiratory failure, more vigorous studies need to be completed.

Finally it is important to state that ventilatory muscle training, specially with resistive or threshold loading may be deleterious. It has been shown that breathing a high PI/PI_{max} or prolonged TI/Ttot may induce muscle fatigue [18]. Both factors are an intrinsic part of this form of training, hence it is possible that if an intense enough program is enforced, fatigue may actually be precipitated. This may help explain why some programs have shown a large non-compliance group when VMT has been used. This morbid consequences may be even more important in the most obstructed of these patients who may be in a borderline fatigue state.

Conclusion

There are more unresolved questions than absolute facts in the area of training and respiratory muscle function. A wealth of information remains to be gained if systematic scientific analysis is applied to answer those questions. More importantly, once the disease is fixed and chronic, we cannot change the lung itself, elucidation of the most effective, less costly and best tolerated form of training, may provide an alternate or complementary form of therapy to chronic oxygen, pharmacotherapy or lung transplant.

References

1. Roussos C, Macklem PT (1982) The respiratory muscles. N Engl J Med 307:786–797
2. Rochester DF (1985) The diaphragm: contractile properties and fatigue. J Clin Invest 75:1397–1402
3. Celli BR (1986) Respiratory muscle function. Clin Chest Med 7:567–583
4. Mead J (1979) Functional significance of the area of apposition of diaphragm to ribcage. Am Rev Respir Dis 119:31–32
5. Tobin M (1988) Respiratory muscles in diseases. Clin Chest Med 9:263–286
6. Sharp JT (1985) Therapeutic considerations in respiratory muscle function. Chest 88(2):118–123
7. Supinsky GS, Kelsen SG (1982) Effects of elastase-induced emphysema on the force-generating ability of the diaphragm. J Clin Invest 70:978–988
8. Farkas G, Roussos C (1982) Adaptatility of the hamster's diaphragm to emphysema and/or exercise. J Appl Physiol 53:1263–1271
9. De Troyer A, Estenne M (1984) Coordination between ribcage muscles and diaphragm during quiet breathing in humans. J Appl Physiol 57(3):899–906
10. Farkas GA, Decramer M, Rochester DF, et al (1985) contractile properties of intercostal muscles and their functional significance. J Appl Physiol 59(2):528–535
11. Celli BR (1988) Arm exercise and ventilation. Chest 93:673–674
12. Banzett R, Topulos G, Leith D, Natios C (1983) Bracing arms increases the capacity for sustained hyperpnea. Am Rev Respir Dis 133:106–109
13. Maestro L, Dohnage T, Avendano MA, Goldstein R (1990) Influence of arm position in ventilation during incremental exercise in healthy individuals, Chest 98(2):113(S)
14. Celli, BR, Rassulo J, Make B (1986) Dyssynchronous breathing during arm but not leg exercise in patients with chronic airflow obstruction. N Engl J Med 314:1485–1490
15. De Troyer A, Sampson M, Sigrist S, et al (1983) How the abdominal muscles act on the ribcage. J Appl Physiol 54(2):465–469
16. Martinez F, Couser J, Celli B (1990) Factors influencing ventilatory muscle recruitment in patients with chronic airflow obstruction. Am Rev Respir Dis 142:276–282
17. Sieck GC (1988) Diaphragm muscle: structural and functional organization. Clin Chest Med 9:195–210
18. Bellemare F, Grassino A (1982) Evaluation of diaphragmatic fatigue. J Appl Physiol 53:1196–1206
19. Moltke E, Skouby AP (1963) The influence of tonic neck reflexes on the activity of some muscles of the trunk in patients with asthma and emphysema. Acta Med Scand 173:299–305
20. Sant' Ambrogio G, Widdicombe J (1965) Respiratory reflexes acting on the diaphragm and inspiratory intercostal muscles on the rabbit. J Physiol 180:766–779
21. Sharp JT (1983) The inspiratory muscles in emphysema. Clin Chest Med 4:421–432
22. Sinclair DJ, Ingram CG (1980) Controlled trial of supervised exercise training in chronic bronchitis. Br Med J 1:519–521
23. Cockroft AE, Saunders MJ, Berry G (1981) Randomized controlled trial of rehabilitation in chronic respiratory disability. Thorax 36:200–203
24. Paez PN, Phillipson EA, Mosangkay M, et al (1967) The physiological basis of training patients with emphysema. Am Rev Respir Dis 95:944–953
25. Mohsenifar Z, Horak D, Brown H, et al (1983) Sensitive indices of improvement in a pulmonary rehabilitation program. Chest 83:189–192
26. Belman M, Kendregan BA (1981) Exercise training fails to increase skeletal muscle enzymes in patients with chronic obstructive pulmonary disease. Am Rev Respir Dis 123:256–261
27. Tangri S, Wolf CR (1973) The breathing pattern in chronic obstructive lung disease during the performance of some common daily activities. Chest 63:126–127
28. Lake FR, Hendersen K, Briffa T, et al (1990) Upper limb and lower limb exercise training in patients with chronic airflow obstruction. Chest 97:1077–1082
29. Keens TG, Krastins B, Wannamaker EM, et al (1977) Ventilatory muscle endurance training in normal subjects and patients with cystic fibrosis. Am Rev Respir Dis 116:853–860

30. Ries, AL, Ellis B, Hawkins RW (1988) Upper extremity exercise training in chronic obstructive pulmonary disease. Chest 93:688–692
31. Epstein S, Breslin E, Roa J, Celli B (1991) Impact of unsupported arm training (AT) and ventilatory muscle training (VMT) on the metabolic and ventilatory consequences of unsupported arm elevation (UAE) and exercise (UAEX) in patients with chronic airflow obstruction (CAO). (in press)
32. Cherniack NS, Altose M (1987) Mechanisms of dyspnea. Clin Chest Med 8:207–214
33. Killian KJ, Gandevia SC, Summers, et al (1984) Effect of increased lung volume on perception of breathlessness effort and tension. J Appl Physiol 57:686–691
34. Ward ME, Eidelman D, Stubbing DG, et al (1988) Respiratory sensation and pattern of respiratory muscle activation during fatigue. J Appl Physiol 65:2181–2189
35. Breslin E, Garroutte B, Kohlman-Carrieri V, Celli B (1990) Correlations between dyspnea, diaphragm and sternomastoid recruitment during inspiratory resistance breathing in normal subjects. Chest 98:298–302
36. Casciari R, Fairshter R, Harrison A, et al (1981) Effects of breathing retraining in patients with chronic obstructive pulmonary disease. Chest 79:393–398
37. Cherniack R (1959) The oxygen consumption and efficiency of the respiratory muscles in health and emphysema. J Clin Invest 38:494–499
38. Benditt, J, Pollock M, Breslin E, et al (1990) Comprehensive pulmonary rehabilitation decreases the work of breathing during leg cycle ergometry in patients with severe chronic airflow obstruction (CAO). Am Rev Respir Dis 141(2):A509
39. Leith DE, Bradley M (1976) Ventilatory muscle strength and endurance training. J Appl Physiol 4:508–516
40. Lecog A, Delhez L, Janssens S, et al (1970) Réentraînement de la fonction motrice ventilatoire chez des insuffisants respiratoires chroniques. Acta Tuberc Pneumol Bel 61:63–69
41. Reid WD, Warren CP (1984) Ventilatory muscle strength and endurance training in elderly subjects and patients with chronic airflow limitation: a pilot study. Physio Canada 36:305–311
42. Pardy R, Livingston R, Despas P, et al (1981) Inspiratory muscle training compared with physiotherapy in patients with chronic airflow limitation. Am Rev Respir Dis 123:421–425
43. Larson JL, Kim MJ, Sharp JT (1988) Inspiratory muscle training with a pressure threshold breathing device in patients with chronic obstructive pulmonary disease. Am Rev Respir Dis 138:689–696
44. Harver A, Mahler D, Daubenspeck J (1989) Targeted inspiratory muscle training improves respiratory muscle function and reduces dyspnea in patients with chronic obstructive pulmonary disease. Am Intern Med 111:117–124
45. Belman M, Shadmehr R (1988) Targeted resistive ventilatory muscle training in chronic obstructive pulmonary disease. J Appl Physiol 65:2726–2735
46. Chen H, Dukes R, Martin B (1985) Inspiratory muscle training in patients with chronic obstructive pulmonary disease. Am Rev Respir Dis 131:251–255
47. Bjerre-Jempsen K, Secher N, Kok-Jensen A (1981) Inspiratory resistance training in severe chronic obstructive pulmonary disease. Eur J Respir Dis 62:405–411
48. Falk P, Eriksen AM, Kolliker K, et al (1985) Relieving dyspnea with an inexpensive and simple method in patients with severe chronic airflow limitation. Eur J Respir Dis 66:181–186
49. Noseda A, Carpiaux J, Vandeput N, et al (1987) Resistive inspiratory muscle training and exercise performance in COPD patients. A comparative study with conventional breathing retraining. Bull Eur Physiopathol Respir 23:457–463
50. Jones DT, Thomson RA, Sears MR (1985) Physical exercise and resistive breathing training in severe chronic airways obstruction. Are they effective? Eur J Respir Dis 67:159–166
51. Belman M, Mittman C (1980) Ventilatory muscle training improves exercise capacity in chronic obstructive pulmonary disease patients. Am Rev Respir Dis 121:273–280
52. Ries AL, Moser KM (1986) Comparison of isocapneic hyperventilation and walking exercise training at home in pulmonary rehabilitation. Chest 90:285–289
53. Levine S, Weiser P, Gillen J (1986) Evaluation of a ventilatory muscle endurance training program in the rehabilitation of patients with chronic obstructive pulmonary disease. Am Rev Respir Dis 133:400–406

54. Belman MJ (1981) Respiratory failure treated by ventilatory muscle training (VMT): A report of two cases. Eur J Respir Dis 62:391–393
55. Aldrich TK, Karpel JP, Uhrlass RM, et al (1989) Weaning from mechanical ventilation: Adjunctive use of inspiratory muscle resistive training. Crit Care 17:143–147
56. Scheinhom DJ, Ho C (1991) Avoiding home mechanical ventilation; the regional weaning center. Proceeding International Conference on Pulm Rehab and Home Vent 3:A35

Pharmacotherapy of the Respiratory Muscle

M. Aubier

Introduction

The respiratory system consists of a gas-exchanging organ, the lungs and a pump that ventilates them. The pump consists of the chest wall, which includes the rib cage, the respiratory muscles, and the respiratory centers in the central nervous system which control the diaphragm and the muscles used to expand the chest wall during breathing. The pump is the working or active part of the respiratory system, the lungs being merely passively inflated when the respiratory muscles contracts. The pump is just as vital as the heart, since without it, the lungs would obviously be unable to function, and arterial blood gas homeostasis would not be maintained.

In the past few years, it has been shown that respiratory muscle dysfunction may occur in patients with chronic obstructive pulmonary disease (COPD) [1], as well as in patients with cardiovascular disease [2]. Since respiratory muscle dysfunction can lead to ventilatory failure, its recognition in respiratory diseases will have important therapeutic implications. In some instances such as acute respiratory failure (ARF), the primary goal will be to reduce the load imposed on the respiratory muscles. This can be accomplished by removing the underlying obstruction by using bronchodilators as in asthma. However, in chronic respiratory system disorders, such as COPD, it may be difficult to reduce the load on the respiratory muscles. Therefore, drugs that improve respiratory muscle contractility may prove clinically useful.

This chapter will deal with a new aspect of pharmacological treatment of respiratory insufficiency which is represented by respiratory muscle pharmacotherapy. It should be noted, however, that respiratory muscle pharmacotherapy is still in its infancy and evolving. We will therefore focus on the drugs that are proven to have a positive effect on respiratory muscles.

Elements of Respiratory Muscle Contraction

Respiratory muscle function can be modulated by acting at two levels:

1. the excitation-contraction coupling process, and
2. the energy supply to the muscles.

Excitation-Contraction Coupling

Among the group of skeletal muscles, the diaphragm presents some unique features. It must contract phasically during life and thus functionally appears to be closer to the myocardium than to limb muscles. In view of this functional similarity between the heart and the diaphragm, there should also be some similarities in their cellular contractile mechanisms and particularly, their excitation-contraction coupling processes. This hypothesis has been supported by recent experimental evidence. Indeed, although the central role of calcium in the excitation-contraction coupling of skeletal muscle is well established, the cellular mechanisms by which calcium is made available to the contractile proteins during excitation to elicit contraction of the muscle remain unclear. It is generally thought that the activation of the contractile elements is essentially independent of extracellular calcium [3], the cyclic nature of Ca^{2+} fluxes in skeletal muscle during excitation-contraction coupling being regarded strictly as intracellular and independent of extracellular calcium. In the cardiac muscle, on the contrary, the passage of calcium across the cell membrane is of major importance because without it there would be insufficient calcium from the sarcoplasmic reticulum to initiate contraction.

Recent studies *in vivo* [4] and *in vitro* [5] have challenged these classical notions (Fig. 1) It has been found that, in calcium-free medium, isolated diaphragmatic fibers obtained from rats behaved similarly to single papillary muscle fibers observed from the same animal. Indeed, a striking similarity was observed between diaphragmatic and papillary muscle fibers' contractile responses to extracellular calcium deprivation: in both cases complete twitch abolition was observed. On the contrary, no twitch abolition was observed with single soleus or extensor digitorium longus fibers, a slow and fast peripheral skeletal muscle, when exposed to 3 h

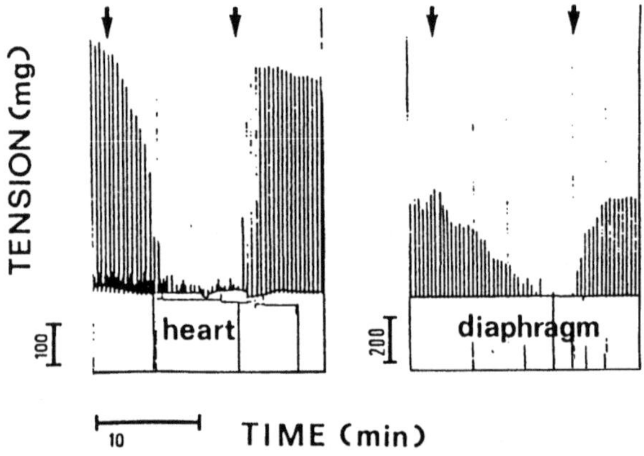

Fig. 1. Typical continuous recordings of papillary twitches *(left)* and diaphragmatic twitches *(right)* obtained during supramaximal stimulations of a single papillary and diaphragmatic fibers preparation during control (Krebs-perfusing solution) and during Ca^{2+} free perfusion solution. First arrow indicates time at which preparations were perfused with the Krebs solution depleted of Ca^{2+}. Second arrow indicates time at which preparations were reperfused with Krebs solution containing Ca^{2+}

of calcium-free medium. These data have also been confirmed in the dog *in vivo* [4] when the animal was rendered hypocalcemic by infusion of Ca^{2+} chelator (ethylene-glycolbis (β-aminoethylether)-N, N′-tetra acetic acid), which led to a decrease in ionized extracellular calcium. In these animals, a marked depression in diaphragmactic contractility was noted with hypocalcemia, whereas the sartorius, a peripheral skeletal muscle of similar histochemical profile, was not affected. Therefore, it appears that the diaphragm is a unique skeletal muscle that resembles cardiac muscle. These results provide new insight on the mechanisms of diaphragmatic contraction, notably by underlining the particularity of the diaphragm with respect to the other striated skeletal muscles. They also have important pharmacological implications: owing to the similarities between diaphragmatic and cardiac muscle fiber's reliance on extracellular Ca^{2+} it is conceivable that drugs or agents that exert a direct inotropic positive or negative effect on the myocardium may have similar action on the diaphragm.

Energy Supply

Besides the fact that respiratory muscle dysfunction may result from an impairment of calcium movement at the respiratory muscle cell level, respiratory muscle dysfunction will also occur when the supply of nutrients to the respiratory muscles is insufficient to meet the metabolic demand [6]. During breathing, the oxygen requirements of the respiratory muscles, and especially the diaphragm, are met primarily by increased diaphragmatic blood flow [7], which is related to cardiac output during unobstructed hyperventilation [8], hypoxia, and exercise [9]. It seems possible that when blood flow to the muscle is insufficient, lack of oxygen leads to a shift in anaerobic glycolytic pathways of high-energy phosphate generation. This shift would increase the acid accumulation associated with a given level of ATP turnover, impairing sarcoplasmic reticulum function and reducing the force generating capability of the diaphragm.

Some evidence [10] also suggests that blood flow may play a role in "washing out" the by-products of cellular metabolism. Thus, it is possible that increased diaphragmatic blood flow may increase the washout of toxic by-products of cellular metabolism concomitantly to an improvement in diaphragmatic energetics.

Whatever the mechanism, because respiratory muscle function, and particularly diaphragmatic function, are tightly linked to the level of muscle blood flow, it may be possible to improve diaphragmatic function by administering pharmacologic agents that augment diaphragmatic blood flow in patients in whom diaphragmatic blood flow is diminished or not high enough to meet the energy demands of breathing.

We will first review the drugs which act on the respiratory muscles and essentially the diaphragm, the main inspiratory muscle, by acting on the excitation coupling process. We will also review the drugs which improve diaphragmatic function by acting on its energy supply.

Drugs Acting at the Level of Excitation-Contraction Coupling

Digitalis

Digitalis preparations are well known for their inotropic effect on cardiac muscle, whereas they have practically no effect on peripheral skeletal muscle [11, 12]. This phenomenon could be accounted for by differences in excitation-contraction cou-

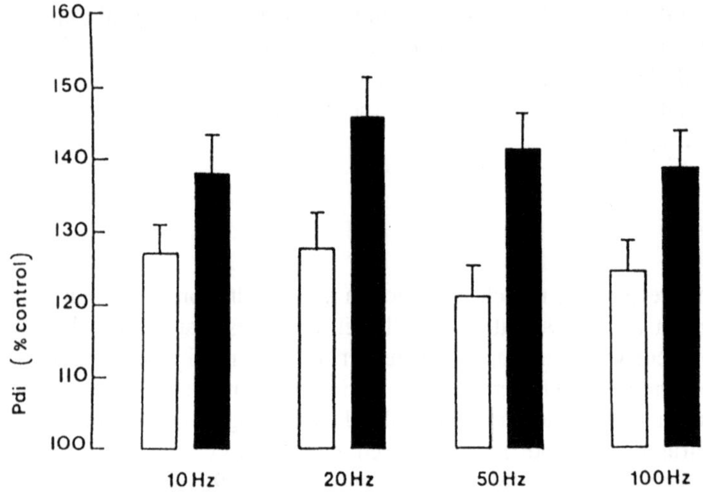

Fig. 2. Mean percent changes in transdiaphragmatic pressure (Pdi) for 10 dogs with diaphragmatic stimulation at 10, 20, 50, and 100 Hz, 60 min after administration of 0.04 mg/kg of digoxin (open bars) and 0.2 mg/kg of digoxin (closed bars). Pdi is expressed in percent of mean control value. Bars represent ± SE

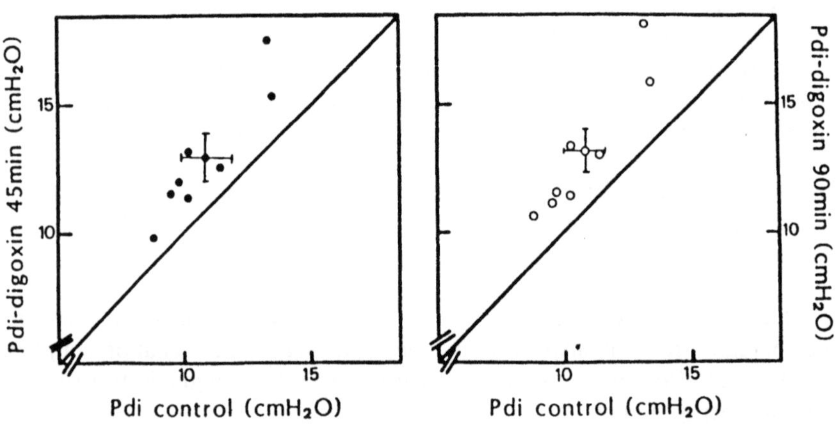

Fig. 3. Individual and mean changes in transdiaphragmatic pressure (Pdi) generated during phrenic stimulation 45 min (left panel) and 90 min (right panel) after digoxin administration in the 8 patients studied. The solid line represents the line of identity. Bars represent ± SE

pling in the two types of muscle. Indeed, digitalis is known to inhibit NA^+K^+ adenosine triphosphatase at the cell membrane level, which indirectly will augment cell entry of calcium [13]. This influx of calcium will then increase contraction strength by increasing the concentration of this cation in the vicinity of the myofibrils. Because the action of digitalis appears to be strongly related to cell membrane transport of calcium, and owing to the similarities between the myocardium and the diaphragm concerning the role of extracellular calcium in their contractile processes, recent studies have evaluated the effects of digoxin on diaphragmatic strength generation in dogs (Fig. 2) [14, 15] and in COPD patients (Fig. 3) during ARF. In both studies, a strong inotropic effect of digoxin was found without any change in cardiac output or diaphragmatic blood flow, which was measured in the animal study [16, 17]. This suggests that digoxin had a direct inotropic effect on diaphragmatic contractility. Furthermore, in the animal study, it was found that in the same animal, digoxin had no effect on a peripherial skeletal muscle, the sartorius, confirming the differences in the mechanisms of contraction of the diaphragm and the peripheral skeletal muscles. These data strongly suggest that, contrary to that in the hindlimb muscle, extracellular calcium is, as for the heart, necessary for diaphragmatic muscle contraction. This similarity in the importance of extra-cellular calcium in the diaphragm and the heart's contractile processes probably explains the inotropic effect of digoxin on the diaphragm.

Xanthines

Mechanism of action. In a recent study [18], is has been demonstrated in dogs *in vivo* that although theophylline, at therapeutic doses, increased the force of contraction of the diaphragm, its action was affected by prior administration of verapamil. This substance blocked the potential effect of theophylline, suggesting that theophylline may affect calcium channels located at the cell membrane levels, because verapamil is believed to inhibit the slow inward calcium currents. How this increased calcium influx produced by theophylline may increase muscle contraction is not yet clear. There are two possible explanations: because the quantity of calcium entering the cell during a normal action potential is insufficient to activate the contractile proteins directly, a theory of calcium-induced calcium release has been proposed. The theory suggests that the small amount of calcium crossing the sarcolemma during an action potential does not activate the myofilaments directly, but induces a release of calcium from the sarcoplasmic reticulum that is sufficient for activation. Alternatively, under some circumstances, the magnitude of calcium influx might be increased such that the sarcoplasmic reticulum could be bypassed and the contractile proteins activated directly [19]. The mechanism by which theophylline affects the cell membrane to increase the influx of calcium is not fully understood. Theophylline, which potentiates muscle contractility only in the presence of calcium in the medium, is a potent antagonist of adenosine; adenosine, however, has been shown to decrease calcium influx in frog skeletal muscle [20]. Therefore, it is possible that theophylline might block adenosine receptor. Convincing support for this hypothesis comes from a study [21] which found that the concentration of theophylline required to show antagonism to adenosine was substantially lower than that required to demonstrate other effects (for example phosphodiesterase inhibition and intracellular Ca^{+} translocation) that have been suggested to explain the drug's actions. Furthermore, it has been shown that the effects of theophylline and enprofylline, a xanthine derivative with no antiadenosine effect, had different actions on the human diaphragm, i.e. no inotropic effect was observed with enprofylline [21].

Effects of theophylline on respiratory muscle: *In vitro studies.* In isolated preparations, theophylline has been shown to strengthen the contractions of skeletal muscle that are elicited by direct and indirect electrical stimulation, an action caused by a potentiation of twitch tension [22]. This effect has also been well documented in isolated phrenic nerve diaphragm preparation of rats [23]. Indeed theophylline, in concentrations ranging from 25 to 100 µg/ml, was found to increase both tension development and the maximum rate of rise of tension during electrical stimulation of the diaphragm. The increase in tension of the nerve-stimulated preparation observed with theophylline was not significantly different from the increase observed when the diaphragm was stimulated directly. This suggests that theophylline has a direct inotropic effect on the diaphragmatic fiber. It should be noted that all the experiments that demonstrated an inotropic effect of theophylline on skeletal muscle or isolated diaphragm tissue were performed with doses much higher than the therapeutic doses used in humans. It therefore has been argued that theophylline had no effect on the diaphragm at therapeutic doses in humans or that the effects observed *in vivo,* are primarily the result of a secondary action of the drug, such as an increased muscle blood flow by metabolic effects, or both. One of the major problems with the *in vitro* preparations used for the experiments in this study is that large strips of muscle devoid of blood supply are used. This inherently limits the drug's diffusion into the tissues and could explain the lack of sensitivity of these preparations to a therapeutic dose of theophylline.

Recently, using an *in vitro* model of isolated diaphragmatic fibers, we have demonstrated that theophylline produced a dose-dependent increase in peak-twitch tension, [24] which, at a concentration of theophylline equivalent to a therapeutic dose of 15 mg/l, amounted to $111 \pm 1{,}5\%$ of control ($p < 0{,}05$). On the other hand, theophylline had no effect on a hemidiaphragm preparation until a dose of 250 mg/l was given. These findings demonstrate, therefore, that theophylline has an inotropic effect on isolated diaphragmatic fibers at therapeutic dose level and also suggest that the effects of theophylline on diaphragmatic contractility are caused by a direct action of the drug on the contractile properties of the diaphragmatic fibers. It should also be noted that theophylline has been shown *in vitro* to improve the contractility in fatigued skeletal muscles in similar way to that in the fresh muscles.

Human studies. In normal human subjects, theophylline, at the usual therapeutic dose (the dose used for a bronchodilator effect), has a potent effect on diaphragmatic contractility, confirming *in vitro* findings. During voluntary graded inspiratory efforts, the transdiaphragmatic pressure following aminophylline infusion increases significantly, with an average of 15% at any given electrical activity [25].

Theophylline has been known to be effective against skeletal muscle fatigue for many years. We recently extended this observation to the fatigued diaphragm. Fatigue was produced in two groups of subjects by resistive loaded breathing. Aminophylline was infused either before the fatigue run and maintained throughout the recovery period, or injected IV after the fatiguing procedure. When aminophylline was injected before the fatigue run, transdiaphragmatic pressure recovered rapidly after fatigue at all frequencies of stimulation. When aminophylline was administered after the fatigue run, theophylline (mean plasma level 14 ± 2 mg/l Pdi) increased significantly as compared to placebo [16].

Patients. The clinical benefit of theophylline in COPD patients is not clear-cut, however. Indeed, conflicting data are reported in the literature. Eaton et al. [26] reported that aminophylline did not affect dyspnea at rest and that it did not significantly improve 12 min walk or progressive cycle ergometry performance of COPD patients. By contrast, Nietrzeba et al. [27] found that aminophylline improved maximal inspiratory pressure and peak inspiratory flow rate as well as exercice performance in COPD patients, and Malher et al. [28] found that it had a benefical effect on the sensation of dyspnea. In acute exacerbations of COPD patients, no significant additional benefits were observed when theophylline was added to an otherwise standard treatment (inhaled metaproterenol, ampicillin, and supplemental oxygen). It should be noted, however, that these studies were generally performed on a few patients and over a relatively short time. To solve that problem, Murciano et al. who had previously demonstrated an effect on diaphragmatic contractility and fatigue on COPD [29] have recently studied 60 severe COPD patients [30]. All patients were studied in stable state and were severely obstructive, with a mean FEV_1 amounting $29 \pm 10\%$ of predicted and mean PaO_2, and $PaCO_2$ 61 ± 10 mm Hg and 51 ± 8 mm Hg, respectively, while breathing room air. Dyspnea was evaluated by a visual analog scale. Respiratory muscle performance was evaluated by the ratio of pleural pressure production of fatigue, the transdiaphragmatic pressure obtained after drug infusion exceeded preinfusion values. No significant change in the mechanical properties of the respiratory system was noted after Ppl over minimal pleural pressure (Pplmin) at functional residual capacity. The patients received sustained release theophylline or placebo during a 2 month period. This was a randomized cross-over single blind study with a wash-out period of 15 days between the theophylline and placebo periods. After 2 months of theophylline administration (mean plasmatic level 15 mg ± 3 mg/ml), minute ventilation (VE) increased from 10 ± 25 to 12 ± 25 l/min ($P < 0.001$). This increase in VE was secondary to a significant increase in tidal volume (VT), whereas respiratory frequency (f) was not significantly affected. These changes were accompagnied by a significant improvement in arterial blood gases, with PaO_2 increasing by 5 mm Hg ($P < 0.0001$), and $PaCO_2$ decreasing by 6 mm Hg ($P < 0.0001$) on the average. Dyspnea was reduced significantly and Ppl/Pplmin amounted 0.43 ± 0.17 and 0.27 ± 0.11 ($P < 0.0001$) after 2 months of placebo and 2 months of theophylline, respectively, suggesting that respiratory muscle reserve was markedly enhanced in these patients (Fig. 4). No significant change in lung function data was observed after 2 months of theophylline administration. At the end of the 2 month placebo period, no significant changes in any of the above parameters were noted. These data clearly demonstrate that in severe COPD patients, theophylline improves

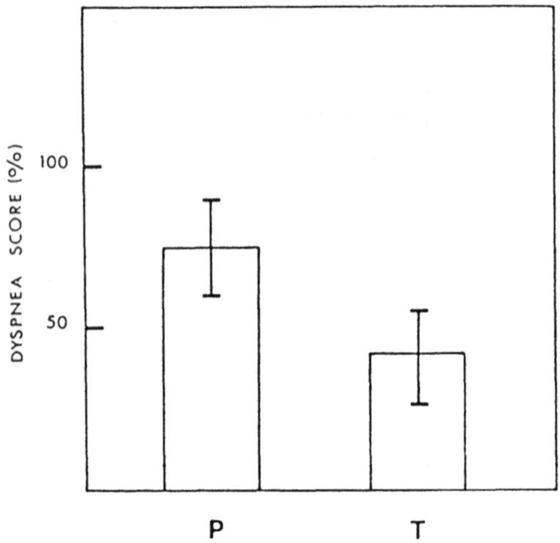

Fig. 4. Mean values in dyspnea score for the 60 patients studied after 2 months of placebo (P) and 2 months of theophylline (T). Dyspnea score is expressed in percent, 100% representing maximal dyspnea, and 0% no dyspnea. Bars represent ± SE

dyspnea and arterial blood gases, with these improvements being probably related to an enhancement of respiratory muscle performance. Long-term administration of theophylline therefore appears to be clinically useful in these patients.

Drugs Acting on Respiratory Muscle Energy Supply

Dopamine, a vasoactive drug widely used in patients with hypoperfusion syndrome, increases myocardial contractility, visceral and particularly renal and splanchnic blood flow, thus possibly also increasing diaphragmatic blood flow. We investigated the effects of dopamine on diaphragmatic function in patients with COPD during ARF secondary to pulmonary infection [31]. The changes in transdiaphragmatic pressure during electrical bilateral supramaximal stimulation of the phrenic nerve were evaluated in 8 patients with COPD during ARF. In 3 patients, changes in diaphragmatic pressure, cardiac output (CO) evaluated with a Swan Ganz catheter, and diaphragmatic blood flow evaluated by timed volume collections of left phrenic venous effluent (a catheter was introduced into the right femoral vein and advanced into the left inferior phrenic vein) were measured before dopamine infusion, 10 min after the onset of dopamine infusion (10 µg/kg body weight/min during 30 min) and 15 min after the end of dopamine infusion. Arterial blood gases and pH were measured before and at the end of dopamine infusion. Arterial blood gases and pH were maintained within normal range by mechanical ventilation (MV) throughout the study. With dopamine infusion, heart rate increased by 17% ($P<0.001$) and CO by 40% ($p<0.001$), on the average. The increase in CO was accompanied by a marked increase in diaphragmatic blood flow (30% on the average) in the 3 patients in whom it was measured ($P<0.001$) (Fig. 1). Diaphragmatic strenght also increased significantly during dopamine administration. Transdiaphragmatic pressure for an identical phrenic stimulation increased by 30% ($p<0.001$) on the average (Fig. 5). The changes in CO, diaphragmatic blood flow, and transdiaphragmatic pressure persisted throughout the infusion period; all values returned to control values 15 min after the end of dopamine administration. The results show that diaphragmatic function can be markedly improved by administering dopamine to these patients. The data also suggest that the beneficial effect of dopamine on the diaphragm is the result of increased diaphragmatic blood flow.

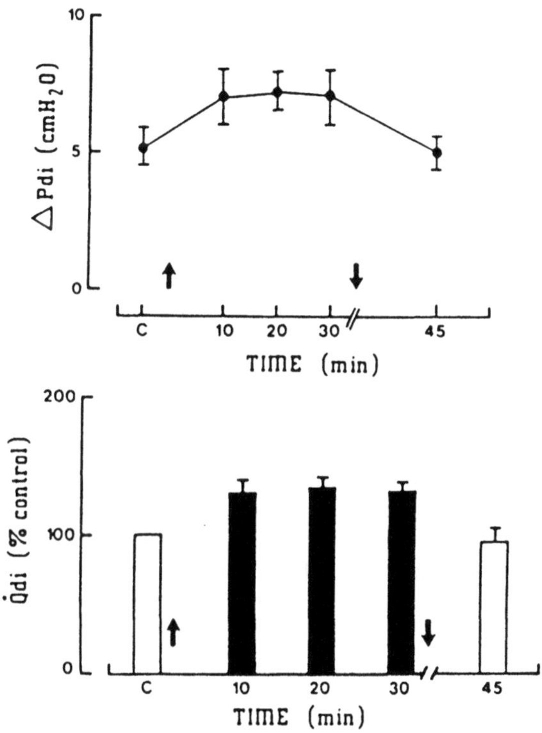

Fig. 5. The *top panel* shows the time course of the mean changes in transdiaphragmatic pressure (Pdi) generated during phrenic stimulation during control (C), throughout dopamine administration, and 15 min after the end of dopamine administration in 8 patients. The first arrow indicates the onset of dopamine administration, and the second arrow the end of dopamine administration. The open triangle represents variations in Pdi between control and dopamine. The *bottom panel* shows the time course of the mean changes in diaphragmatic blood flow (Qdi) during control (C), throughout dopamine administration for 3 patients. The first arrow indicates the onset of dopamine administration and the second arrow the end of dopamine administration. Diaphragmatic blood flow is expressed in percent of control values (i.e. before dopamine administration). Bars represent ± SE

Metabolic Disorders

Although an important goal in air pump failure is to improve the contractility and endurance of the respiratory muscles by pharmacological agents, another one is also to recognize and treat electrolyte disturbances which by themselves can compromise muscle function.

Acidosis

Metabolic acidosis. Metabolic acidosis has been shown to be an important determinant in the contractile process of skeletal muscle. Indeed, *in vitro,* an excellent correlation has been found between the degree of acidosis and the decrease in contractile force [32]. The same phenomenon has also been recently demonstrated in the dog *in vivo* [33].

Respiratory acidosis. Juan et al. [34] have recently studied, in normal subjects, the effect of acute changes in partial pressure of arterial carbon dioxide on diaphragmatic contractility. This was achieved by measuring the ability of the diaphragm to generate pressure at a given level of excitation by determining the relation between the electrical activity of the diaphragm and transdiaphragmatic pressure during a voluntary quasi-isometric inspiratory effort carried out at different levels of end-tidal carbon dioxide. They found that acute respiratory acidosis equivalent to an arterial carbon dioxide tension of about 54 mm Hg decreases the contractility and endurance time of the diaphragm in human beings.

Electrolyte disorders. How various electrolyte disorders influence the contractility of the respiratory muscles is still almost unknown. We recently studied the effect of hypophosphatemia, a frequent laboratory findings in patients with respiratory illness, in 8 patients with ARF who were artificially ventilated [35]. Diaphragmatic

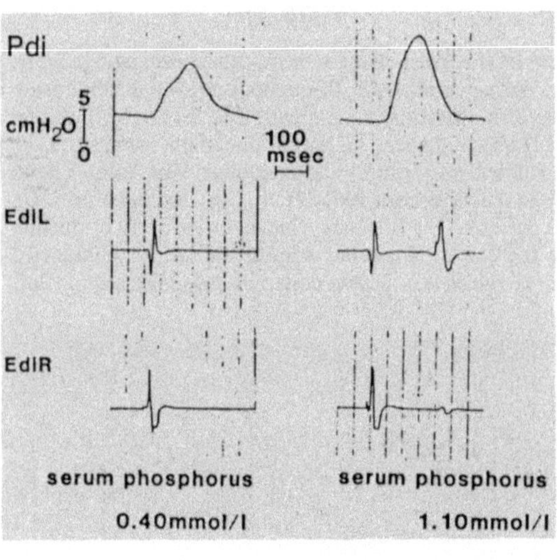

Fig. 6. Typical tracings of transdiaphragmatic pressure (Pdi) and electrical activity of the left hemidiaphragm (EdiL), and the right hemidiaphragm (EdiR) generated during phrenic stimulation in one patient before (left panel) and after (right panel) correction of hypophosphatemia

function was evaluated in each patient before and after correction of hypophosphatemia, the contractile properties of the diaphragm being assessed by measuring the transdiaphragmatic pressure generated at functional residual capacity during bilateral supramaximal electrical stimulation of the phrenic nerves. In all patients, the increase in serum phosphorus was accompanied by a marked increase in transdiaphragmatic pressure after phrenic stimulation, the mean increase in transdiaphragmatic pressure for the 8 patients averaging 70% (Fig. 6). These results clearly demonstrate that diaphragmatic function is impaired by hypophosphatemia, which may lead to weaning difficulties and thus may prolong artifical ventilation. This illustrates therefore, the importance of the treatment of metabolic disorders in the critically ill patients, disorders which may, by themselves, induce respiratory muscle dysfunction. Once all the metabolic disorders have been corrected, drugs which potentiate respiratory muscle contraction by bearing a direct influence on muscle contractility could be beneficial in patients with ARF.

Conclusion

Certainly many compounds may interfere with the contractile processes of the respiratory muscle and particularly the diaphragm. These compounds act by different mechanisms, either at the level of the excitation-contraction coupling process or/and by modulating respiratory muscle blood flow. A review of all the agents capable of improving respiratory muscle function is not possible because only very few compounds have been tested so far. However, because the respiratory muscles seem to play an important role in the pathogenesis of dyspnea and respiratory failure, further research in the pharmacotherapy of the respiratory muscles is certainly needed.

References

1. Rochester DF (1980) Respiratory disease: Attention turns to the pump. Am J Med 81:803–805
2. De Troyer A, Estenne M, Yenault JC (1980) Disturbance of respiratory muscle function in patients with mitral valve disease. Am J Med 69:867–873
3. Adams RJ, Schwartz A (1980) Comparative mechanisms for concentration of cardiac skeletal muscle. Chest 78:123–133
4. Aubier M, Viires N, Piquet J, et al (1985) Effects of hypocalcemia on diaphragmatic strength generation. J Appl Physiol 58:2053–2061
5. Viires N, Murciano D, Seta JP, Dureuil B, Pariente R, Aubier M (1988) Effects of Ca^{2+} withdrawal on diaphragmatic fiber tension generation. J Appl Physiol 64:15–19
6. Macklem PT, Roussos C (1977) Respiratory muscle fatigue: a cause of respiratory failure? Clin Sci Mol Med 53:419–422
7. Robertson CM Jr, Foster GH, Johson RL Jr (1977) The relationship of respiratory failure to the oxygen consumption of, lactate production by, and distribution of blood flow among respiratory muscle during increasing inspiratory resistance. J Clin Invest 59:31–42
8. Rochester DF, Pradel-Guena F (1973) Measurement of diaphragmatic blood flow in dogs from xenon 133 clearance. J Appl Physiol 34:68–74
9. Adachi H, Strauss W, Ochi H, Wagner HN Jr (1976) The effects of hypoxia on the regional distribution of cardiac output in the dog. Cir Res 39:314–319

10. Mortimer JJ, Magnusson R, Peterson I (1970) Conduction velocity in ischemic muscle: effect on EMG frequency spectrum. Am J Physiol 219:1324–1329
11. Moran N (1972) The effects of cardiac glycosides on mechanical properties of heart muscle. In: Marks BM, Weisler AM (eds) Basic and Clinical Pharmacology of Digitalis. Springfield, Illinois, Thomas, pp. 94–117
12. Smith TW, Maber F (1973) Digitalis. N Engl J Med 289:945–952
13. Katz AM, Repke DI (1973) Calcium - membrane interaction in the myocardium: Effects of ouabain, epinephrine and 3′5′-cyclic adenosine monophosphate. Am J Cardiol 31:193–201
14. Aubier M, Viires N, Murciano D, et al (1986) Effects of digoxin on diaphragmatic strength generation. J Appl Physiol 61:1767–1774
15. Kikuchi Y, Hid W, Shindoh C, et al (1987) Effects of digitalis on the diaphragm in anesthetized dogs. J Appl Physiol 63:277–284
16. Aubier M, Viires N, Murciano D, Seta JP, Pariente R (1986) Effects of digoxin on diaphragmatic strength generation. J Appl Physiol 61:1767–1774
17. Aubier M, Murciano D, Viires N, et al (1987) Effects of digoxin on diaphragmatic strength generation in patients with chronic obstructive pulmonary disease during acute respiratory failure. Am Rev Respir Dis 135:544–548
18. Aubier M, Murciano D, Viires N, Lecoguic Y, Pariente R (1985) Diaphragmatic contractility enhanced by aminophylline: role of extracellular calcium. J App Physiol 54:460–464
19. Potreau D, Raymond G (1979) Calcium-dependent electrical activity and contraction of voltage clamped frog single muscle fibers. J Physiol (London) 307:9–22
20. Prosdocini M, Bianchi CP (1981) Effect of adenosine on oxygen uptake and electrolyte content of frog muscle. J Pharmacol Exp Ther 218:87–96
21. Sawynok J, Thamandas KH (1976) Inhibition of acetylcholine release from cholinergic nerves by adenosine, adenine nucleotides and morphine: Antagonism by theophylline. J Pharmacol Exp Ther 197:379–390
22. Jones DA, Howell S, Roussos C, et al (1982) Low frequency fatigue in isolated skeletal muscles and the effects of methylxanthines. Clin Sci 63:161–167
23. Kentera D, Varagic VM (1975) The effects of cyclic N-2-0 dibutyryl-adenosine 3′5′-monophosphate, adrenaline and mainophylline on the isometric contractility of the isolated diaphragm of the rat. Br J Pharmacol 54:375–381
24. Viires N, Aubier M, Murciano D, Marty C, Pariente R (1986) Effects of theophylline on isolated diaphragmatic fibers: a model for pharmacological studies on diaphragmatic contractility. Am Rev Respir Dis 133:1060–1064
25. Aubier M, De Troyer A, Sampson M, Macklem PT, Roussos C (1981) Aminophylline improves diaphragmatic contractility. N Engl J Med 305:249–252
26. Eaton M, Green BA, Church TR, Mc Gowan T, Nievoehner DF (1980) Efficacy of theophylline in "irreversible" airflow obstruction. Ann Intern Med 92:758–761
27. Nietrzeba RM, Elliott GG, Adams TD, Yeh MP, Yanowitz FG (1984) Effects of aminophylline upon the exercise performance of patients with stable respiration. Eur J Resp Dis 20:361–367
28. Malher DA, Matthay RA, Snyder PE, Wells CK, Loke J (1985) Sustained-release theophylline reduces dyspnea in non-reversible obstructive airway disease. Am Rev Respir Dis 131:22–25
29. Murciano D, Aubier M, Viires N, Mal M, Pariente R (1987) Effects of theophylline and enprophylline on diaphragmatic contractility. J Appl Physiol 63:51–57
30. Murciano D, Auclair MH, Pariente R, Aubier M (1989) A randomized controlled trial of theophylline in patients with severe chronic obstructive pulmonary disease. N Engl J Med 320:1521–1525
31. Aubier M, Murciano D, Menu Y, Boczkowski J, Mal H, Pariente R (1989) Dopamine effects on diaphragmatic strength during acute respiratory failure in chronic obstructive pulmonary disease. Ann Intern Med 110:107–123
32. Fitts RH, Holloszy O (1976) Lactate and contractile force in frog muscle during development of fatigue and recovery. Am J Physiol 231:430–433
33. Schader JH, Juan G, Hawell S, Fitzgerald R, Roussos C (1985) Arterial CO_2 partial pressure effects diaphragmatic function. J Appl Physiol 58:823–829

34. Juan G, Calverey P, Talamo C, Schnader JY, Roussos C (1984) Effect of carbon dioxide on diaphragmatic function in human beings. N Engl J Med 310:74–79
35. Aubier M, Murciano D, Lecoguic Y, et al (1985) Effect of hypophosphatemia on diaphragmatic contractility in patients with acute respiratory failure. N Engl J Med 313:420–424

Nutrition and Ventilatory Failure

S.K. Pingleton

Introduction

Ventilatory failure results from a variety of etiologies including lung diseases, chest wall abnormalities and neuromuscular disorders. Malnutrition can also cause or worsen ventilatory failure. Adverse effects of malnutrition upon thoraco-pulmonary function that may cause ventilatory failure include impairment of respiratory muscle function, decreased ventilatory drive and altered pulmonary defense mechanisms [1]. This chapter will focus on the effect of protein-calorie malnutrition on the respiratory system with special emphasis on respiratory muscle function. Other nutritional disorders such as electrolyte abnormalities which also impact on respiratory muscle function will be discussed. Finally, the effect of nutritional repletion on respiratory system function will be detailed.

Malnutrition

Investigators in the late 1960's first noted the association between weight loss and increased mortality in COPD [2, 3]. More recently, weight loss was found in 70% of patients hospitalized with COPD and anthropomorphic measurements were abnormal in half of these patients [4]. Data from the recent large COPD population enrolled in the Intermittent Partial Pressure Breathing Trial evaluated the frequency of protein-calorie malnutrition in patients with COPD population [5]. Approximately 25% of the patients enrolled in the study were malnourished as defined by <90% ideal body weight. The frequency of malnutrition increased to 35% in those patients with severe airflow obstruction (FeV_1 <30% predicted). The study confirmed an independent effect of weight loss on mortality.

The frequency of malnutrition has also been examined in respiratory failure patients. Driver assessed nutritional status of patients with COPD in respiratory failure [6]. Ideal body weight, anthropomorphic measurements, and visceral measurements of nutritional status were less in respiratory failure patients than those from a control group of 18 patients without respiratory failure. They concluded malnutrition should be suspected in any patient with COPD and respiratory failure. In a preliminary study, nutritional status of 80 consecutive respiratory ICU patients was evaluated [7]. Weight loss (<80% ideal body weight) was noted in 24%. Anthropomorphic measurements of triceps skin-fold thickness and mid-arm muscle circumference were abnormal in almost one-half of the patients. Although poor nutritional status did not appear to predispose to the need for mechanical ventilation

(MV); malnourished patients who require MV had a significantly higher mortality than well-nourished patients requiring MV. Thus, malnutrition is a common problem in patients with chronic lung disease and acute respiratory failure (ARF).

Hospitalized patients may also experience deterioration in nutritional status during their stay. In a retrospective study of 26 patients, Driver and LeBrun [8] found inadequate nutritional support in 23. They suggest inadequate nutrition on an iatrogenic basis occurs in ventilated patients. Similar results were found when nutritional therapy was retrospectively assessed in respiratory ICU patients over a one year period of time [9]. Calorie, protein and carbohydrate requirements were met in only 70, 26 and 51% of ICU days, respectively. Patients with ARF are at risk for worsening nutritional status without appropriate nutritional support.

The Effect of Malnutrition on Thoracopulmonary Function

Poor nutritional status can adversely affect thoracopulmonary function by impairment of respiratory muscle function, ventilatory drive, and pulmonary defense mechanisms (Table 1) [1]. The adverse effects of malnutrition occur independently of the presence or absence of primary lung disease. However, malnutrition's adverse effects could be additive in some patients with ARF such as those with respiratory failure caused by COPD. In COPD, primary abnormalities of decreased inspiratory pressure and increased work of breathing are found. Inspiratory muscle weakness as assessed by maximal inspiratory pressure results from both mechanical disadvantage to inspiratory muscles consequent to hyperinflation and generalized muscle weakness [10, 11]. In COPD, inspiratory muscle weakness must be severe for hypercapnia to occur. In patients with myopathy, hypercapnia occurs when inspiratory pressure are less than one-third [12]. However, hypercapnia was found in 13 of 18 patients with COPD when inspiratory pressures were only less than half normal [13]. Thus, hypercapnia occurs with much less respiratory muscle weakness when other mechanical abnormalities are present that increase the work of breathing. While none of these studies have addressed the patient critically ill with COPD, they do suggest malnutrition may further compromise an already compromised lung function. Hypercapnic respiratory failure and/or difficulty in weaning from MV may be more easily precipitated in the malnourished patient with COPD than in the normally nourished patient with COPD.

In simple starvation or undernutrition, fat and protein are lost, but the loss of protein is minimized by reducing the need to use it as a source of energy [14]. Nitrogen loss is modified by mobilization of fat and enhanced fat oxidation is the principle source of energy in the starving individual. Some protein wasting does occur despite the availability of fat as a source of energy and it becomes markedly

Table 1. Adverse effects of malnutrition upon thoracopulmonary function

- Decreased respiratory muscle function
- Altered ventilatory drive
- Impaired pulmonary defense mechanisms

accelerated when fat stores are used up. In critical illness, protein catabolism occurs to provide energy. With inadequate caloric intake in critically ill patients, energy sources are derived from protein breakdown and gluconeogenesis. Of various protein "pools" available, the muscle protein pool is susceptible to catabolism to provide fuel [15]. Inspiratory and expiratory respiratory muscles, primarily the diaphragm and intercostals, are skeletal muscles and therefore susceptible to this catabolic effect. Because the diaphragm is the critical respiratory muscle, the following discussion will focus on it, although these considerations are generally valid for all respiratory muscles. It is important to note that little if any data exist directly examining respiratory muscle function and malnutrition in the critically ill patient with respiratory failure.

Malnutrition reduces diaphragmatic muscle mass in health and disease [16, 17]. Thurlbeck [16] correlated low diaphragmatic mass with low body weight in patients with emphysema. The diaphragmatic weight was lower than predicted from body weight, suggesting that additional factors are operative. In a necropsy study, Arora and Rochester [17] evaluated diaphragmatic muscle mass, thickness, and area in normal-weight patients dying suddenly, and underweight patients dying of a variety of diseases (Table 2). Body weight and diaphragmatic muscle mass were reduced to 70 and 60% of normal in poorly nourished patients. A further study quantitated the contribution of reduced diaphragmatic muscle mass to transdiaphragmatic pressures, an index of diaphragmatic muscle strength [18]. Compared with values in normal subjects, transdiaphragmatic pressures were reduced by 66%, whereas diaphragmatic muscle thickness was reduced by 25%. This suggests that transdiaphragmatic pressure is reduced in part because there is less muscle but also because the remaining muscle is weaker.

Animal studies confirm the loss of diaphragmatic strength in prolonged nutritional deprivation. In an *in vitro* hamster model where food was reduced by 33⅓% for four weeks, body weight was reduced to 75% of the control values [19]. Diaphragm weight and muscle thickness were similarly reduced to 73% and 70% of controls, respectively. Caloric restriction produced changes in diaphragm muscle fiber composition and muscle fiber size. The percentage of fast twitch glycolytic and oxidative fibers decreased (−4% and −2%) slightly. More dramatic changes were found in the muscle fiber size. The cross-section area of fast twitch fibers (Type II) were reduced to 77 and 76% compared to normal. The cross-sectional

Table 2. Values for diaphragm muscle mass, thickness and area

Category	Group	n	DMM	DMT	DMA
Normals	N	27	262 (49)	0.35 (0.05)	754 (123)
	M	6	432 (89)[a]	0.45 (0.05)[a]	944 (120)[a]
Patients	W	23	218 (65)[a]	0.32 (0.06)	684 (123)
	U	14	150 (48)[a]	0.26 (0.06)[a]	580 (90)[a]

DMM: Diaphragmatic muscle length; *DMT:* diaphragmatic muscle thickness; *DMA:* diaphragmative area; *N* and *M:* normal weight and increased weight subjects; *W* and *U:* normal weight and underweight patients, respectively. (From [17] with permission)

[a] $p<0.01$

area of slow oxidative (Type I) fibers was unchanged. Maximum isometric tension was reduced by 73% in undernourished controls. Likewise, using isolated diaphragmatic strips from rats, Lewis et al. [20] evaluated the contractile and fatigue properties of the diaphragm when food was restricted until the body weight of the nutritionally deprived animals was 50% of the controls. The diaphragmatic strength as assessed by peak twitch tension was reduced by 50 and 41%, respectively (Fig. 1). When these were corrected for diaphragmatic weight, no difference between malnourished and normally nourished animals were found. The shape of the force-frequency curve was generally similar between the two groups except at 5 and 10 pulses/sec where greater relative tension was produced in diaphragms from the nutritionally deprived animals.

These observations in the chronically malnourished state are explained on the basis of the relatively greater extent of fast-twitch fiber atrophy which was also found. The cross-sectional area of both fast and slow-twitch fibers was decreased, but the decrease in cross-sectional area was significantly greater for fast-twitch fibers (Fig. 2). This in effect would result in a proportional increase in the contribution of slow-twitch fibers to the contractile response. Because slow-twitch fibers contract and relax more slowly and thus tetanize at lower stimulation frequency, malnutrition would shift the force-frequency curve to the left. Interestingly, endurance time (defined as the time required for tension to fall to 50% of the control value) of diaphragms from nutritionally deprived animals was prolonged in nutritionally deprived animals (56 ± 13 sec) compared to controls (43 ± 4 sec) at 20 pulses/sec. The explanation for apparent increased fatigue endurance is not known with certainty; however, later work in an acute starvation model from the same laboratory found endurance tests were different after direct muscle stimulation as compared to phrenic nerve stimulation [21]. No difference in diaphragmatic fatiguability was noted in acute starvation after direct muscle stimulation while nerve stimulation resulted in an almost 30% decrease in the fatigue index. Acute nutritional deprivation appears to increase the susceptibility of the diaphragm to neurotransmission failure.

Drew et al. [22] also studied diaphragmatic function in a hamster model of chronic visceral leishmaniasis. Animals were divided into control, infected and ca-

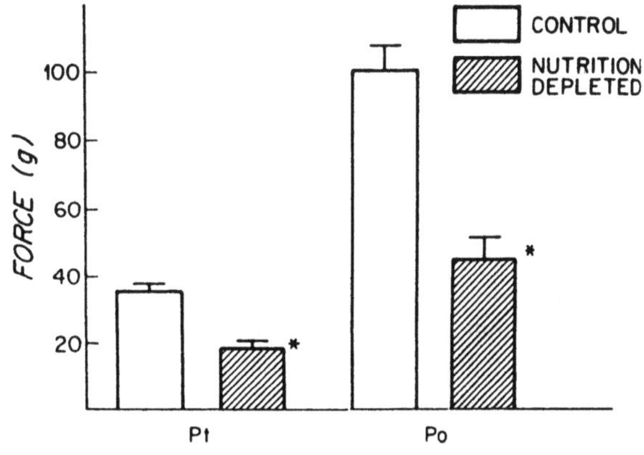

Fig. 1. Peak twitch (P_t) and peak tetanic (P_o) tension represented as mean force in g ± SE. Significant difference between groups ($P < 0.01$) (From [20] with permission)

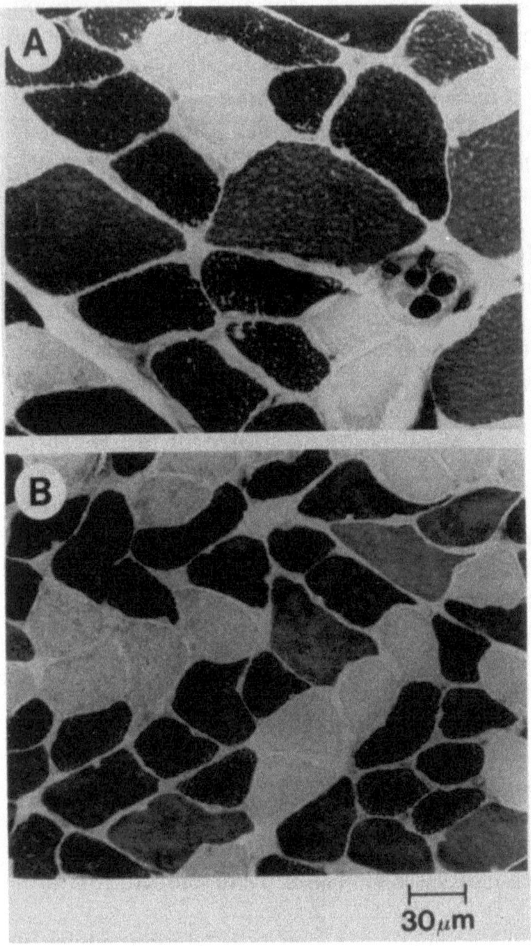

Fig. 2. Cross-sections of diaphragm muscle stained for myosin ATPase (alkaline preincubation). Darkly staining fibers are fast-twitch; lightly staining fibers are slow-twitch. The section shown in A is from a control animal and that shown in B is from a nutritionally deprived (ND) animal. Note that both fast- and slow-twitch fibers are smaller in diaphragm from ND animal. (From [20] with permission)

lorie-deprived group in an attempt to distinguish the skeletal muscle effect of a chronic wasting infection (7–12 weeks) as compared to those of simple caloric restriction. Diaphragmatic peak tetanic tension was decreased (50.8 ± 3.1 g) compared to controls (80.1 ± 3.1 g), but when normalized to muscle wet weight, tension was not different. Thus, in chronic nutritional deprivation leading to malnutrition, diaphragmatic strength is reduced in proportion to diaphragmatic and body weight loss. The reduction in diaphragmatic tension appears to be explained primarily by loss of muscle mass and cross-sectional area. The loss of muscle mass appears to represent a decrease in fiber size rather than fiber number.

The effects of acute nutritional deprivation on diaphragmatic function in acute starvation are less clear. In an *in vivo* rat model of acute four day starvation where body weight and diaphragm weight significantly decreased (19% and 16%, respectively), Dureuil et al. [23] found decreased transdiaphragmatic pressures (Pdi) in the starved group (Fig. 3) which normalized when corrected for the difference in diaphragm muscle weight (Fig. 4). The endurance index in this model of direct

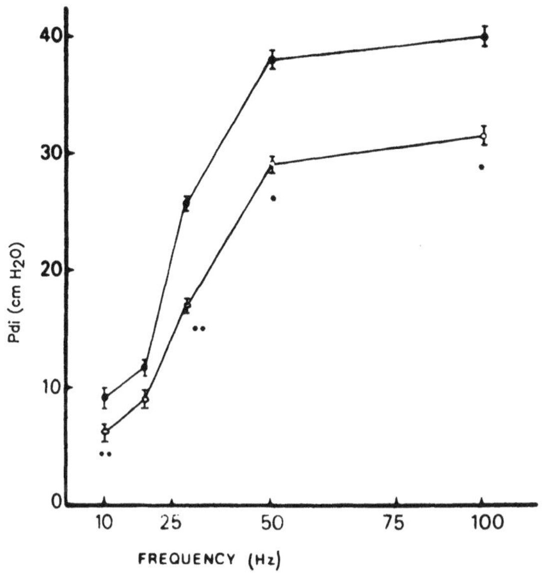

Fig. 3. Relationship between frequency of stimulation and transdiaphragmatic pressure (Pdi) in control (●) and starved (○) animals. Each points represents the x ± SEM.
*Significantly different from control animals, $p < 0.05$;
**significantly different from control animals, $p < 0.001$.
(From [23] with permission)

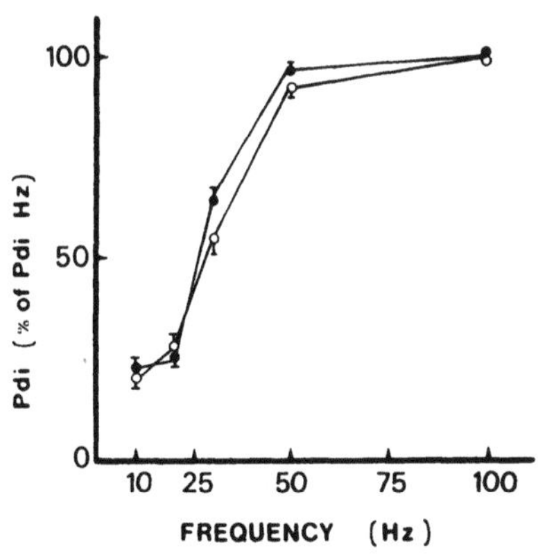

Fig. 4. Normalized frequency-pressure curves showing relative response to changes in stimulation frequency in control (●) and starved (○) animals. Each point is the mean value expressed as a percent of 100 Hz transdiaphragmatic pressure (% Pdi 100 Hz); bars ± SEM. (From [23] with permission)

phrenic nerve stimulation was reduced in starved animals (0.63 ± 0.01 as compared to normal 1.4 ± 0.02). Lewis and Sieck [21] evaluated contractile and fatigue properties of an *in vitro* nerve-muscle strip preparation after 90 h of starvation. Contractions were evoked by using phrenic nerve preparation (left hemidiaphragm) or direct muscle stimulation (right hemidiaphragm). Despite a 20% reduction in body weight, no significant change in diaphragmatic weights was found. When corrected for body weight, peak twitch and tetanic tensions were not reduced. The fatigue index was reduced only with nerve stimulation. The proportion of Type I and II muscle fibers of the diaphragm was similar in both groups and no difference in diaphragmatic cross-sectional areas were noted for either Type I or Type II fibers. The disparency between these studies may relate to the greater severity of starvation as defined by the significantly decreased body and diaphragm weight found in the Dureuil et al. study [23].

Respiratory muscle function is also impaired in poorly nourished humans. When malnourished adult patients without lung disease were studied, respiratory muscle strength, maximum voluntary ventilation and vital capacity were reduced by 37, 41, and 63%, respectively, of the values in the well-nourished patients [24]. The data interpretation is clouded by the fact that the patient's malnutrition was due to malignancy. Given the nature of this systemic disease, the authors could not rule out catabolic factors other than malnutrition contributing to respiratory muscle weakness. Respiratory muscle strength in poorly nourished pediatric and young adults with cystic fibrosis (CF) is controversial. Normal or even greater than normal inspiratory pressures, despite severe malnutrition have been found in CF [25]. In contrast, inspiratory pressures were decreased in a homogenous group of malnourished CF patients [26]. CF is characterized by both malnutrition and chronic hyperinflation. Hyperinflation places the diaphragm at mechanical disadvantage so it can no longer operate according to its optimal force-length relationship. Conflicting data in the CF studies may arise over the appropriate correction factor for hyperinflation [11]. Recently Lands et al. [11] found the decreased respiratory muscle strength in CF was due to the mechanical disadvantage placed on the diaphragm by the marked hyperinflation. Respiratory muscle strength was mildly influenced by nutritional status but not to any degree of clinical significance. It could be speculated, however, that further impairment of respiratory function, even mild, could jeopardize respiratory muscle strength during periods of exacerbation.

Respiratory muscle strength in patients without systemic disease or hyperinflation is decreased. Kelly et al. [27] studied respiratory muscle strength and body composition in adult patients hospitalized on a surgical service. Maximal inspiratory pressures were lower (33 ± 3 cm H_2O) in malnourished patients than those who were normal (45 ± 5 cm H_2O). Diaphragmatic strength is decreased in patients without systemic disease or hyperinflation. Transdiaphragmatic pressures were decreased (stimulated Pdi 16 ± 5 cm H_2O) in ten patients with anorexia nervosa, a relatively pure model of malnutrition without systemic disease [28]. Thus, the human data suggest malnutrition alone does decrease respiratory muscle strength. Alterations in respiratory muscle strength in diseases complicated by hyperinflation and malnutrition may result more from hyperinflation than malnutrition. Underweight patients with reduction of diaphragmatic mass may have contractile forced reduction out of proportion to the reduction in muscle mass [4, 18]. This suggests multiple other factors could contribute to the diaphragmatic muscle dysfunction. These factors include mineral and electrolyte deficiencies [29, 30], impaired muscle membrane function [31], reduction of critical high energy metabolic stores [32] and infection including sepsis and viral infections [33, 34].

Mineral and electrolyte deficiencies can impair respiratory muscle function. Hypophosphatemia reduces diaphragmatic contractile strength as measured by transdiaphragmatic pressure (Pdi) in mechanically ventilated patients with ARF [29]. Hypophosphatemia developing in non-ventilated patients can precipitate ARF [35]. Likewise hypocalcemia is associated with decreased diaphragmatic function [36]. When hypocalcemia was induced by EGTA infusion in dogs, Pdi decreased to $74 \pm 5\%$ and $79 \pm 6\%$ for low and high frequencies as compared to control. Maintenance of the observed decrease in blood pressure and cardiac output with dextran infusion did not ameliorate the decrease in diaphragmatic function. Thus, extracellular calcium plays a role in diaphragmatic strength generation and the decreased diaphragmatic strength is not related to change in cardiac output. Hypomagnesium can also cause decrease in respiratory muscle strength [30]. Improvement in respiratory muscle function was found in 17 hypomagnesemic patients (serum magnesium 0.56 ± 0.3 mmol/l) after institution of magnesium replacement.

Malnutrition also affects ventilatory drive. Zwillich et al. [37] suggested that the interaction of nutrition and ventilatory drive seems to be a direct function of the influence of nutrition on metabolic rate. In general, conditions which reduce metabolic rate reduce ventilatory drive. A decrease in metabolic rate occurs with starvation [38]. Doekel et al. [39] demonstrated a parallel fall in metabolic rate and hypoxic ventilatory response which returned towards normal with refeeding. Studies of hospitalized patients receiving total parenteral nutrition demonstrated a marked effect of protein intake on the ventilatory response to CO_2 [40]. This effect could be detrimental, however, in patients with limited pulmonary reserve leading to an unnecessary increase in respiratory effort.

Malnutrition has also been shown to alter immune function. Protein calorie malnutrition is the most frequent cause of acquired immunodeficiency in humans [41]. Polymorphonuclear leukocytes are normal in number; chemotaxis, opsonic function and phagocytic function usually remain or are mildly depressed while intracellular killing decreases [42]. Thymus, spleen and lymph nodes become markedly atrophic, and lymphocytes may decrease. While immunoglobulins remain normal or slightly increased, antibody response may be depressed [42].

Although death from starvation is frequently accompanied by pneumonia, it is unclear whether this is an immune deficit or a defect in the respiratory system predisposing the patient to infection. Rosenbaum et al. [43] have demonstrated a marked decrease in "sighing" in hospitalized patients with malnutrition. Studies of patients with chest wall weakness due to muscle disease or from submaximal paralyzing doses of curare have demonstrated a decrease in functional residual capacity [44–45]. This reported decrease may predispose the patient to atelectasis and infection providing one possible mechanism for the increased respiratory morbidity associated with starvation.

Renutrition

Nutrition repletion can improve diminished respiratory muscle strength in some patients. A 37% increase in maximal inspiratory pressure and a 12% increase in body cell mass was noted in 21 of 29 hospitalized patients given parental nutrition for 2–4 weeks [27]. The other 8 patients had a 10% decrease in body cell mass and a similar but not significant decrease in maximum inspiratory pressure. Improvement in respiratory muscle function with orally administered nutritional repletion in COPD patients appears to depend on the presence of weight gain. Wilson et al. [46] administered oral nutrition repletion for 2 weeks in 6 ambulatory patients with COPD. Body weight increased by 6% with maximum inspiratory pressures and maximum transdiaphragmatic pressures increasing by 41%. In contrast, when

8 weeks of nutritional supplementation in 21 malnourished COPD patients produced no change in weight, no change in respiratory muscle function was found [47]. Short term refeeding in malnourished COPD patients can also improve respiratory muscle function. With the administration of nocturnal nasoenterally administered calories in a controlled study, Whitaker et al. [48] found significant weight gain and improved maximum expiratory pressures after 16 days of refeeding. Maximum inspiratory pressures increased by 19% after feeding, but this was not significant. Renutrition also has been found to improve diaphragmatic contractility in a more "pure" model of malnutrition, that of anorexia nervosa [28]. After one month of enteral nutrition (weight gain 15%) stimulated Pdi was increased from 16 ± 5 cm H_2O to 23 ± 7 cm H_2O suggesting compromised diaphragmatic function is reversible with renutrition.

The mechanism of improved muscle performance with renutrition is not known with certainty. It has been shown in animals and human studies that chronic hypocaloric dieting produces changes in skeletal muscle that may be important in the genesis of muscle dysfunction. In addition to protein catabolism, these changes include depletion of glycolytic and oxidative enzymes, reduction in high energy phosphate stores and increase in intracellular calcium. Severe malnutrition depresses muscle glycolytic energy activity, thus reducing the availability of energy from glycolysis during contraction [49]. Succinate dehydrogenase (SH), phosphofructokinase and hydroxyacyl-CoA-dehydrogenase were reduced in skeletal muscle homogenates of malnourished rats [50]. Energy stores are also decreased in severe undernutrition. Creatine phosphate fell in a 2-day fasting rat model which was associated with a loss of muscle total creatinine [51]. Thus the reserves of energy phosphorus were decreased and the calculated free ADP rose suggesting deficient oxidative phosphorylation. These findings suggest reduced glycolytic and oxidative enzymes such as phosphofructokinase and succinate dehydrogenase may limit the flux of glycolytic and oxidative pathways. Succinate dehydrogenase activity, when quantified in individual muscle fibers does not appear to be altered in diaphragmative muscle in chronic undernutrition [52]. Oxidative muscle activity may depend in part on fiber type and exercise activity of a particular muscle. The electrophysiological properties of the muscle can also be altered by modification of the cell membrane properties which decreases the sodium potassium pump activity, alters ionic permeability and thus unbalance the intercellular electrolyte composition [53]. These data suggest alteration in muscle contractile and endurance properties are not simply or solely due to changes in lean tissue. Indeed, renutrition studies in hypocaloric dieting and fasting, severe starvation of anorexia nervosa patients, document improvement in muscle performance at a time when significant changes in body composition could not be detected [54]. In anorexia nervosa patients, maximal peripheral muscle force (adductor pollicus) increased significantly by 18% and muscle fatiguability decreased to normal after 4 weeks of refeeding. In contrast, body weight, although significant increased by 11% at 4 weeks and 19% after 8 weeks, was still only 76% of mean ideal body weight at 8 weeks. Three of four aspects of muscle function were restored at a time when body weight was only 71% ideal body, total body nitrogen $<85\%$ of normal and anergy still observed in half of the 6 anorexia nervosa patients. Thus refeeding restored muscle function at a time when other aspects of body composition was still markedly abnormal. The authors suggest changes in intracellular electrolytes may be responsible for early improvement in muscle contractile and endurance properties.

Appropriate nutritional support requires information regarding energy needs in malnourished patients with weight loss. Based on starvation studies in normals, weight loss has been proposed to be an adaptive mechanism to decrease oxygen consumption ($\dot{V}O_2$) and lessen metabolic demands [55]. Recently, data suggest that in malnourished COPD patients, weight loss results from a hypermetabolic state due in part to an increased work of breathing. Wilson et al. [56] measured resting energy expenditure (REE) in normals, adequately nourished and undernourished COPD patients by indirect calorimetry. Measured REE was higher (1.15 ± 0.02) as compared to the adequately nourished COPD (0.99 ± 0.03) and normal groups (0.93 ± 0.02) (Fig. 5). They concluded that malnourished COPD patients are hypermetabolic in comparison to normally nourished controls. Further work from the same group evaluated the oxygen cost of augmenting ventilation (O_2 cost) in controls, normally nourished and malnourished COPD patients [57]. Oxygen cost was significantly elevated in the malnourished group with COPD (4.28 ± 0.98 ml O_2/l) relative to the normally nourished COPD group (2.61 ± 1.07) and the normal controls (1.23 ± 0.51) (Fig. 6). The malnourished population was characterized by a greater degree of hyperinflation and inspiratory muscle weakness than in the other two groups. Thus, malnourished COPD patients are hypermetabolic and require

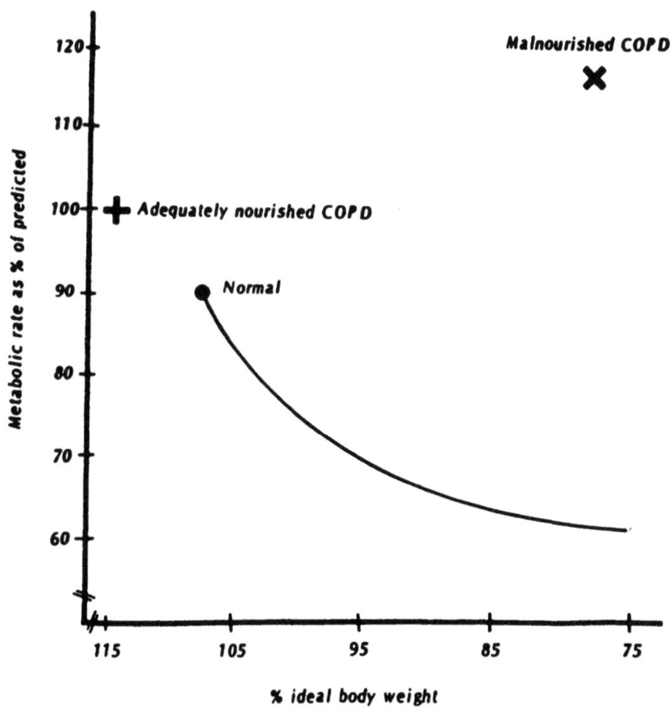

Fig. 5. Metabolic rate (REE) as % of predicted is plotted against ideal body weight. The normal curve is adapted from the Minnesota study. (From [56] with permission)

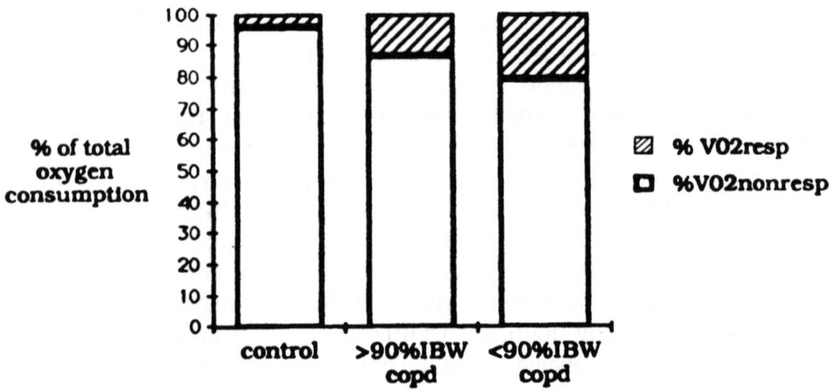

Fig. 6. Comparison of respiratory muscle and nonrespiratory muscle oxygen consumption ($\dot{V}O_2$resp and $\dot{V}O_2$non-resp) during dead space-stimulated ventilation for the three study populations. Measurements are expressed as a percentage of the subjects' total oxygen consumption. (From [57] with permission)

increased energy expenditure due to an increased mechanical work load associated with severe COPD and a reduced ventilatory muscle efficiency.

Energy requirements needed for body weight maintenance can be estimated or assessed by several ways. Indirect calorimetry is one method to assess energy requirements. By measuring oxygen consumption ($\dot{V}O_2$) and carbon dioxide production ($\dot{V}CO_2$) using bag collection, metabolic cart, or cardiac output, total energy is calculated using the Weir equation: Total Calories $= (3.94 \cdot VO_2 + 1.11 \cdot \dot{V}CO_2 \cdot 1.44)$.

Once total energy requirements are determined, the proportion to be given as protein, carbohydrates, and fat are determined. Protein needs for hypercatabolic critically ill patients may reach 1 to 2 g/kg/d or 80 to 150 mg/24 h (0.08 to 0.15 g/d) of total protein, which may require up to 20% of total energy given as protein. The remaining 80% of energy intake can be given as carbohydrates and fat. Nonprotein energy spares utilization of protein for energy. Glucose may spare protein breakdown more than fat but a potential disadvantage of administering 70% to 80% of energy intake as carbohydrates is increased carbon dioxide production. Carbon dioxide production is increased because energy intake in excess of energy needs results in lipogenesis, and a notably increased respiratory quotient (RQ). The RQ is defined as the ratio of carbon dioxide production to oxygen consumption during substrate utilization. For example, when one molecule of glucose is oxidized, six oxygen molecules are necessary for the oxidative process and six molecules of carbon dioxide are produced. Therefore, the RQ of glucose is 1.0. The RQ of lipogenesis is approximately 8.0, reflecting the much greater production of carbon dioxide relative to oxygen consumed [58]. Hypercapnia from increased carbon dioxide production is avoided in normal persons by a compensatory increase in ventilation. Patients with compromised ventilatory status (e.g. COPD or weak respiratory muscles) may be unable to increase ventilation appropriately and hypercapnia may result. The practical significance of this potential complication varies with the patient population. Certainly not all patients with lung disease are susceptible to nutritionally associated hypercapnia in that many patients can increase ventilation thereby avoiding hypercapnia. Although carbon dioxide production was increased in a COPD population after receiving a glucose load, Griske et al. [59] found no significant elevation of arterial carbon dioxide pressure. Brown et al. [60] found a timed walking distance to be 47 m less in 14 of 15 patients with COPD after a large liquid carbohydrate load. Clinical sequelae of nutritionally associated hypercapnia in critically ill patients do include precipitation of hypercapnic respiratory failure or difficulty weaning from MV [61, 62]. Avoiding nutritionally associated increases in carbon dioxide production in critically ill patients is best accomplished by avoiding high or excess total calories. Decreasing the carbohydrate percentage of total calories of feeding formulation does not appear to lower carbon dioxide production [63]. Quantitation of carbon dioxide production can be easily accomplished by analyzing a timed collection of expired air as well as by indirect calorimetry measurements.

Conclusion

Disorders of nutrition, especially prolonged protein-calorie malnutrition can precipitate or worsen ventilatory failure. Respiratory muscle strength and ventilatory drive are decreased with malnutrition. Electrolyte abnormalities, notably hypophosphatemia, hypocalcemia and hypomagnesemia also diminish respiratory muscle strength independent of malnutrition. Nutritional repletion improves respiratory muscle strength although the mechanism of recovery is not known with certainty. Much work remains, especially in critically ill patients, to directly examine and study the effect of malnutrition and refeeding on ventilatory failure.

References

1. Rochester DF, Esau SA (1984) Malnutrition and respiratory system. Chest 85:411–415
2. Vandenburgh E, Van de Woestigne K, Gyselen A (1967) Weight changes in the terminal stages of chronic obstructive lung disease. Am Rev Respir Dis 96:556–565
3. Renzetti AD, McClement JH, Litt BD (1966) The Veterans Administration cooperative study of pulmonary function. Mortality in relation to respiratory function in chronic obstructive pulmonary disease. Am J Med 41:115–129
4. Hunter AMB, Carey MA, Larsh HU (1981) The nutritional status of patients with chronic obstructive pulmonary disease. Am Rev Respir Dis 124:376–381
5. Wilson D, Wright E, Rogers R, Anthonisen N (1987) Body weight in COPD. Am Rev Respir Dis (abstract) 135:A144
6. Driver AG, McAlvey MT, Smith JL (1982) Nutritional assessment of patients with chronic obstructive pulmonary disease and acute respiratory failure. Chest 82:568–571
7. Pingleton SK, Eulberg M (1983) Nutritional analysis of acute respiratory failure. Chest (abstract) 84:A343
8. Driver AG, LeBrun M (1980) Iatrogenic malnutrition in patients receiving ventilatory support. JAMA 244:2195–2196
9. Harmon G, Pingleton SK, Hanson FN, Schloerb PK, Kerby GR (1985) Computer-assisted nutritional therapy (CANT) in the intensive care unit. Am Rev Respir Dis (abstract) 131:A152
10. Weiner P, Suo J, Fernandez E, Cherniack RM (1990) The effect of hyperinflation on respi-

ratory muscle strength and efficiency in healthy subjects and patients with asthma. Am Rev Respir Dis 141:1501–1505
11. Lands L, Desmond KJ, Demizio D, Pavilanis A, Coates AL (1990) The effects of nutritional status and hyperinflation on respiratory muscle strength in children and young adults. Am Rev Respir Dis 141:1506–1509
12. Braun NMT, Arora NS, Rochester DF (1983) Respiratory muscle and pulmonary function in proximal myopathies. Thorax 38:616–623
13. Rochester DF, Braun NMT (1985) Determinants of maximal inspiratory pressure in chronic obstructive pulmonary disease. Am Rev Respir Dis 132:42–47
14. Cahill G (1970) Starvation in man. N Engl J Med 282:668–675
15. Long CL, Birkham RH, Geiger JW (1981) Contribution of skeletal muscle protein in elevated rates of whole body protein catabolism in trauma patients. Am J Clin Nutr 34:1087–1093
16. Thurlbeck WM (1978) Diaphragm and body weight in emphysema. Thorax 33:483–487
17. Arora NS, Rochester DF (1982) Effect of body weight and muscularity on human diaphragm muscle mass, thickness and area. J Appl Physiol 52:64–70
18. Rochester DF, Arora NS, Braun NMT (1981) Maximum contractile force of human diaphragm muscle, determined in vivo. Trans Am Clin Climatol Assoc 82:200–208
19. Kelsen SG, Ference M, Kapoor S (1985) Effects of prolonged undernutrition on structure and function of the diaphragm. J Appl Physiol 58:1354–1359
20. Lewis MI, Sieck GC, Fournier M, Belman MJ (1986) Effect of nutritional deprivation on diaphragm contractility and muscle fiber size. J Appl Physiol 60:596–603
21. Lewis MI, Sieck GC (1990) Effect of acute nutritional deprivation on diaphragm structure and function. J Appl Physiol 68:1938–1944
22. Drew JS, Farkas GA, Pearson RD, Rochester DF (1988) Effects of a chronic wasting infection on skeletal muscle size and contracile properties. J Appl Physiol 64:460–468
23. Dureuil B, Viires N, Veber B, et al. (1989) Acute diaphragmatic changes induced by starvation in rats. Am J Clin Nutr 49:738–744
24. Arora NS, Rochester DF (1982) Respiratory muscle strength and maximal voluntary ventilation in undernourished patients. Am Rev Respir Dis 126:5–8
25. O'Neill S, Leahy F, Pasterkamp H, Tal A (1983) The effects of chronic hyperinflation, nutritional status and posture on respiratory muscle strength in cystic fibrosis. Am Rev Respir Dis 128:1051–1054
26. Szeinbers A, England S, Mindorff C, Fraser IM, Levison H (1985) Maximal inspiratory and expiratory pressures are reduced in hyperinflated, malnourished, young adult males with cystic fibrosis. Am Rev Respir Dis 132:766–769
27. Kelly SM, Rosa A, Field S, Coughlin M, Shizgal HM, Macklem PT (1984) Inspiratory muscle strength and body composition in patients receiving total parenteral nutrition therapy. Am Rev Respir Dis 130:33–37
28. Murciano D, Armengauk MH, Rigaud D, Pariente R, Aubier M (1990) Effect of renutrition on respiratory and diaphragmatic function in patients with severe mental anorexia. Am Rev Respir Dis 141:A547
29. Aubier M, Murciano D, Lecoguic Y, Viires N, Squara P, Pariente R (1985) Effects of hypophosphatemia on diaphragmatic contractility in patients with acute respiratory failure. N Engl J Med 313:420–424
30. Molloy DW, Dhingra S, Solven F, Wilson A, McCarthy DS (1984) Hypomagnesium and respiratory muscle power. Am Rev Resp Dis 129:497–498
31. Cunningham JN Jr, Carter NW, Rector FC Jr, Seldin DW (1970) Resting transmembrane potential difference of skeletal muscle in normal subjects and severely ill patients. J Clin Invest 50:49–59
32. Gertz I, Hedenstierna G, Hellers G, Wahren J (1977) Muscle metabolism in patients with chronic obstructive lung disease and acute respiratory failure. Clin Sci Mol Med 52:395–403
33. Boczkowski, Dureuil B, Branger C, et al (1988) Effects of sepsis on diaphragmatic function in rats. Am Rev Respir Dis 138:260–265
34. Mier-Jedrzejowicz A, Brophy C, Green M (1988) Respiratory muscle weakness during upper respiratory tract infections. Am Rev Respir Dis 138:5–7

35. Newman JH, Neff TA, Ziporin P (1977) Acute respiratory failure associated with hypophosphatemia. N Engl J Med 296:1101–1103
36. Aubier M, Viires N, Piquet J, et al (1985) Effects of hypocalcemia on diaphragmatic strength generation. J Appl Physiol 58:2054–2061
37. Zwillich CW, Sahn SA, Weil JV (1977) Effects of hypermetabolism on ventilation and chemosensitivity. J Clin Invest 60:900–906
38. Keys A, Brozek J, Henschel A, et al (1950) Biology of Human Starvation. Minneapolis, University of Minnesota Press
39. Doekel RC Jr, Zwillich CW, Scoggin CH (1976) Clinical semi-starvation: Depression of hypoxic ventilatory response. N Engl J Med 295:358–361
40. Askanazi J, Rosenbaum SH, Hyman AI, et al (1980) Effects of parenteral nutrition on ventilatory drive. Anesthesiology 53 (Suppl 1):185
41. Chandra RK (1983) Malnutrition. In: Chandra RK (ed) Primary and secondary immunodeficiency disorders. New York, Churchill Livingstone, pp 187
42. Shizgal HM (1981) Nutrition and immune function. Surg Ann 12:15–29
43. Rosenbaum SH, Askanazi J, Hyman AI, et al (1979) Respiratory patterns in profound nutrition depletion. Anesthesiology 51 (Suppl 1):366
44. De Troyer A, Bastenier-Geens J (1979) Effects of neuromuscular blockade on respiratory mechanics in conscious man. J Appl Physiol 47:1162–1168
45. Gibson GJ, Pride NB, Newsom Davis J (1978) Pulmonary mechanics in patients with respiratory muscle weakness. Am Rev Respir Dis 118:373
46. Wilson DO, Rogers RM, Sanders MH, Penvoch BE, Reilly JJ (1986) Nutritional intervention in malnourished patients with emphysema. Am Rev Respir Dis 134:672–677
47. Lewis MI, Belman MJ, Dorr-Uyemural L (1987) Nutritional supplementation in ambulatory patients with chronic obstructive pulmonary disease. Am Rev Respir Dis 125:1062–1068
48. Whittaker JS, Ryan CF, Buckley PA, Road JD (1990) The effects of refeeding on peripheral and respiratory muscle function in malnourished chronic obstructive pulmonary disease patients. Am Rev Respir Dis 142:283–288
49. Layman DKM, Merdian-Bender M, Hegarty PVJ, Swan PB (1981) Changes in aerobic and anaerobic metabolism in rat cardiac and skeletal muscles after total or partial dietary restrictions. J Nutr 111:994–1000
50. McRussell DR, Atwood HL, Whittaker JS, et al (1984) The effect of fasting and hypocaloric diets on the functional and metabolic characteristics of rat gastrocoremius muscle. Clin Sci Lond 67:185–194
51. Pichard C, Vaughan C, Struk R, Armstrong RL, Jeejeebhoy KN (1988) Effect of dietary manipulations (fasting, hypocaloric feeding and subsequent refeeding) on rat muscle energetics as assessed by nuclear magnetic resonance spectroscope. J Clin Invest 82:895–901
52. Sieck GC, Lewis MI, Blanco CE (1989) Effects of under-nutrition on diaphragm fiber size, SDH activity, and fatigue resistance. J Appl Physiol 66:2196–2205
53. Pichard C, Jeejeebhoy KN (1988) Muscle dysfunction in malnourished patients. Quart J Med 260:1021–1045
54. McRussell DR, Pendergast PJ, Darby PL, Garfinkel PE, Whitwell J, Jeejeebhoy KN (1983) A comparison between muscle function and body composition in anorexia nervosa; the effect of refeeding. Am J Clin Nutr 38:229–237
55. Keys A, Brozek J, Henschel A, Michelsen O, Taylor HL (1950) The biology of human starvation. Minneopolis, Minnesota Press
56. Wilson DO, Donahoe M, Rogers RM, Pennock BE (1990) Metabolic rate and weight loss in chronic obstructive lung disease. JPEN 14:7–11
57. Donahoe M, Rogers RM, Wilson DO, Pennock BE (1989) Oxygen consumption of the respiratory muscles in normal and malnourished patients with chronic obstructive lung disease. Am Rev Respir Dis 140:385–391
58. Elwyn DH, Kinney JM (1980) A unique approach to measuring total energy expenditure by indirect calorimetry advances. In: Kinney JM (ed) Assessment of energy metabolism in health and disease: report of the First Ross Conference on Medical Research. Columbus, Ohio, Ross Laboratories, pp 59–62
59. Griske T, Gurnshanthorgh G, Glauser FL (1977) Effects of carbohydrates on carbon dioxide excretion in patients with airway disease. Chest 71:55–58

60. Brown SE, Nagendran RC, McHugh JW, et al (1985) Effects of a large carbohydrate load on walking performance in chronic air-flow obstruction. Am Rev Respir Dis 132:960–962
61. Dark DS, Pingleton SK, Kerby GR (1985) Hypercapnia during weaning: A complication of nutritional support. Chest 88:141–143
62. Covelli HD, Black JW, Olsen MS, et al (1981) Respiratory failure precipitated by high carbohydrate loads. Ann Intern Med 95:579–581
63. Pingleton SK, Lohr G (1991) Nutritionally associated increased carbon dioxide production: Excess total calories versus high proportion of carbohydrate calories. (in press)

Dynamic Hyperinflation

A. Rossi, G. Polese, and G. Brandi

Introduction

Pulmonary hyperinflation is defined by an increase in the functional residual capacity (FRC), which is the amount of gas in the lungs and the airways at the end of a spontaneous expiration. Under normal circumstances and also in some abnormal conditions, the elastic energy stored in the respiratory system during the preceding inspiration is sufficient to breathe out, and the FRC is determined by the opposing elastic forces of the lungs and the chest wall, such that it corresponds to the static equilibrium volume of the total respiratory system (Vr, relaxation volume) [1]. Assuming the quiet breathing of an adult, healthy subject in the standing or sitting position as the control situation, there are several physiological as well as pathological events which can modify the FRC. One of these events is an abnormal increase of FRC above Vr because of dynamic forces, i.e. dynamic hyperinflation [2, 3].

In normal subjects, shifting from the upright or sitting position to the supine position decreases Vr because of the effect of gravity on the abdomen-diaphragm compartment [1]. During anesthesia, Vr is decreased by mean of about 0.5 l compared to the awake subject lying supine, though the mechanism (e.g. changes in muscle tone, atelectasis, etc.) of this further reduction has not been fully elucidated yet [4]. In patients with either an increased inward elastic recoil of the lung, e.g. interstitial pulmonary fibrosis, or a decreased outward elastic recoil of the chest wall, e.g. kyphoscoliosis and marked obesity, Vr is generally at low lung volume. In contrast, patients with chronic obstructive pulmonary disease (COPD) are compelled to breathe at high lung volume because the loss of lung elastic recoil rises Vr up to the static equilibrium point of the chest wall.

In all the above mentioned conditions, the changes in FRC are primarily determined by changes in Vr due to alterations of the volume-pressure characteristics of either the lung or the chest wall [5]. However, other mechanisms can determine changes in FRC. In patients with pulmonary edema, FRC is abnormally small because the intrapulmonary gas is replaced by diffuse airspaces flooding [6, 7], while the pressure-volume characteristics of the thorax can remain unchanged compared to the pre-edema condition, as it has been shown in dogs with oleic acid induced pulmonary edema [8]. Gattinoni et al. [7] defined the injured lung as a "small lung" rather than a "stiff lung". This is, in our opinion, a more appropriate definition, which implies that small tidal volume (VT) should be used to ventilate patients with acute respiratory failure (ARF) due to the acute lung injury in order to prevent the risk of barotrauma.

If dynamic forces are present at the end of the expiration, Vr is not the most important determinant of the level of FRC. Either passive events, such as increased flow resistance, or active forces, such as changes in the timing and pattern of respiratory muscles activation, can adjust FRC at a lung volume different from Vr [2]. For example, during exercise, activation of the expiratory muscles decreases the FRC below Vr [9]. In infants, a combination of several factors like the high frequency of breathing, the persistent post-inspiratory inspiratory muscle activity, and glottis movements prevents breathing at the low Vr determined by the simultaneous presence of a floppy chest wall and a stiff lung [1, 10]. The mechanisms by which all these conditions cause a change in FRC are by themselves physiologically and clinically important: for instance an increase in FRC due to a persistent activation of the inspiratory muscles during expiration produces a decrease in pleural and mediastinal pressure and favor in this way venous return to the heart. At the opposite, airway restrictions at any level (glottis, large and small bronchi) are inevitably accompanied by an increased mediastinal pressure. The interest of FRC is, from this side, linked with the effects of the primary change. At the contrary, FRC or lung volume in general may be viewed as a primary parameter. For this approach only two sets of information are available.

1. the increase of lung volume takes place against a feed-back given by the Hering-Breuer reflex, and
2. changes of Vr induced in healthy subjects by positive or negative pressure breathing are not followed by equal changes in FRC.

For example with a 10 mm Hg negative pressure breathing, a decrease of Vr of about 20% can be calculated while FRC is reduced only by 10%. In other words, against the choice of

1. maintaining constant the pattern of activation of the respiratory muscles and accepting a reduction in FRC equal to that of Vr, or
2. maintaining constant FRC, healthy subjects follow a compromise between 1 and 2: inspiratory muscles are used more but not more enough to maintain FRC constant.

This means that there are mechanisms of stability of lung volume *per se* which are not 100% effective, but are strong enough to modify rather deeply the activation of the respiratory muscles. Therefore, whereas Vr is merely dependent from the passive elastic properties of the lungs and the chest wall, FRC is a more complex variable which can influence the pattern of the respiratory muscle activation. This is not surprising if one considers that lung volume *per se* determines the Hering-Breuer reflex.

Dynamic pulmonary hyperinflation is defined by an increase in FRC above Vr due to dynamic factors. Basically, three mechanisms can determine dynamic hyperinflation:

1. airway constriction at any level;
2. an increase in the post-inspiratory muscle activity;
3. a short expiratory time [11].

In normal subjects, during quiet breathing, the time available between two inspiratory efforts is generally sufficient to complete the tidal expiration as it is indicated by the presence of an appreciable end-expiratory pause. However, FRC can be voluntarily adjusted well above Vr by increasing either the frequency of breathing or the TI/Ttot (TI = inspiratory time; Ttot = total breathing cycle duration), thus shortening the expiratory time (TE) and preventing complete exhalation to Vr. Indeed, tachypnea is one of the mechanisms to uphold FRC in order to improve airway patency and ventilation distribution in infants [10]. However, this pattern of breathing in infants is the only known physiological condition in which FRC is maintained above Vr through a marked reduction in the duration of expiration. In contrast, it has been recognized for a long time that an increase in flow resistance is by far the chief mechanism which can prevent the complete expiration to Vr. Indeed, an increased flow resistance abnormally lengthens the respiratory time constant and therefore the time required to breathe out [2, 11]. Under these circumstances, the final low-flow rate portion of the expiration is cancelled by the sudden onset of the inspiration and a sharp change of the end-expiratory flow pattern replaces the usual end-expiratory pause [12–14]. Although this has been known for many years, some important implications of this occurrence, particularly in critically ill patients, have been more extensively elucidated only by recent work.

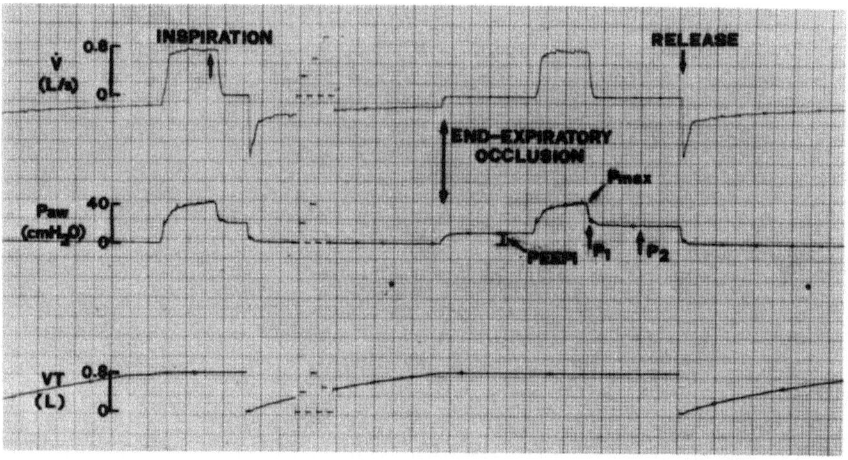

Fig. 1. Records of flow (V), airway pressure (Paw) and volume (VT) in a mechanically ventilated patient. At the end of the tidal expiration, expiratory port is occluded (1 to 2 sec) using the end-expiratory hold button of the ventilator. Positive plateau in Paw provides direct measurement of PEEPi. The occlusion is released for mechanical pulmonary inflation, and the end-inspiratory hold button of the ventilator (Siemens Servo 900 C). During the occlusion, Paw immediately drops from its maximum value (Pmax) to a lower value (P1), followed by a gradual decrease until apparent plateau is achieved. End-inspiratory plateau pressure (P2) respresents the elastic recoil of the respiratory system at end-inflation pulmonary volume; P1 is measured at a point where Paw sharply changes from rapid to slow decrease. Autocalibration of ventilator, which occurred every 10 sec is apparent on the tracings. (From [19] with permission)

Dynamic Pulmonary Hyperinflation and Mechanical Ventilation

There can be little doubt that if flow is present at the end of the expiration, the end-expiratory alveolar pressure must be positive to drive the flow through the conducting airway. In the absence of expiratory muscles activity, the expiratory driving pressure is provided by the elastic recoil pressure of the total respiratory system

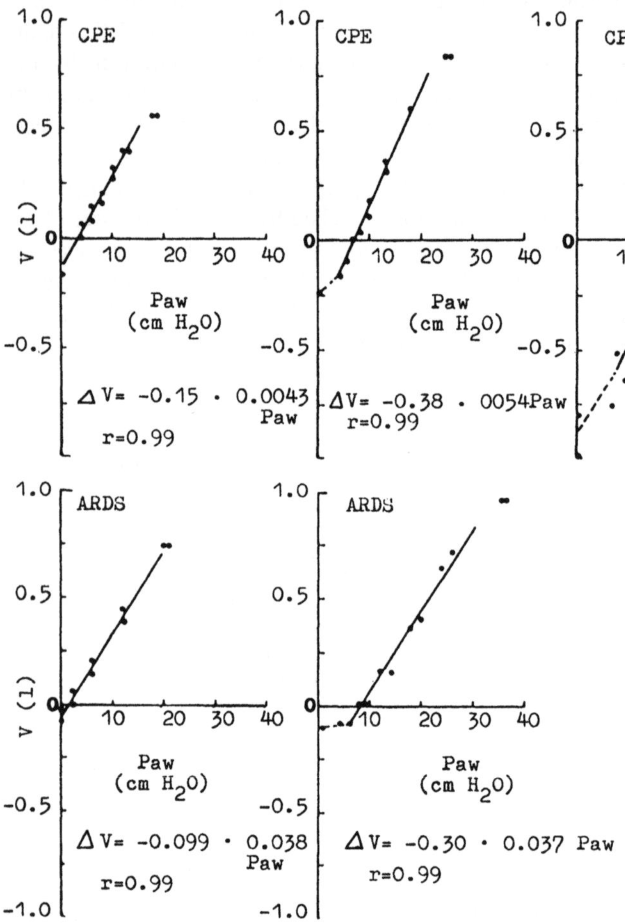

Fig. 2. Static volume pressure (V-P) relationship in 5 representative, mechanically ventilated patients (*CPE* = cardiogenic pulmonary edema; *ARDS* = adult respiratory distress syndrome; *CAO* = chronic airway obstruction). *VT* = 0 is the end-expiratory lung volume during tidal mechanical ventilation.
Closed circles are measurements obtained with the interrupter technique ( ) from two relaxed exhalations in each patient. The solid lines are the regression lines computed over the linear portion of the V-P relationship, the slope respresenting the deflation respiratory compliance. At VT = 0, a positive Paw reflecting PEEPi was observed. Above VT = 0 the V-P relationship was linear except for the end-inspiratory points. The difference between VT = 0 and the intercept on the Y-axis represents the amount of dynamic hyperinflation. A few points toward this intercept deviated from the line because of airway closure. (From [18] with permission)

(Pel, rs), stored with the preceding lung inflation. This was reported for mechanically ventilated patients by Jonson et al. in 1975 [15]. However, it was in 1982 that Pepe and Marini [16] pointed out the importance of this phenomenon in the clinical intensive care setting. Indeed, they made the brilliant observation that the unexpected drop in cardiac output and in systemic arterial blood pressure in some mechanically ventilated patients without any positive end-expiratory pressure (PEEP) set by the ventilator, was associated with a slow and persistent filling of the expiratory bell of the Bennet MA-1 ventilator throughout the expiratory period, until interrupted suddenly by the onset of the mechanical inflation. A brief occlusion of the expiratory port of the ventilator at the end of the tidal expiration, while the patient was relaxed, documented the presence of a positive end-expiratory alveolar pressure by showing a rapid increase in the recorded pressure at the airway opening up to 26 cm H_2O [16]. This positive end-expiratory pressure, due to the end-expiratory Pel, rs because of the incomplete lung emptying, was termed "occult, auto or intrinsic - PEEP" (PEEPi), in order do differentiate it from the PEEP set by the ventilator (Fig. 1) [12, 16, 17]. Not surprisingly, further work has demonstrated dynamic hyperinflation and PEEPi to be a systematic finding in mechanically ventilated patients with acute exacerbation of COPD, in the early phases of ARF [18, 19] as well as after several days of mechanical ventilation (MV) (Fig. 2) [12, 17, 20]. In these patients, in fact, because of the abnormally increased airway resistance and expiratory flow limitation during tidal expiration, a long time, e.g. more than 20 sec, is required to breathe out to Vr [16, 21]. Clearly, such an expiratory duration cannot be used in any ventilatory setting and by necessity the slow progress of

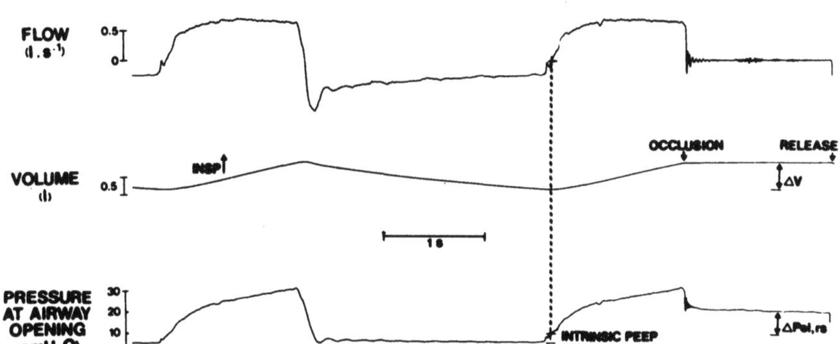

Fig. 3. Tracings of flow, volume and pressure at the airway opening in a mechanically ventilated patient with COPD, with PEEP of 5.5 cm H_2O. Arrows and symbols as in Fig. 1 Note that in this patient, expiratory flow continues throughout expiration, and inspiratory flow starts only after a pressure change of 4.5 cm H_2O is applied by the ventilator, as indicated by the broken line. This pressure is required to overcome the end-expiratory elastic recoil, i.e. PEEPi. This figure illustrates the implications of PEEPi on measurement of static compliance. This latter is conventionally obtained as the ratio of inflation volume to the difference between the plateau end-inspiratory pressure and the PEEP set by the ventilator. Clearly, the end-expiratory elastic recoil pressure of the respiratory system (i.e. PEEPi) must also be subtracted from the end-inspiratory plateau in order to obtain the correct value of δPEL, rs. In this example, uncorrected compliance amounted to 0.055 l/cm H_2O, whereas after correction for PEEPi the corresponding value was increased to 0.082 l/cm H_2O. (From [12] with permission)

expiration is suddenly cut by the onset of the mechanical inflation, i.e. dynamic hyperinflation occurs. This was indeed documented by continuous recording of flow and pressure at the airway opening as well as by means of expiratory flow/volume curves (Fig. 3 and 4) [12, 17, 22, 23]. In the early days of MV, with commonly used ventilatory settings, FRC can be 1 l or even more above Vr in COPD patients and PEEPi can be as high as 22 cm H_2O (Fig. 2) [18]. Clearly such high values of PEEPi can have deleterious effects on cardiac output and oxygen transport [16], such that it is necessary to set, in these patients, a TE as long as it is compatible with an adequate gas exchange and patient's comfort. In this connection, it should be noted that the use of ventilatory settings with high inspiratory flow rates and long expiratory duration not only reduces the undesired hemodynamic effects of high levels of the "occult PEEP" (PEEPi), but it can also improve gas exchange, allowing a better lung emptying [24].

Dynamic pulmonary hyperinflation and PEEPi can be significantly reduced by some bronchodilators, e.g. methylxantines and adrenergic agents which decrease airway resistance because of their relaxant effects on bronchial smooth muscle, thus improving the rate of lung emptying [19, 25]. Using simple and non-invasive techniques, frequent measurements of respiratory mechanics before and after administration of the drugs can help to optimize the dose as well as the timing of administration (Fig. 5).

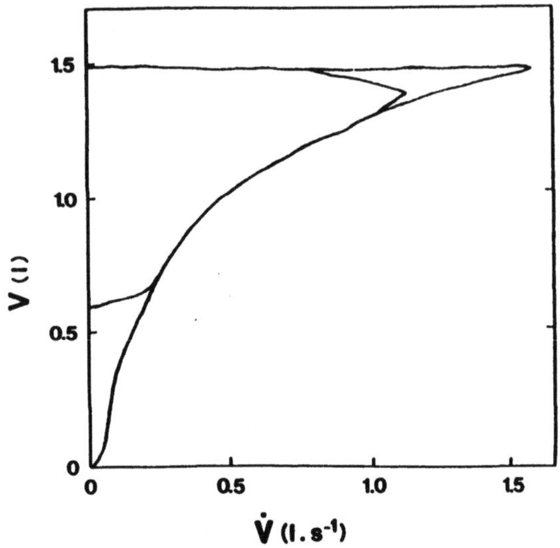

Fig. 4. Relaxed expiratory volume-flow curves in a mechanically ventilated patient with PEEP set by the ventilator at 4 cm H_2O (smaller loop) and without PEEP (outer loop). With 4 cm H_2O PEEP, the intrinsic PEEP was 7.5 cm H_2O. During expiration with PEEP of 4 cm H_2O, the flow volume loop exhibited a characteristic truncated appearance due to the onset of the next mechanical inflation before expiration could be completed, i.e. the patient was dynamically hyperinflated. Complete relaxed expiration against atmospheric pressure resulted in a reduction of the end-expiratory lung volume, but during most of expiration the rate of lung emptying was unchanged due to pre-existing dynamic expiratory flow limitation, such that removal of PEEP did not affect the effective expiratory driving pressure. (From [22] with permission)

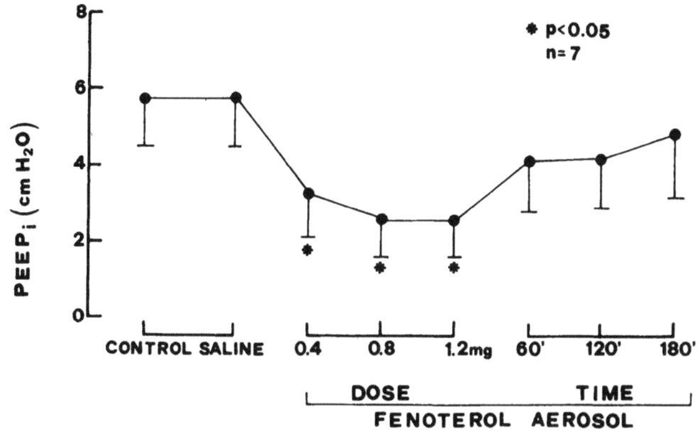

Fig. 5. Effect of fenoterol on PEEPi, measured by means of the end-expiratory occlusion as shown in Fig. 1 in seven mechanically ventilated patients with acute exacerbation of chronic airflow obstruction. Filled circles show mean values from the seven patients and bars the standard error. ANOVA was significant ($p<0.05$), then all values were compared to control using the Wilcoxon's test for paired data. These patients, at the time of the study, were receiving continuous amynophylline infusion at a constant rate, so that the effect of fenoterol was on top of the effect of aminophylline. (From [25] with permission)

An interesting clinical observation has been reported by Conti et al. [26] in a mechanically ventilated COPD patient, in whom an isorhythmic atrioventricular dissociation was associated with dynamic hyperinflation during intermittent positive pressure ventilation (IPPV) and intermittent mandatory ventilation (IMV), PEEPi amounting to 12 and 17 cm H_2O, respectively; the cardiac arrhythmia was successfully reversed by applying 20 cm H_2O of pressure support ventilation (PSV), which by decreasing the respiratory rate, reduced PEEPi to 7 cm H_2O. The presence of a marked dynamic hyperinflation during IMV has been reported also by Braschi et al. [27].

Beside its hemodynamic effects, which are similar to an equivalent level of external PEEP, PEEPi introduces a significant error in the computation of static respiratory compliance (Cst, rs) if it is computed according to the traditional formula: Cst, rs = VT / (Pel, rs - PEEP), where VT is the tidal volume and Pel, rs is the plateau pressure at the airway opening after 1.5–2.0 sec of end-inspiratory occlusion), instead of the correct formula:

$$\text{Cst, rs} = \text{VT} / (\text{Pel, rs} - \text{PEEP} - \text{PEEPi}) \ [12, 18, 20].$$

It is noteworthy, in this connection, that the corrected compliance (i.e. corrected for PEEPi) was found to be significantly correlated with gas exchange impairment (the A-aO_2 difference), whereas the uncorrected compliance was not [18].

We would like to stress, in this connection that even modern microprocessor equipped mechanical ventilators, which can display the "on-line" computation of Crs, do not take PEEPi into account, thus providing an incorrect and therefore useless information. In fact, the error in the computation of compliance due to PEEPi is poorly predictable because the magnitude of PEEPi depends from several

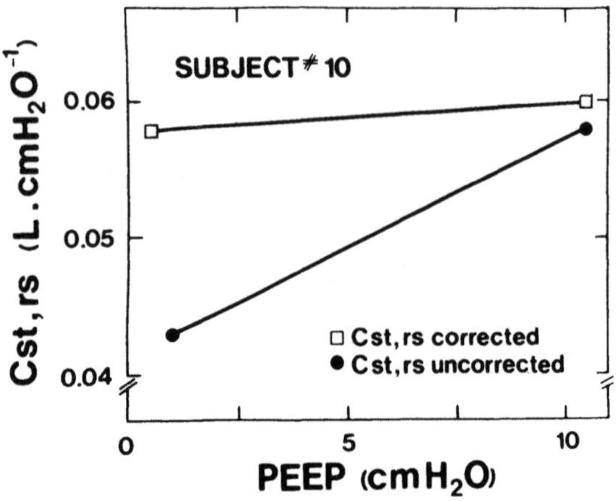

Fig. 6. Relationsship between static respiratory compliance (Cst, rs) and PEEP in a representative, mechanically ventilated patient. Although the true (corrected) compliance is only minimally affected by the level of PEEP, the uncorrected Cst, rs varies substantially with PEEP. (From [12] with permission)

factors, for example the patient's characteristic (resistance and compliance) which can change with the rapid evolution of the underlying disease, and the ventilatory setting (TE and PEEP) as well as the size of the endotracheal tube, which are generally different between patients. Furthermore, because external PEEP can replace PEEPi and not be added to it (see another chapter in this book), the error in the computation of Cst, rs with application of PEEP can provide a misleading clinical information (Fig. 6).

Recently, we have partitioned the total respiratory system mechanics into lung and chest wall components in mechanically ventilated patients [29]. We have found that PEEPi, rs, i.e. the end-expiratory Pel, rs, was mainly due to lung [1] recoil, i.e. PEEPi, 1, though there was also a small end-expiratory inward recoil of the chest wall (PEEPi,w) which on the average was abouth 16% of PEEPi, rs, but which amounted to 2.3 cm H_2O in a COPD patient. The evidence of a positive pleural pressure throughout expiration in all the examined COPD patients is important to explain the expiratory flow limitation during tidal expiration in these patients, at least during MV [21].

Dynamic Pulmonary Hyperinflation and ARDS

It seems contradictory to use the word hyperinflation, though "dynamic", in patients with the adult respiratory distress syndrome (ARDS) in whom the marked reduction in FRC is reported as a characteristic [6]. Indeed, the amount of gas in the injured lung is undoubtedly reduced compared to the normal lung [7]. However, recent work by our group showed that a variable degree of dynamic increase in FRC can be present also in mechanically ventilated patients without COPD, particularly in patients with cardiogenic pulmonary edema (CPE) and in patients with ARDS, at least in early phases and during controlled MV (Fig. 2) [18, 20, 28], as reported in Table 1.

Dynamic hyperinflation and PEEPi in patients with ARDS and pulmonary edema may be surprising if one considers the high driving pressure for expiration pro-

Table 1. Range and prevalence of PEEPi and dynamic hyperinflation in 95 consecutive mechanically ventilated patients

Diagnosis	No.	PEEPi (cmH_2O) range	Prevalence
COPD	47	2.6–22	47/47 (100%)
ARDS	28	1.0– 8.1	15/28 (58%)
CPE	10	1.0– 6.0	8/10 (80%)
Other	10	1.0– 4.1	5/10 (50%)

PEEPi: intrinsic positive end-expiratory pressure; *COPD* = chronic obstructive pulmonary disease; *ARDS* = adult respiratory distress syndrome; *CPE* = cardiogenic pulmonary edema; *Other* = patients with acute respiratory failure of extrapulmonary origin

vided by the low respiratory compliance [6]. However, a first mechanism which can retard the expiratory flow in mechanically ventilated patients even without COPD is an increase in respiratory flow resistance. This has been reported recently for both CPE [18] and ARDS patients [18, 28, 30]. Second, expiration can be unduly slowed also by the added resistance of narrow bore endotracheal tubes plus ventilator tubings and devices [28]. This added resistance was found to average 13.2 ± 2.9 $cm\ H_2O \cdot l^{-1} \cdot s$ with a common ventilatory setting using *in vitro* calculated values [28]. However, it has to be considered that the pressure/flow relationship of the endotracheal tubes is markedly curvilinear [17], and therefore it can be significantly affected by changes in the inspiratory flow rate, i.e. it increases with higher flows. Besides, the resistance of the endotracheal tube *in situ* can be higher than values predicted using *in vitro* measurements, because of kinking and compression of the tube as well as because of secretions in the lumen [29, 31]. Nevertheless, because of the increased driving pressure due to the abnormally low respiratory compliance, the amount of dynamic hyperinflation and PEEPi was found to be much lower in patients with pulmonary edema (and ARDS) than in mechanically ventilated COPD patients [18, 20, 28]. Apparently, the magnitude of dynamic hyperinflation and PEEPi is far from being troublesome in mechanically ventilated patients with CPE and ARDS as it can be in COPD patients, who usually exhibit much higher values [12, 18, 19, 20, 25]. Nevertheless, the presence of dynamic hyperinflation in patients with pulmonary edema has important implications both in terms of MV and gas exchange as well as in terms of spontaneous breathing and ventilatory modes requiring patient's cooperation (see below).

Dynamic Hyperinflation, PEEPi, and Gas Exchange

Dynamic hyperinflation is likely to be a systematic corollary of the inverse ratio MV (IRV), which is a particular ventilatory setting with a long TI followed by a short TE. IRV has been suggested as an alternative ventilatory support technique for patients with severe hypoxemia who do not respond to the conventional volume controlled MV [32, 33]. Indeed, some physiological and clinical studies are encouraging. It has been also suggested that improved oxygenation can be achieved with IRV using lower levels of Pmax, i.e. the peak cycling pressure, and PEEP than with conventional MV [34]. Therefore IRV has been invoked to reduce the risk of barotrauma in mechanically ventilated patients. However, there can be little doubt that during IRV, the short TE is likely to be associated with an incomplete expiration and hence with dynamic hyperinflation and PEEPi. Indeed, in seven mechanically ventilated patients with pulmonary edema and without COPD, we were able to elicit dynamic hyperinflation by shortening TE from 3.2 sec - 1.2 sec, on the average, while VT and the ventilatory frequency (f) were kept essentially constant: PEEPi went from 1 - 8.6 cm H_2O, and FRC adjusted about 0.45 l above Vr, on the average [35]. In that study, switching our patients from the traditional controlled MV to IRV, we observed a slight improvement in PaO_2, associated with a significant drop in cardiac output, i.e. 0.6 l on the average, which was of the same amount as the drop in cardiac output caused by 8 cm H_2O of externally applied PEEP in the same patients [35]. Surprisingly, PEEPi is not commonly reported in other IRV studies, though the presence of PEEPi might help to explain the improvement in PaO_2 as well as the drop in cardiac filling observed in some patients when implemented with IRV. It has to be mentioned that in our study neither 8 cm H_2O PEEP nor the 8.6 cm H_2O PEEPi improved the oxygen delivery [35]. However, while it may not be unexpected that equivalent levels of PEEP and PEEPi can have the same effect on cardiac output, the effects of PEEP and PEEPi on the overall gas exchange are more difficult to predict. In fact, while PEEP is probably distributed homogeneously within the lung, the distribution of PEEPi is likely to be uneven because of time constant inequalities between lung units. The magnitude of PEEPi ought to be higher in the units with a long time constant, probably the more "diseased" though still ventilating units, than in those with a short time constant. As a consequence, with PEEP lung inflation will start while all lung units are at their elastic equilibrium volume, whereas with dynamic hyperinflation and PEEPi, the short time constant units will be filling from the onset of lung inflation while the long time constant units will be still emptying. In this latter condition, the distribution of the inspired gas is likely to be more inhomogeneous. This could explain why PaO_2 increased in 6 out of 7 patients of our study with PEEP, and only in 4 patients of the same group with PEEPi and IRV-induced dynamic hyperinflation. On the other hand, one could think that the distribution of PEEPi, compared to PEEP, should be more favorable for the deranged lung. In fact, according to the theory, PEEPi should be higher in some "diseased" part of the lung, where PEEP to prevent collapse is probably needed. However, whether the use of an induced PEEPi instead of an equivalent level of externally applied PEEP might be of some benefit to improve gas exchange in some mechanically ventilated patients remains to be established because the distribution of ventilation and blood flow in injured lungs is too complex to allow definite predictions.

The documented dynamic pulmonary hyperinflation induced by IRV implies that the observed reduction in the peak cycling pressure might not be as important as previously thought in terms of safety. In the clinical setting, a decrease in Pmax is generally considered to herald a reduced risk of barotrauma [36]. However, Pmax includes the resistive pressure to drive flow through the endotracheal tube and the central airway, which is unlikely to produce alveolar disruption. Using the end-inspiratory occlusion technique, we have partitioned Pmax into its resistive and elastic components [37]. As expected, the end-inspiratory recoil pressure measured during the 1.5–2 sec of airway occlusion, which reflects more closely alveolar pressure, was higher during IRV than with IPPV, and comparable to that obtained with external application of an equivalent level of PEEP [35].

In this connection, it could be mentioned that, beside IRV, the high frequency jet ventilation (HFJV) is another form of ventilatory induced dynamic hyperinflation because the shortness of the expiratory time setting determines an incomplete expiration. Recently, in six COPD patients, Conti et al. [38] have shown that at similar conditions of gas exchange in HFJV and IPPV, average values of PEEPi and δFRC were comparable, i.e. 8.9 ± 3.8 vs 8.8 ± 4.7 cm H_2O and 0.56 ± 0.19 vs 0.54 ± 0.21 l, respectively. These data suggest that the mechanism through which some ventilatory modes like IRV and HFJV "work" might be determined, at least in part, by the induced dynamic hyperinflation and PEEPi rather than by more complex mechanisms related to the shape of the inspiratory flow (rapidly decaying or constant) and the pattern of the distribution of ventilation. This problem deserves some further investigation because of its relevance for gas exchange during mechanical ventilatory support.

We have reported here that dynamic hyperinflation and its systematic corollary, i.e. PEEPi, is rather common in mechanically ventilated patients with and without COPD, though much larger in the former than in the latter, and also with different modes of MV like CMV, IRV, IMV, HFJV. Because of their implications in terms of mechanics, gas exchange, and hemodynamics, detection and measurement of dynamic pulmonary hyperinflation and PEEPi should be part of the routine assessment of respiratory function in all mechanically ventilated patients. This can be done easily during any mode of controlled MV, when the respiratory muscles are relaxed, by means of two simple maneuvers suitable for bedside use. First, PEEPi can be measured with a brief end-expiratory airway occlusion as described elsewhere (Fig. 1) [16, 28, 35]. Second, the δFRC, i.e. the difference between the FRC during tidal MV and Vr, can be measured by disconnecting the patient from the ventilator just for the time of one complete (or almost complete) relaxed expiration (Fig. 2) [18, 21]. As mentioned above, these simple measurements might help to improve pharmachological therapy as well as the use of PEEP.

Dynamic Hyperinflation, Inspiratory Effort, and Weaning

Another aspect of PEEPi, which is of primary clinical importance, is its adverse effects on the inspiratory efforts expanded by the patients during assisted modes of MV as well as during weaning and spontaneous ventilation. Although the dynamic increase of FRC has been known for a long time, this particular implication has been pointed out only in recent years [12, 21, 39, 40]. Briefly, in order to create a negative pressure in the central airways to start the inspiratory flow, PEEPi has to be counterbalanced first. Therefore, with ventilatory modes requiring patient's effort (e.g. not only the classic assist-control ventilation, but also newer ventilatory modes like the pressure support ventilation [41]), PEEPi is added to the "triggering" pressure (generally set at 1–2 cm H_2O) so that the total pressure which has to be developed by the inspiratory muscles to initiate the mechanical breath is markedly increased. In other words, PEEPi acts as an "inspiratory threshold load". Also during weaning, PEEPi is an inspiratory threshold load which has to be offset by the contracting inspiratory muscles [42]. This aspect of dynamic hyperinflation in critically ill COPD patients as well as the possible benefit of the external application of low levels of PEEP to reduce PEEPi has been recently reviewed [22] and will be discussed in other chapters of this book. However, there are some other aspects which can deserve a few further words.

Dynamic hyperinflation and PEEPi has been reported in some ARDS patients during MV with common ventilatory setting (TE averaging 2.2 sec) and in all the ARDS patients examined during IRV (TE averaging 1.2 sec), but it has not been addressed yet in spontaneously breathing ARDS patients, although the increased respiratory resistance could prevent a complete expiration to Vr in these patients. In this connection, it has to be emphasized that all patients with early ARDS invariably exhibit the rapid shallow breathing, possibly due to stimulation of J-type pulmonary receptors [6]. Under those circumstances, PEEPi is likely to exist and could provide an important extra load for the respiratory muscles in ARDS patients, in whom the work of breathing is already increased by the abnormally low compliance, while the respiratory muscle contractility can be impaired by factors like sepsis or shock. Whether ARDS patients are at risk to develop respiratory muscle fatigue for these reasons remains to be established [43]. A better understanding of the pathophysilogical events of early ARDS, particularly of the mechanism leading to ventilatory impairment, could have important implications for the management and the ventilatory support of these patients. For example, Brochard et al. [44] have recently published the possibility of non-invasive ventilatory support for COPD patients with ARF. The same possibility might be explored for ARDS patients, for example as a mean to prevent the frequent, lifethreatening, ventilator-associated infections [45, 46].

The fact that pulmonary hyperinflation is determined, at least in part, by fast-developing dynamic factors can be crucial for the respiratory muscles. It is well recognized that hyperinflation profoundly alters respiratory muscle function, though it may have the beneficial effect of improving airway patency, thereby allowing a better distribution of ventilation and an increase in minute ventilation (VE) in patients who are using their maximal expiratory flow rate during tidal breathing [2, 11, 47]. At high lung volumes, inspiratory muscles are shorter and displaced to a less advantageous position of their length-tension curve [1]. However, it has been suggested that an important distinction should be made between the chronic slow-developing static hyperinflation due to the loss of lung elastic recoil and the acute fast-developing dynamic hyperinflation due to bronchoconstriction and/or respiratory tract infection, or to an abnormally increased frequency of breathing (e.g. the rapid shallow breathing invariably exhibited by patients with ARF) [47]. In fact, it has been shown that changes in the inspiratory muscle characteristics can compensate for the decrease in the operating length determined by hyperinflation. In emphysematous hamsters, the diaphragm drops out sarcomers, resulting in a shift of the whole length-tension curve to a shorter length, such that the muscle adapts to the shorter operating length [43]. Whether this adaptation occurs also in humans is not clear, however that observation suggests that the sudden rise in FRC which occurs with the dynamic hyperinflation (e.g. because of a rapid rise in airway resistance) could be much more deleterious for the respiratory muscles action than the chronic hyperinflation due to the loss of lung elastic recoil.

Dynamic Hyperinflation and ARF in COPD Patients

Recent work by our group [13] as well as from other investigators [14, 48] has shown that a slight degree of dynamic hyperinflation is present in COPD patients

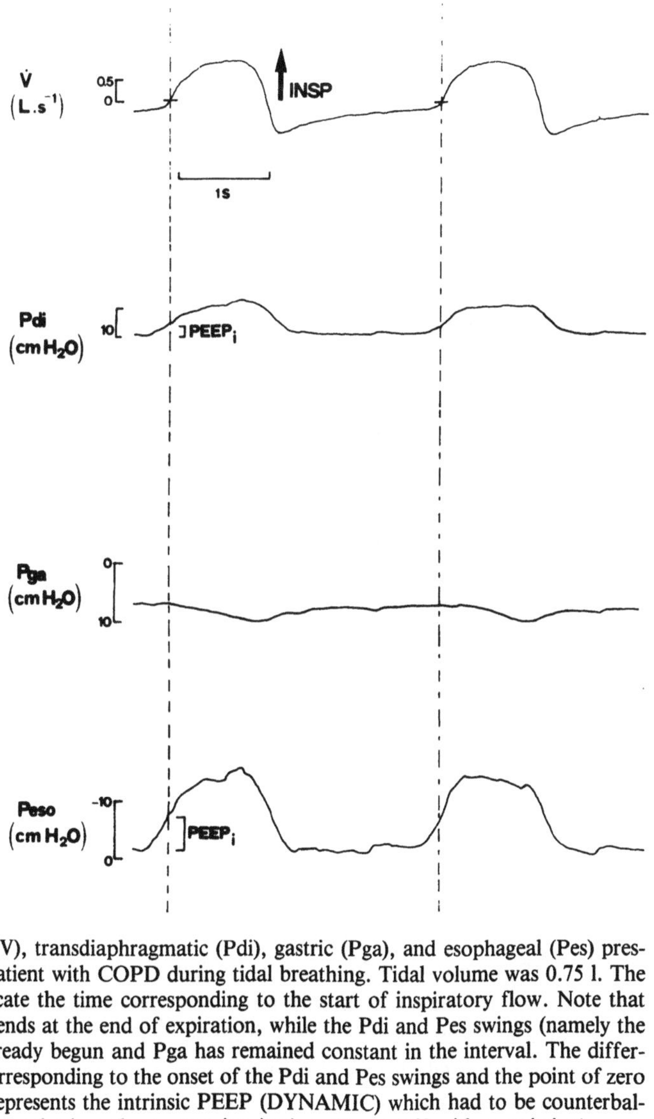

Fig. 7. Tracings of flow (V), transdiaphragmatic (Pdi), gastric (Pga), and esophageal (Pes) pressure in a representative patient with COPD during tidal breathing. Tidal volume was 0.75 l. The vertical dashed lines indicate the time corresponding to the start of inspiratory flow. Note that expiratory flow abruptly ends at the end of expiration, while the Pdi and Pes swings (namely the inspiratory effort) had already begun and Pga has remained constant in the interval. The difference between the point corresponding to the onset of the Pdi and Pes swings and the point of zero flow on the Pes tracing represents the intrinsic PEEP (DYNAMIC) which had to be counterbalanced by the inspiratory muscles in order to start inspiration. (From [13] with permission)

not only during ARF but also in stable condition. The extravolume between Vr and FRC has not been measured directly, however dynamic hyperinflation has been inferred by the pattern of the end-expiratory flow [14] and by the systematic presence of PEEPi [13, 14, 48]. This latter has been measured on the esophageal (pleural) pressure tracing as the difference between the onset of the negative deflection and the point corresponding to the beginning of the inspiratory flow (Fig. 7). This measurement of PEEPi is indirect. Direct measurement of PEEPi, by means of the brief end-expiratory airway occlusion can be performed quite easily in mechanically ventilated patients, whereas it is less suitable to give reliable results during spontaneous breathing. Indeed, the respiratory muscles are often relaxed during MV, particularly in the expiratory time, such that when the airway is occluded at the end of the expiration, a nice plateau in airway pressure provides the value of the end-expiratory recoil pressure, i.e. PEEPi when present, as well as the evidence of respiratory muscle relaxation and equilibration between alveolar and mouth pressure. In contrast, spontaneously breathing patients often react to airway occlusion thus preventing the plateau in mouth pressure. Our indirect measurement of PEEPi, however, is probably valid, provided that the expiratory muscles are relaxed during expiration. In fact, the expiratory muscles could contract until almost the end of expiration and then relax suddenly, such that the initial decrease in Pes might be due to the relaxation of the expiratory muscles rather than to the contraction of the inspiratory muscles. This possibility can be assessed by measurement of gastric pressure (Pga) in order to detect whether the decrease in Pes is associated with a decrease in Pga, indicating expiratory muscles decontraction. We have shown that in our stable COPD patients, Pga remained constant throughout most of the tidal expiration after the initial post-inspiratory decay, thus supporting our technique to measure PEEPi [13]. However, it has to be recognized that PEEPi measured on the Pes deflection as previously described can underestimate the true degree of dynamic hyperinflation, because it corresponds to the dynamic PEEPi, which is the minimum PEEPi when the first lung units with the relatively shorter time constant start filling. Dynamic PEEPi was found to be about 60–70% of the static PEEPi, measured by means of the end-expiratory airway occlusion after equilibration between all the lung units, at least in COPD patients recovering from acute exacerbation [49].

The existence of a slight degree of dynamic hyperinflation in COPD patients in stable condition, and the evidence of a protective mechanism of the diaphragmatic length-tension properties in emphysematous hamsters, support the hypothesis that dynamic pulmonary hyperinflation can play a key role in the development of ARF in these patients. Indeed, respiratory tract infection, which is by far the most common cause of acute exacerbation, and ARF in COPD patients, increase airway resistance by means of the inflammatory process leading to abnormal mucus production and thickening of bronchial wall as well as to the reflex bronchoconstriction [50]. The expiratory flow rate is unduly slowed by the reduced bronchial caliber while the frequency of breathing is increased because of stimulation of irritant receptors and fever. Under these circumstances, the discrepancy between a long time needed to breathe out and the short TE of the rapid and shallow breathing pattern increases progressively, ensuing dynamic hyperinflation and rising PEEPi. Indeed, PEEPi averaged 2.5 ± 1.5 cm H_2O in stable COPD patients [13], 8.8 ± 2.3

cm H_2O in acutely ill, spontaneously breathing COPD patients [51], and 4.5 ± 0.6 cm H_2O in COPD patients during weaning [49]. The increment of PEEPi from the stable to the acute condition clearly increases the ventilatory load upon the respiratory muscles while the work of breathing is already enhanced by the high resistance and elastance [51]. On the other hand, dynamic hyperinflation reduces the respiratory muscle efficiency as pressure generators because of the sudden, uncompensated, shorter operating length plus other factors [47]. Indeed, we have found that the minimum pleural pressure during a Mueller maneuver averaged 77 ± 16 cm H_2O in 60 consecutive stable COPD patients and 40 ± 6 cm H_2O in 8 COPD patients with ARF and difficult weaning. Under these circumstances, i.e. increased workload and decreased inspiratory muscle strength, the decrease in VT can become a mandatory choice to minimize the elastic work of breathing, while a further increase in f is required to defend VE [52]. With the worsening of the underlying pathology, the pattern of breathing becomes progressively more rapid and shallow, thus generating a sort of vicious circle leading to respiratory muscle fatigue and acute ventilatory failure [50].

Dynamic Hyperinflation and Asthma

An increase in lung volumes is usually observed in asthmatic patients during an acute attack. The residual volume can increase because of gas trapping due to premature airway closure [53]. The total lung capacity has been observed to increase significantly when measured correctly by means of chest X-ray (avoiding potential errors of both the plethysmographic and the helium dilution techniques) [54] though the underlying mechanism has not been fully understood (changes in surface elastic properties of the lung lining fluid?). Vr has been found to increase significantly during acute bronchoconstriction in asthmatics because of changes in the position of the pressure-volume curve of the lung [55]. The increase in FRC can be in part the consequence of these changes and in part it can be determined by dynamic events like the increase in airway resistance (see above) and in the post-inspiratory inspiratory muscles activity (PIIA) [53]. This latter mechanism has been investigated by Martin et al. in an elegant series of publications [3]. They have shown that during histamine induced bronchoconstriction, there was a significant PIIA which resulted in a retardation of expiratory flow and enhanced hyperinflation [3]. Since the diaphragm relaxed earlier in expiration compared to pre-bronchoconstriction status, it was concluded that the PIIA was attributable to rib cage musculature and that the increase in FRC was, at least in part, accounted for by inspiratory displacement of the rib cage compartment of the chest wall. This finding in asthmatics may be surprising in view of the increased rate of decay of PIIA observed in COPD patients at any given TE, compared to normals [14, 56]. In fact, it seems reasonable the expiratory braking action of the PIIA to be reduced when expiration is already retarded by other factors, i.e. increased flow resistance and expiratory flows limitation [14]. However, this increased PIIA in asthmatics might well represent another difference between the acute and the chronic development of airway obstruction and pulmonary hyperinflation. Teleologically, one might think that an increased PIIA during acute bronchoconstriction might help to keep a negative pleural pressure which otherwise would be positive at high lung volumes (FRC during acute bronchoconstriction can exceed the predicted TLC) with detrimental effects not only on the expiratory flow rate (i.e. a positive pleural pressure favors flow limitation), but also on venous return and cardiac filling.

Recently, Wheatley et al. [55] raised the possibility that hyperinflation in asthmatics might be advantageous not only by improving the airway patency and inspired gas distribution while decreasing the inspiratory flow-resistive work, but also by minimizing the total respiratory muscle work and hence minimizing the energy expenditure. This is a quiet stimulating hypothesis in view of the diffuse idea that hyperinflation increases severely the elastic component of inspiratory muscle work. Those authors have found that the increase in the elastic work was offset by the decrease in the resistive one, while the expiratory work was markedly reduced [55].

In this connection, we would like to report here some preliminary results of measurements of respiratory mechanics in a few asthmatic patients during MV because of ARF due to the severity of the attack (Table 2).

These data show that increased respiratory resistance and a high PEEPi, frequently associated with a low respiratory compliance, are a common finding in asthmatic patients requiring MV. The interest of these numbers stems from the fact that, to our knowledge, there is no other systematic report of respiratory mechanics in mechanically ventilated asthmatics in the literature, while sophisticated measurements have been performed for gas exchange [57]. This latter study by Rodriguez-Roisin et al. [57] helped to explain hypoxemia in asthmatics. Our data support the idea that asthmatic patients can be at risk to develop respiratory muscle fatigue, alveolar hypoventilation, and hypercapnia, because of a rapid and severe dynamic hyperinflation (see above) which can be the life-threatening characteristic of a severe asthmatic attack [58]. Detection and measurement of PEEPi is important in the management of severe asthma for two reasons, at least:

Table 2. Respiratory mechanics in three young asthmatic patients during the first day of mechanical ventilation in the control mode

Variable	A.F. (f, 36)	B.S. (f, 17)	O.G. (f, 28)
$\dot{V}E$ (l/min)	8.4	9.5	9.6
f (b/min)	12.0	13.0	12.0
VT (l)	0.70	0.73	0.80
TE (s)	3.1	2.9	3.7
PEEPi (cmH_2O)	12.9	13.6	8.0
δFRC (l)	0.81	0.30	0.48
Cst, rs (l/cmH_2O)	0.044	0.060	0.040
Rrs ($cmH_2O/l/s$)	36.5	17.8	33.1

$\dot{V}E$ = minute ventilation; f = ventilatory frequency; *VT* = inflation volume; *TE* = expiratory time; *PEEPi* = intrinsic positive end-expiratory pressure; δFRC = difference between the static equilibrium volume of the respiratory system and the functional residual capacity during mechanical ventilation; *Cst, rs* = static respiratory compliance; *Rrs* = respiratory resistance after subtraction of endotracheal tube and measuring equipment

1. application of an external PEEP lower than the measured PEEPi might help to unload the respiratory muscles and to prevent tracheal intubation [59], and
2. optimization of mechanical ventilatory setting could be achieved in order to minimize PEEPi and its adverse hemodynamic, cardiac, and mechanical effects.

We believe that because of its therapeutic implications, the mechanism(s) of pulmonary hyperinflation in bronchial asthma deserves further attention by respiratory physiologists, not only because bronchial asthma is one of the most common respiratory diseases, but also because acute asthmatic attack can be a life-threatening condition particularly in young patients [60].

Conclusions

In summary we have discussed in this review that:

1. dynamic pulmonary hyperinflation due to increased airflow resistance can be a common event in mechanically ventilated patients even in patients without COPD. In all these patients, intrinsic PEEP (PEEPi) is a systematic corollary of dynamic hyperinflation and has some important implications:
   - PEEPi can have the same adverse cardiovascular effects as an equivalent level of external application of PEEP;
   - the undetected PEEPi indroduces a significant error in the computation of respiratory static compliance; the error is up to 100% in COPD patients and to 30% in ARDS patients;
   - dynamic hyperinflation and PEEPi might help to explain the improvement in PaO_2 as well as the drop in cardiac filling when patients are implemented with the inverse ratio MV.
   - PEEPi acts as an inspiratory threshold load which adds to the triggering pressure during assisted MV modes.
2. The fast-developing dynamic hyperinflation due to acute bronchoconstriction, respiratory tract infection, and/or high frequency of breathing can play a key role in the development of respiratory muscle fatigue and ventilatory failure as well as in difficult weaning; indeed, PEEPi provides an extra-burden for the respiratory muscles while their capability as pressure generators is impaired by the shorter operational length and a less favorable geometrical arrangement because of the high and growing FRC.
3. In asthmatic patients, dynamic hyperinflation might be due not only to increased flow resistance, but also to increased PIIA of the rib cage inspiratory muscles. However, PEEPi was found systematically in asthmatic patients during MV because of a severe attack. A further definition of the mechanisms leading to pulmonary hyperinflation in asthma could help to prevent tracheal intubation as well as to optimize the mode and setting of MV when needed.

References

1. Agostoni E, Mead J (1964) Statics of the Respiratory System. In: Fenn WO, Rahn H (eds), Handbook of physiology. Section 3: Respiration. Vol I. Washington DC, American Physiological Society, pp 387–409
2. Macklem PT (1984) Hyperinflation. Am Rev Respir Dis 129:1–2
3. Martin JG, De Troyer A (1985) The thorax and control of functional residual capacity. In: Roussos C, Macklem PT (eds), Lung biology in health and disease, the thorax, Vol. 29, Part B. Dekker Marcel Inc., New York, pp 899–921
4. Reder K, Marsh HM (1986) Respiratory mechanics during anesthesia and mechanical ventilation. In: Macklem PT, Mead J (eds), Handbook of physiology. Section 3: Respiration. Vol III. Washington DC, American Physiological Society, pp. 737–752
5. Pride NB, Macklem PT (1986) Lung mechanics in disease. In: Macklem PT, Mead J (eds) Handbook of physiology. Section 3: Respiration, Vol III. Washington DC, American Physiological Society, pp 659–692
6. Suter PM (1985) Assessment of respiratory mechanics in ARDS In: Zapol ZM, Falke KJ (eds) Acute respiratory failure. Vol. 24; Lung biology in health and disease. Marcel Dekker Inc, New York, pp 899–921
7. Gattinoni L, Pesenti A, Avalli L, Rossi F, Bombino M (1987) Pressure-volume curve of total respiratory system in acute respiratory failure. Computed tomographic scan study. Am Rev Respir Dis 136:730–736
8. Slutsky AS, Scharf SM, Brown R, Ingram RH Jr (1980) The effect of oleic acid-induced pulmonary edema on pulmonary and chest wall mechanics in dogs. Am Rev Respir Dis 121:91–96
9. Whipp BJ, Pardy RL (1986) Breathing during exercise. In: Macklem PT, Mead J (eds) Handbook of physiology. Section 3: Respiration. Vol III. Washington DC, American Physiological Society, pp 605–629
10. Mortola JP (1983) Dynamic of breathing in newborn mammals. Physiological Review 67:187–243
11. Demedts M (1990) Mechanism and consequences of hyperinflation. Eur Respir J 3:617–619
12. Rossi A, Gottfried SB, Zocchi L et al (1985) Measurement of static compliance of total respiratory system in patients with acute respiratory failure during mechanical ventilation. Am Rev Respir Dis 131:672–678
13. Dal Vecchio L, Polese G, Poggi R, Rossi A (1990) "Intrinsic" positive end-expiratory pressure in stable patients with chronic obstructive pulmonary disease. Eur Respir J 3:74–80
14. Morris, MJ, Lane DJ (1981) Tidal expiratory flow patterns in patients with airflow obstruction. Thorax 36:135–142
15. Jonson B, Nordstrom L, Olsson SG, Akerback D (1975) Monitoring of ventilation and lung mechanics during automatic ventilation. A new device. Bull Eur Physiopathol Respir 11:729–743
16. Pepe PE, Marini JJ (1982) Occult positive end-expiratory pressure in mechanically ventilated patients with airflow obstruction. Am Rev Respir Dis 126:166–170
17. Gottfried SB, Rossi A, Higgs BD et al. (1985) Noninvasive determination of respiratory system mechanics during mechanical ventilation for acute respiratory failure. Am Rev Respir Dis 131:414–420
18. Broseghini C, Brandolese R, Poggi R et al. (1988) Respiratory mechanics during the first day of mechanical ventilation in patients with pulmonary edema and chronic airway obstruction. Am Rev Respir Dis 138:355–361
19. Poggi R, Brandolese R, Bernasconi M, Manzin E, Rossi A (1989) Doxofylline and respiratory mechanics. Short term effects in mechanically ventilated patients with airflow obstruction and respiratory failure. Chest 96:772–778
20. Bernasconi M, Ploysongsang Y, Gottfried SB, Milic-Emili J, Rossi A (1988) Respiratory compliance and resistance in mechanically ventilated patients with acute respiratory failure. Intensive Care Med 14:547–553
21. Kimball WR, Leith DE, Robins AG (1982) Dynamic hyperinflation and ventilator dependence in chronic obstructive pulmonary disease. Am Rev Respir Dis 126:991–995

22. Rossi A, Brandolese R, Milic-Emili J, Gottfried SB (1990) The role of PEEP in patients with chronic obstructive pulmonary disease during assisted ventilation. Eur Resp J 3:816–822
23. Saetta M, Rossi A, Gottfried SB et al. (1985) Expiratory volume-flow relationship during mechanical ventilation in patients with acute respiratory failure. Am Rev Respir Dis 131:A132
24. Connors AF Jr, McCaffree DR, Gray BA (1981) Effect of inspiratory flow rate on gas exchange during mechanical ventilation. Am Rev Respir Dis 124:537–543
25. Bernasconi M, Brandolese R, Poggi R, Manzin E, Rossi A (1990) Dose-response effects and time course of effects of inhaled fenoterol on respiratory mechanics and arterial oxygen tension in mechanically ventilated patients with chronic airflow obstruction. Intensive Care Med 16:108–114
26. Conti G, Bufi M, Antonelli M, Rocco M, Gasparetto A (1989) Pressure support ventilation (PSV) reverses hyperinflation induced isorhythmic A-V dissociation. Intensive Care Med 15:319–321
27. Braschi A, Iotti G, Rodi G, Emmi V, Sala Gallini G (1988) Dynamic pulmonary hyperinflation during intermittent mandatory ventilation. Intensive Care Med 14:284
28. Broseghini C, Brandolese R, Poggi R, Bernasconi M, Manzin E, Rossi A (1988) Respiratory resistance and intrinsic positive end-expiratory pressure (PEEP) in patients with the adult respiratory distress syndrome (ARDS). Eur Respir J 1:726–731
29. Polese G, Rossi A, Brandi G et al. (1990) Partitioning of respiratory mechanics in mechanically ventilated COPD patients. Eur Respir J 2:337s
30. Wright PE, Barnard GR (1989) The role of airflow resistance in patients with the adult respiratory distress syndrome. Am Rev Respir Dis 139:1169–1174
31. Wright PE, Marini JJ, Bernard GR (1989) In vitro versus in vivo comparison on endotracheal tube airflow resistance. Am Rev Respir Dis 10:10–16
32. Gurevitch MJ, Van Dyke JV, Young ES, Jackson K (1986) Improved oxygenation and lower peak airway pressure in severe adult respiratory distress syndrome. Chest 2:211–213
33. Abraham E, Yoshihara G (1989) Cardiorespiratory effects of pressure controlled inverse ratio ventilation in severe respiratory failure. Chest 96:1356–1359
34. Gattinoni L, Marcolin R, Caspani ML, Fumagalli R, Mascheroni D, Pesenti A (1985) Constant mean airway pressure with different patterns of positive pressure breathing during the adult respiratory distress syndrome. Bull Eur Physiopathol Respir 21:275–279
35. Brandolese R, Broseghini C, Polese G, Milic-Emili J, Brandi G, Rossi A (1991) Effect of intrinsic PEEP on pulmonary gas exchange in mechanically ventilated patients with pulmonary edema (in press)
36. Haake R, Schlichtig R, Ulstad DR, Henschen R (1987) Barotrauma. Pathophysiology, risk factors, and prevention. Chest 91:608–613
37. Rossi A, Gottfried SB, Higgs BD, Zocchi L, Grassino A, Milic-Emili J (1985) Respiratory mechanics in mechanically ventilated patients with respiratory failure. J Appl Physiol 58:1849–1858
38. Conti G, Bufi M, Rocco M et al (1990) Auto-PEEP and dynamic hyperinflation in COPD patients during controlled mechanical ventilation and high frequency jet ventilation. Intensive Care Med 16:81–84
39. Smith TC, Marini JJ (1988) Impact of PEEP on lung mechanics and work of breathing in severe airflow obstruction. J Appl Physiol 65:1488–1499
40. Gottfried SB, Rossi A, Milic-Emili J (1986) Dynamic hyperinflation, intrinsic PEEP, and the mechanically ventilated patient. Intensive Crit Care Dig 5:30–33
41. Brochard L, Harf A, Lorino H, Lemaire F (1989) Inspiratory pressure support prevents diaphragmatic fatigue during weaning from mechanical ventilation. Am Rev Respir Dis 139:513–521
42. Milic-Emili J (1986) Is weaning an art or a science? Am Rev Respir Dis 134:1107–1108
43. Roussos C, Macklem PT (1986) Inspiratory muscle fatigue. In: Macklem PT, Mead J (eds) Handbook of physiology. Section 3: Respiration, Vol III. American Physiological Society. Washington DC, pp 511–527
44. Brochard L, Isabey D, Piquet J et al. (1990) Reversal of acute exacerbation of chronic obstructive lung disease by inspiratory assistance with a face mask. N Engl J Med 323:1523–1530

45. Meduri GU (1990) Ventilator-associated pneumonia in patients with respiratory failure. A diagnostic approach. Chest 97:1208–1219
46. Pingleton SK (1988) Complications of acute respiratory failure. Am Rev Respir Dis 137:1463–1493
47. Decramer M (1989) Effects of hyperinflation on the respiratory muscle. Eur Respir J 2:299–302
48. Haluszka J, Chartrand DA, Grassino AE, Milic-Emili J (1990) Intrinsic PEEP and arterial PCO_2 in stable patients with chronic obstructive pulmonary disease. Am Rev Respir Dis 141:1194–1197
49. Petroff BJ, Legare M, Goldberg P, Milic-Emili J, Gottfried SB (1990) Continuous positive airway pressure reduces work of breathing and dyspnea during weaning from mechanical ventilation in severe chronic obstructive pulmonary disease. Am Rev Respir Dis 141:281–289
50. Derenne JP, Fleury B, Pariente R (1988) Acute respiratory failure of chronic obstructive pulmonary disease. Am Rev Respir Dis 138:1006–1033
51. Fleury B, Murciano D, Talamo C, Aubier M, Pariente R, Milici-Emili J (1985) Work of breathing in patients with chronic obstructive pulmonary disease in acute respiratory failure. Am Rev Respir Dis 132:822–827
52. Roussos C (1985) Energetics. In: Roussos C, Macklem PT (eds) Lung biology in health and disease, Vol 29, the thorax, part A. Marcel Dekker Inc, New York, pp 437–492
53. Cormier Y, Lecours R, Legris C (1990) Mechanism of hyperinflation in asthma. Eur Respir J 3:619–624
54. Blackie SP, Al-Majed S, Staples CA, Hilliam C, Pare PD (1990) Changes in total lung capacity during acute spontaneous asthma. Am Rev Respir Dis 142:79–83
55. Wheatley JR, West S, Cala SJ, Engel LA (1990) The effect of hyperinflation on respiratory muscle work in acute induced asthma. Eur Respir J 3:625–632
56. Citterio G, Agostoni E, Del Santo A, Marazzini L (1981) Decay of inspiratory muscle activity in chronic airway obstruction. J Appl Physiol 51:1388–1397
57. Rodriguez-Roisin R, Ballester E, Roca J, Torres A, Wagner PD (1989) Mechanism of hypoxemia in patients with status asthmaticus requiring mechanical ventilation. Am Rev Respir Dis 139:732–739
58. Perret C (1989) Sudden asphyxia in asthma. In: Vincent JL (ed) Update in intensive care and emergency medicine, Vol 12. Springer, Berlin Heidelberg New York, pp 86–90
59. Branthwaite MA (1990) An update on mechanical ventilation for severe acute asthma. Clinical Intensive Care 1:4–6
60. Luksza AR, Smith P, Coakley J, Gordan IJ, Atherton ST (1986) Acute severe asthma treated by mechanical ventilation: 10 years' experience from a district general hospital. Thorax 41:459–463

Disorders of the Chest Wall: Implications for Respiratory Failure

S. E. Eveloff and F. D. McCool

Introduction

The chest wall is a major component of the inspiratory pump and consists of the bony structures of the rib cage, the spine and its articulations, and the respiratory muscles and their nerves. The respiratory muscles are broadly categorized as either inspiratory or expiratory. The inspiratory muscles are essential for maintaining ventilation as well as for performing non-respiratory tasks. The major muscles of inspiration include the diaphragm, external intercostal muscles, parasternals, and other accessory muscles. Expiration in quiet breathing is usually passive but active deflation can occur by activating the abdominal or internal intercostal muscles. A variety of diseases can involve the respiratory muscles or any of the components of the chest wall. These diseases may by themselves, or in combination with other disease processes, cause acute (ARF) or chronic respiratory failure. This chapter will not attempt to review all these disease processes, but will instead focus on selected pathological processes involving the muscles (bilateral diaphragm paralysis), spine and its articulations (kyphoscoliosis), and bones of the rib cage (flail chest).

Bilateral Diaphragm Paralysis

Respiratory failure as a consequence of bilateral diaphragm paralysis (BDP) or extreme diaphragm weakness is an uncommon clinical condition. BDP may occur as a result of an isolated defect along the neuromuscular axis serving the diaphragm, or may be an isolated manifestation of a systemic neuromuscular disease. In either case, a reasonable index of suspicion for this entity should be maintained in the appropriate clinical context, as definitive diagnosis requires specialized testing and may have specific prognostic implications.

Detailed analysis of BDP as a discrete entity has existed only since 1976, when Newsom-Davis et al. [1] first evaluated a series of such patients using transdiaphragmatic pressure monitoring. Despite several studies since then, certain aspects of BDP still remain controversial. Specific issues remaining unresolved include which parameter of transdiaphragmatic pressure monitoring offers the most reliable assessment of function [1–5], the degree of sensitivity and specificity of fluoroscopy in evaluating BDP [6–9], whether isolated BDP in the absence of other respiratory muscle weakness leads to acute and/or chronic respiratory failure [1, 2, 9–11], and the compensatory mechanisms of inspiration used by patients with this condition.

Etiology

BDP or extreme weakness most commonly occurs in association with systemic disease causing generalized muscle weakness. However, isolated diaphragm dysfunction may rarely be the initial or predominant manifestation of systemic diseases (Table 1). Recently, the increasing frequency of cardiac surgery, improvements in recognition and treatment of thoracic neoplastic disease [9], and the improvements in acute salvage of trauma victims are contributing to iatrogenic and traumatic phrenic nerve injury as a growing cause of BDP. For example, phrenic nerve injury after open-heart surgery occurs up to 10% of the time, and may be secondary to thermal injury, actual nerve transsection, nerve traction, or ischemic injury, especially with internal mammary artery grafting [7, 12, 13]. An appropriate index of suspicion must be maintained in patients with these antecedent histories, as phrenic nerve dysfunction in these settings may have more subtle manifestations than when associated with more generalized diseases.

Table 1. Causes of diaphragmatic weakness or paralysis

Cervical spinal cord lesions
Traumatic syringomyelia
Carcinomatous encephalomyelitis
Spinal cord tumors
Anterior horn cell lesions (C_3-C_4)
Amyotrophic lateral sclerosis
Spinal muscular atrophy
Poliomyelitis
Phrenic neuropathies
Trauma, surgery ("phrenic frostbite")
Herpes zoster
Immunologic (e.g. Guillain-Barré syndrome)
Infection (e.g. diphtheria)
Tumor (direct phrenic invasion, metastatic)
Metabolic (e.g. porphyrias)
Endocrine (e.g. diabetes)
Toxic (e.g. arsenic, organophosphates)
Idiopathic
Neuromuscular
Myasthenia gravis
Lambert-Eaton myasthenic syndrome
Toxins (botulism)
Muscular dystrophies (Duchenne's, limb girdle)
Myotonic dystrophy
Endocrine disorders (thyrotoxicosis, Cushing's disease, myxedema)
Metabolic disorders (malnutrition, hypophosphatemia)
Immunologic (polymyositis, dermatomyositis, systemic lupus erythematosus)
Trichinosis
Idiopathic

Clinical Presentation

Bedside evaluations of symptoms and signs of patients with suspected bilateral diaphragm paralysis is a sensitive but somewhat non-specific means of assessing diaphragm dysfunction (Table 2). When considered in a suggestive clinical context, recognition of such symptoms and signs provide the clinician with the opportunity to initiate appropriate studies while avoiding a prolonged period of fruitless testing and patient discomfort.

Many patients with respiratory failure, including those with diaphragm dysfunction, will complain of dyspnea. Orthopnea, in the absence of congestive heart failure, provides better diagnostic sensitivity and is almost invariably present in patients with BDP. Discomfort even while being examined in the supine position may be the initial suggestion of diaphragmatic impairment. Dyspnea on immersion, although uncommon, has also been reported [14].

The most important aspect of physical examination in these patients is observation and recognition of specific breathing pattern abnormalities. In patients with BDP or with severe diaphragm weakness, inspiration results in inward or paradoxical motion of the abdomen. This pattern may be better appreciated in patients by simultaneous palpation of the rib cage and abdominal wall during inspiration. Paradoxical abdominal movement is most obvious in the supine position, and may resolve totally when the patient is upright. There is even some evidence to suggest that this paradoxical movement may actually offer quantitative information of diaphragm function [5]. In a large series of patients with varying degrees of diaphragm dysfunction who had transdiaphragmatic pressure monitoring in the upright and supine positions, both orthopnea and abdominal paradox in the supine position were always present when transdiaphragmatic pressure change during a sniff maneuver was less than 30 cm H_2O. This assessment, however, was not 100% sensitive or specific in the patients studied, and was based on a sniff Pdi maneuver, which differs from transdiaphragmatic pressure generated by a tidal volume (VT) or total lung capacity (TLC) maneuver. However, it does suggest that abdominal paradox may reliably predict severe diaphragm dysfunction.

This particular breathing pattern and its subjective correlate, orthopnea, can be

Table 2. Clinical assessment of diaphragm dysfunction

Screening for diaphragm dysfunction
Presence of orthopnea
Paradoxical motion of rib cage and abdomen
TLC $<$ 70% predicted
MIP $<$ 60 cm H_2O
ΔVC from supine to prone $>$ 30%
Diagnostic tests for diaphragm dysfunction
Pdi during breath to TLC $<$ 25 cm H_2O
Pdi during maximal Mueller maneuver $<$ 60 cm H_2O
Pdi during maximal sniff maneuver $<$ 70 cm H_2O

Abbreviations: *TLC:* total lung capacity; *MIP:* maximal static inspiratory pressure; *ΔVC:* change in vital capacity; *Pdi:* transdiaphragmatic pressure

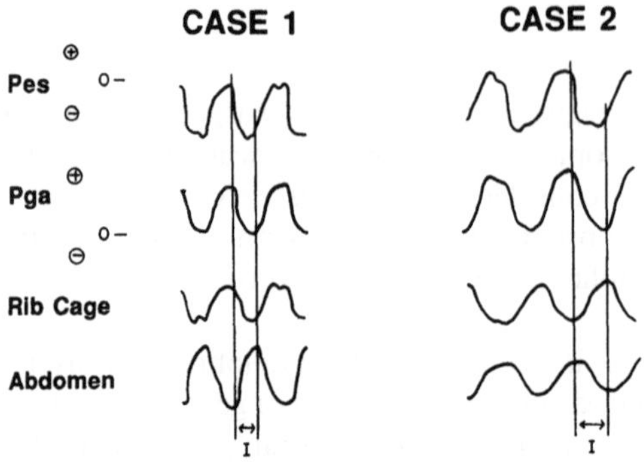

Fig. 1. Tracings of esophageal and gastric pressure in two patients with bilateral diaphragm paralysis. As in normals esophageal pressure becomes more negative during inspiration. In contrast to normal, gastric pressure becomes more negative and parallels the change in Pes. Patients with bilateral diaphragm paralysis may use two strategies to inhale. Case 1 utilizes a strategy whereby the abdominal muscles are recruited to actively exhale below FRC and inspiration (I) is accomplished by the passive recoil of the respiratory system. With this strategy there is outward motion of the abdomen and inward motion of the rib cage during inspiration. Case 2 utilizes the inspiratory muscles of the rib cage to inhale. There is outward displacement of the rib cage and inward motion of the abdomen during inspiration

explained by gravitational effects on abdominal contents. In BDP, the diaphragm behaves as a flaccid, passive membrane separating the thoracic and abdominal compartments. One strategy that these patients can use to inhale is recruitment of the muscles of the rib cage. When upright, the intercostal and accessory muscles will elevate the rib cage and displace the abdominal contents cephalad, thereby shifting the support of these contents from the abdominal wall to the diaphragm. This shift in support reduces the pressure below both hemidiaphragms. This more negative subdiaphragmatic pressure is transmitted across the diaphragm to assist with lung inflation. In contrast, when supine, the muscles of the rib cage are ineffective in lowering subdiaphragmatic pressure and gravity enhances displacement of the abdominal contents into the thorax. Such cephalad movement of the passive diaphragm makes inspiration extremely inefficient and uncomfortable in the supine position [14]. An alternate strategy that may be utilized by patients with BDP is recruitment of the abdominal muscles to actively exhale below functional residual capacity (FRC) and then relaxing them to passively inhale. The implications of the two strategies on abdominal wall displacements are opposite. The abdominal muscle relaxation technique requires inward displacement of the belly wall during expiration and outward displacement during inspiration; whereas the rib cage muscle recruitment mechanism requires inward displacement of the abdomen during inspiration (Fig. 1).

Diagnostic Tests

Lung volumes. Patients with BDP typically have restrictive disease with a reduction of their vital capacity (VC) and TLC to less than 70% of predicted when upright.

More importantly, however, VC may then decrease further by 30–50% measured in the supine position. This marked positional reduction in VC was first described by McCredie et al. [15] in 1962 in three patients. In contrast, changes in VC in normal subjects on assumption of the supine posture ranges from 10% [16] to 20% [17]. A decrease in FRC and TLC has also been described with BDP paralysis [2, 9, 10, 11, 15], and one case report [11] further describes a 30% decrease in FRC on assumption of the supine position. Given the lack of additional diagnostic sensitivity and specificity, these measurements are not considered as important as the measurements change in VC with the supine position in these patients. Furthermore, measurements of VC can be performed at the bedside in both intubated and spontaneously breathing patients. Therefore, a critical observation in patients with suspected BDP or even in patients with unexplained respiratory failure is a positional dependency of dyspnea, abdominal paradoxical movement especially in the supine position, and the pronounced reduction of VC in the supine position.

Maximal inspiratory pressures. Maximal static inspiratory pressure (PImax) can also be helpful in assessing the presence of BDP and can be easily obtained at the bedside. However, PImax has to be interpreted cautiously. Because the maximal static inspiratory pressure is the result of diaphragmatic, intercostal, and accessory muscle activation, the PImax is an indication of global inspiratory muscle strength and it does not assess diaphragm activity specifically. Furthermore, PImax is by lung volume dependent, effort dependent, and subject to a great deal of variability as a result of age and sex differences [18, 19]. Thus, serial testing needs to be performed

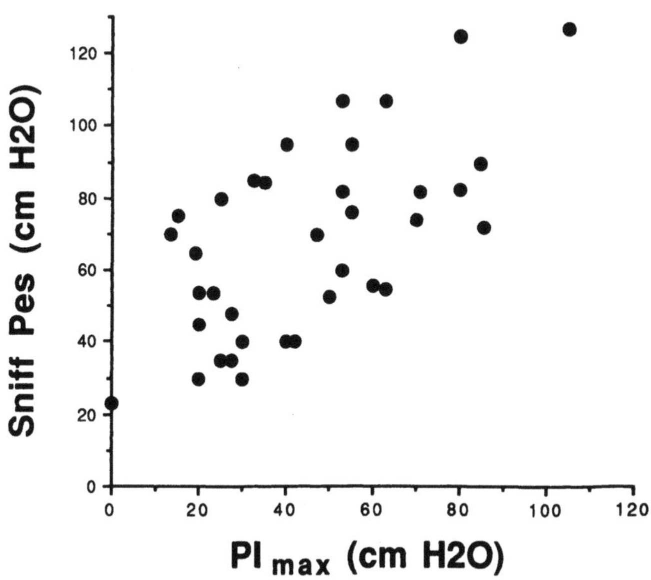

Fig. 2. Values of Pes obtained during the sniff maneuver (Sniff Pes) are generally greater than pressure obtained during the maximal Mueller efforts (PImax) in patients evaluated for respiratory muscle weakness.

with maximal efforts at comparable lung volumes. However, if careful attention is given to these technical details, PImax is a useful and reliable initial screening test for BDP. If PImax is normal, BDP is unlikely. However, if PImax is less than 60% of predicted, BDP should be suspected. Indeed, Abd et al. [8] found that all subjects with BDP as a consequence of coronary artery bypass grafting had a PImax less than 30% of predicted. Most recently, the sniff maneuver has been advocated as a test to assess respiratory muscle performance [5] since it is easy to perform and the changes in esophageal pressure during a maximal sniff were as great as those obtained during a maximal Mueller (PImax) effort (Fig. 2). Properly conducted, assessment of global inspiratory muscle strength by either PImax or sniff maneuvers should be considered an important aspect of the initial bedside screening in patients with suspected diaphragm paralysis.

Radiography. Chest radiographs generally demonstrate bilaterally elevated hemidiaphragms with reduced lung volumes. However, this finding is not specific for BDP since low lung volumes may be attributed to other restrictive processes or to poor inspiratory efforts.

Evaluation of diaphragm motion by fluoroscopy has also been used to assess diaphragm dysfunction but is limited when evaluating BDP. First, paradoxical diaphragm motion may be elicited in normal individuals. Alexander [6] found that most normals have unequal excursion of right and left diaphragm movement on inspiration. Furthermore, 6% of the patients demonstrated paradoxical movement of one diaphragm on performing a sniff maneuver. Second, patients with bilateral diaphragm paralysis may exhibit normal caudal displacement of the diaphragm when inhaling. Patients with BDP may actively contract the abdominal muscles and displace the diaphragm cephalad during expiration. By relaxing the abdominal wall at end-expiration, the diaphragm can descend and inspiration can be achieved by the passive recoil of the respiratory system. The use of the rib cage muscles to lower subdiaphragmatic pressure during inspiration may also promote caudal motion of the diaphragm. Therefore, even though some studies still use fluoroscopy to diagnose BDP [8], it should be considered the least reliable objective test available, and can usually be omitted. Neither direction [1, 6, 20] or absolute excursion [6] of the diaphragm provide improved diagnostic accuracy.

Transdiaphragmatic pressure monitoring. BDP can be confirmed by measuring transdiaphragmatic pressure (Pdi; Pdi = Pga - Pes). Diaphragm descent produces a transdiaphragmatic pressure change such that pleural pressure falls and abdominal pressure increases. The measurement of Pdi is much more specific for diaphragmatic dysfunction than the tests previously discussed. It can be performed at the bedside using commercially available esophageal and gastric balloon-catheter systems, pressure transducers, and recording devices found in many intensive care units. Details concerning the apparatus and the specific insertion and monitoring procedure have been well described [1, 21–23].

With BDP, one would expect changes in Pes and Pga to parallel one another during tidal breathing and therefore produce no change in Pdi. This pattern may also be seen during a maximal Mueller maneuver (Fig. 3). However, controversy exists as to which inspiratory maneuver provides the most reliable and specific in-

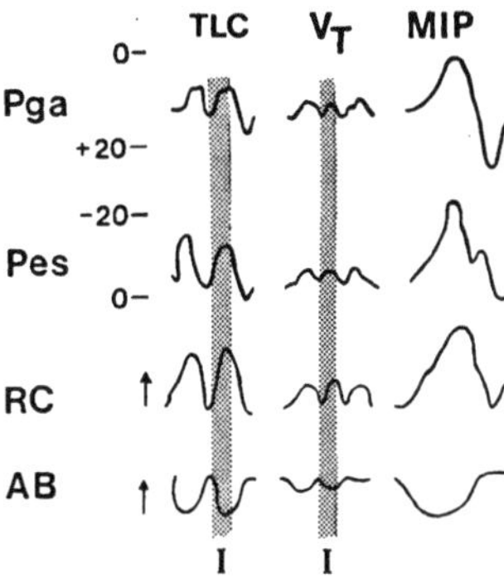

Fig. 3. Changes in esophageal (Pes) and gastric (Pga) pressures and anteroposterior rib cage dimensions (RC) and anteroposterior abdominal dimensions (Ab) during inspiration to TLC, tidal breathing (VT) and maximum static inspiratory efforts (MIP) in a patient with bilateral diaphragm paralysis. Arrow indicates increasing rib cage and abdomen dimensions; I denotes inspiratory phase of the breathing cycle in this patient with BDP

formation during transdiaphragmatic pressure monitoring. Three maneuvers have been utilized: a maximal inspiration to TLC (PdiTLC), a maximal static inspiratory maneuver (Pdimax), and a maximal inspiratory sniff (Pdisniff).

Normal values for PdiTLC usually exceed 25 cm H_2O [1]. However, this test is limited because the static pressure the diaphragm is capable of generating is much greater than the pressures that are required to achieve TLC, thus possibly reducing the sensitivity of this test [24]. There is also wide variability in normal values reported for this test and occasional very low values are obtained [23, 24].

A better assessment of the maximal pressure-generating capacity of the diaphragm can be obtained by measuring Pdi during a maximal inspiratory effort. The magnitude of Pdi during this maneuver will depend upon the same factors that influence PImax (i.e. volume and degree of activation). Normal Pdimax during a Mueller maneuver is variable, and ranges from 80–140 cm H_2O [22, 23]. However, if Pes and Pga become more negative to a similar degree (Pdi = 0), BDP is certainly present, and if Pdi is less than 40 cm H_2O, diaphragm dysfunction is likely present.

A third maneuver utilizing transdiaphragmatic pressure monitoring is the sniff maneuver. Overall, it has been found to give more reproducible results, less intersubject variability, and has better defined lower limits [24]. It produces a greater Pdi than performance of Pdimax despite it being a dynamic maneuver, possibly because of greater diaphragm activation or because of more uniform activation of the diaphragm with other muscles [24]. It is also a very simple maneuver to perform. Pdisniff values are higher, and range from mean values of 120–150 cm H_2O with a lower limit of normal being approximately 70–80 cm H_2O. In the studies that have compared Pdisniff to the other maneuvers in patients with diaphragm dysfunction [2, 5], Pdisniff correlated well with both PdiTLC and Pdimax. There was better reproducibility of Pdisniff between different trials in one study [5] but all three maneuvers appeared to offer equivalent information regarding the degree of diaphragm dysfunction when compared to historical controls or normal values.

In summary, the constellation of a reduced TLC, PImax, greater than 30% reduction in VC when assuming the supine position, and paradoxical rib cage or abdomen motion during inspiration should raise the possibility of BDP. Assessing specific diaphragm strength with transdiaphragmatic pressure monitoring remains the best means of determining BDP. The patient should be monitored during a maximal static inspiratory maneuver (Mueller maneuver), and during a maximal sniff maneuver. Pdi values for any of the maneuvers of 0 cm H_2O indicate total flaccidity of the diaphragm and confirm BDP. Other low but non-zero values need to be interpreted in light of the above normal values, although accurate distinction between low normal values and abnormal values have yet to be established with certainty. Well controlled studies comparing each of these maneuvers in normals and in patients with diaphragm weakness or paralysis are needed to further standardize these tests, and to determine the relative reliability of each.

Course and Prognosis

As the diaphragm is the principle respiratory muscle in man, loss of diaphragm function would be expected to cause a profound reduction in inspiratory volume, leading to severe dyspnea and respiratory failure [25]. This has indeed proven to be the case in many published case reports and series. Respiratory failure, characterized by hypoventilation and/or the need for assisted ventilation, has been described with BDP [1, 8, 9, 11] (Table 3). Where arterial blood gas values were reported, these patients had mild to moderate hypoxemia and CO_2 retention, either supine, or both upright and supine. Additionally, all patients had significant dyspnea or orthopnea, fatigue, or sleep disturbances.

Other reports, however, have suggested a more benign course [2, 10, 15]. In these patients, CO_2 retention did not occur at any time during the course of illness, assisted ventilation was not required (except for transient ventilation in one patient [15]), and there was no evidence of nocturnal hypoventilation. Even in some of the reports supporting the occurrence of respiratory failure, CO_2 retention did not occur despite the need for assisted ventilation [8, 11]. Laroche et al, [2] followed six patients with well documented bilateral diaphragm paralysis and found no evidence of nocturnal or awake hypoventilation or requirement for assisted ventilation. They explained this discrepancy between their study and others on the basis of weakness of other respiratory muscles in patients with respiratory failure, as opposed to the isolated diaphragm paralysis found in all six of their patients.

An equally important determinant of the occurrence of hypoventilation may be

Table 3. Bilateral diaphragm paralysis. Clinical course

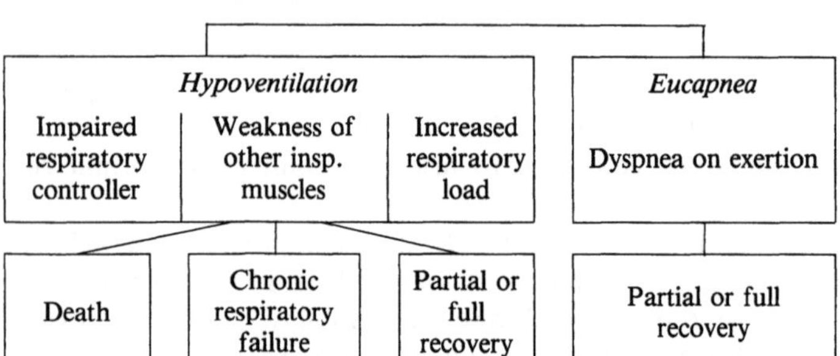

disturbed central responsiveness. Goldman [26] suggested that the diaphragm receives the major portion of central respiratory drive during quiet breathing. Paralysis of the diaphragm with consequent dependence on secondary muscles of inspiration would theoretically be associated with a lessened central drive and greater derangement of CO_2 regulation. BDP, therefore, does not invariability lead to hypoventilation or to the need for assisted ventilation. In such patients hypoventilation may occur only in a subset of patients with impairment of central regulation of breathing, weakness of other muscles, or increased respiratory loading.

Regardless of etiology or the presence or absence of respiratory failure, in general the prognosis of BDP is favorable. Even many patients initially requiring maximal ventilatory support can be successfully weaned of assisted ventilation totally or may be weaned to the point of requiring only intermittent, non-invasive ventilatory support [2, 8, 9, 11, 12, 15]. Hypoventilation with and without disordered sleep and daytime fatigue may be similarly managed non invasively at home [1].

The extent to which etiology of the diaphragm dysfunction determines prognosis for recovery is unclear. Improvement in BDP when it is a manifestation of a more generalized neuromuscular disorder will generally parallel the response to treatment of the overall disease process [27, 28]. An increasingly recognized cause of BDP, post-surgical phrenic nerve damage, generally has a favorable outcome, although recovery is typically prolonged and non-invasive ventilatory support may be necessary on a chronic basis [8, 12]. Clinical recovery with other types of phrenic nerve injury can be expected in most cases, although to varying degrees [9, 10, 11, 15].

In conclusion, therapy of BDP in the absence of specific generalized neuromuscular syndromes consists of ventilatory support and serial assessment for the return of function, which can be expected in many cases. Either mechanical ventilation or non-invasive ventilation [1, 8, 9] can significantly alleviate subjective symptoms such as orthopnea, disordered sleep, and can ameliorate blood gas abnormalities. Avoidance of the supine position will also help symptomatically.

Kyphoscoliosis

Kyphoscoliosis is a disease that affect the spine and its articulations. By its very nature, severe kyphoscoliosis is an easily recognizable cause of respiratory failure in afflicted patients. Many aspects of cardiorespiratory failure in kyphoscoliosis continue to require further explanation despite decades of observation of these subjects. Identification of characteristics that determine progression to cardiorespiratory failure, formulation of mechanisms of cardiac and ventilatory failure, and the impact of nocturnal or sleep events on the clinical couse are only some of the aspects of kyphoscoliosis still requiring further investigation. The area of much current research, however, and the focus of this section is the treatment of cardiorespiratory failure secondary to kyphoscoliosis.

Diagnosis and Etiology

Kyphoscoliosis is simply defined as the deformation of spine involving lateral displacement or curvature (scoliosis) or an anteroposterior angulation (kyphosis). Scoliosis of the spine is almost always associated with kyphosis (usually mild), whereas kyphosis may exist as an isolated deformity when associated with destruction or compression of the vertebral bodies. Furthermore, in addition to lateral displacement and kyphosis, scoliosis is invariably associated with rotation of the spine around its long axis. The lateral and rotatory movement may create severe distortion of the ribs. On the convex aspect of the spinal curvature the ribs are widely separated and rotated posteriorly; on the concave side the ribs are crowded together and rotated anteriorly (Fig. 4). [29] The hump that is noted on examination of these patients is therefore made up of the posteriorly angulated ribs as opposed to the spine. Finally, the severity of scoliosis is based on the angle formed by both limbs of the convex primary curvature known as the Cobb angle (Fig. 5)

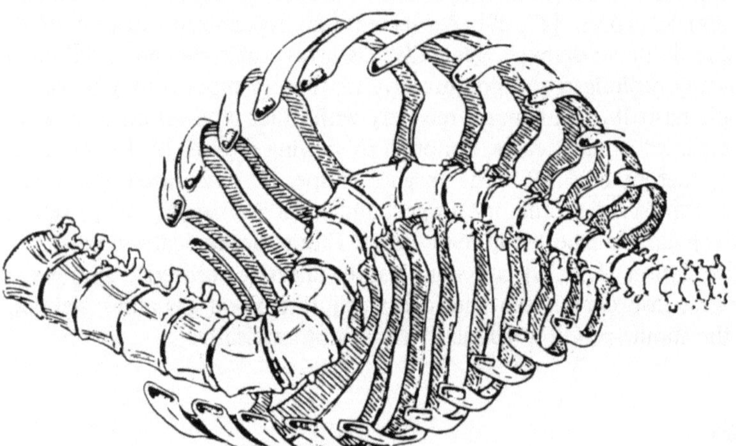

Fig. 4. Schematic representation of the rotation of the spine and rib cage seen with scoliosis. (From [66] with permission)

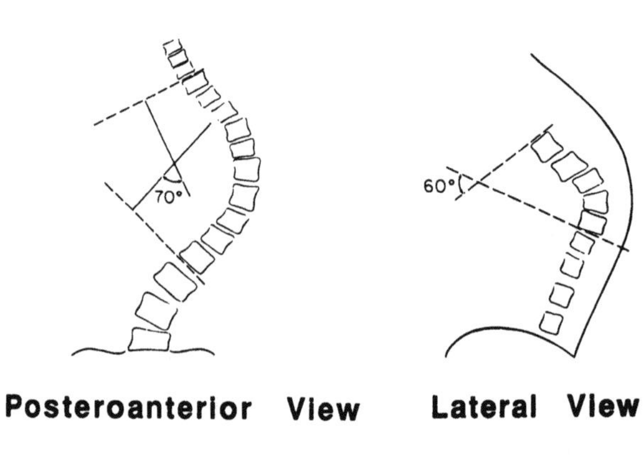

Fig. 5. Schematic of the posteroanterior radiograph depicting the lines constructed to measure the Cobb angle of scoliosis and lines drawn on the lateral radiograph to measure the Cobb angle of kyphosis. (From [66] with permission)

[30]. The most common form of kyphoscoliosis is idiopathic, often beginning in early childhood. Secondary kyphoscoliosis is a sequelae of various neuromuscular diseases, diseases of vertebrae and connective tissue, and of therapeutic interventions such as thoracoplasty and recurrent pneumothorax (Table 4) [31, 32].

Diagnostic Tests

Bergovsky et al. [29] have best summarized the derangements of pulmonary function produced by kyphoscoliosis. Their description has been confirmed more recently by other investigators [33, 34]. Kyphoscoliosis produces a characteristic pattern of restrictive lung disease; VC is decreased, sometimes dramatically, with relative preservation of residual volume (RV). In severe cases, the RV/TLC ratio becomes abnormally high, sometimes increasing to 50%. The most likely physiological explanation of lung volume changes in kyphoscoliosis involves decreased chest wall compliance and consequently a diminished resting position of the chest wall [33]. This would result in a reduction of FRC. The diminished chest wall compliance

Table 4. Causes of kyphoscoliosis

Idiopathic neuromuscular disease
Muscular dystrophy
Poliomyelitis
Cerebral palsy
Friedreich's ataxia
Vertebral disease
Osteoporosis
Osteomalacia
Vitamin D-resistant rickets
Tuberculosis spondylitis
Neurofibromatosis
Syndromes affecting connective tissue
Marfan's syndrome
Ehlers-Danlos syndrome
Morquio's syndrome
Thoracic cage abnormalities
Thoracoplasty

Table 5. Respiratory mechanics in kyphoscoliosis

Decreased chest wall compliance
↓
Decreased lung compliance → Decreased TLC
↓
Increased elastic load
↓
Increased work of breathing

would also decrease TLC. Lung compliance appears to be relatively normal. The reduced lung and chest wall compliances would increase the elastic load on the respiratory muscles and increase the work of breathing (Table 5).

Clinical Course

Cardiorespiratory failure is briefly defined as a severe gas exchange defect or severe ventilatory defect of the respiratory system resulting in hypoxemia and/or hypercarbia, with or without cor pulmonale. The occurrence or such physiological derangements as a direct consequence of kyphoscoliosis is quite variable. Perhaps because of this variability, characterization of predictors of and mechanisms leading to cardiorespiratory failure has been difficult (Fig. 6).

Bergovsky et al. [29] found the degree of spinal deformity as measured by the Cobb angle was the most important prognostic factor for cardiorespiratory failure. An angle of at least 100° was indicative of a significant risk for progression of cardiorespiratory failure. They also found that the effects of kyphosis and scoliosis were additive in terms of impairing respiratory function. Severe scoliosis without significant kyphosis did not usually impart as poor a prognosis. They postulated that the increased elastic load secondary to reduced chest wall compliance increased the work of breathing. To minimize the elastic work per breath, these patients altered their breathing pattern by taking smaller, more frequent breaths. This could lead to greater dead space ventilation, alveolar hypoventilation, hypoxemia, and cor pulmonale.

Some recent studies have disputed the importance of the relationship between the severity of the spinal deformity and clinical course in kyphoscoliosis. Rom et al. [35] described 10 patients surviving into their 7th decade with minimal or mild cardiorespiratory impairment despite Cobb angles greater than 105°. Others have found no correlation between inspiratory muscle strength as assessed by PImax and Pdimax and spinal curvature [34]. A large retrospective review [36] found that an alternate predictor of eventual cardiorespiratory failure was the age of onset of scoliosis. Specifics of spinal curvature in these subjects were not given, although it

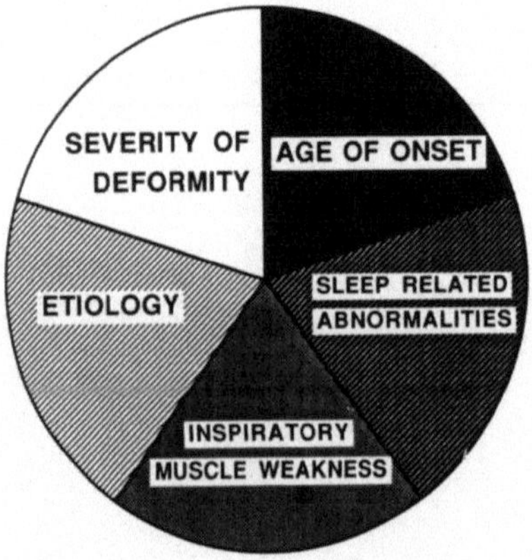

Fig. 6. Factors predisposing patients with kyphoscoliosis to respiratory failure

was implied that curvature was equally severe among patients with and without cardiorespiratory failure.

Controversy also exists as to whether the etiology of kyphoscoliosis is a predictor of the development of respiratory failure. While some studies [29, 37] have found a correlation between etiology and respiratory failure, others have not [34, 36]. Respiratory muscle dysfunction in patients with paralytic kyphoscoliosis as opposed to non-paralytic kyphoscoliosis may possibly contribute to a more progressive course, but this remains poorly documented since increased age and more severe spinal curvature were also evident in this study [29].

Finally, several recent studies have found that sleep related abnormalities may significantly impact on the clinical course of patients with kyphoscoliosis [38–41]. The influence of sleep related events on cardiorespiratory failure on kyphoscoliosis should be emphasized, as it is a factor that is potentially treatable or reversible. Several studies have documented significant nocturnal hypoventilation and arterial oxygen desaturation in kyphoscoliotic patients during sleep, especially through the REM stage of sleep (Fig. 7) [38–41]. Nocturnal hypoventilation and arterial desaturation may be due to reduced chest wall movement or obstructive apneas [38, 39, 41]. First, chest wall motion may be diminished because of its stiffness and because the action of the diaphragm on the rib cage may be ineffective. To compensate for this, the intercostal and accessory muscles are recruited to enhance inspiration [34]. During REM sleep, the activity of the intercostal and accessory muscles decreases more than the diaphragm. Because patients with kyphoscoliosis are more dependent on these muscles to maintain ventilation, REM-induced hypoventilation occurs. Second, distortion of upper airway anatomy in kyphoscoliosis may also predispose

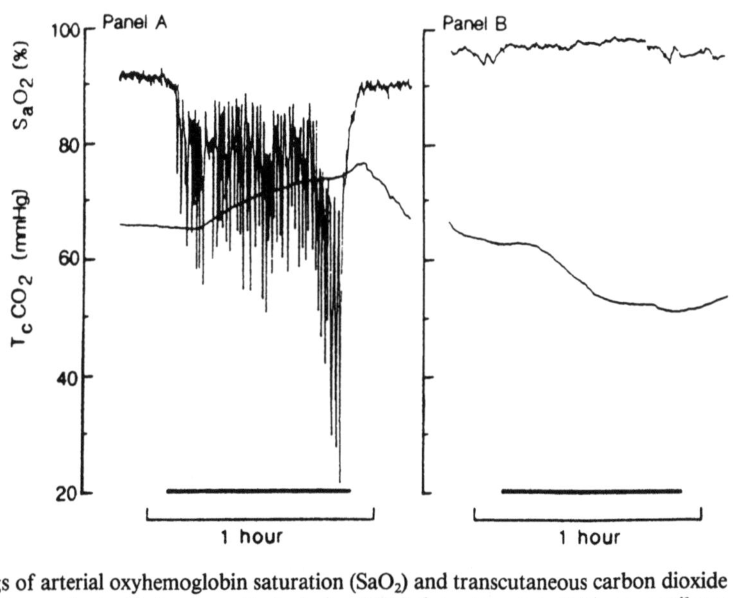

Fig. 7. Recordings of arterial oxyhemoglobin saturation (SaO_2) and transcutaneous carbon dioxide tension ($TcCO_2$) in a patient with kyphoscoliosis during REM sleep. *Panel A:* With no ventilator support, there is oxyhemoglobin desaturation and CO_2 retention. *Panel B:* With nasal positive pressure ventilation these changes are reversed (From [67] with permission)

these patients to intermittent airway obstruction during REM-induced hypotonia of the pharyngeal muscles. Regardless of the exact mechanisms, recurrent hypercarbia and hypoxemia during sleep may set in motion or potentiate the development of hypercarbia, cor pulmonale, and respiratory muscle dysfunction [38].

Treatment and Prognosis

In general, most people with varying degrees of kyphoscoliosis have an excellent prognosis, with little impairment of breathing or overall lifestyle [29]. However, once cor pulmonale develops, the prognosis worsens considerably and death generally occurs within a year if untreated [29]. Recently the prognosis for many patients with severe kyphoscoliosis has been improved, in part because of improved methods of treating hypoventilation [35, 42, 43].

In the decompensated patient with hypercarbia and cor pulmonale, initial conservative therapy with oxygen, chest physiotherapy, bronchodilators, and diuretics may result in significant clinical improvement [29, 43]. In one study, two third of patients requiring ICU care for cardiorespiratory failure associated with kyphoscoliosis responded to conservative therapy alone.

The use of intermittent positive pressure ventilation (IPPV) should also be considered an important addition to the conservative therapy of these patients. Shinha and Bergovsky [44] found in six patients that five minutes of IPPV resulted in a 70% increase in lung compliance, a decreased work of breathing (WOB), improved PCO_2, and variably improved PO_2. This improvement persisted for 2–3 h after the treatment. IPPV, however, has not been shown to be as efficacious in other diseases associated with diminished respiratory system compliance [45].

In cases of respiratory failure refractory to the measures described above, mechanical ventilation (MV) should be initiated. This can be delivered either by positive or negative pressure devices [36, 37, 43]. However, the standard of care for acute respiratory failure remains MV and positive pressure ventilation with a volume-cycled ventilator [43]. Positive pressure ventilation can also be used as chronic therapy of kyphoscoliosis to avert respiratory decompensation. For example, long-term ventilation at night has resulted in improvement in gas exchange, ventilation, cardiac function, and daytime activities (Fig. 7) [42].

The most recent developments in treatment of cardiorespiratory failure in kyphoscoliosis have involved the application of continuous or nocturnal positive pressure ventilation via non-invasive means [41, 48, 49]. As with more traditional means of assisted ventilation, non-invasive ventilation via a nasal mask is accomplished by delivering an increased VT and thus improving alveolar ventilation while reducing WOB. These are likely predisposing factors for respiratory failure in kyphoscoliotic patients [48]. Their amelioration by nasal ventilation has been documented by decreased diaphragmatic EMG activity, a reduction in negative esophageal pressure swings, improved synchronization between rib cage and abdominal motion, and by small decreases in end-tidal CO_2.

Other studies [41, 49] also suggest that non-invasive positive pressure ventilation improves daytime function and ameliorates hypoventilation in decompensated kyphoscoliotics. In addition, ventilation at night benefits these patients by reducing sleep-related events, both obstructive and non-obstructive [48]. These studies and others support an increasing reliance on non-invasive positive pressure ventilation, especially nocturnally, for alleviation of cardiorespiratory failure in kyphoscoliosis. Better controlled clinical trials in both acute and chronic states of decompensation are still needed to better define the role of this intervention.

In summary, people with kyphoscoliosis may progress to respiratory failure and cor pulmonale. There is no clear consensus on which specific characteristics reliably predict such a progression, although the degree of spinal distortion certainly plays a significant role. Respiratory failure is primarily due to altered respiratory compliance and atelectasis leading to an increased WOB. Central ventilatory control defects, respiratory muscle fatigue, and sleep-related breathing dysfunction also contribute. Cor pulmonale and pulmonary hypertension in this disease are caused by alveolar hypoventilation, medial proliferation secondary to chronic hypoxemia, and a reduction of the pulmonary vascular bed by mechanical compression. Even after the development of cardiorespiratory failure, prognosis may not be as grim as previously thought. Conservative measures coupled with IPPV, negative pressure ventilators, or standard tracheostomy and positive pressure ventilation can improve symptoms. Non-invasive delivery of positive pressure ventilation is an appealing alternative to these other more cumbersome interventions, and should be considered in all decompensated patients.

Flail Chest

Flail chest occurs in approximately 20% of patients with blunt chest wall trauma [50] and the accompanying mortality may be as high as 30–40% [51]. Flail chest is producted by double fractures of three or more contiguous ribs or combined sternal and rib fractures. The etiology of the rib fractures is usually traumatic. However, flail chest may also occur when there are pathological fractures of the ribs such as those due to multiple myeloma. As a result of blunt chest trauma, there may be also underlying pulmonary contusion.

Pathophysiology

The physiological changes that occur with flail chest depend upon two factors:

1. ineffective ventilation related to paradoxical motion of the flail segment which results in increased energy demands of the respiration muscles, and
2. hypoxia secondary to the underlying pulmonary contusion which results in decreased energy supplies (Table 6).

The paradoxical motion of the chest wall secondary to loss of the structural integrity of the rib cage likely reflects changes in underlying pleural pressure. Normally, several major forces act on the rib cage during quiet breathing that permit it to expand in a uniform fashion. These forces include the passive recoil of the rib cage, the insertional actions of the intercostal muscles and diaphragm, and transthoracic

Table 6. Pathophysiology of flail chest

<table>
<tr><th colspan="5">Increased energy demands</th><th>Reduced energy supplies</th></tr>
<tr><td colspan="2">Increased work of breathing</td><td colspan="3">Decreased efficiency of breathing</td><td>Hypoxia</td></tr>
<tr><td rowspan="2">Increased force of muscle contraction</td><td rowspan="2">Increased distance of muscle shortening</td><td rowspan="2">Shorter diaphragm operational length</td><td colspan="2">Ineffective chest wall motion</td><td>Pulmonary contusion</td></tr>
<tr><td>Uncoupling from insertional actions of the diaphragm and rib cage muscles</td><td>More negative swings in pleural pressure</td><td></td></tr>
</table>

and abdominal pressures [52]. An imbalance of these forces may result in rib cage distortion. In patients with flail chest, the same forces act on the rib cage. However, the rib cage is more readily distorted in this instance. For example, rib fractures may uncouple a part of the chest wall from the inspiratory (rib cage expanding) actions of the intercostal muscles. Consequently, during inspiration the collapsing influence of negative intrathoracic pressure may be unapposed and thus cause inward displacement of a localized part of the rib cage. During expiration as pleural pressure becomes more positive, the flail segment moves outward. The paradoxical motion of the flail segment may be further enhanced when transthoracic pressure swings during inspiration become more negative because of decreased lung compliance. Lung contusion or microatelectasis secondary to pain and splinting are factors that would promote such changes in lung compliance and worsen paradoxical chest wall motion.

Different patterns of chest wall (rib cage and abdomen) and rib cage distortion can be seen in patients with flail chest [53]. These patterns include: 1) inward displacement of the lower rib cage as the transverse rib cage and abdomen are expanding, 2) inward displacement of transverse rib cage as the lower rib cage and abdomen are expanding, and 3) inward displacement of the lower rib cage and abdomen as the transverse rib cage is expanding. The pattern of paradox may reflect either the location of the rib fractures, or altered recruitment patterns of the respiratory muscles (Fig. 8).

WOB is increased in patients with flail chest. Because of the paradoxical motion of the chest wall, the inspiratory muscles must shorten more for a given VT. Since work is the product of force and distance shortened, the extra shortening results in increased work performed by the inspiratory muscles [54]. Furthermore, the inspiratory muscles are operating at shorter lengths. Accordingly, they are less efficient [55, 56]. Thus the combination of increased work and decreased efficiency would increase the energy demands of the muscles and would predispose them to fatigue.

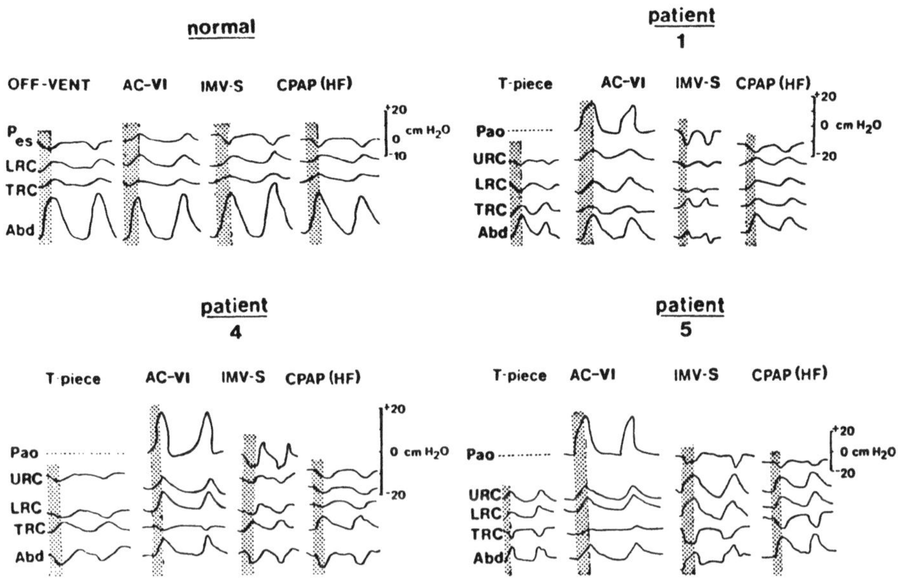

Fig. 8. Representative tracings of chest wall dimensions and pressure versus time for a normal subject and three patients with flail chest. Note little difference in chest wall configuration among ventilator (assisted) and spontaneous breaths in the normal subject. Each of the three patients with flail chest shows a distinct pattern of chest wall distortion. The shaded area represents inspiration. During spontaneous breaths on an IMV circuit (IMV-S) there is distortion of the chest wall in all patients. This distortion is partially reversed while spontaneously breathing on a high flow CPAP circuit (CPAP-HF) in patient one. (From [53] with permission)

In addition, energy supplies to the muscles may be reduced because of hypoxia secondary to atelectasis or contusion. The reduced energy supplies may further predispose these patients to developing inspiratory muscle fatigue.

Treatment

The major thrust of therapy with flail chest includes measures to control pain and assistance with ventilation when necessary. Pain relief can be accomplished by intercostal nerve blocks or by the use of epidural anesthesia either with morphine or 0.5% bupivacaine [57]. Adequate pain relief will result in improved VT, VC, and a more effective cough.

Although as argued above, the ineffective ventilation secondary to the flail segment may result in respiratory failure, the need for stabilizing the flail segment is controversial. Fixing the flail segment was initially accomplished by the use of tape, strappings, and external devices [58]. With the advent of positive pressure ventilators, internal splinting via positive pressure was recommended [59]. This treatment included tracheostomy and a prolonged 3–5 week period of MV. This mode of therapy did not significantly alter mortality [60] and subjected patients to the complications of tracheostomy and prolonged MV. In 1975, Trinkle [61] contended that the flail segment itself was unimportant and that the ventilator management would only be appropriate if respiratory failure accompanied flail chest. However, the importance of the flail segment in the pathogenesis of respiratory failure still remains controversial and others have once again proposed externally fixating the chest wall to avoid prolonged periods of MV [62, 63].

The general consensus regarding treatment is that optimal pain control is important in managing these patients and that chest physiotherapy and incentive spirometry coordinated with periods of optimal pain control is beneficial. In instances where these patients become progressively tachypneic and hypoxic, MV is indicated. However, the mode of MV chosen should be one that does not promote negative swings in pleural pressure. The resistive and elastic loads imposed by mechanical ventilators [64] will make pleural pressure more negative, worsen the chest wall distorsion in these patients, and increase the oxygen cost of breathing during spontaneous or assisted breaths. The IMV mode has frequently been used as a means of ventilating patients with flail chest [65] but it can also be one of the modes that imposes the greatest resistive load on the respiratory system. Therefore, spontaneous breaths on this mode may aggravate chest wall distortion. Tzelepis et al. [53] found that a low-impedance, high-flow CPAP system resulted in less distortion when compared to spontaneous breaths on an IMV circuit. They speculated that this mode may reduce the likelihood of developing inspiratory muscle fatigue and thus be preferred for weaning.

To summarize, there are individual differences in the pattern of chest wall distortion in patients with flail chest. Greater chest wall distortion increases the inspiratory muscle displacement for a given VT which in turn increases WOB. There also is a decrease in the efficiency of breathing which results in an increased oxygen cost of breathing. These are all factors that may predispose to respiratory failure or may impair weaning.

References

1. Newsom Davis J, Goldman M, Loh L, Carson M (1976) Diaphragm function and alevolar hypoventilation. Quarterly J Med 45:87–100
2. Laroche CM, Carroll N, Moxham J, Green M (1988) Clinical significance of severe isolated diaphragm weakness. Am Rev Resp Dis 138:862–866
3. Wilcox PG, Pardy RL (1989) Diaphragmatic weakness and paralysis. Lung 167:323–341
4. Gibson GJ (1989) Diaphragmatic paresis: Pathophysiology, clinical features, and investigation. Thorax 44:960–970
5. Mier-Jedrzejowicz A, Brophy C, Moxham J, Green M (1988) Assessment of diaphragm weakness. Am Rev Resp Dis 137:877–883
6. Alexander C (1966) Diaphragm movements and diagnosis of diaphragmatic paralysis. Clin Radiol 17:79–83
7. Loh L, Goldman M, Newsom Davis J (1977) The assessment of diaphragm paralysis. Medicine 56:165–189
8. Abd AG, Braun NMT, Baskin MI, O'Sullivan MM, Alkaitis DA (1989) Diaphragmatic dysfunction after open heart surgery: Treatment with a rocking bed. Ann Int Med 111:881–886
9. Kreitzer SM, Feldman NT, Saunders NA, Ingram RH (1978) Dilateral diaphragmatic paralysis with hypercapnic respiratory failure. Am J Med 65:89–95

10. Camfferman F, Bogaard JM, van der Meche FGA, Hilvering C (1985) Idiopathic bilateral diaphragmatic paralysis. Eur J Respir Dis 66:65–71
11. Sandham JD, Shaw DT, Guenter CA (1977) Acute supine respiratory failure due to bilateral diaphragmatic paralysis. Chest 72:96–98
12. Matthay MA, Wiener-Kronish JP (1989) Respiratory management after cardiac surgery. Chest 95:424–434
13. Wilcox P, Baile EM, Hards J et al. (1988) Phrenic nerve function and its relationship to atelectasis after coronary artery bypass surgery. Chest 93:693–698
14. McCool FD, Mead J (1989) Dyspnea on immersion: Mechanisms in patients with bilateral diaphragm paralysis. Am Rev Resp Dis 139:275–276
15. McCredie M, Lovejoy FW Jr, Kaltreider NL (1962) Pulmonary function in diaphragmatic paralysis. Thorax 17:213–217
16. Agostoni E, Mead J (1964) Status of the respiratory system. In: Fenn WD, Rahn H (eds), Handbook of Physiology, Sec. 3, Vol. 1. Respiration. Am Physiol Society, Washington, DC, p. 387
17. Allen SM, Hunt B, Green M (1985) Fall in vital capacity with posture. Br J Dis Chest 79:267–271
18. Black LF, Hyatt RE (1969) Maximal respiratory pressures: Normal values and relationships to age and sex. Am Rev Resp Dis 99:696–702
19. De Troyer A, Yernault JC (1980) Inspiratory muscle force in normal subjects and patients with interstitial lung disease. Thorax 35:92–100
20. Tarver RD, Dewey JC, Cory DA, Vix VA (1989) Imaging the diaphragm and its disorders. J Thoracic Imag 4(1):1–18
21. Agostoni E, Rahn H (1960) Abdominal and thoracic pressures at different lung volumes. J Appl Physiol 15:1087–1092
22. Laporta D, Grassino A (1985) Assessment of transdiaphragmatic pressure in humans. J Appl Physiol 58:1469–1476
23. De Troyer A, Estenne M (1981) Limitations of measurement of transdiaphragmatic pressure in detecting diaphragmatic weakness. Thorax 36:169–174
24. Miller JM, Moxham J, Green M (1985) The maximal sniff in the assessment of diaphragm function in man. Clin Sci 69:91–96
25. Roussos CS, Macklem PT (1982) The respiratory muscles. N Engl J Med 307:786–797
26. Goldman M (1970) Mechanical coupling of the diaphragm and rib cage. In: Pergelly LD, Rebuck AS, Campbell EJM, (eds) Loaded Breathing, Longman, Canada, Ltd., p 50
27. Mier-Jedrezejowicz AK, Brophy C, Green M (1988) Respiratory muscle function in myasthenia gravis. Am Rev Resp Dir 138:867–873
28. Harrison BDW, Collens JV, Brown KGE, Clark TJH (1971) Respiratory failure in neuromuscular diseases. Thorax 26:579–584
29. Bergofsky EH, Tureno GM, Fishman AP (1959) Cardiorespiratory failure in kyphoscoliosis. Medicine (Baltimore) 38:263–317
30. Cobb JR (1948) Outline for the study of scoliosis. Instructional course Lecture, Am Academy of Orthopedic Surgeons 5:261
31. Bredin CP (1989) Pulmonary function in long-term survivors of thoracoplasty. Chest 95:18–20
32. Philips MS, Kinnear WJM, Shneerson JM (1987) Late sequelae of pulmonary tuberculosis treated by thoracoplasty. Thorax 42:445–451
33. Bergofsky EH (1979) Respiratory failure in disorders of the thoracic cage. Am Rev Res Dis 119:643–669
34. Lisboa C, Moreno R, Fava M, Ferretti R, Cruz E (1985) Inspiratory muscle function in patient with severe kyphoscoliosis. Am Rev Resp Dis 132:48–52
35. Rom WN, Miller A (1978) Unexpected longevity in patients with severe kyphoscoliosis. Thorax 33:106–110
36. Branthwaite MR (1986) Cardiorespiratory consequences of unfused idiopathic scoliosis. Br J Dis Chest 80:360–369
37. Editorial (1985) Respiratory function in scoliosis. Lancet 1(8420):84–85
38. Sawicka EH, Branthwaite MA (1987) Respiration during sleep in kyphoscoliosis. Thorax 42:801–808

39. Meyon BL, West P, Israels J, Kryger M (1980) Sleep breathing abnormalities in kyphoscoliosis. Am Rev Resp Dis 122:617–621
40. Guilleminault C, Kurlan G, Wirkle R, Miles LE (1981) Severe kyphoscoliosis, breathing, and sleep. Chest 79:626–630
41. Celles ER, Grundstein RR, Chan S, Bye PTP, Sullivan CE (1988) Noninvasive ventilatory support during sleep improves respiratory failure in kyphoscoliosis. Chest 94:811–815
42. Hoeppner VH, Cockcroft DW, Dosman JA, Cotton DJ (1984) Nighttime ventilation improves respiratory failure in secondary kyphoscoliosis. Am Rev Resp Dis 129:240–243
43. Libby DM, Briscoe WA, Boyce B, Smith JP (1982) Acute respiratory failure in scoliosis or kyphosis. Am J Med 73:532–538
44. Sinha R, Bergofsky EH (1972) Prolonged alteration of lung mechanisms in kyphoscoliosis by positive-pressure hyperinflation. Am Rev Resp Dis 106:47–57
45. McCool FD, Mayewski RJ, Shayne DS, Gibson CJ, Grigg RC, Hyde RW (1986) Intermittent positive pressure breathing in patients with respiratory muscle weakness: alterations in total respiratory system compliance. Chest 90:546–552
46. Wiers PWJ, Le Coultre R, Dallinga OT, Van Dyl W, Merinez AF, Sluiter HJ (1977) Cuirass respirator treatment of chronic respiratory failure in scoliotic patients. Thorax 32:221–228
47. Sawicka EH, Spencer GT, Branthwaite MA (1986) Management of respiratory failure complicating pregnancy in severe kyphoscoliosis: a new use for an old technique. Br J Dis Chest 80:191–196
48. Carrey Z, Gottfried SG, Levy RD (1990) Ventilatory muscle support in respiratory failure with nasal positive-pressure ventilation. Chest 97:150–158
49. Bach JR, Alba AS (1990) Management of chronic alveolar hypoventilation by nasal ventilation. Chest 97:52–57
50. Richardson JD, Adams L, Flint LM (1980) Selective management of flail chest and pulmonary contusion. Ann Surg 196:481–487
51. Todd TRJ, Shamji F (1985) Pathophysiology of chest wall trauma. In: Roussos C, Macklem PT (eds) The thorax. Part B. Marcel Dekker, New York, pp. 979–997
52. Loring SH, Mead J (1982) Action of the diaphragm on the rib cage inferred from a force balance analysis. J Appl Physiol 53:956–960
53. Tzelepis GE, McCool FD, Hoppin FG Jr (1989) Chest wall distortion in patients with flail chest. Am Rev Resp Dis 140:31–37
54. Goldman MD, Grimby A, Mead J (1976) Mechanical work of breathing derived from rib cage and abdominal V-P partitioning. J Appl Physiol 41:752–763
55. Collett PW, Engel LA (1986) Influence of lung volume on oxygen cost of resistive breathing. J Appl Physiol 61:16–24
56. McCool FD, Tzelepsis GE, Leith DE, Hoppin FG Jr (1989) Oxygen cost of breathing during fatiguing inspiratory resistive loads. J Appl Physiol 66:2045–2055
57. Shackford SR (1986) Blunt chest trauma: the intensiveness perspective. J Intensive Care Med 1:125–136
58. Cohen EA (1955) Treatment of flail chest by towel clip traction. Am J Surg 90:517–519
59. Avery EE, Morch ET, Benson DW (1956) Critically crushed chests: a new method of treatment with continuous mechanical hyperventilation to produce alkalotic apnea and internal pneumatic stabilizations. J Thorac Surg 32:291–298
60. Shackford SR, Smith DE, Zarins CD, et al (1976) The management of flail chest: a comparison of ventilatory and nonventilatory treatment. Am J Surg 132:759–762
61. Trinkle JK, Richardson JD, Franz JL, Grover FL, Arom KV, Holmstrom FM (1975) Management of flail chest without mechanical ventilation. Ann Thorac Surg 19:355–363
62. Thomas AN, Blaisdell WF, Lewis FR, Scholbohm RM (1978) Operative stabilization of flail chest after blunt trauma. J Thorac Cardiovasc Surg 75:793–801
63. Moore BP (1975) Operative stabilization of non-penetrating chest injuries. J Thorac Cardiovasc Surg 70:619–630
64. Marini JJ, Rodriguez RM, Lamb V (1986) The inspiratory work load of patient-initiated mechanical ventilation. Am Rev Resp Dis 134:902–909
65. Cullen P, Modell JH, Dirby RR, Klein EF, Long W (1985) Treatment of flail chest. Use of intermittent mandatory ventilation and positive end-expiratory pressure. Arch Surg 110:1099–1103

66. Rochester DF, Findley MJ (1988) The lungs and neuromuscular and chest wall diseases. In: Murray, Nadel (eds) Textbook of respiratory medicine. WB Saunders pp 1942–1971
67. Ellis ER, Grunstein RR, Chan S, et al (1988) Noninvasive ventilatory support during sleep improves respiratory failure in kyphoscoliosis. Chest 94:811–815

Pathophysiology of Ventilatory Failure in Patients with Neuromyopathies

M. Estenne

Introduction

Acute ventilatory failure manifested by hypercapnia and respiratory acidosis may develop in all conditions causing severe weakness of the respiratory muscles. These conditions include neurological disorders which produce dysfunction at any level in the pathways connecting "the respiratory centers" and the respiratory muscles [1]. For example, acute ventilatory failure may be observed in the acute inflammatory stage of poliomyelitis and in amyotrophic lateral sclerosis (involving the neurons of the anterior horns of the spinal cord), in the early phase of the Guillain-Barré syndrome (involving peripheral nerves), in an acute episode of myasthenia gravis (involving the neuromuscular junction), or in diseases involving the muscles themselves like muscular dystrophy or acid-maltase deficiency. In addition, acute dysfunction of the respiratory muscles may also occur in non-neurological disorders like cardiogenic [2, 3] or septic [4] shock, acidosis [5], abnormalities in serum electrolytes [6], steroid-induced myopathy [7], or may be produced by an impressive number of pharmacological agents and naturally occurring toxins or venoms [1]. Whatever its cause, acute and severe respiratory muscle weakness may lead to acute ventilatory failure and respiratory acidosis, and may eventually equire mechanical ventilation (MV).

In a large number of patients with muscle weakness due to neurological disor-

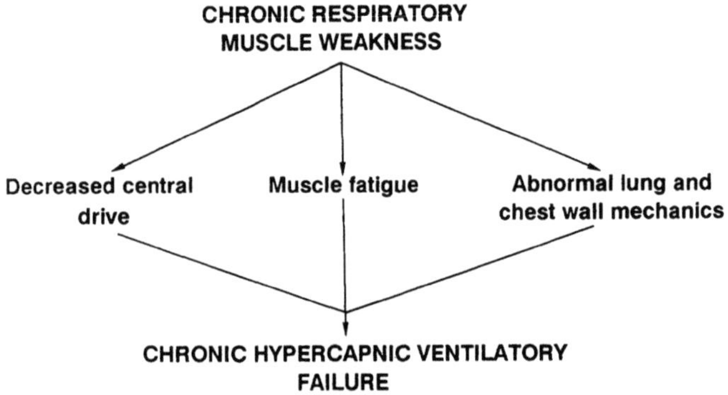

Fig. 1. Three groups of factors may contribute to the development of hypercapnic ventilatory failure when there is chronic weakness of the respiratory muscles: 1) decreased central ventilatory drive; 2) muscle fatigue; 3) alterations in lung and chest wall mechanics

ders, however, ventilatory failure has an insidious progression and develops in the absence of any obvious precipitating factor and with only limited symptoms. Interestingly, the degree of hypercapnia in patients with this type of chronic ventilatory failure is not tightly coupled to the severity of the respiratory muscle weakness [8]. This suggests that alveolar hypoventilation occurring in this context is not simply due to the direct effect of weakness of the respiratory muscles leading to inability to inflate the lungs fully. In fact, a variety of additional pathogenic mechanisms may be involved (Fig. 1). These include

1. alterations in the mechanical properties of the lungs and chest wall,
2. development of fatigue in the respiratory muscles, and
3. alterations in the central regulation of breathing.

Although numerous neurological diseases are capable of producing chronic weakness of the respiratory muscles, the general pattern of pathophysiological mechanisms leading to chronic ventilatory failure is common to a range of disorders. In the present chapter, we will give a general account of these mechanisms when there is severe, chronic muscle weakness involving both inspiratory and expiratory muscles; this is largely based on studies in patients with muscular dystrophies [9] and traumatic tetraplegia [10] which have been more extensively studied than other disorders. When appropriate, we will draw attention to features which are more specific of some individual disorders. In the last section of this review, we will discuss the mechanisms by which nocturnal assisted ventilation operates to reverse chronic ventilatory failure in these patients.

Alterations in the Mechanical Properties of the Respiratory System

Early studies on poliomyelitic patients [11–13] have all reported decreases in vital capacity (VC) and its two components, inspiratory capacity (IC) and expiratory

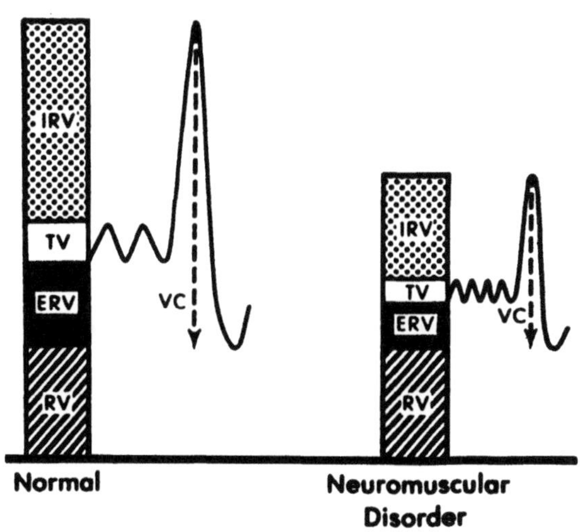

Fig. 2. Lung volumes and vital capacity determinations in a typical patient with chronic neuromuscular disorder and moderate respiratory muscle weakness, and in a healthy subject of similar age and height. *VC* indicates vital capacity; *IRV:* inspiratory reserve volume; *VT:* tidal volume; *ERV:* expiratory reserve volume; and *RV:* residual volume. (From [9] with permission)

reserve volume (ERV). Subsequently, numerous studies on various neuromuscular disorders have amply confirmed that VC is reduced as a consequence of respiratory muscle weakness (Fig. 2), that the relative reduction in IC and ERV reflects the distribution of the weakness among the inspiratory versus the expiratory muscles, and that VC decreases regularly with progression of the disease [9, 10, 14–17].

The reduction in VC was initially attributed to the direct effect of respiratory muscle weakness. However, because of the sigmoid shape of the pressure-volume curve of the normal relaxed respiratory system, so that at the extremes of the VC large changes in pressure produce only small changes in volume, VC would be expected to be relatively well preserved until muscle weakness becomes very severe. For example, when a 40% decrease in respiratory muscle strength is produced acutely by partial curarization in normal humans, VC shows only a 15% reduction [18]. In patients with chronic respiratory muscle weakness, however, reductions in VC are usually greater than anticipated for the degree of muscle weakness [19, 20]. This is illustrated in Fig. 3 which shows the relationship between respiratory muscle strength and VC in 25 patients with long-standing neuromuscular disorders as well as the theoretical effect of respiratory muscle weakness on VC (solid curve). Although VC is highly correlated with respiratory muscle strength, the reductions in VC are disproportionate to the degree of muscle weakness.

Scoliosis, heart failure, or bronchopneumonia may all contribute to the loss of VC in some patients, but a disproportionate loss of lung volume may be present without any of these complications. Recent studies have demonstrated that alterations in the mechanical properties of the lung and chest wall significantly contribute to the loss of lung volume in patients with chronic weakness of the respiratory muscles.

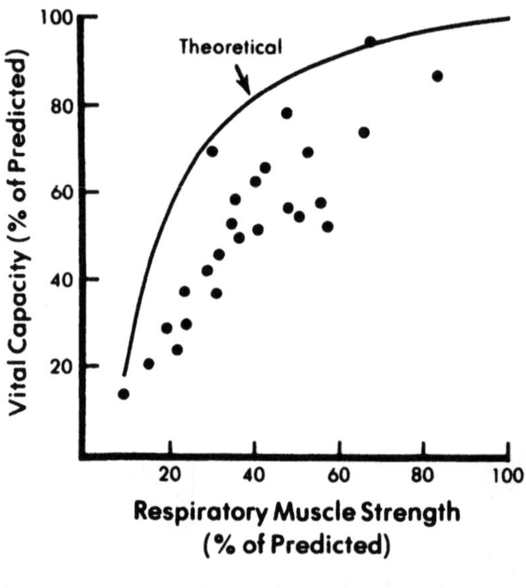

Fig. 3. Relationships between respiratory muscle strength and vital capacity in 25 patients with long-standing neuromuscular disorders. The solid curve indicates the theoretical effect of respiratory muscle weakness on vital capacity. This relationship is calculated from the standard maximal pressure-volume curve, assuming that respiratory system recoil in such patients is the same as that measured in normal subjects. Note that the reductions in vital capacity are disproportionate to the degree of muscle weakness. (From [20] with permission)

Pulmonary Mechanics

Since the position of full inflation is set by a balance between the lung recoil pressure (Pst, L) and the most negative pleural pressure which can be generated by the inspiratory muscles (Ppl min) [21, 22], weakness of the inspiratory muscles prevents a normal Pst, L from being developed in the lung at full inflation and so truncates the upper part of the static pressure-volume (PV) curve of the lung. However, in patients with long-standing and severe respiratory muscle weakness, the inability to expand the lungs fully is associated with further changes in the lung PV curve [9, 10, 23–25]. As shown in Fig. 4, not only is the Pst, L at full inflation low in relation to the normal value, but Pst, L is increased at any absolute lung volume, pulmonary compliance is reduced, and Pst, L at functional residual capacity (FRC) is normal or decreased.

Three factors are theoretically capable of decreasing lung compliance in otherwise normal lungs when weakness of the respiratory muscles exists. One is dispersed alveolar collapse which may be undetected by conventional radiographic techniques [26]. These atelectasis would be related to the inability of the patients to expand the lungs fully. Although the available data are limited, the lungs of patients with severe respiratory muscle weakness usually show patchy atelectasis at necropsy [27]. A second mechanism is a generalized increase in the surface tension of the alveolar lining layer, due to breathing at low lung volume [28, 29]. A third possibility is that the reduction in lung compliance results from shortening and stif-

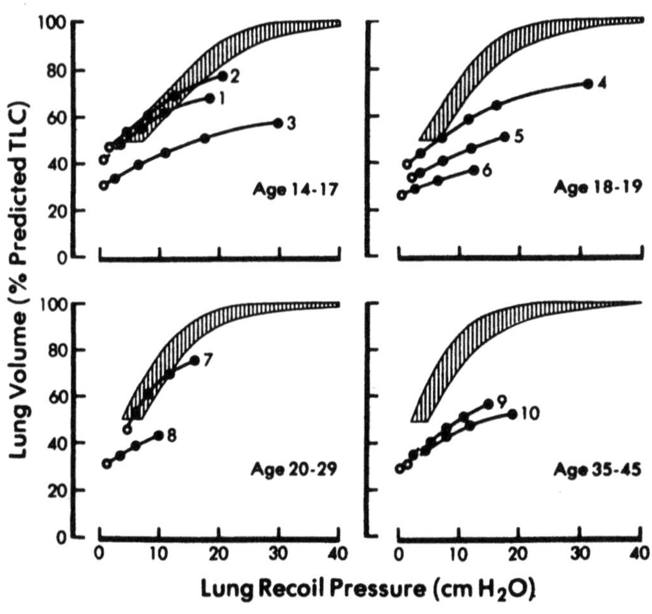

Fig. 4. Static expiratory pressure-volume curves of the lungs in 10 patients with chronic respiratory muscle weakness. The open circles denote the position of functional residual capacity. The hatched area represents ± 1 SD of normal values. Volume is expressed as percent of predicted TLC to allow for differences in patient size (From [25] with permission)

fening of the elastic fibers within the lungs. Because of their chronically limited range of activity, it is possible that patients with neuromuscular disorders do not stretch the respiratory structures enough, resulting in changes in the elastic properties of lung tissue.

In an attempt to define the relative role played by these different mechanisms, we have recently performed high resolution computerized tomographic (CT) scanners of the lungs in a few patients with traumatic transection of the lower cervical cord. All the patients had marked respiratory muscle weakness and reductions in both VC and lung compliance. In none of them, however, did the scanner show areas of atelectasis. In fact, the lung parenchyma appeared normal. Although these results need to be confirmed in a larger group of patients with a variety of chronic neuromuscular disorders, they suggest that the reduction in lung compliance which develops when the respiratory muscles are chronically weakened is due to alterations in surface forces or in the elastic properties of lung tissue and not to atelectasis.

Chest wall Mechanics

Dynamics. Patients with neuromuscular disorders often show marked distortion of the chest wall during quiet breathing. This is well illustrated by patients with traumatic tetraplegia [30–33] or bilateral diaphragmatic paralysis [34–36]. Fig. 5 shows the changes in the anteroposterior (AP) diameters of the abdomen, the lower rib

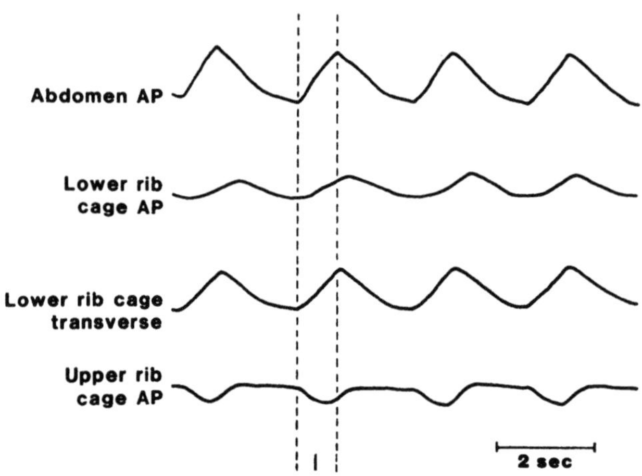

Fig. 5. Pattern of rib cage motion in a representative C5 tetraplegic subject breathing at rest in the seated posture. The respiratory changes in anteroposterior (AP) diameters of the abdomen, lower rib cage, and upper rib cage are shown as well as the changes in transverse diameter of the lower rib cage. In all traces, an upward deflection corresponds to an increase in diameter, and a downward deflection corresponds to a decrease in diameter. I indicates the duration of inspiration. Note that during inspiration, the lower rib cage expands more along the transverse than the AP diameter, and that the AP diameter of the upper rib cage decreases. (From [10] with permission)

cage (5th costal cartilage) and the upper rib cage (manubrium sterni) as well as the changes in the transverse diameter of the lower rib cage in a tetraplegic subject with a complete cord transection at the C_5 level breathing at rest in the seated posture. Two abnormalities in the pattern of chest wall motion are apparent. First, unlike in a normal subject, the increase in the AP diameter of the lower rib cage during inspiration is smaller than the increase in the AP diameter of the abdomen, and in addition, the rib cage expansion is delayed relative to the abdominal expansion. Second, while during inspiration the lower rib cage expands along both its AP and transverse dimension, there is a decrease in the AP diameter of the upper rib cage. These alterations are due to the fact that the inspiratory intercostal muscles and the scalenes are paralyzed [32]. During inspiration, the diaphragm produces some expansion of the lower rib cage through its insertions on the lower ribs and the increase in abdominal pressure which acts in the area of apposition. In contrast, the upper rib cage is mainly driven by the intrathoracic pressure when all rib cage inspiratory muscles are paralyzed. As a result, it moves paradoxically inward during isolated contraction of the diaphragm.

Distortion of the chest wall during breathing is also a prominent feature of bilateral diaphragmatic paralysis. When the diaphragm is paralyzed, the inspiratory intercostal and the neck muscles are the only muscles active during inspiration. As a result, the rib cage expands during inspiration but, since no transdiaphragmatic pressure is developed, abdominal pressure remains equal to pleural pressure and falls. As a result, the abdomen moves paradoxically inward during inspiration and opposes inflation of the lungs [34–36].

Statics. In addition to distortions of the chest wall during breathing, patients with neuromuscular disorders may show marked alterations in the static mechanical properties of the chest wall. Direct measurements of chest wall compliance have been performed in patients with chronic respiratory muscle weakness using the cycling tidal volume (VT) method [13] which provides values of dynamic compliance, or using the midposition shift method [37] which provides values of static compliance. The two methods have yielded virtually identical results and demonstrate that in patients with chronic neuromuscular disorders chest wall compliance is decreased to about two-thirds of normal values [13, 38, 39].

By using pairs of linearized magnetometers, Estenne and De Troyer [39] were able to partition chest wall compliance into its rib cage and abdominal components in 20 subjects in the late stages of traumatic tetraplegia. Individual values of rib cage and abdominal compliance obtained in these subjects are compared with the normal range in Fig. 6. Eighteen of 20 subjects had values of rib cage compliance at least 1 standard error of the estimate (SEE) below normal, whereas 13 of 20 subjects had values of abdominal compliance at least 1 SEE above normal. On the average, rib cage compliance amounted to 55% of normal while abdominal compliance amounted to 170% of normal. Thus, if the chest wall is stiffer than normal after cervical cord injury, this is because the rib cage compartment is abnormally stiff.

To the extent that the elastic properties of a system are in part determined by the stresses to which the system is subjected, the elastic properties of the rib cage in tetraplegic subjects may change because the extensive paralysis of the inspiratory

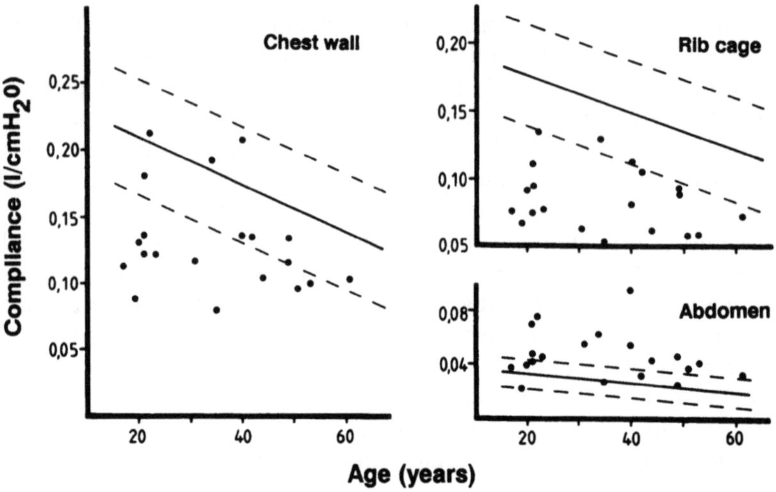

Fig. 6. Values of chest wall, rib cage, and abdominal compliance in 20 seated tetraplegic subjects. Full and dashed lines represent regression equations ± 1 SEE in 61 healthy adults (Estenne et al. (1985) J Appl Physiol 59:1842–1848). Rib cage compliance is below the normal range in most tetraplegic subjects. (From [39] with permission)

muscles reduces markedly the range of rib cage motion (Fig. 5). There are good reasons to believe, therefore, that traumatic transection of the cervical cord leads to gradual stiffening of rib cage tissues (tendons and ligaments) and ankylosis in the costosternal and costovertebral articulations.

Although rib cage compliance has not been specifically investigated in patients with chronic neuromuscular disorders other than traumatic tetraplegia, it is likely that similar alterations in rib cage distensibility develop, in particular when the inspiratory muscles of the rib cage are involved. In addition, the development of scoliosis, which is a frequent occurrence in patients in the latter stages of muscular dystrophy, may also contribute to decrease rib cage and chest wall compliance.

Physiological Consequences

In patients with chronic weakness of the respiratory muscles, a number of factors thus act in combination to augment the lung volume restriction resulting from the loss of distending pressure *per se*. These factors include the decreased pulmonary compliance and the rib cage stiffness (Fig. 7), and the paradoxical displacements of the chest wall. In addition to increasing the loss of lung volume, these alterations increase the elastic work of breathing and enhance the metabolic cost of lowering pleural pressure and inflating the lungs. In so doing, they thus increase the load against which the inspiratory muscles must contract and place at an even greater disadvantage these patients who have already less respiratory muscle power than normal persons.

As often observed in conditions which produce an increase in the elastic work of

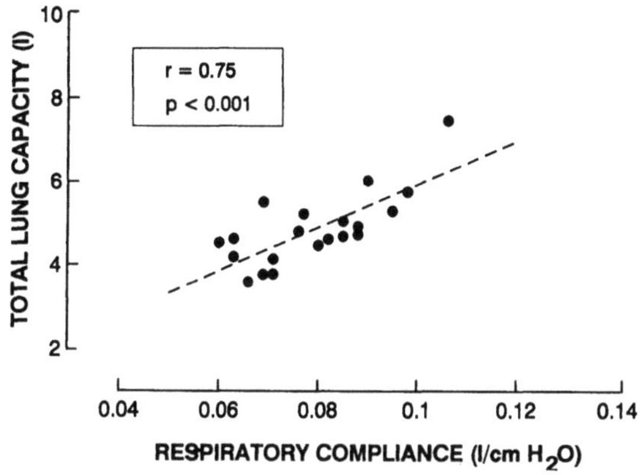

Fig. 7. Relationships between respiratory compliance and total lung capacity in 20 tetraplegic subjects. The dashed line is the line of regression. The close relationship suggests that the decreased distensibility of the respiratory system really is an important determinant of the reduced lung volume (From [10] with permission)

breathing, patients with neuromuscular disorders tend to breathe faster and with a smaller VT than healthy subjects (Fig. 2) [23, 34, 40]. The receptors responsible for this altered pattern of breathing are uncertain. It could reflexly be elicited by vagal pulmonary receptors sensing the changes in pulmonary compliance. Alternatively, it could be related to afferent signals arising in the chest wall or in the weakened respiratory muscles themselves. Whatever its mechanism, this inefficient pattern of breathing will result in a decreased alveolar ventilation and in CO_2 retention if there is no compensatory increase in inspiratory effort.

Fatigue of the Respiratory Muscles

The pathophysiology of respiratory muscle fatigue and its possible contribution to the development of ventilatory failure have been reviewed in a preceding chapter of this volume. To avoid undue repetition, we will thus only discuss the problem of respiratory muscle fatigue in the context of neuromuscular disorders.

There is general agreement that fatigue develops when the energy demand of the inspiratory muscles exceeds the energy supply [41]. Such imbalance may occur in patients with neuromuscular disorders for a number of reasons. First, the energy demand is likely to be augmented because the work of breathing is greater than normal and because the strength of the respiratory muscles is reduced. Each of these factors increases the fraction of maximum pressure developed by the inspiratory muscles and hence increases their energy requirements. In addition, the energy demand may be augmented because the efficiency of the inspiratory muscles is reduced. This may be due to the increased respiratory load, to paradoxical motion of the rib cage or abdominal wall, and to changes in the operating length of the inspiratory muscles. All these factors will contribute to make the energy demand of the inspiratory muscles greater than normal.

In muscular dystrophies which involve the heart, the cardiac output is often substantially reduced. As a result, blood flow and oxygen supply to the inspiratory muscles may be impaired. This phenomenon can be further amplified when hypoxemia is present, which is a frequent occurrence in patients with neuromuscular disorders. In addition, because these patients frequently have a poor nutritional status, the energy stores in the inspiratory muscles may be depleted. All these factors will contribute to make the energy supply to the inspiratory muscles smaller than normal.

On this basis, one can thus understand why patients with neuromuscular disorders have a reduced ventilatory endurance and why they may be particularly prone to inspiratory muscle fatigue. In this context, two alternative pathways might be proposed to account for the development of ventilatory failure [42]. Because the critical level of power output for muscle fatigue must be exceeded to maintain adequate alveolar ventilation as the disease progresses, the central nervous system may set a lower level of ventilation in order to avoid fatigue. Alternatively, it is possible that the muscles become chronically fatigued such that the decrease in alveolar ventilation is the result of muscle failure. Although each of these pathways could conceivably contribute to chronic ventilatory failure in patients with neuromuscular disorders, none of them has been readily demonstrated. This, however, may simply reflect the fact that at present it is difficult to test for respiratory muscle fatigue. The observation that daytime hypercapnia is markedly improved when nocturnal assisted ventilation is instituted has been taken as indirect evidence that chronic fatigue contributes significantly to ventilatory failure, i.e. the primary effect of assisted ventilation would be to rest the inspiratory muscles and thereby to improve their function. Although this is an attractive hypothesis, other mechanisms than muscle rest *per se* may account for the beneficial effects of assisted ventilation (see below).

Alterations in the Central Control of Breathing

Specific dysfunction of the respiratory centers undoubtedly occurs in bulbar poliomyelitis, in which there is gross irregularity of the rate of respiration and incoordination of the respiratory muscles in the absence of anterior horn cell disease. Alterations in the central control mechanisms of respiration have also been repeatedly suggested in a number of patients with other neuromuscular disorders like myotonic dystrophy [43] or acid maltase deficiency [44].

Alterations in the central respiratory control may also develop in patients with neuromuscular disorders which do not produce specific dysfunction of the respiratory centers. These alterations might be related to sleep-induced hypoventilation. Early studies in patients with severely weak or completely paralyzed diaphragm have documented severe degrees of hypoxemia and hypercapnia during sleep, in particular during rapid eye movement (REM) phases [45–50]. Subsequently, numerous studies on various neuromuscular disorders have extensively confirmed that sleep is accompanied by early deteriorations in blood gas data. The sleep pattern is usually grossly disorganized and fragmented, and although adequate ventilation may be maintained during wakefulness and non-REM sleep, oxygen desaturation and hypercapnia typically develop during REM sleep (Fig. 8). In a recent study of 20 patients with various neuromuscular disorders [50], it was found that minimum oxygen saturation during REM sleep is directly correlated with VC and daytime ar-

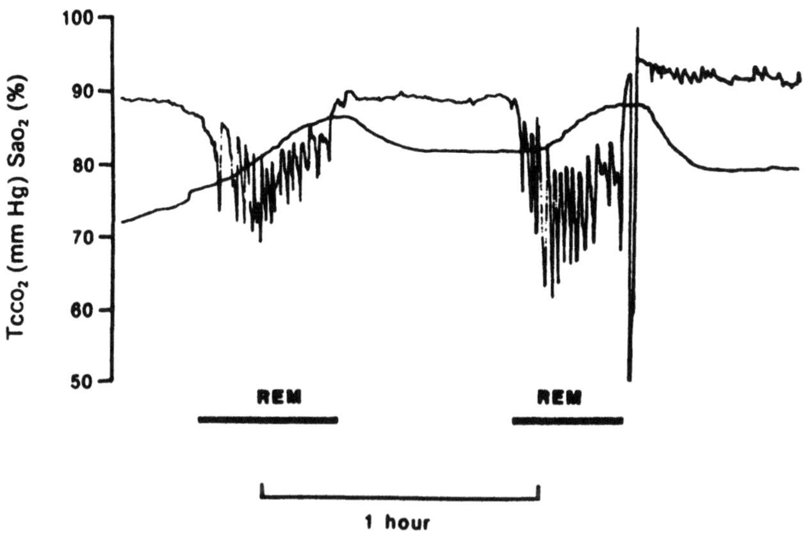

Fig. 8. Part of the recording from the all night sleep study in a patient with acid maltase deficiency. Arterial hemoglobin oxygen saturation (SaO_2) and transcutaneous carbon dioxide ($TcCO_2$) are shown. Note the desaturation and hypercapnia in REM sleep. (From [50] with permission)

terial oxygen tension, and is inversely correlated with daytime carbon dioxide tension.

In contrast, the degree of sleep hypoxemia is not correlated with the severity of respiratory muscle weakness [49, 50]. This may in part reflect the major role played by the distribution of respiratory muscle dysfunction between the rib cage muscles and the diaphragm in determining the adequacy of ventilation during sleep. There is convincing evidence that hypoventilation and arterial desaturation are more pronounced when the diaphragm is involved. This is due to the physiological inhibition of intercostal and accessory muscle inspiratory activity which occurs during REM sleep and leaves alone a weak diaphragm, unable to sustain adequate alveolar ventilation [44]. In addition to this mechanism, a number of other factors could contribute to the sleep-induced deteriorations in gas exchange [48]. These include the narrowing of the upper airways due to pharyngeal muscle weakness, the suppression of the stimulatory effect of wakefulness on ventilatory drive, the fall in FRC in the supine posture, the rapid shallow breathing pattern typical of REM sleep, and the reduction in chemoresponses associated with REM sleep.

Although the relative importance of these factors is likely to vary among patients and in the same patient during the night, they will all promote the occurrence of repeated episodes of hypoxemia and hypercapnia during sleep. These alterations, in turn, may lead to decrease the sensitivity of central and peripheral chemoreceptors in a manner analogous to what occurs in hypercapnic patients with obstructive sleep apnea syndromes [51]. The presence of sleep-induced hypoventilation in patients with neuromuscular disorders would thus play a primary role in the development of daytime ventilatory failure.

Effects of Nocturnal Assisted Ventilation

Nocturnal assisted ventilation has been extensively applied in patients with chronic neuromuscular disorders using negative pressure ventilation (tank, cuirass) or positive pressure ventilation through a tracheostomy or a nasal mask [52–62]. Following initiation of this treatment, virtually all patients report marked improvement in their clinical condition with reversal of the morning headaches and daytime hypersomnolence, improved intellectual performance, increased ability to perform activities of daily living, and clearing of systemic signs of venous congestion. These improvements are achieved within a few weeks after the onset of nighttime ventilation and can be sustained in the long-term provided the treatment is continued. The physiological counterpart is an improvement of arterial blood gas values during daytime. There is a rapid decrease in arterial carbon dioxide tensions, and in some patients the values eventually fall within the normal range.

The mechanisms by which nocturnal assisted ventilation is able to reverse daytime ventilatory failure remain speculative. By inflating the respiratory system with larger tidal volumes than those used by the patients during spontaneous breathing, assisted ventilation may reexpand collapsed areas within the lungs and increase pulmonary compliance. Similarly, it may decrease the stiffening of rib cage tissues and increase chest wall compliance. In so doing, assisted ventilation may reduce the work of breathing and hence decrease the load placed on the inspiratory muscles. Another mechanism might involve an improvement in inspiratory muscle function. Ventilating the patients several hours a day could conceivably rest the fatigued inspiratory muscles and improve their strength and endurance. Finally, improving nocturnal blood gases could result in a resetting of central control with an increase in chemosensitivity.

The available studies do not provide much information regarding the relative role played by these different mechanisms but it should be stressed that the reversal of chronic ventilatory failure may occur without any concomitant improvement in pulmonary function [54]. This suggests that changes in lung and chest wall mechanics are not the primary mechanism of improvement. Increases in inspiratory and expiratory muscle strength have been reported [48, 55] but these improvements are usually small in magnitude. Further studies will thus be required to get a better understanding of how nocturnal assisted ventilation operates to reverse chronic ventilatory failure in patients with neuromuscular disorders. Results of these studies should also offer a number of insights into the pathophysiological mechanisms of the ventilatory failure.

Conclusions

The development of chronic ventilatory failure in patients with long-standing neuromuscular disorders is not simply due to the direct effect of weakness of the respiratory muscles.

The following pathophysiological mechanisms may also be involved (Fig. 9):

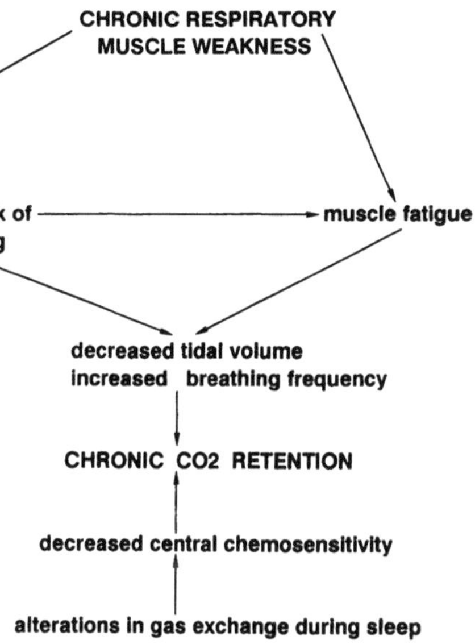

Fig. 9. Diagram illustrating the pathophysiological mechanisms that may contribute to chronic ventilatory failure in patients with chronic weakness of the respiratory muscles. *Crs* = respiratory compliance

1. stiffening of the lungs and rib cage, and distortion of the chest wall during breathing which increase the load placed on the inspiratory muscles;
2. imbalance between the energy demand of the inspiratory muscles and the energy supply leading to a reduced ventilatory endurance and to the development of muscle fatigue; and
3. sleep-induced hypoventilation producing a decrease in chemosensitivity.

The relative role played by these mechanisms is likely to vary among patients according to the type and the severity of their disease but each of these abnormalities is susceptible to be improved by assisted nocturnal ventilation. This is probably why this treatment is so effective in reversing chronic ventilatory failure in patients with neuromuscular disorders.

Acknowledgments. The authors are indebted to Ms. G. Basile for typing the manuscript. Supported in part by research grants from the Association Française contre les Myopathies and the Fonds National de la Recherche Scientifique (1.5.049. 89 F).

References

1. Kaminski MJ, Young RR (1985) Neuromuscular and neurological disorders affecting respiration. In: Roussos C, Macklem PT (eds) The Thorax, Part B. Marcel Dekker Inc, New York, pp 1023–1087
2. Aubier M, Trippenbach T, Roussos C (1981) Respiratory muscle fatigue during cardiogenic shock. J Appl Physiol 51:499–508
3. Estenne M, Yernault JC (1984) The mechanism of CO_2 retention in cardiac pulmonary edema. Chest 86:936–938

4. Hussain SNA, Simkus G, Roussos C (1985) Respiratory muscle fatigue: a cause of ventilatory failure in septic shock. J Appl Physiol 58:2033–2040
5. Juan G, Calverley P, Talamo C, Schnader J, Roussos C (1984) Effect of carbon dioxide on diaphragmatic function in human beings. N Eng J Med 310:874–879
6. Aubier G, Murciano D, Lecocguic Y, et al (1985) Effect of hypophosphatemia on diaphragmatic contractility in patients with acute respiratory failure. N Engl J Med 313:420–424
7. Janssens S, Decramer M (1989) Corticosteroid-induced myopathy and the respiratory muscles. Chest 95:1160–1162
8. Braun NMT, Arora NS, Rochester DF (1983) Respiratory muscle and pulmonary function in polyomyositis and other proximal myopathies. Thorax 38:616–623
9. De Troyer A, Pride NB (1985) The respiratory system in neuromuscular disorders. In: Roussos C, Macklem PT (eds) The Thorax, Part B. Marcel Dekker Inc, New York, pp 1089–1121
10. Estenne M, De Troyer A (1990) Respiratory muscle involvement in tetraplegia. In: Tobin MJ (ed) Problems in respiratory care: the respiratory muscles. JB Lippincott Company, Philadelphia, pp 360–374
11. Affeldt JE (1965) Neuromotor paralysis. In: Fenn WO, Rahn H (eds) Handbood of Physiology, Section 3: Respiration, Volume 2. American Physiological Society, Washington DC, pp 1509–1518
12. Lukas DS, Plum F (1952) Pulmonary function in patients convalescing from acute poliomyelitis with respiratory paralysis. Am J Med 12:388–396
13. Ferris BG, Mead J, Whittenberger JL, Saxton GA (1952) Pulmonary function in convalescent poliomyelitis patients. III. Compliance of the lungs and thorax. New Engl J Med 247:390–393
14. Keltz H (1965) The effect of respiratory muscle dysfunction on pulmonary function. Studies in patients with neuromuscular disease. Am Rev Respir Dis 91:934–938
15. Hapke EJ, Meek CJ, Jacobs J (1972) Pulmonary function in progressive muscular dystrophy. Chest 61:41–47
16. Inkley SR, Oldenburg FC, Vignos PJ (1974) Pulmonary function in Duchenne muscular distrophy related to stage of disease. Am J Med 56:297–306
17. Burke SS, Grove NM, Houser CR, Johnson DM (1977) Respiratory aspects of pseudo-hypertrophic muscular dystrophy. Am J Dis Child 121:230–234
18. Gal TJ, Goldberg SK (1981) Relationship between respiratory muscle strength and vital capacity during partial curarization in awake humans. Anesthesiology 54:141–147
19. Gibson GJ, Pride NB (1979) Lung mechanics in diaphragmatic paralysis. Am Rev Respir Dis 119:119–120
20. De Troyer A, Borenstein S, Cordier R (1980) Analysis of lung volume restriction in patients with respiratory muscle weakness. Thorax 35:603–610
21. Gibson GJ, Pride NB, O'Cain C, Quagliato R (1976) Sex and age differences in pulmonary mechanics in normal nonsmoking subjects. J Appl Physiol 41:20–25
22. De Troyer A, Estenne M, Yernault JC (1980) Disturbance of respiratory muscle function in patients with mitral valve disease. Am J Med 69:867–873
23. Gibson GJ, Pride NB, Newsom Davis J, Loh LC (1977) Pulmonary mechanics in patients with respiratory muscle weakness. Am Rev Respir Dis 115:389–395
24. De Troyer A, Heilporn A (1980) Respiratory mechanics in quadriplegia. The respiratory function of the intercostal muscles. Am Rev Respir Dis 122:591–600
25. De Troyer A, Deisser P (1981) The effects of intermittent positive pressure breathing on patients with respiratory muscle weakness. Am Rev Respir Dis 124:132–137
26. Prys-Roberts C, Nunn JF, Dobson RH, Robinson RH, Greenbaum R, Harris RS (1967) Radiologically undetectable pulmonary collapse in the supine position. Lancet 2:399–401
27. Blossom RA, Affeldt JE (1956) Chronic poliomyelitic respirator deaths. Am J Med 20:77–87
28. Mead J, Collier C (1959) Relation of volume history of lungs to respiratory mechanics in anesthetized dogs. J Appl Physiol 14:669–678
29. Young SL, Tierney DF, Clements JA (1970) Mechanism of compliance change in excised rat lungs at low transpulmonary pressure. J Appl Physiol 29:780–785

30. Mortola JP, Sant'Ambrogio G (1978) Motion of the rib cage and the abdomen in tetraplegic patients. Clin Sci 54:25–32
31. Danon J, Druz WS, Goldberg NB, Sharp JT (1979) Function of the isolated paced diaphragm and the cervical accessory muscles in C_1 quadriplegics. Am Rev Respir Dis 119:909–919
32. Estenne M, De Troyer A (1985) Relationship between respiratory muscle electromyogram and rib cage motion in tetraplegia. Am Rev Respir Dis 132:53–59
33. De Troyer A, Estenne M, Vincken W (1986) Rib cage motion and muscle use in high tetraplegics. Am Rev Respir Dis 133:1115–1119
34. Newsom Davis J, Goldman M, Loh L, Casson M (1976) Diaphragm function and alveolar hypoventilation. Q J Med 45:87–100
35. Higenbottam T, Allen D, Loh L, Clark TJH (1977) Abdominal wall movement in normals and patients with hemidiaphragmatic and bilateral diaphragmatic palsy. Thorax 32:589–595
36. Kreitzer SM, Feldman NT, Saunders NA, Ingram RH (1978) Bilateral diaphragmatic paralysis with hypercapnic respiratory failure. A physiologic assessment. Am J Med 65:89–95
37. Heaf PDJ, Prime FJ (1956) Compliance of the thorax in normal human subjects. Clin Sci 15:319–327
38. Estenne M, Heilporn A, Delhez L, Yernault JC, De Troyer A (1983) Chest wall stiffness in patients with chronic respiratory muscle weakness. Am Rev Respir Dis 198:1002–1007
39. Estenne M, De Troyer A (1986) The effects of tetraplegia on chest wall statics. Am Rev Respir Dis 134:121–124
40. Bégin R, Bureau MA, Lupien L, Lemieux B (1980) Control and modulation of respiration in Steinert's myotonic dystrophy. Am Rev Respir Dis 121:281–289
41. Roussos C, Moxham J (1985) Respiratory muscle fatigue. In: Roussos C, Macklem PT (eds) The Thorax, Part B. Marcel Dekker Inc, New York, pp 829–870
42. Roussos C (1985) Ventilatory failure and respiratory muscles. In: Roussos C, Macklem PT (eds) The Thorax, Part B. Marcel Dekker Inc, New York, pp 1253–1279
43. Kilburn KH, Eagan JT, Sieker HO, Heyman A (1959) Cardiopulmonary insufficiency in myotonic and progressive muscular dystrophy. N Engl J Med 261:1089–1096
44. Rosenow EC, Engel AG (1978) Acid maltase deficiency in adults presenting as respiratory failure. Am J Med 64:485–491
45. Loh L, Hughes JMB, Newsom Davis J (1979) Gas exchange problems in bilateral diaphragm paralysis. Bull Eur Physiopathol Respir 15:137–141
46. Skatrud J, Iber C, McHugh W, Rasmussen H, Nichols D (1980) Determinants of hypoventilation during wakefulness and sleep in diaphragmatic paralysis. Am Rev Respir Dis 121:537–593
47. Ellis ER, Bye PTP, Bruderer JW, Sullivan CE (1987) Treatment of respiratory failure during sleep in patients with neuromuscular disease. Positive-pressure ventilation through a nose mask. Am Rev Respir Dis 135:148–152
48. Goldstein RS, Molotiu N, Skrastins R, et al (1987) Reversal of sleep-induced hypoventilation and chronic respiratory failure by nocturnal negative pressure ventilation in patients with restrictive ventilatory impairment. Am Rev Respir Dis 135:1049–1055
49. Smith PEM, Calverley PMA, Edwards RHT (1988) Hypoxemia during sleep in Duchenne muscular dystrophy. Am Rev Respir Dis 137:884–888
50. Bye PTP, Ellis ER, Issa FG, Donnelly PM, Sullivan CE (1990) Respiratory failure and sleep in neuromuscular disease. Thorax 45:241–247
51. Sullivan CE, Issa FG, Berthon-Jones M, Saunders NA (1984) Pathophysiology of sleep apnea. In: Saunders NA, Sullivan CE (eds) Sleep and breathing. Marcel Dekker Inc, New York, pp 299–363
52. Garay S, Turino GT, Goldring R (1981) Sustained reversal of chronic hypercapnia in patients with alveolar hypoventilation syndromes: long-term maintenance with noninvasive nocturnal mechanical ventilation. Am J Med 70:269–274
53. Sullivan CE, Issa FG, Berthon-Jones M, Eves L (1981) Reversal of obstructive sleep apnea by continuous positive airway pressure applied through the nares. Lancet 2:862–865
54. Curran FJ (1981) Night ventilation by body respirators for patients in chronic respiratory failure due to late stage Duchenne muscular dystrophy. Arch Phys Med Rehab 62:270–274

55. Marino W, Braun NMT (1982) Reversal of the clinical sequelae of respiratory muscle fatigue by intermittent mechanical ventilation. Am Rev Respir Dis 125:85
56. Kerby GR, Mayer LS, Pingleton SK (1987) Nocturnal positive pressure ventilation via a nasal mask. Am Rev Respir Dis 135:738–740
57. Driver AG, Blackburn BB, Marcuard SP, Austin EM (1987) Bilateral diaphragm paralysis treated with cuirass ventilation. Chest 92:683–685
58. Braun NMT (1987) Nocturnal ventilation - A new method. Am Rev Respir Dis 135:523–524
59. Caroll N, Branthwaite MA (1988) Control of nocturnal hypoventilation by nasal intermittent positive pressure ventilation. Thorax 43:349–353
60. Kinnear W, Hockley S, Harvey J, Shneerson (1988) The effects of one year nocturnal cuirass-assisted ventilation in chest wall disease. Eur Respir J 1:204–208
61. Mohr CH, Hill NS (1990) Long-term follow-up of nocturnal ventilatory assistance in patients with respiratory failure due to Duchenne-type muscular dystrophy. Chest 97:91–96
62. Branthwaite MA (1990) Home mechanical ventilation. Eur Respir J 3:743–745

Risk Factors for Ventilatory Failure in Infants and Children

C. Gaultier

Introduction

In newborns, infants and children a variety of diseases can rapidly lead to ventilatory failure: neonatal distress syndrome, bronchopulmonary dysplasia, bronchiolitis due to viral infection, upper airway obstruction, and acute exacerbations of chronic obstructive pulmonary diseases (COPD). In the early period of life, the ventilatory response to respiratory disease is limited and risk factors for ventilatory failure are related to the immaturity of the developing respiratory system. Newborns and infants have limitations in their ability to substain breathing and defend blood gas homeostasis. Compared with adults, these limitations are principally related to the compliant rib cage, the small force reserve of the respiratory muscles, and reduced O_2 stores with a high metabolic rate.

Mechanical Properties of the Chest Wall

During development, the shape of the thorax changes significantly. At birth, the ribs are mainly cartilage and extend almost at right angles from the vertebral column. As a result, the rib cage is more circular than in the adult (Fig. 1) [1], and

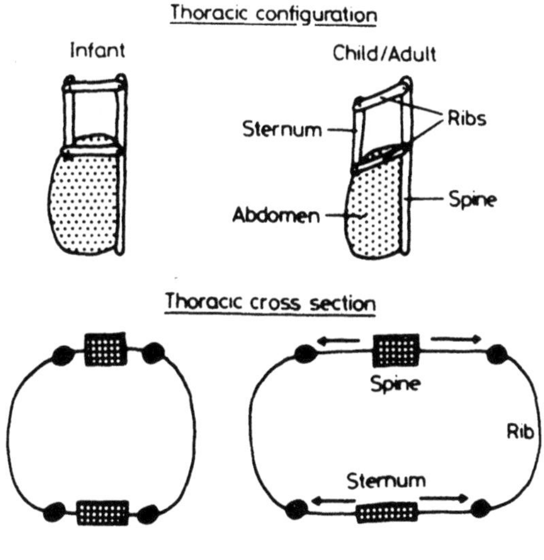

Fig. 1. Observed changes in configuration and cross sectional shape of the thorax from infancy to early childhood. Upper panel: infantile and adult rib cage configuration. Lower panel: how rib growth at costochondral junctions and posterior rib angles could explain the observed changes in cross sectional shape of the thorax. (From [3] with permission)

this is mechanically inefficient. In adults, the volume of the rib cage can be increased by elevating the ribs. In infants, the ribs are already elevated and this may be one reason why motion of the rib cage during room air breathing contributes little to tidal volume (VT). Using calibrated respiratory inductance plethysmography, the contribution of the rib cage to tidal breathing at 1 month of age was estimated to be 34% during non-rapid-eye-movements (NREM) sleep [2]. Moreover, the angle of insertion of the diaphragm is different in adults and infants: nearly horizontal in infants, while it is obliquely cephaled in adults.

With age changes in rib cage geometry occur (Fig. 1) [1, 2]. The thoracic index (ratio of the anteroposterior over the lateral diameter of the thorax) dramatically decreases during the first two years of life [3]. Concurrently, there is progressive mineralization of the ribs. These changes in shape and structure are of major importance in improving the stiffness of the rib cage. Changes in posture from supine to upright position at the end of the first year of life may lead to changes in chest wall shape. With time, gravitational forces operating on the rib cage together with the effects of rib growth would be expected to result in the observed changes in rib cage geometry. Concurrently with changes in rib cage shape, the contribution of the rib cage to tidal breathing during NREM sleep significantly increases during infancy, approaching that found in adolescents [4], after the first year of age (Fig. 2) [2].

A high chest wall compliance (Cw) relative to lung compliance is an inherent characteristic of the newborn mammal [5]. Cw has been measured in preterm and full-term human newborns [6], and in children and adolescents [7]. In the 32 week preterm neonate, Cw is 6.4 ml/cm H_2O/kg and decreases to 4.2 ml/cm H_2O/kg in the full-term neonate. By adolescence, the chest wall has become much more rigid

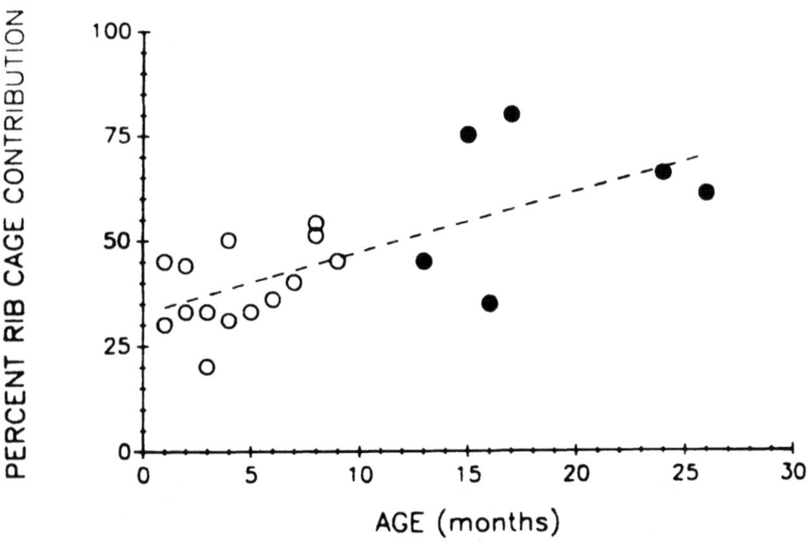

Fig. 2. Relationship between age and percent rib cage contribution to tidal volume (% RC). % RC increases with age prior to one year of age: % RC = 1.4 × age (months) + 33 (r = 0.69, p<0.01). After one year of age (closed circles), % RC is similar to that found in quietly sleeping adolescents [66]. (From [2] with permission)

with a mean Cw of 2.5 ml/cm H_2O/kg [7]. Chest wall muscles augment the rigidity of the relatively compliant infant rib cage by their tonic contraction. This fixates the chest wall which would otherwise be pulled inwards by diaphragmatic contraction. The compliant rib cage of newborns and infants is easily deformed by the effect of large diaphragmatic effort, or when the stabilizing effect of intercostal muscles is inhibited, such as during REM sleep. It must be emphasized that full-term newborns spend up to 70% of their total sleep time in REM sleep and that REM sleep is even more prominent in premature infants [8].

During REM sleep with inhibition of the intercostal muscles, the effect of phasic inspiratory diaphragmatic contraction causes the rib cage to move inward rather than to expand (Fig. 3) [9].

During the rib cage distortion associated with REM sleep, several mechanical derangements have been observed:

1. decrease in functional residual capacity [10];
2. decrease in transcutaneous partial pressure of O_2 [11];
3. increase in the diaphragmatic work of breathing [12, 13];
4. decrease in the high/low ratio of the diaphragmatic electromyogram (EMG) suggesting diaphragmatic fatigue [14].

In preterm human newborns, Guslits et al. [12] assessed diaphragmatic work utilizing measurements of transdiaphragmatic pressure and abdominal volume displacement. During periods of minimal rib cage distortion, inspiratory diaphragmatic work averaged 5.9 g/cm/ml. This increased to an average of 12 g/cm/ml during

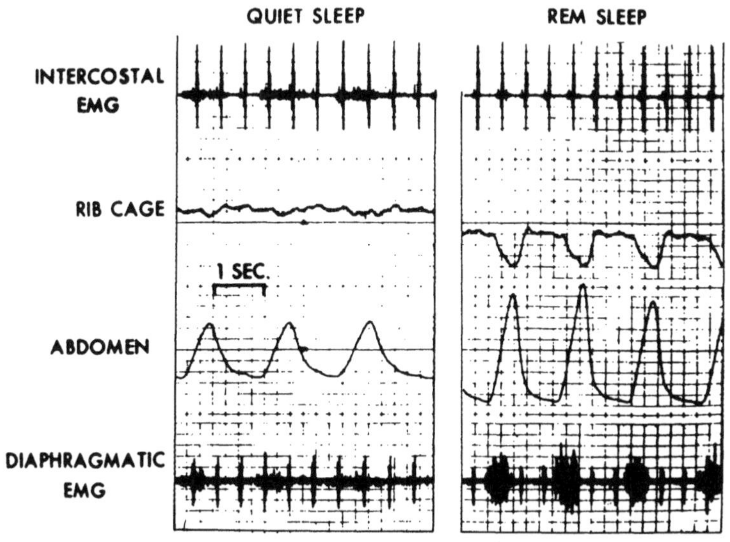

Fig. 3. Surface intercostal and diaphragmatic EMG and motion of rib cage and abdomen (magnetometer) in an infant in non-REM (quiet) and REM sleep. Note the almost complete suppression of the intercostal EMG and the marked increase in the diaphragmatic EMG in REM sleep. Also note the paradoxical motion of the rib cage and increase in abdominal motion in REM. (From [14] with permission)

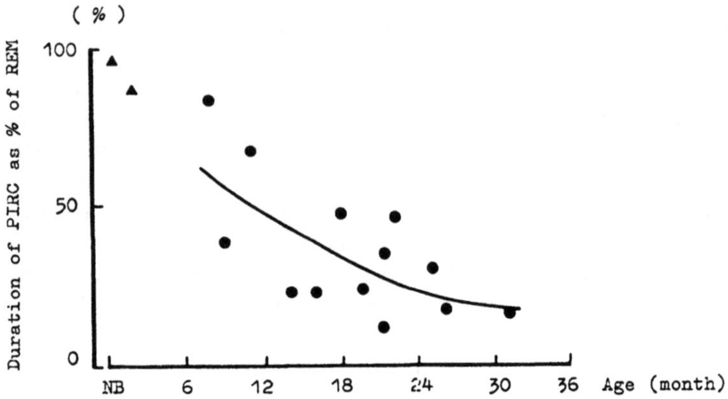

Fig. 4. Duration of paradoxical inward rib cage (PIRC) motion on inspiration expressed as a percentage of rapid eye movement sleep (REM) time as a function of age (NB = newborns). Circles are individual values of PIRC in infants from 7 to 31 months of age. Duration of PIRC decreased significantly with age as a power function ($r = -0.66$, $p<0.02$). Triangles are previously published values if PIRC during REM sleep in neonates [9]. (From [15] with permission)

periods of paradoxical rib cage motion. This estimated diaphragmatic work of breathing may represent a significant expenditure of calories and may contribute to the development of diaphragmatic fatigue and ventilatory failure. With advancing age and changes in rib cage geometry, the duration of paradoxical rib cage motion during REM sleep decreases and becomes little or none at all after three years of age (Fig. 4) [15].

In the case of respiratory disease with impairment of lung mechanics [16] as in bronchopulmonary dysplasia [17, 18], or with upper airway obstruction [19], substantial asynchrony between rib cage and abdominal wall motion during tidal breathing has been observed during NREM sleep. Rib cage and abdominal motion asynchrony can be objectively quantified by phase-angle measurement from a non-calibrated respiratory inductance plethysmography [19].

Respiratory Muscles

With growth, there is a progressive increase in the bulk of the muscle attached to the rib cage. Coinciding with the increase in muscle bulk, there is an increase in maximal static inspiratory and expiratory pressures with a substantial difference between sexes in children and adolescents [20, 21]. Maximal static inspiratory pressure (PImax) at functional residual capacity (FRC) approximates 70 cm H_2O in 7–8 years old boys and 60 cm H_2O in age-matched girls (Fig. 5) [20, 21]. Newborn infants have been reported to generate large dynamic pressures (-70 cm H_2O) during the first breath [22]. In healthy infants from 1.7 months to 12 months, maximal transdiaphragmatic pressure (Pdi) was recorded while crying against an occluded airway [23]. Maximal Pdi was equal to 55 ± 8 cm H_2O at 2 months of age, and to 62 ± 16 cm H_2O at 8.6 months. The maximum pressures exerted by infants are sur-

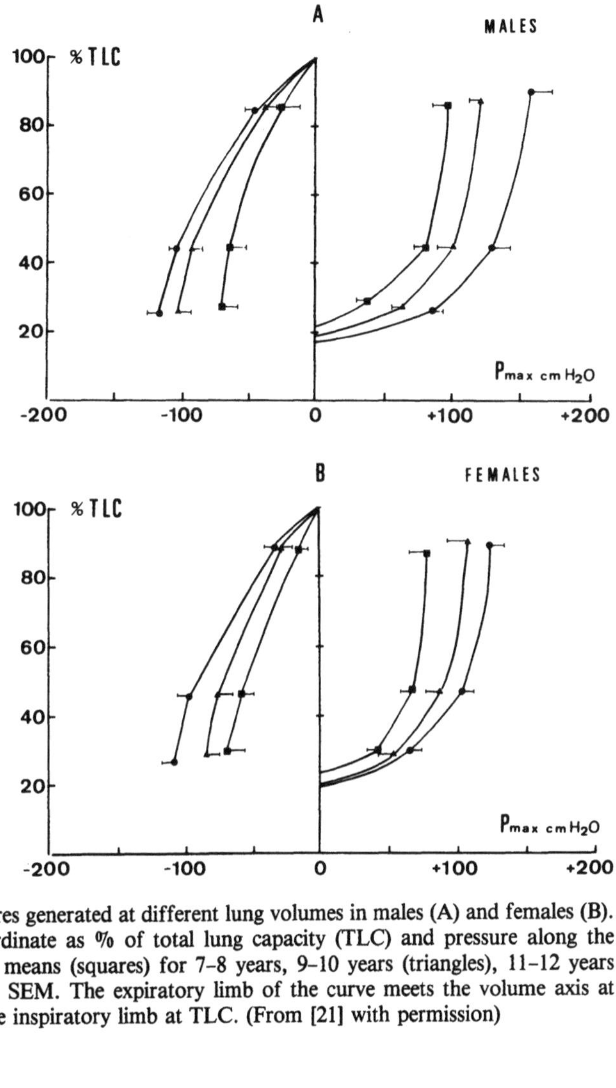

Fig. 5. Maximal static pressures generated at different lung volumes in males (A) and females (B). Volume is plotted on the ordinate as % of total lung capacity (TLC) and pressure along the abscissa. The values are the means (squares) for 7–8 years, 9–10 years (triangles), 11–12 years (circles). The bars indicate 1 SEM. The expiratory limb of the curve meets the volume axis at residual volume (RV) and the inspiratory limb at TLC. (From [21] with permission)

prisingly high compared with adults. This is probably related to the small radius of curvature of the rib cage, diaphragm, and abdomen, which by the Laplace relationship, will convert small tensions developed by the infant into relatively large pressures.

Despite relatively high maximal static inspiratory pressure, the inspiratory force reserve of the respiratory muscles is reduced with respect to adults because inspiratory pressure demand at rest is greater [24]. In children over 4 years of age, the inspiratory pressure demand has been estimated from measurements of the mouth occlusion pressure (P0.1) and the inspiratory time (TI) assuming that the pressure developed by the respiratory muscles increases linearly during inspiration. The ratio of mean inspiratory pressure (PI) to PImax at FRC amounts 0.20 at 7 years of age (Fig. 6); this is more than twice the value in adults for the ratio of Pdi over Pdimax

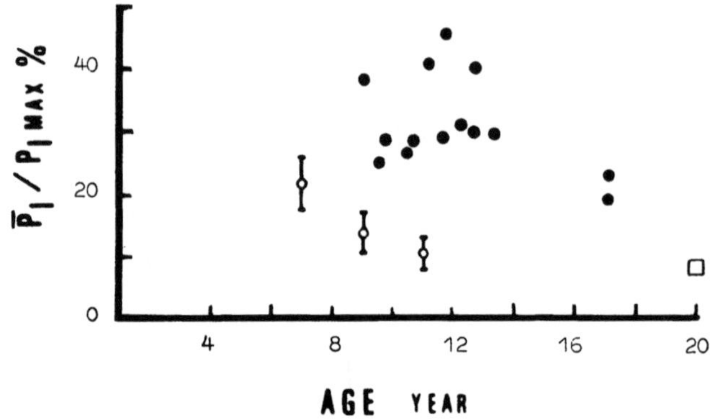

Fig. 6. The fraction of maximal inspiratory static pressure (PImax) used for breathing at rest (plotted as the ratio of the mean inspiratory pressure (PI) to PImax) as a function of age. Open circles represent mean values in healthy children [21, 24], and the bars represent 1 SD. The square indicates the mean predicted values in adult [25]. Filled circles are values in children with COPD. Increased PI/PImax in children with COPD is evident. (From [32] with permission)

at FRC, i.e. 0.07 [25]. Taking into account data for P0.1 in newborn infants and TI [26, 27], Milic-Emili [28] estimated resting Pdi to amount to 14 cm H_2O in newborns. High pressure demand in newborns is related to high minute ventilation (VE) (410 ml/min/kg [27] vs 110 ml/min/kg in the adult), and to high metabolic rate [29]. Considering the Pdimax reported at 2 months of age [23], the Pdi/Pdimax ratio should be estimated to be equal to 0.22 during the early period of life. Therefore, it appears that despite relatively high maximal pressure developed the infant has a small inspiratory force reserve.

Bellemare and Grassino [30, 31] analyzed diaphragmatic fatiguability in humans. In normal adults, there is a fatigue threshold which is reached when the so-called tension-time index of the diaphragm (TTdi) exceeds 0.15. TTdi is the product of TI over the total duration (Ttot) of the respiratory cycle (TI/Ttot) multiplied by the Pdi/Pdimax ratio. In adults at rest, TTdi is equal to 0.03. Since this TTdi is far

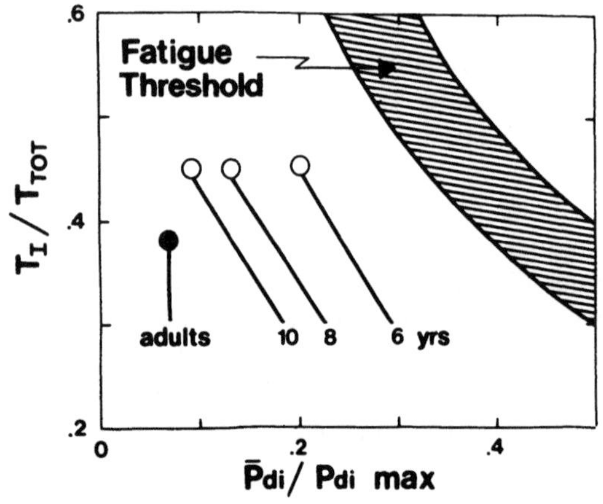

Fig. 7. Relationship between TI/Ttot and Pdi/Pdimax. The hatched area defines the fatigue threshold, and corresponds to tension time index of the diaphragm = 0.15 [30, 31]. Closed circle: average value for normal young adult during resting breathing. Open circles: average value for children (10.8 and 6 years old). Bars indicate ± 1 SD.
(From [25] with permission)

from the fatigue threshold, normal adults have a large respiratory reserve in terms of fatiguability of the diaphragm. Figure 7 shows that, in 6-year old children, the respiratory reserve is relatively small but approaches the adult value by the age of 10 years [25].

In cases of impairment of lung mechanics as in COPD, the PI developed by the respiratory muscles for breathing at rest increases. Furthermore in children with COPD, PImax generated at the end-expiratory level is low because of hyperinflation [32]. Therefore, the PI/PImax ratio increases and can reach values as high as 0.40 (Fig. 6) [32]. Children with COPD may decrease TI/Ttot presumably as a strategy to breathe below the fatigue threshold of the respiratory muscles. We observed an inverse correlation between PI/PImax and TI/Ttot (Fig. 8) [32]. Young children with COPD manifest a lower TI/Ttot than older ones during breathing at rest, presumably to spare the fraction of their lower inspiratory force reserve [33]. A similar breathing strategy has been also observed in children with increased elastic load [34]. Therefore in children with respiratory disease, minimal changes is breathing pattern which cause an increase in TI/Ttot may expose them to respiratory muscle fatigue and ventilatory failure. Any life condition in which an increase in the breathing load occurs, as during exercise [35] or sleep [36], limits the possibilities of adaptation of the breathing pattern. The younger the child, the greater the limitation.

In addition to small inspiratory muscle reserve, young infants and especially preterm ones are exposed to fatigue because they have a very low percentage (< 10%) of type I fibers (slow-twitch high oxidative fibers) in the diaphragm and in the intercostal muscles [37]. The type I fibers increase rapidly to about 30% at term and continue to increase throughout the first year of life, when they reach adult values of about 50–60%.

There are a number of approaches to the diagnosis of respiratory muscle fatigue, but one easily adaptable to sick infants is spectral frequency analysis of the diaphragmatic EMG. On-line spectral frequency analysis of the surface diaphragmatic EMG can be done at the bedside in the neonatal intensive care unit [38]. Increase in the low frequency and decrease in the high frequency power in the EMG (H/L ratio) has been shown to precede the loss of force in a muscle developing high-frequency fatigue [39]. Muller et al. [14] showed that these changes occur in the

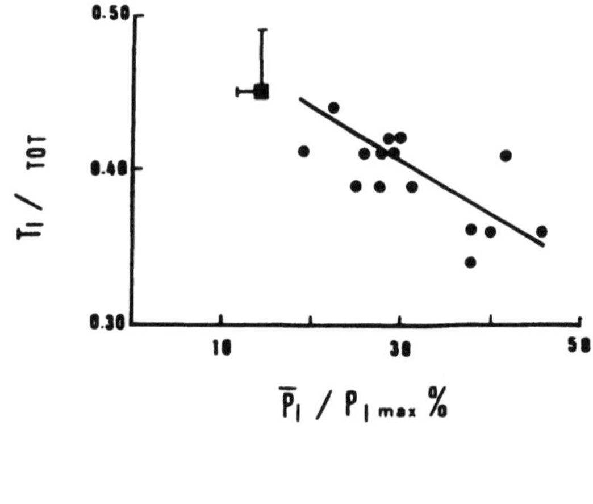

Fig. 8. Duty cycle (TI/Ttot) as a function of the fraction of maximal inspiratory static pressure used for breathing at rest (PI/PImax). The square indicates the mean predicted value for age-matched normal children; bars are 1 SD. Full circles are values obtained in children with COPD. The solid line is the regression line between PI/PImax and TI/Ttot in children with COPD (TI/Ttot = 2.6^{-3} PI/PImax % + 0.48, r = −0.64, p = 0.01). (From [32] with permission)

surface diaphragmatic EMG in healthy preterm infants during periods of marked chest wall distortion.

In infants with respiratory disease, a fall in the H/L ratio was invariably associated with increasing end-tidal CO_2 [4]. In preterm infants, Lopes et al. [41] found EMG evidence of diaphragmatic fatigue preceding episodes of apnea, suggesting that apnea was a strategy used to allow the diaphragm to recover. However, infants are able to use other respiratory muscles to unload (rest) the diaphragm. In case of increases respiratory drive due to CO_2 breathing or to increased upper airway resistance, infants and children recruit intercostals and/or abdominal muscles [42–44]. However, this protective muscle recruitment to prevent an increase in diaphragmatic work of breathing and diaphragmatic fatigue is suppressed during REM sleep [43, 44].

Oxygen Stores and Gas Exchange

The oxygen (O_2) stores can be estimated from the volume of the lungs, venous and arterial blood. In the infant, there are about 8 ml (16%) in the lungs, and 43 ml (84%) in the blood; in the adult, about 250 ml (24%) in the lungs and 800 ml (70%) in the blood. Therefore, the newborn has small O_2 stores in the lungs in relation to its high metabolic rate [29].

During resting breathing, the volume of gas in the lungs at FRC represents lung O_2 stores. FRC is determined by the static passive balance of forces between the lung and chest wall. In the infant, the outward recoil of the chest wall is very small and the inward recoil of the lung slightly lower than in the adult [45]. Consequently, the static passive balance of forces would dictate a very low FRC relative to total lung capacity (TLC) ratio in infants, which would be inadequate for gas exchange. From the measured FRC and estimated TLC in infants [46], the dynamic FRC/TLC ratio appears to be about 40%, that is similar to that in the supine adult. Thus, there are compelling reasons to believe that in newborns and infants with a low outward recoil of the chest wall, the dynamic end-expiratory volume is substantially above the passively determined FRC.

It has been shown that in the infant, in contrast to the adult, expiration is terminated at substantial flow rates [47]. This suggests an active interruption of a relaxed expiration. The newborn may use two mechanisms to actively slow expiration and maintain FRC. These mechanisms include post-inspiratory activity of the diaphragm [48], and laryngeal narrowing during expiration [49] which, in the extreme, is the "grunting" observed in the newborn with respiratory distress syndrome. Laryngeal braking of expiration acts as an auto-PEEP effect to increase FRC. In the lamb, Harding et al. [50] have shown that adductor of the larynx acts as an expiratory brake in awake, NREM sleep but not in REM sleep. During REM sleep, disappearance of active laryngeal braking may explain in part the fall in FRC observed in healthy newborns [10]. Transition from dynamically maintained end-expiratory lung volume to passively determined occurs in the second half of the first year of life [51, 52].

Hypoxemia develops more rapidly during apnea in the infant compared with the adult since metabolic O_2 consumption is 2 to 3 fold greater in relation to the available O_2 stores. In REM sleep, with reduction of O_2 stores in the lung [10] and an increase in O_2 consumption [53], hypoxemia will be accelerated during apnea.

The risk for occurrence of severe hypoxemia and reduction on O_2 delivery to tissue is greater in infant than in the adult. In the newborn, the arterial oxygen pressure (PaO_2) is approximatively 70 torr [54]. The alveolo-arterial difference in partial pressure of O_2 (A-a PO_2) is about 30 torr during air breathing and 120 torr during O_2 breathing [53]. During infancy and childhood, PaO_2 measured in arterialized blood samples rises rapidly during the first two years of age, and then slowly up to the age of 8 (Fig. 9) [56, 57]. In children after the age of 8, PAO_2 does not change with age and reaches adult values [54].

The lung volume at which some of the small intrapulmonary airways are closed (closing volume (CV)) is an index of suspectibility to hypoxemia, and closing capacity, i.e. CV plus residual volume, decreases with age. Infants and young children may have a closing capacity greater than FRC, and some areas of the lung may be closed throughout part or all the VE with consequent impairment of gas exchange. At 8 years, the closing capacity is close to FRC. Children of 8 years of age have a higher closing volume compared with adolescents [58, 59].

The mechanism for improvement in pulmonary gas exchange during growth has been more fully investigated in piglets than in humans. Using the multiple gas technique in the awake growing piglet, Escourrou et al. [60] have shown that low PaO_2 at a young age was due to two mechanisms: ventilation-perfusion mismatch, and diffusion limitation for O_2 [60]. The exact morphological basis for this limitation is not fully established. However in young animals and humans, a double capillary layer has been demonstrated that halves the effective capillary surface in contact with alveolar gas [61, 62]. Thus the available surface for diffusion is presumably lower in the growing lung during the persistence of a double capillary layer compared with later one. A double capillary layer is no longer seen after 2–3 years of age in humans [62]. In addition, the capillary blood volume is lower at birth, increasing from <22% of septal volume at birth to 42% in the adult lung. This may also be a limiting factor for diffusion [62]. Finally, the overall pulmonary diffusing capacity for O_2 increases 30–35 times from infancy to adulthood and rises at a higher rate than body mass. In newborn, the ratio of pulmonary diffusing capacity

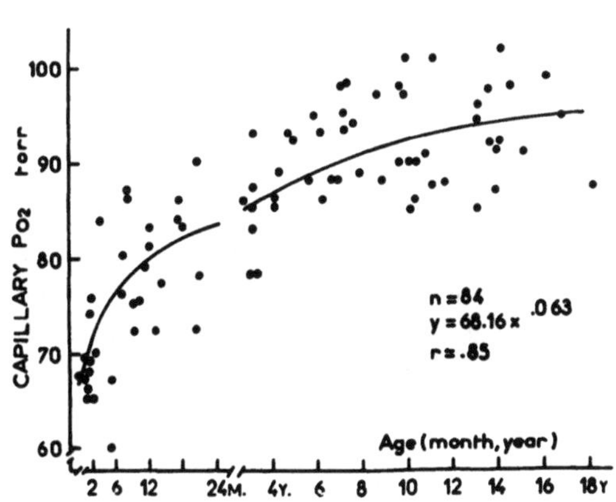

Fig. 9. Capillary PO_2 in 84 infants and children aged from 20 days to 18 years plotted against age. (From [57] with permission)

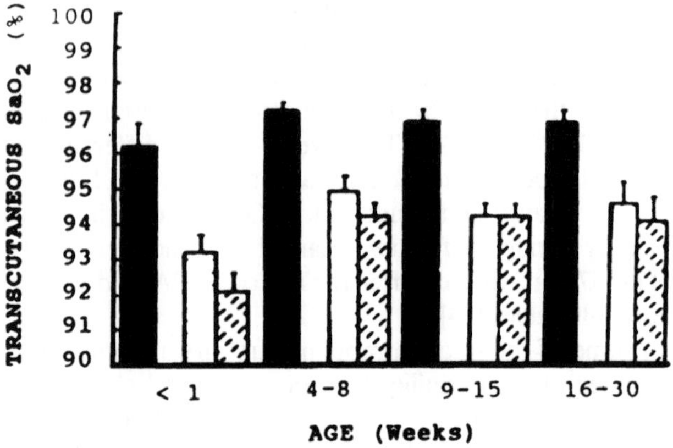

Fig. 10. Mean transcutaneous oxygen saturation (SaO_2), measured by pulse oximetry, is displayed on the abscisa and age in weeks on the ordinate. Full columns refer to wakefulness, open columns to NREM sleep and hatched columns to REM sleep. Bars are 1 SEM. (From [65] with permission)

to FRC is close to that obtained in 11–13 years old boy during submaximal exercise, i.e. 20 ml/torr/min per liter of FRC [63]. Therefore in newborns, the capillary surface available for gas exchange is nearly maximal, and reserve capillary surface is extremely limited.

The relative low PaO_2 in infants and young children places them close to the steep part of the oxyhemoglobin dissociation curve. And further decrease in PaO_2 may induce severe oxygen desaturation. During sleep, especially REM sleep, falls in O_2 saturation to <90% have been shown in healthy full-term infants (Fig. 10) [64]. With advancing age, the occurrence of fall in O_2 saturation to <90% decreases and such desaturations are not observed in healthy children over age 9 years [65, 67]. This improvement of oxygenation during sleep is associated with a decrease in the occurrence of sleep-related apneas [66]. Infants and children with impairment of gas exchange during wakefulness secondary to respiratory disease are exposed to severe O_2 desaturation during sleep, especially during REM sleep [36, 68, 69]. Thus, management of these patients must include 24h monitoring of O_2 saturation, and treatment must take into account the exacerbation of respiratory disturbances during sleep.

Conclusion

During the early period of life, there are some limitations to maintenance of adequate alveolar ventilation to appropriate age-related high metabolic requirement. The younger the subject, the higher the limitations. The greater highly compliant rib cage is a mechanical disadvantage in the infant for coping with any abnormal condition of loaded breathing. The biochemical composition of diaphragmatic fibers exposes the infant to diaphragmatic fatigue. Their small inspiratory muscle reserve places infants and young children close to the fatigue threshold. This renders them suspectible to development of ventilatory failure following small changes in mechanical load. Finally, their relatively low PaO_2 compared with older children plays a role in rapid O_2 desturation especially during sleep. However, newborns appear to utilize breathing strategies which maintain adequate ventilation, and defend blood gas homeostasis in both health and disease conditions. Recruitment of accessory muscles occurrence and laryngeal braking of expiration act to decrease the work to the diaphragm, recruit new alveoli by an auto-PEEP effect, increase FRC, and improve gas exchange by an increase in capillary surface area. However, it must be emphasized that these breathing strategies are depressed during REM sleep, which is most prominent sleep state in the newborn. With advancing age, improvement in the mechanical properties of the chest wall, increase in inspiratory muscle reserve and improvement in gas exchange, all help to decrease the contraints limiting the adaptation to loaded breathing.

Acknowledgments. The author thank M. Goldman (Clamart) on sabbatical leave from Philadelphia (USA) for his help and criticisms and L. Piche for typing the manuscript.

References

1. Takahashi E, Atsumi H (1955) Age differences in thoracic form as indicated by the Thoracic Index. Human Biol 27:65–74
2. Hershenson MB, Colin AA, Wohl MEB, Stark AR (1990) Change in the contribution of the rib cage to total breathing during infancy. Am Rev Respir Dis 141:922–925
3. Openshaw P, Edwards S, Helms P (1984) Changes in rib cage geometry during childhood. Thorax 39:624–627
4. Tabachnik E, Muller NL, Bryan AC, Levison H (1982) Changes in ventilation and chest wall mechanics during sleep in normal adolescents. J Appl Physiol 51:557–564
5. Agostoni E (1959) Volume-pressure relationship to the thorax and lung in the newborn. J Appl Physiol 14:909–913
6. Gerhart T, Bancalari E (1980) Chest wall compliance in full-term and premature infants. Acta Paediatr Scand 69:359–364
7. Sharp M, Druz W, Balgot R, Bandelin V, Damon J (1970) Total respiratory compliance in infants and children. J Appl Physiol 2:775–779
8. Anders TF, Emde R, Parmelee A (1971) A manual of standardized terminology. Techniques and criteria for scoring of states of sleep and wakefulness in newborn infants. UCLA Brain information service/BRI Publications Office, Los Angeles
9. Curzi-Dascalova L (1978) Thoracico-abdominal respiratory correlations in infants: constancy and variability in different sleep states. Early Hum Dev 2:25–38
10. Henderson-Smart DJ, Read DJC (1979) Reduced lung volume during behavioral active sleep in the newborn. J Appl Physiol 46:1081–1085
11. Martin RJ, Okken A, Rubin D (1979) Arterial oxygen tension during active and quiet sleep. J Pediatr 94:271–274
12. Guslits BG, Gaston SE, Bryan MH, England SJ, Bryan AC (1987) Diaphragmatic work of breathing in premature human infants. J Appl Physiol 62:1410–1415
13. Heldt GP, Mc Ilroy MB (1987) Distortion of chest wall and work of diaphragm in preterm infants. J Appl Physiol 62:164–169
14. Muller NL, Gulston G, Cade D, Whitton J, Froese AB, Bryan MH, Bryan AC (1979) Diaphragmatic muscle fatigue in the newborn. J Appl Physiol 46:688–695

15. Gaultier CL, Praud JP, Canet E, Delaperche MF, D'Allest AM (1987) Paradoxical inward rib cage motion during rapid eye movement sleep in infants and young children. J Dev Physiol 9:391-397
16. Sivan Y, Deakers TW, Newth CJL (1990) Thoracoabdominal asynchrony in acute upper airway obstruction in small children. Am Rev Respir 142:540-544
17. Rome ES, Miller MJ, Goldthwait DA, Osorio IO, Fanaroff AA, Martin RJ (1987) Effect of sleep state on chest wall movements and gas exchange in infants with resolving bronchopulmonary dysplasia. Pediatr Pulmonol 3:259-263
18. Allen J, Greenspan J, Deoras K, Keklekian E, Wolfson M, Shaffer T (1989) Thoracoabdominal asynchrony in infants with bronchopulmonary dysplasia. Pediatr Res 25:363 A
19. Allen JL, Wolfson MR, McDowell K, Shaffer TH (1990) Thoracoabdominal asynchrony in infants with airway obstruction. Am Rev Respir Dis 141:337-342
20. Cook CD, Sutherland JM, Segal S et al (1957) Studies of respiratory physiology in the newborn infant. III. Measurements of mechanics of respiration. J Clin Invest 36:440-418
21. Gaultier CL, Zinman R (1983) Maximal static pressure in healthy children. Respir Physiol 51:45-61
22. Karlberg P, Koch G (1962) Respiratory studies in newborns. Acta Paediatr Scand 105 (Suppl):439-448
23. Scott CB, Nickerson BG, Sargent CW, Platzker AC, Warburton D, Keens TG (1983) Developmental pattern of maximal transdiaphragmatic pressure in infants during crying. Pediatr Res 17:707-709
24. Gaultier CL, Perret L, Boule M, Buvry A, Girard F (1981) Occlusion pressure and breathing pattern in healthy children. Respir Physiol 46:71-80
25. Milic-Emili J (1984) Respiratory muscle fatigue in children. In: Prakash O (ed) Critical care of the child. Martinus Nijhoff, Dordrecht:87-94
26. Fisher JT, Mortola JP, Smith JB, Fox GS, Weeks S (1982) Respiration in newborns, development of the control of breathing. Am Rev Respir Dis 125:650-657
27. Mortola JP, Fisher JT, Smith B, Fox G, Weeks S (1982) Dynamics of breathing in infants. J Appl Physiol 52:1209-1215
28. Milic-Emili J (1983) Respiratory muscle fatigue and its implication in respiratory distress syndrome. In: Cosmi EV, Scarpelli EM (eds), Pulmonary Surfactant System. Elsevier Science, Rome, pp. 135-141
29. Robertson JO, Reid DD (1952) Standards for the basal metabolism of normal people in Britain. Lancet 1:940-943
30. Bellemare F, Grassino A (1982) Effects of pressure and timing of contraction on the human diaphragm fatigue. J Appl Physiol 53:1190-1193
31. Bellemare F, Grassino A (1982) Evaluation of human diaphragmatic fatigue. J Appl Physiol 53:1196-1206
32. Gaultier CL, Boule M, Tournier G, Girard F (1985) Inspiratory force reserve of the respiratory muscles in children with chronic obstructive pulmonary disease. Am Rev Respir Dis 131:811-815
33. Gaultier CL, Perret L, Boule M, Baculard A, Grimfeld A, Girard F (1982) Occlusion pressure and breathing pattern in children with chronic obstructive pulmonary disease. Bull Eur Physiopath Respir 18:851-862
34. Gaultier CL, Perret L, Boule M, Tournier G, Girard F (1982) Control of breathing in children with interstitial lung disease. Pediatr Res 16:779-783
35. Boule M, Gaultier CL, Tournier G, Girard F (1991) Limited exercise-related increase in duty-cycle in children with chronic obstructive pulmonary disease (in press)
36. Gaultier CL, Praud JP, Clement A et al (1985) respiration during sleep in children with chronic obstructive pulmonary disease. Chest 87:168-173
37. Keens JG, Bryan AC, Levison H, Ianuzzo CD (1978) Developmental pattern of muscle fiber types in human ventilatory muscle. J Appl Physiol 44:909-913
38. Chambille B, Vardon G, Monrigal JP, Dehan M, Gaultier CL (1989) Technique of on-line analysis of diaphragmatic electromyogram activity in the newborn. Eur Resp J 2:883-886
39. Bigland-Ritchie B, Donovan EF, Roussos C (1981) Conduction velocity and EMG power spectrum changes in fatigue of substained maximal efforts. J Appl Physiol 51:1300-1305

40. Muller NL, Volgyesi G, Bryan MH, Bryan AC (1979) The concept of diaphragmatic muscle fatigue in the newborn infant. J Pediatr 95:793–797
41. Lopes JM, Muller NL, Bryan MH, Bryan AC (1981) Synergistic behavior of inspiratory muscles after diaphragmatic fatigue in the newborn. J Appl Physiol 51:547–551
42. Hershenson MB, Stark AR, Mead J (1989) Action of the inspiratory muscles of the rib cage during breathing in newborns. Am Rev Respir Dis 139:1207–1212
43. Praud JP, Egreteau L, Benlabed M, Curzi-Dascalova L, Nedelcoux H, Gaultier CL (1991) Abdominal muscle activity during CO_2 rebreathing in sleeping neonates. J Appl Physiol (in press)
44. Praud JP, D'Allest AM, Nedelcoux H, Curzi-Dascalova L, Guilleminault C, Gaultier CL (1989) Sleep-related abdominal muscle behavior during partial or complete obstructed breathing in prepubertal children. Pediatr Res 26:347–350
45. Fagan DG (1976) Shape changes in static V.P loops for children's lungs related to growth. Thorax 31:534–543
46. Gaultier CL, Boule M, Allaire Y, Clement A, Girard F (1979) Growth of lung volumes during the first three years of life. Bull Eur Physiopathol Respir 15:1103–1116
47. Kosch PC, Stark AR (1983) Dynamic maintenance of end-expiratory lung volume in full-term infants. J Appl Physiol 54:773–777
48. Mortola JP, Milic-Emili J, Noworaj A, Smith B, Fox G, Weeks S (1984) Muscle pressure and flow during expiration in infants. Am Rev Respir Dis 129:49–53
49. Kosch PC, Hutchinson AA, Wozniak JA, Carlo WA, Stark AR (1988) Posterior cricoarytenoid and diaphragm activities during tidal breathing in neonates. J Appl Physiol 64:1968–1978
50. Harding R, Johnson P, McClelland ME (1980) Respiratory function of the larynx in developing sheep and the influence of sleep state. Respir Physiol 40:165–179
51. Colin AA, Wohl MEB, Mead J, Ratjen FA, Glass G, Stark AR (1989) Transition from dynamically maintained to relaxed end-expiratory volume in human infants. J Appl Physiol 67:2107–2111
52. Ratjen FA, Colin AA, Stark AR, Mead J, Wohl MEB (1989) Changes of time constants during infancy and early childhood. J Appl Physiol 67:2112–2115
53. Stothers JK, Warner RM (1978) Oxygen consumption and neonatal sleep states. J Physiol 278:435–440
54. Koch G (1968) Alveolar ventilation, diffusion capacity and the (A-a) PO_2 difference in the newborn infant. Respir Physiol 4:168–192
55. Levison HEA, Featherby EA, Weng TR (1970) Arterial blood gases, alveolar-arterial oxygen difference, and physiologic dead space in children and young adults. Am Rev Respir Dis 101:972–974
56. Gaultier CL, Boule M, Allaire Y, Clement A, Buvry A, Girard F (1978) Determination of capillary oxygen tension in infants and children. Bull Eur Physiopath Respir 14:287–297
57. Dong SH, Lik HM, Song GW, Rong ZP, Wy YP (1985) Arterialized capillary blood gases and acid-base studies in normal individuals 29 days to 24 years of age. Am J Dis Child 139:1019–1022
58. Mansell A, Bryan AC, Levison H (1972) Airway closure in children. J Appl Physiol 33:711–714
59. Gaultier CL, Allaire Y, Pappo A, Girard F (1975) Etude du volume de fermeture chez l'enfant sain et atteint d'obstruction bronchique. In: Hatzfeld (ed) Distribution of pulmonary gas exchanges. Colloque INSERM 51, Paris pp 365–372
60. Escourrou PJL, Teisseire BP, Herigault RA, Vallez MO, Dupeyrat AJ, Gaultier CL (1988) Mechanism of improvement in pulmonary gas exchange during growth in awake piglets. J Appl Physiol 65:1055–1061
61. Burri PH (1986) Development and growth of the human lung. In: Fishman AP (ed), Handbook of Physiology, the respiratory system, circulation and nonrespiratory functions. Am Physiol Soc, Bethesda, sect 3, vol 1, chap 1:pp 1–45
62. Zeltner TB, Caduff JH, Gehr P, Pfenninger J, Burri PH (1987) The postnatal development and growth of the human lung. I. Morphometry. Respir Physiol 67:247–267

63. Koch G, Eriksson BO (1973) Effect of physical training on anatomical R.L shunt at rest and pulmonary diffusing capacity during near maximal exercise in boys 11–13 years old. Scand J Clin Lab Invest 31:95–103
64. Mok JY, McLaughlin FJ, Pintar M, Hak H, Amazo-Galvez R, Levison H (1986) Transcutaneous monitoring of oxygenation. What is normal? J Pediatr 118:365–371
65. Chipps BE, Mak H, Schuberth KC, Talamo JH, Menkes HA (1980) Nocturnal oxygen saturation in normal and asthmatic children. Pediatrics 65:1157–1160
66. Tabachnik E, Muller NL, Bryan AC, Levison H (1981) Changes in ventilation and chest wall mechanics during sleep in normal adolescents. J Appl Physiol 51:557–564
67. Gaultier CL (1985) Breathing and sleep during growth: physiology and pathology. Bull Eur Physiopathol respir 21:55–112
68. Garg M, Kurzner SI, Bautista DB, Keens TG (1988) Clinically unsuspected hypoxia during sleep and feeding in infants with bronchopulmonary dysplasia. Pediatrics 81:635–642
69. Muller NL, Francis PW, Gurwitz D, Levison H, Bryan AC (1980) Mechanism of hemoglobin desaturation during rapid-eye-movement sleep in normal subjects and in patients with cystic fibrosis. Am Rev Respir Dis 121:463–469

Controlled Ventilation: Targets, Hazards and Options

J.J. Marini

Introduction

Controlled mechanical ventilation (CMV) is intended to assure adequate gas exchange without incurring adverse effects related to ventilatory support. In recent years, numerous options for controlling ventilation have been proposed, most geared to the objectives of improving oxygenation and minimizing barotrauma. To choose rationally among these alternatives, it is crucial both to identify appropriate therapeutic endpoints for ventilatory support and to avoid iatrogenic misadventures. The purpose of this chapter is to examine the physiologic targets, hazards and options that characterize controlled ventilation of the critically ill patient.

Definition of Controlled Ventilation

By definition, controlling ventilation implies that all ventilatory support is provided mechanically and that the patient's efforts to breathe have been effectively silenced. Although any form of pressure assisted breathing (such as assist/control, synchronized mandatory ventilation, or pressure support) can be used to provide a major fraction of the power required to accomplish the breathing workload, the patient's effort during these cycles may be highly variable with substantially different physiological implications [1, 2]. Therefore, attention here will focus on only that setting in which airway pressure accounts for the entire inspiratory transpulmonary pressure gradient.

Why Control Ventilation?

The need to control ventilation may arise in the clinical setting for a variety of reasons. All can be classified as needs to manipulate the ventilatory pattern, to reduce agitation and the oxygen cost of breathing, to facilitate treatment or to prevent exaggerated excursions of the injured thorax. Perhaps the most common indication for CMV is to provide maximal support to a patient with such marginal cardiorespiratory reserve that the work of breathing compromises comfort, gas exchange, or cardiac function. In a variety of settings, combative patients often require such deep levels of sedation that ventilatory control is initiated, with or without fully intending to do so. Reducing the oxygen consumption rate of a patient with critical coronary ischemia, for example, may prove a life saving measure, especially in the setting of circulatory shock or acute pulmonary edema. As further example, it has been clearly shown that silencing ventilatory effort can improve arterial oxygenation in agitated patients with acute lung injury (ARDS) [3]. The precise explanation, however, remains in doubt and may well vary among different patients. Almost invariably, cardiac output (CO) falls as ventilatory control is established, in parallel with declining oxygen consumption ($\dot{V}O_2$). Because venous admixture tends to respond directionally in the same fashion as CO, one possibility is that the reduction in blood flow might reduce shunt fraction [4]. A second possibility is that the decline in $\dot{V}O_2$ might occur out of proportion to a decline in CO, thereby restoring appropriate balance between O_2 demand and O_2 delivery [5]. The resultant increase in mixed venous O_2 saturation could account, in part, for an improved arterial oxygen content and apparent improvement in oxygen exchange across the lung. Finally, most patients who experience improvement in gas exchange after instituting controlled ventilation exhibit vigorous use of the expiratory muscles prior to paralysis in an attempt to minimize inspiratory effort through "work sharing" (Fig. 1). Preventing such activity may allow positive end-expiratory pressure (PEEP) to recruit significant lung volume, especially from basilar regions. Whatever the explanation, controlling ventilation may have a positive impact on oxygen exchange.

Apart from it's influence on $\dot{V}O_2$ and it's value in preventing patient effort from interfering with intended patterns of conventional ventilation, establishing ventilatory control greatly facilitates the application of therapeutic but "non-physiological" breathing patterns. Such interventions as inverse ratio ventilation [6, 7], independent lung ventilation [8], low frequency positive pressure ventilation [9], continuous flow ventilation [10], and enforced CO_2 retention ("permissive hypercapnia") [11] require that patient's effort be prevented. Intentional hyperventilation may be the appropriate therapeutic strategy when reduction of cerebral blood volume and intracranial pressure are urgent priorities, as after closed head injury.

Although seldom suffficient reason in itself to undertake deep sedation or paralysis, controlling ventilation greatly facilitates the monitoring of respiratory system

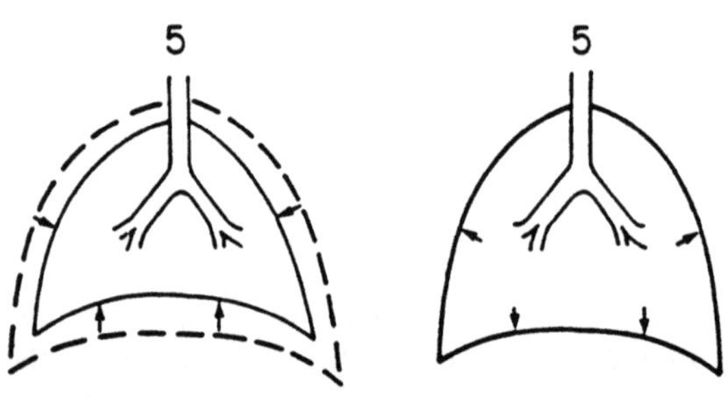

Fig. 1. Mechanism of "inspiratory work sharing". By forcing the chest to a volume below the equilibrium position appropriate to the applied level of end-expiratory pressure (5 cm H_2O), the mechanical advantage of the inspiratory muscles is improved. Furthermore, the potential energy stored in the chest wall during expiration *(left panel)* can be released to aid inflation *(right panel)*. (From [83] with permission)

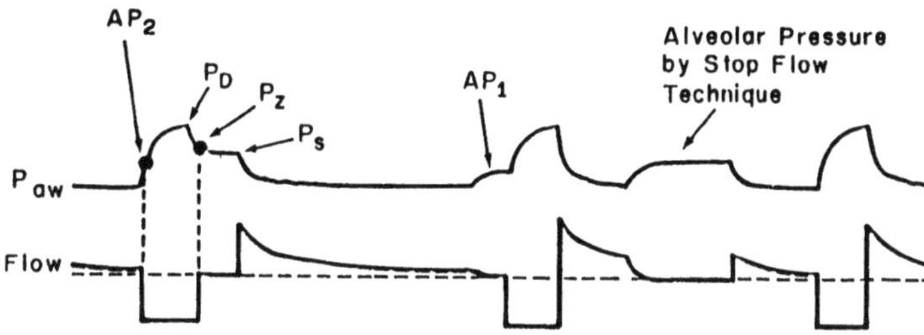

Fig. 2. Simultaneous tracings of airway pressure (Paw) and flow during controlled volume-cycled ventilation in a patient with airflow obstruction. P_D, P_Z and P_S represent the peak inflation pressure during dynamic conditions, the pressure at the point of flow cessation, and the pressure after complete equilibration among all alveolar compartments, respectively. With ventilation controlled, alveolar pressure can also be estimated by the stop flow technique applied in mid-expiration or at end-exhalation (auto-PEEP, AP_1). In addition, auto-PEEP can be estimated as the Paw needed to counterbalance elastic recoil and stop expiratory flow (AP_2)

mechanics (Fig. 2) [12, 13]. Indeed, airway pressure alone does not provide sufficient information to enable the clinician or investigator to assess directly any aspect of respiratory mechanics with precision or confidence, unless controlled conditions are assured. When passive conditions are achieved however, respiratory system impedance and its subcomponents (resistance, compliance, and auto-PEEP), as well as estimates of the mechanical work of spontaneous breathing (and the pressure time product) are readily measured or calculated [12, 13]. The same information can be obtained regarding the lungs when an esophageal balloon catheter is inserted, whether or not controlled ventilation has been established. However, the mechanical properties of the chest wall can only be evaluated under passive conditions.

Requirements for Establishing Ventilatory Control

External control of the breathing rhythm implies cessation of spontaneous breathing efforts. In a normal healthy individual the apneic threshold lies well below the waking CO_2 set point of 40 mm Hg [14, 15]. Typically, this value is approximately 30–32 mm Hg, but there is wide individual variation. These set points have not been well characterized for patients with critical illness, and in many cases are likely to be lower still [15]. Moreover, the apneic threshold might be expected to vary with the rapidly changing levels of metabolism and alertness that characterize this setting. Sedation, often supplemented by protracted skeletal muscle relaxation (paralysis), is almost routinely required for the conscious patient.

Muscle relaxants must be used with careful regard for their important potential for producing psychological as well as physical harm [16]. Muscle relaxants must not be used in the conscious, or lightly sedated patient. Therefore, concomitant and continuous suppression of consciousness with infused midazolam or lorazepam is the standard of practice in most North American intensive care units. Although short term suppression of neuromuscular tone has few if any obvious detrimental

Table 1. Detrimental effects of paralysis

- Accelerated wasting of skeletal muscle
- Electrolyte imbalance/H_2O retention
- Reduced tissue turgor and vascular tone
- Sustained paralytic syndrome
- Dependent infiltration and atelectasis
- Cardiovascular effects
- Obstipation

effects upon their withdrawal, it is clear that protracted therapeutic paralysis is accompanied by undesirable sequelae (Table 1).

Accelerated wasting of skeletal muscle protein, electrolyte depletion, water retention, deterioration of tissue turgor and diminished vascular tone are to be anticipated when paralysis is maintained for longer than three days [17]. It may be important to insure that some neural traffic to the muscle, however diminished, continue during the period over which muscle relaxants are employed. To achieve this end, many practitioners use a percutaneous nerve stimulator to guide the infusion rate of the blocking agent. Others prefer to use boluses of neuromuscular blockers, administered only as needed to suppress signs of arousal. With either technique, total "cutoff" of the muscle from neural stimulation should be prevented. In my view, paralytics should not be initiated at a continuous and unchanging rate without frequently reassessing their impact on the target tissue. Relaxants should be withdrawn when no longer necessary to maintain ventilatory control.

Choice of the agents used in sedation and paralysis should be individualized. For example, it is generally understood that morphine has unparalleled anxiolytic, analgesic, and ventilatory drive suppressing properties. Its venodilating properties, while highly desirable in certain settings (e.g. cardiogenic pulmonary edema), may prove detrimental in others where a high level of vascular tone is needed to preserve venous return. The benzodiazepines generally have less vascular and gut immobilizing effects, but vary in their duration of action. It is not uncommon for sedation to persist for days after attempted reversal. Practitioners should also be aware that protracted paralysis has been noted to occur after use of continuous therapeutic paralysis [18–20]. Many of these reports concern the treatment of patients with status asthma simultaneously given high doses of corticosteroids [18, 19]. Here, myonecrosis and release of muscle enzymes into the blood can be detected in an amazingly high percentage of patients given both types of medication. Although the precise mechanism and role of muscle relaxants is not currently known, this phenomenon does appear to be more frequent with the use of certain agents (e.g. pancuronium) than with others (e.g. atracurium). It is also worth noting that the paralytic agents vary in their metabolic and excretion pathways, as well as in the activity and cumulation rates of their metabolites [20]. Dosages of pancuronium and vecuronium, if not operationally adjusted as advocated above, should be given in doses that reflect the status of their primary route of excretion (renal and hepatic, respectively). Atracurium appears to be degraded primarily by tissue metabolism.

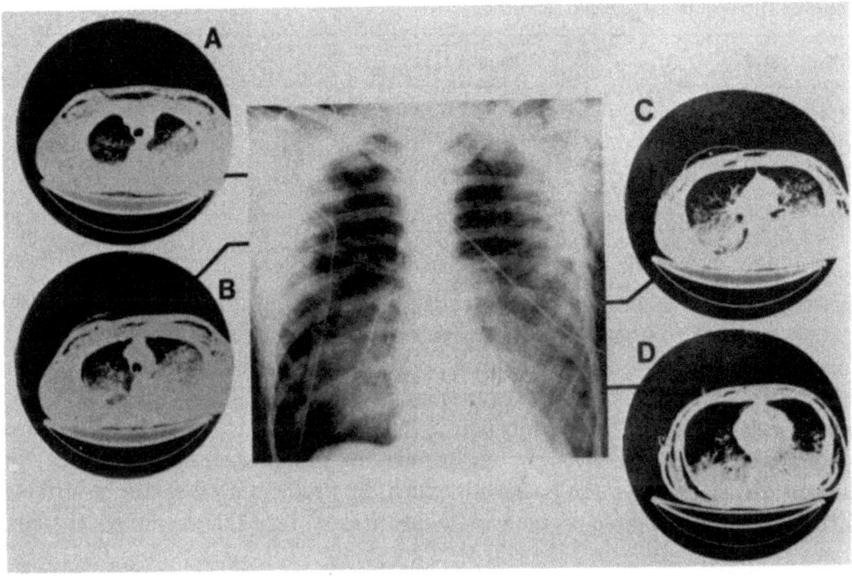

Fig. 3. Standard anteroposterior chest roentgenogram in a patient with ARDS and the corresponding tomographic (CT) images at the levels indicated (A through D). Note lack of homogeneity and tendency toward posterior involvement on the CT images, despite appearance of diffuse, symmetrical movement by the standard chest film. (From [23] with permission)

Perhaps the most predictable and potentially troublesome aspect of protracted suppression of spontaneous breathing for the patient with marginal gas exchange concerns the monotonous breathing pattern associated with CMV, usually in conjunction with impaired cough. As the studies of Gattinoni and others have clearly shown [9, 21–23], infiltrates are usually distributed in a gravity dependent fashion (Fig. 3). This gravitational dependence may help to explain the striking improvement in gas exchange that often accompanies a shift to the prone position [24]. Constancy of position encourages the accumulation of airway secretions in these same dependent regions. Dependent atelectasis and infiltration undoubtedly contribute to shunting in the patient receiving controlled ventilatory support. The lateral decubitus position is associated with a higher *average* FRC than the supine position [25]. Furthermore, the non-dependent lung assumes a resting volume higher than it has in the sitting position while draining secretions more effectively. For these reasons, special effort should be made to vary posture and to maintain the airways bronchodilated and clear of retained secretions.

Appropriate Therapeutic Targets

The therapeutic goals of the ventilatory process are to eliminate metabolic CO_2 at an appropriate rate and to assure adequate arterial oxygen tension. Because both objectives are linked inextricably to the requirement to apply potentially injurious

Table 2. Therapeutic targets

Conservative	(?) Adequate (?)
Hgb > 90% O_2 saturated	Hgb > 80% O_2 saturated
$PaCO_2 \approx 40$ mmHg	$PaCO_2 < 65$ mmHg
$pH_a \approx 7.40$	$pH_a > 7.25$
$FiO_2 < 0.65$	

airway pressure, it is essential to identify the minimum effective levels of PaO_2, $PaCO_2$ and pH compatible with satisfactory organ function. Surprisingly little information is available on these crucial points for normal healthy subjects. Considerably less is known about the tolerance limits of critically ill patients. The intensive care unit is populated by patients whose reserves, tolerance, and disease processes span a wide spectrum. Even among patients of similar age, medical history and current disease process, the pace with which the problem evolves can be strikingly different, allowing ample or, conversely, insufficient time for physiological adaptation.

Because the clinician applies potentially noxious therapy in seeking specific therapeutic results, it seems prudent to question the therapeutic endpoints which drive our current ventilatory strategy (Table 2). Apart from relieving the work of breathing, the clinician focuses on achieving acceptable gas exchange with the lowest levels of applied pressure and inspired oxygen that accomplish this therapeutic objective. Two major questions immediately arise: What is adequate gas exchange? and, What are dangerous levels of applied pressure?

Adequate PaO_2, $PaCO_2$ and pH

Oxygen tension. The oxygen concentrations and pressures applied to the patient with a crisis of oxygenation are both potentially injurious. It appears likely (although unproven) that an inspired oxygen fraction >0.65, if given long enough, will eventually harm the aerated lung parenchyma. It is worth considering that many patients with ARDS have half or more of all lung units collapsed, flooded, or infiltrated, and therefore may in some sense be shielded from long-term O_2 toxicity in those diseased lung units. Normal values for PaO_2 in a healthy patient living at sea level generally fall within a narrow, well defined range. Although PaO_2 declines somewhat with advancing age [26], arterial hemoglobin remains almost entirely saturated with oxygen throughout life. At a normal pH, blood O_2 saturation and content remain nearly normal until PO_2 falls lower than ≈ 60 mm Hg. Several important physiological responses are evoked primarily or exclusively when this saturation threshold has been crossed. These include hypoxic ventilatory response, pulmonary arterial vasoconstriction, and erythropoietin release [27]. Although the physiological significance of desaturation cannot be denied, it is apparent that brief episodes of modest desaturation evoke little in the way of vital organ dysfunction and produce no lasting effect, provided that O_2 delivery can be maintained by a compensatory cardiovascular response. In an otherwise healthy individual with good cardiovascular reserves, overt cerebral dysfunction requires arterial oxygen saturation to fall below 40 mm Hg, and consciousness is lost at levels lower than 30 mm Hg (without ischemia, permanent cerebral damage is unlikely if PO_2 exceeds 20 mm Hg).

People visiting Pike's Peak (Colorado, USA) by automobile ascend rapidly to an altitude of 4300 meters (inspired $PO_2 \approx 91$ torr; normal ≈ 159 torr), many without noticing the slightest symptom (in others, hypoxemia stimulates the drive to breathe sufficiently to produce acute symptomatic respiratory alkalosis). Given a few days to accommodate to the hypoxemia-altitude acclimatization-vigorous work can be accomplished [28]. Indeed, Mount Everest (elevation 8848 meters, inspired $PO_2 \approx 43$ torr) has been scaled without the benefit of supplemental oxygen. The extent to which certain critically ill patients can be made to slowly "acclimatize" to hypoxemia in similar fashion remains an important but unresolved question. Therefore, although something close to full O_2 saturation seems an appropriate clinical objective for a patient with multisystems organ failure [29], it is not entirely clear that high ventilating pressures or toxic O_2 concentrations should be applied in pursuit of this goal to a patient with isolated lung failure, normal hemoglobin concentration, and a healthy heart.

Carbon dioxide. An even more compelling argument can be made in favor of abandoning the normal target for carbon dioxide tension (≈ 40 torr) when insistence on that value requires hazardous treatment. Although carbon dioxide is the major end-product of cellular metabolism, carbon dioxide itself is remarkably free of noxious effects. Most problems associated with CO_2 retention either do not apply to the patient receiving controlled ventilation, or are associated with concomitant plasmatic or cellular acidosis [30]. These latter effects, the great majority of which are produced by the rapid, unbuffered retention of CO_2, include cerebral congestion, central nervous system dysfunction, skeletal muscle weakness, bronchoconstriction, heightened adrenergic activity, and cardiovascular impairment. Because the cellular membrane is much more permeable to carbon dioxide than to $[HCO_3]^-$, disparities can develop between plasmatic and intracellular pH during periods of rapid build-up or elimination of CO_2. Conversely, paradoxical intracellular acidosis can result from overzealous administration of bicarbonate [31–34]. With care taken to allow adjustment of serum bicarbonate, almost all adverse effects of CO_2 can be eliminated by maintaining pH normal and allowing CO_2 retention or elimination to occur slowly.

When CO_2 cumulates slowly enough to allow $[HCO_3]^-$ concentrations to keep pace, few important physiological effects ensue. Although sensitivity of the respiratory drive center to changes in ventilation is blunted by the compensatory elevation in tissue $[HCO_3]^-$ concentration, any acidosis that does result tends to be well buffered [31]. Furthermore, such considerations have little import for the patient receiving controlled ventilation. For the spontaneously breathing patient with a chronically elevated breathing workload, deliberately resetting the "homeostatic set point" for CO_2 appears to be an appropriate strategy without detectable adverse sequelae. With healthy kidneys, renal retention of bicarbonate sufficient to keep pH within normal limits is the rule until the $PaCO_2$ exceeds 65 mm Hg [35] (beyond that concentration of plasmatic CO_2, steps are usually required to expand the buffer base with exogenously administered alkali). Thus, there is some reason to believe that the patient with seriously disordered and compromised lung function might naturally seek or tolerate a higher $PaCO_2$ than that set for him by the well meaning clinician.

Permissive hypercapnia or enforced CO_2 retention (ECR) with compensatory buffering presents an attractive therapeutic strategy. Because fewer breaths and less ventilatory effort are required to maintain hypercapnia, allowing carbon dioxide retention decreases in the work of breathing. Therefore, ECR can be intentionally employed in the management of patients who would otherwise require noxious levels of pressure to achieve sufficient ventilation to maintain $PaCO_2$ concentrations in the normal range. In one of the most intriguing clinical studies of status asthma yet published, Darioli and Perret [11] demonstrated the feasibility of this approach in critically ill ventilated asthmatics, all of whom survived without injury. Such encouraging results suggest that in this reversible condition, the standard therapeutic paradigm itself may present the greatest threat to full recovery.

The need to keep $PaCO_2$ targeted at the normal level must also be questioned in forms of lung disease not usually characterized by CO_2 retention [36]. The therapeutic approach to ARDS has been under intense scrutiny in recent years, with interest piqued by the observations that high transpulmonary pressures may disrupt the delicate alveolar-capillary membranes of normal experimental animals [37, 38] (see below). Strikingly improved survival has been reported when care is taken to prevent exposure to high pressure, either by using extrapulmonary methods of CO_2 removal or by following a strategy of permissive hypercapnia [11, 39–41]. Thus, many European centers, following the lead of the Milan group, have reported similar experience, salvaging 40–50% of patients treated with low pressure mechanical ventilation made possible by extracorporeal CO_2 removal ($ECCO_2R$) (see chapter by Gattinoni in this volume). Interestingly, a study now underway in North America [40] seems to be demonstrating equally encouraging results *without* $ECCO_2R$, provided that ventilatory cycling pressures are held in check.

Very recently, Hickling et al. [41] reported their experience with permissive hypercapnia in patients with ARDS indicating survival rates much higher than expected on the basis of other published experience. All such observations seem internally consistent with the idea that the pathology of ARDS is heterogeneous, and that lung tissue capable of effectively participating in gas exchange is reasonably normal in it's mechanical behavior. Such tissue should not, therefore, be subjected to pressures much beyond those encountered during health. Adherence to this principle often requires that $PaCO_2$ be allowed to rise, buffering CO_2 accumulation, when necessary, to avert significant acidemia. The buffer base can be replenished with bicarbonate, acetate, or synthetic agents, such as tromethamine (Tris buffer) [42].

Hydrogen ion concentration and pH. Whether directly monitored or indirectly indexed by pH, hydrogen ion concentration is closely followed during critical illness. Yet, within rather broad limits, pH is probably more significant as a marker of the underlying disease process than for its inherent physiological actions. Diabetic ketoacidosis, for example, may produce very low pH values without notable cardiovascular problems, once circulating volume has been adequately restored and adrenergic reflexes are intact [43]. That is not to say that severe acidosis is well tolerated by all patients; even mild acidosis (7.20>pH>7.40) accentuates the drive to breathe, alters the O_2 binding affinity of hemoglobin, and acts synergistically with alveolar and mixed venous hypoxia to cause pulmonary vasoconstriction [44] (the strength of this effect in humans is still debated, however [42, 44]). The importance of these effects must be assessed carefully for the specific patient under consideration. Mild acidemia may be well tolerated by the great majority of patients, only to prove problematic for the patient with cor pulmonale. Conversely, even through pH values lower than 7.20 appear to impair normal cardiovacular function, there is considerable uncertainty and scientific debate on this point as well. Intact adrenergic tone may mask all cardiodepressant effects of falling pH until acidosis is extreme.

In my view, insistence on preserving pH at or above 7.40 has no firm basis, either in experimental observation or in clinical practice. When pH falls slowly, quite low levels may be well tolerated. On the other hand, the pressure cost of maintaining a normal pH may be unacceptably high. A patient with severe airflow obstruction, or one being supported with inverse ratio ventilation, may experience greatly accentuated air trapping with comparatively minor increases in the minute ventilation (VE) requirement. As predicted by the Henderson Hasselbach equation:

$$pH = 6.1 + \log\left(\frac{[HCO_3]^-}{0.03\,PaCO_2}\right)$$

a rather minor change in the pH set point may be accompanied by surprising increases or reductions in the VE requirement. Willingness to allow pH to fall to a lower range may allow for markedly reduced and inherently safer pressure, without a serious trade-off.

What are the Consequences of Airway Pressurization?

Consequences of High Pressure

Apart from selecting appropriate therapeutic targets, the clinician undertaking controlled ventilatory support must also be aware of the consequences of pressure application. Neonatologists have long been careful to avoid excessive pressure, noting that infant survival often hinged on their ability to prevent barotrauma [45]. Until recently, comparatively little attention was paid to pressure injury in adults, since clinicians lacked evidence that the alveolar tissues of adult patients are susceptible to the same types of injury encountered by their younger counterparts. Although the frequency of certain types of barotrauma undoubtedly differs with age, it is now recognized that the spectrum of injury is virtually identical.

Over the past decade, interstitial emphysema [46], tension cyst formation [47], and systemic gas embolism [48] have been clearly demonstrated in patients with

ARDS; problems unreported and unsuspected only a short time ago. Moreover, dilatory and destructive changes in the small airways and bronchi that are reminiscent of bronchopulmonary dysplasia can be identified on pathological specimens of adult lungs ventilated for long periods by high pressure [49, 50].

Perhaps the most important observation related to our newer understanding of barotrauma is that pressure-related lung injury is not necessarily a consequence of tissue rupture. As already noted, the disease process in patients with acute lung injury is not as diffusely distributed as once believed. The aerated portions that participate in gas exchange constitute approximately one third of the total volume occupied by these wet partially collapsed and cell-infiltrated lungs [51]. Overall lung and chest wall volumes are approximately normal. The striking gravitational distribution of radiographic infiltrates are consistent with the heterogeneous ventilation/perfusion distributions documented by inert gas analysis [52]. The sum of available information suggests, therefore, that in ARDS we are dealing with an aerable, functioning lung that is not so much stiff as it is undersized [53].

Given the high deadspace fraction and CO_2 production of ARDS, insistence on maintaining normal VT may force this residual lung to sustain repeated exposure to high pressure and to wide tidal excursions of *alveolar* volume. In a normal subject, exposure to a *transmural* pressure of 35 cm H_2O will achieve the alveolar size associated with total lung capacity. It may not be surprising, therefore, that transmural alveolar pressures greater than 35–50 cm H_2O predictably injure normal (let alone fragile) alveolar membranes, rendering them permeable to water and protein [37, 38]. Furthermore, wide tidal excursions themselves overventilate the patent units of the lung, a process which may cause regional alkalosis, deplete surfactant, produce damaging shear stress, or otherwise accentuate tissue injury. According to current understanding, therefore, high tidal pressures and wide tidal excursions are to be avoided (Fig. 4) [54].

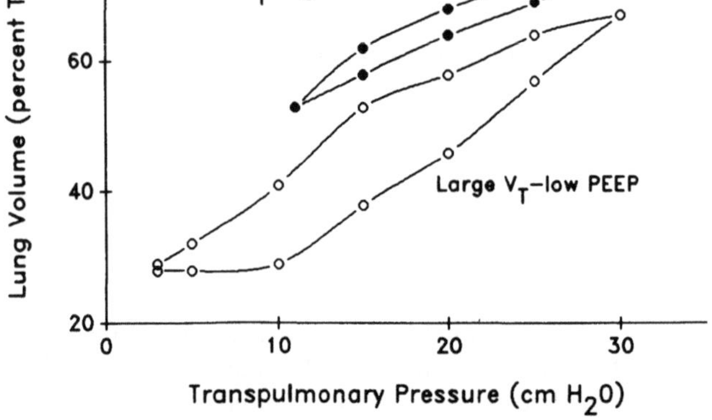

Fig. 4. Lung volume as a function of transpulmonary pressure for two patterns of ventilation in dogs with acute lung injury. Both patterns maintained peak airway pressure <30 cm H_2O. However, the large VT-low PEEP group experienced worse gas exchange and edema. (From [54] with permission)

Consequences of Low Pressure

Recognizing that excessive pressures must be avoided, there is equally convincing data that in certain settings (typified by acute lung injury) tidal *alveolar* pressures must not be allowed to fall too far. A certain minimal pressure, typically in the range of 7–12 cm H_2O, seems to be required in acute lung injury in order to prevent end-expiratory collapse of edematous lung tissue [55, 56] (computed tomographic scans indicate that pressure-mediated recruitment may be most extensive in the heavily infiltrated, dependent areas exposed to the greatest compressive forces). Early in the course of ARDS, failure to provide an adequate level of end-expiratory alveolar pressure (Pex) is often manifest by low compliance and a static pressure-volume curve, hysteresis, and distinct points of inflection [54–56]. These features are made indistinct or entirely obliterated by the addition of sufficient Pex. Over time, the process of tidal recruitment and collapse may cause additional lung injury or permanent de-recruitment, thereby creating an even smaller (and apparently stiffer) lung [56, 57]. Raising Pex can be accomplished either by the application of PEEP, or by encouraging the development of dynamic hyperinflation and "auto-PEEP" (Fig. 5) [6]. Thus,

$$\text{Pex} = \text{PEEP} + \text{Auto-PEEP}$$

These arguments do not apply to the patient mechanically ventilated for severe airflow obstruction. Although the addition of PEEP or CPAP can often help the spontaneously breathing or machine assisted patient cope with the work of breathing [58, 59], there currently is no compelling evidence that the addition of PEEP has any other therapeutic benefit for such patients. Hyperinflation is almost always accentuated when PEEP is added, particularly when PEEP exceeds the original level of auto-PEEP [58, 60]. Although some have suggested that this hyperinflation could have therapeutic benefit, others believe (with good justification) that any additional hyperinflation is likely to be hazardous [58] and poorly tolerated hemody-

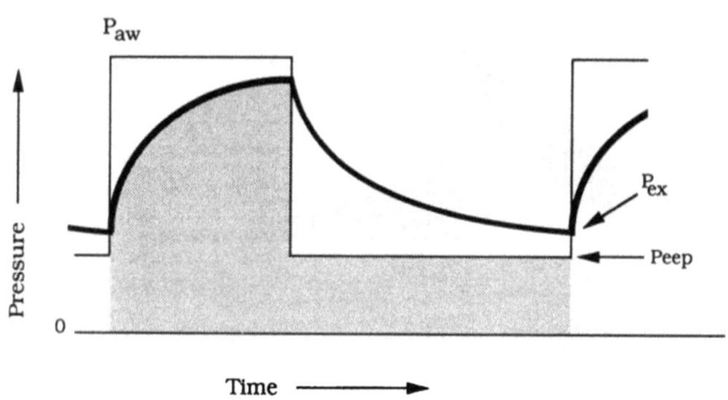

Fig. 5. Airway pressure *(fine line)* and alveolar pressure *(heavy line)* during pressure controlled ventilation, with airtrapping. End-expiratory alveolar pressure (Pex) is the sum of PEEP (the central airway pressure at end-exhalation) and auto-PEEP

namically by the heavily sedated or paralyzed patient receiving controlled ventilation.

Importance of Mean Airway Pressure to Ventilator Adjustment

The preceding discussion has argued that tidal alveolar pressures should neither be driven too high (at end-inspiration), nor in certain settings - exemplified by ARDS - should tidal alveolar pressure dip too low (at end-expiration). Can the objectives of controlled ventilation be achieved within the confines of these guidelines, and if so, how is this accomplished? Formulating the answers to these questions requires careful definition of the appropriate objectives for ventilation (adequate gas exchange, tolerable adverse effects) as well as a clear understanding of the fundamental importance of mean airway pressure to the desired and undesired effects of mechanical ventilation.

Relationship of Mean Airway to Mean Alveolar Pressure

Although the terms "mean *airway* pressure" and "mean *alveolar* pressure" are used almost interchangeably in the medical literature, these terms are not synonymous. More importantly, few clinicians fully understand the exact basis for the relationship between them. At any instant, the pressure applied across the passive respiratory system (equal to pressure at the airway opening) must be entirely accounted for by its conserved (elastic) and dissipated (non-elastic) components (Fig. 6) [61, 62]. During exhalation, alveolar pressure conserved during inflation drives expiratory flow, so that the tidal component of elastic pressure must dissipate before exhalation stops. Using elementary calculus, it can be shown that equivalence between mean airway and mean alveolar pressures depends upon equivalent frictional

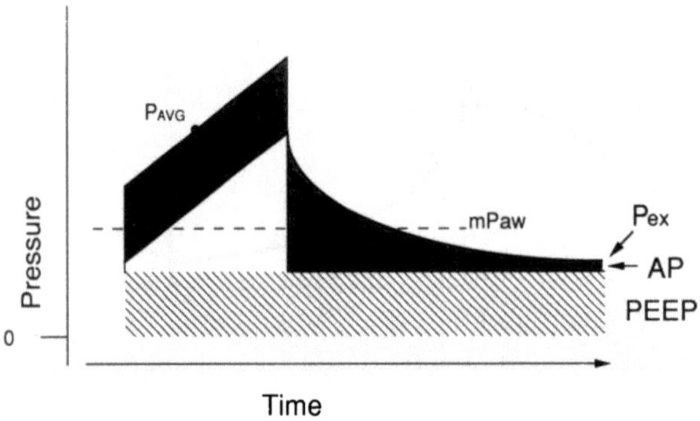

Fig. 6. Hypothetical pressure profile for airway pressure *(fine line)* and alveolar pressure *(heavy line)* during controlled ventilation with constant inspiratory flow. The pressure gradients driving flow (frictional pressures) are shaded. Pavg is the average inspiratory inflation pressure, and mPaw is mean airway pressure over the entire cycle. mPaw = Pavg (Ti/Ttot) + PEEP (Te/Ttot)

("resistive") pressure losses during the inspiratory and expiratory periods. The relevant expression is:

$$mPalv = mPaw + \frac{VE(Rx - Ri)}{60}$$

where mPalv and mPaw are mean alveolar and mean airway pressures, VE is minute ventilation (l/min), and Ri and Rx are volume-averaged values for inspiratory and expiratory "resistance" (the quotient of driving pressure to flow) [62]. Since Rx normally exceeds Ri by a small amount, mean airway pressure tends to provide a good first approximation of mPalv [63]. Equivalence between these two mean pressures is *not* preserved, however, in the setting of severe airflow obstruction, where Rx may be severalfold higher than Ri [58, 64]. As the above equation predicts, such differences are exacerbated by increases in the delivered minute ventilation.

Physiological Significance of Mean Airway Pressure

The concept of mean airway pressure (mPaw), or more precisely, mean alveolar pressure, is central to understanding the benefits and hazards of CMV. mPalv is linked to five key outcomes of ventilatory support:

1. Total ventilation
2. Arterial oxygenation
3. Hemodynamic compromise
4. Fluid retention
5. Barotrauma (?)

In a sense, mPaw can be considered associated with two beneficial actions (ventilation, oxygenation), and three potentially noxious ones (hemodynamic compromise, fluid retention, and barotrauma).

Ventilation, by definition a dynamic process, is driven by pressure differences

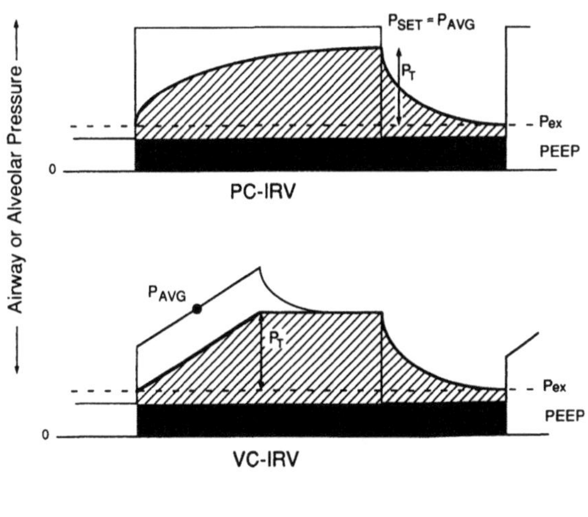

Fig. 7. Airway pressure profile *(outer envelope)* and alveolar pressure profile *(crosshatched and shaded)* during inflation with constant pressure (PC-IRV) and constant flow (VC-IRV). Peak alveolar pressure is the sum of tidal elastic pressure (PT) and Pex

developed between the airway opening and the alveolus. Expansion and contraction of the respiratory system requires power provided by the ventilatory pressures. The average pressure required to inflate the respiratory system during a single tidal cycle (Pavg) can be expressed in terms of a modified "equation of motion" (Fig.7):

$$\text{Pavg} = \text{Ri}\left(\frac{\text{Vt}}{\text{ti}}\right) + \frac{\text{Vavg}}{\text{C}} + \text{Pex}$$

where Ri is inspiratory resistance; ti is inspiratory flow duration; Vavg is average volume above FRC, respectively. Here, the first term is the flow resistive pressure, the second is the average inspiratory *tidal* elastic pressure, and Pex is the *static* elastic pressure, the sum of PEEP and auto-PEEP. When rewritten in terms of VE the expression becomes:

$$\text{Pavg} = \text{Rx}\left(\frac{\text{VE}}{60\text{D}}\right) + \frac{\text{Vavg}}{\text{C}} + \frac{\text{VE}}{\text{C}\left(e^{60(1-\text{D})/\text{fRxC}}\right)}$$

where D is inspiratory duty cycle, Ti/Ttot; Rx is expiratory resistance; f is frequency, respectively. This equation emphasizes that mean airway pressure (mPaw = Pavg × D) is an approximately linear function of ventilation ... and *vice versa*.

mPalv closely indexed by mPaw, relates directly to mean alveolar volume, and therefore to oxygen exchange across the lung. In keeping with this idea, several experimental and clinical studies of acute lung injury have demonstrated an approximately linear correspondence between mPaw and indices of pulmonary O_2 exchange, once some critical value of end-expiratory or mPalv is exceeded [65–67]. The application of PEEP and the use of inverse ratio ventilation may enhance arterial oxygenation largely through their associated increases of average lung volume and mPalv.

The place of mPalv in the generation of barotrauma is less clear. Although mPaw correlates reasonably well with the incidence of rupture forms of pressure injury, it is not certain that mPalv itself (separated from concomitant increases of peak alveolar pressure) poses an independent risk, at least, not at the pressure levels commonly employed in critical care [68]. My own view is that peak alveolar pressure, an indicator of the maximal stretching forces applied to distensible alveoli, is much more important in *causing* the injury. Once rupture has occurred, however, a high level of mean alveolar pressure may be instrumental in *exacerbating* the damage or *accentuating* gas leakage through rents in the alveolar tissues, i.e. in bringing barotrauma to clinical attention.

Whatever the uncertainty related to mPaw and barotrauma, it seems quite apparent that mPaw is a close and easily measurable correlate of adverse hemodynamic sequelae [69]. Raising mPalv during passive ventilation increases both lung and chest volume by similar amounts. Lung expansion tends to increase right ventricular afterload – which already poses a life-threatening problem for many patients with ARF. More importantly, the increase of intrapleural pressure acts to raise right atrial pressure, thereby impeding venous return [70]. Rising backpressure is made even more significant by the impaired systemic venous tone and tissue turgor consequent to sedation/paralysis (discussed above).

Fluid retention during MV is not always a manifestation of a failing heart. Indeed, sodium and water retention was one of the first complications recognized in the modern era of ventilator management [71]. Dysfunction of this type seems to correlate with the magnitude of average airway (and therefore alveolar and intrapleural) pressure, and can be reliably elicited by using PEEP [72]. The mechanism remains uncertain, but could involve reflex mediated corticomedullary shunting, globally reduced renal perfusion, or interference with the humoral control of renal-fluid adjustment [73].

A Strategy for Implementing Controlled Ventilation

As the foregoing discussion has emphasized, airway pressure is a "two edged sword", crucial to achieving the objectives of ventilation, but dangerous when applied to excess. In formulating a rational strategy for implementing *controlled* ventilation that is based on current data, one overarching principle serves to guide setting selection:

"The clinician should apply only those pressure levels absolutely required to meet unequivocally important clinical objectives."

Consistent with this principle, VE requirement should be minimized by treating fever, sepsis, metabolic acidosis, and agitation while avoiding excessive calorie administration or carbohydrate loading. Full recruitment of lung volume should be assured by attention to fluid status, position changes, secretion clearance, and application of sufficient end-expiratory pressure to maximize compliance. For patients with acute lung injury, a minimum of 7 cm H_2O is usually required; for patients with acute airflow obstruction, no added PEEP may be needed or desirable during controlled ventilation. PEEP should not be added beyond levels which cause compliance to deteriorate or maximal transpulmonary pressure to exceed safe limits. This upper target level for *transpulmonary* pressure should approximate 35 cm H_2O, a value that corresponds to a maximal static airway pressure ("plateau pressure") of 40–50 cm H_2O, depending on the stiffness or flexibility of the chest wall. With these requirements satisfied, mPalv should be raised just enough to assure adequate O_2 exchange across the lung at safe concentrations of inspired oxygen. In making this judgement, I rely on standard methods for assessing vital organ function (e.g. urine flow), supplemented by such metabolic indicators as the serum anion gap and the arterial lactate concentration.

For patients with single organ (lung) failure – whether acute lung injury, asthma or decompensated COPD – my threshold for increasing ventilator pressures to support gas exchange is considerably higher than for those with cardiac dysfunction, shock, or multisystem organ failure (in the latter cases, adequate reserves and compensatory mechanism that ensure adequate oxygen extraction cannot be assumed intact). Rather arbitrarily, I permit pH to remain as low as 7.25, provided that acidemia is clearly produced by my deliberate attempt to reduce applied pressure, that pH falls gradually and thereafter remains stable, and that acidemia is not accompanied by worsened pulmonary hypertension or vital organ compromise. Bicarbonate infusion is a rational adjunct to this strategy when the salt and water load can be easily dealt with. Dialysis or hemofiltration may be required when they cannot.

It is generally recognized that a $PaCO_2$ of 40 mm Hg should not be the goal for an acutely ill patient with airflow obstruction or neuromuscular weakness who normally maintains hypercapnia. Indeed, a $PaCO_2$ level somewhat higher than normal may be more compatible with successful machine withdrawal later on. It should also be recognized that a normal $PaCO_2$ is not necessarily an appropriate target value to set for patients with acute lung injury (ARDS), who have small volume, seriously compromised lungs. With this in mind, my personal strategy for the most critically ill patients with high pressure requirements (whatever the etiology) is to deliberately raise $PaCO_2$ by gradual "hypoventilation", allowing $PaCO_2$ to climb by approximately 5 mm Hg each day that clear signs of improved radiographic, clinical, and oxygen exchange status are not observed.

Options for Controlled Ventilation – Mode and Machine Settings

Within the general framework of the strategy just developed, the clinician must choose the mode of machine cycling (the inspiratory "offswitch"), the VT and cycling frequency, the inspiratory flow waveform, the end-inflation pause length, and the duration of the inspiratory duty cycle.

Tidal Volume and Cycling Frequency

The selected VT should not be so small as to markedly increase the deadspace fraction, nor so large that the end-inspiratory alveolar pressure exceeds safe limits. The traditional guideline of 10–15 ml/kg of lean body weight is often too high for patients with severe lung injury or profound air trapping; a selection of 6–8 ml/kg is often more feasible. In my practice, I use VT of up to 10 ml/kg, so long as peak static airway pressure (plateau pressure) does not exceed 40–50 cm H_2O, depending on estimated chest wall stiffness. Under passive conditions, chest wall compliance can be crudely approximated as the quotient of VT and the inspiratory swing of central venous pressure (CVP), expressed in cm H_2O. CVP fluctuations tend to parallel those occurring in the pleural space. In similar fashion, the tidal swing in transalveolar pressure is estimated by subtracting the respiratory CVP fluctuation from the peak static airway pressure. With VT selected, frequency is adjusted to keep $PaCO_2$ at the desired level (dictated by pH and the need to keep peak and mean cycling pressures within acceptable bounds).

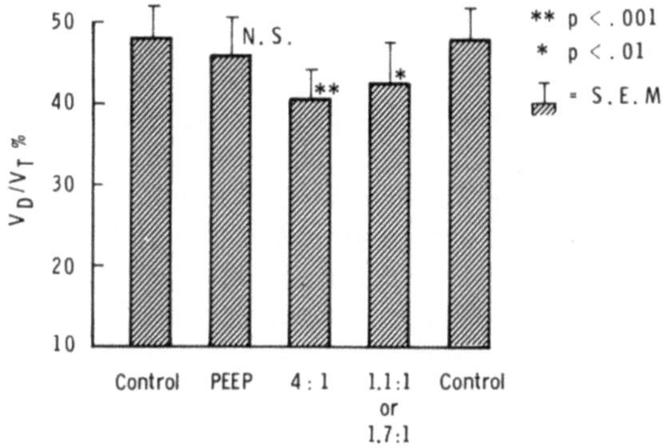

Fig. 8. Dead space fraction (VD/VT%) in patients with acute lung injury treated without PEEP (control), with PEEP, and with inverse ratio ventilation (4:1, 1:1, or 1.7:1). (From [75] with permission)

Flow Magnitude and Waveform

In the setting of severe airflow obstruction, where the principal problem is achieving alveolar ventilation, rapid inspiratory flows (60–100 l/min) permit sufficient time for exhalation to minimize dynamic hyperinflation, thereby improving gas exchange [74]. Using a decelerating flow profile may or may not improve the ventilation homogeneity achieved by a constant flow profile of similar duration. Rational choices for mean flow rate and waveform may be somewhat different in the setting of ARDS. It is generally true that the shape of the inspiratory flow waveform has little impact on oxygen exchange, once mean airway pressure and duty cycle length are taken into account. For such patients, there now seems to be good evidence, however, that slowing end-inspiratory flow improves the distribution of ventilation and reduces the deadspace fraction, enhancing the efficiency of ventilation [75, 76] (Fig. 8). End-inspiratory flow deceleration can be achieved with constant pressure ventilation, or by adding a brief end-inspiratory pause to a constant flow, volume cycled pattern [76]. Many ventilators now offer linearly decelerating flow profiles as an option for volume cycled ventilation as well.

Duty Cycle and Extended (Inverse) Ratio Ventilation

Inverse ratio ventilation (IRV), a form of ventilatory support introduced more than twenty years ago to the care of neonates with the infant respiratory distress syndrome [7], has been the recent subject of great interest and controversy among clinicians treating ARDS [6, 75, 77–79]. In this form of treatment, the duty cycle is prolonged to a much greater extent than the traditional 0.20 to 0.33 guideline would allow. Mean inspiratory flow rate (the quotient of tidal volume and inspiratory time) is much lower than conventionally prescribed. IRV has been used with duty cycles ranging from 0.5 (the lower limit consistent with its definition) to 0.8, often with dramatic effect.

Extending the duty cycle appears to improve oxygenation primarily by increasing the mean airway pressure [78, 80]. It has also been argued that prolonged traction with high pressure enables recruitment of lung units that would otherwise remain collapsed. Consistent with this notion, several investigators have noted improved chest compliance after the institution of IRV, as well as an apparent time dependence to this phenomenon [6, 79]. Ventilatory efficiency also tends to improve, as expected for a waveform that inherently decelerates flow and automatically provides an end-inspiratory pause. Although the comparative data are meager, it appears that IRV may be somewhat more effective than conventional ventilation using PEEP to provide an identical mean airway pressure [81].

Extending the duty cycle is a logical means of raising mean airway pressure once the lower and upper bounds of the tidal cycle have been adjusted to their safe limits. To raise end-expiratory pressure further causes peak alveolar pressure to encroach on the upper ceiling, forcing a reduction in VT. Lengthening the duty cycle usually achieves the desired mPaw without this potentially undesired effect. Thus, I consider *extending* the duty cycle to be a logical extension of the ventilatory strategy already outlined, at least for the patient with acute lung injury. In my practice, I only *invert* the ratio (beyond an I/E ratio of 1/1) when I need to further elevate the mean airway pressure, and then only to the extent necessary to achieve the desired result. Pressure controlled ventilation allows direct selection of the inspiratory time fraction (Fig. 9). During volume cycled ventilation (constant or linearly decelerating flow profile), the options for duty cycle extension include adding a pause, increasing the cycling frequency (thereby slowing the *relative* rate of inspiratory flow), or choosing a lower peak inspiratory flow setting (for an identical Ti/Ttot, the decelerating flow algorithm causes a greater increase in mPalv than does constant flow).

In my view, the published experience with IRV has fueled a controversy that distracts attention from the logic of the underlying strategy, obscuring the potential

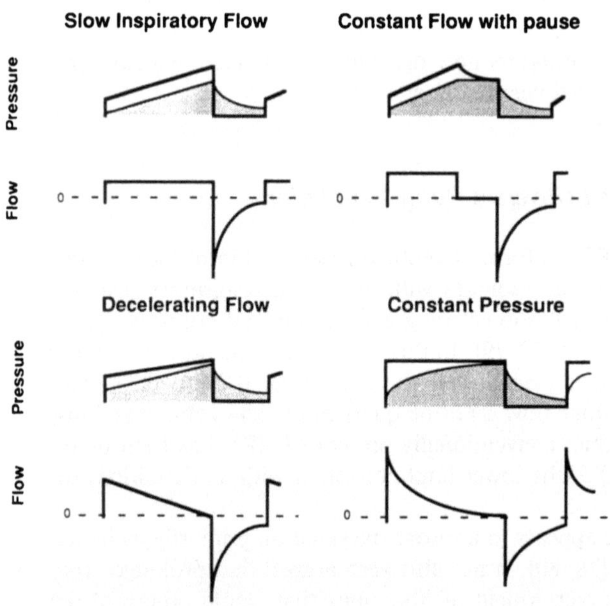

Fig. 9. Three flow controlled, volume cycled methods of delivering inverse ratio ventilation, compared with constant pressure IRV. Note the similarity of alveolar pressure waveforms (shaded)

value of the pressure monitored, extended ratio approach. Several of the most widely quoted papers advocate the use of VT that invariably result in peak alveolar pressures well in excess of those now considered prudent [6, 79]. As a result, both the published and anecdotal clinical experience with this technique have been beset with a discouraging incidence of barotrauma. With appropriate targets for $PaCO_2$, pH, PaO_2, and peak alveolar pressure, extended ratio ventilation forms an integral part of the ventilatory approach I now advocate.

Extending the duty cycle to the point of inverting the inspiratory/expiratory ratio would appear to be a hazardous and counterproductive intervention for the patient with severe airflow obstruction. Here, where unnecessary elevations of mean airway pressure often present serious clinical problems, ratio inversion would appear to have little rationale. Indeed, for these patients, it is now generally accepted practice to use relatively rapid inspiratory flow rates and short inspiratory time fractions to maximize the time available for exhalation [74].

Selection of "Controlled" Parameter during Controlled Ventilation

The equation of motion of the respiratory system indicates that the clinician has the option of controlling flow and VT or applied pressure and VT - but not all three at once. Traditionally, flow controlled, volume cycled modes have been selected, an option which guarantees VE but allows airway and alveolar pressures to rise when impedance deteriorates. With our newer understanding of pressure-related tissue injury, however, interest has refocused on the pressure controlled, time cycled modes of ventilation. Although this strategy effectively controls peak and mean airway pressures, the relationship between ventilation and the clinician set variables (frequency, applied pressure, and duty cycle) is neither intuitive nor straightforward (Fig. 10) [82]. For both flow controlled and pressure controlled strategies, therefore, close pressure and volume monitoring is essential.

Future Directions in Controlled Mechanical Ventilation

Valuable data gathered in recent years by numerous investigators from a variety of sources emphasize the need to limit pressure exposure in the ventilated lung. Certain adjuncts to pulmonary ventilation, such as intratracheal insufflation of fresh gas or intracaval gas exchange by hollow fiber catheter appear especially promising (see chapters elsewhere in this volume by Slutsky and Mortensen). Experimental and clinical evidence strongly suggest that a spectrum of innovative techniques ranging in invasiveness from extracororeal oxygenation and CO_2 removal to retargeting of the fundamental goals of MV themselves may allow controlled ventilation to achieve its full potential as a life support technique.

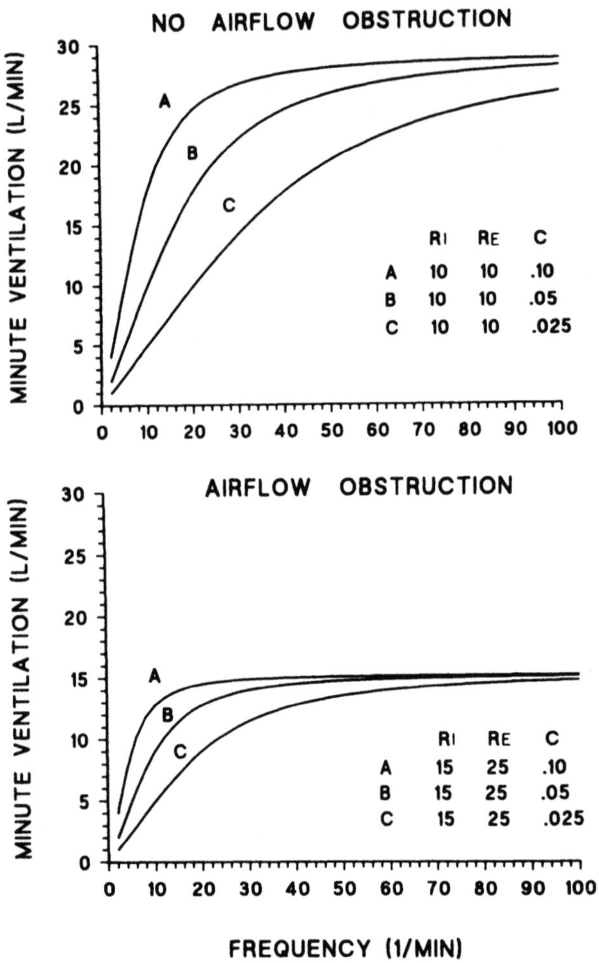

Fig. 10. *Top panel:* Minute ventilation ($\dot{V}E$) as a function of frequency for three values of respiratory system compliance, with RI = RE and no major degree of airflow obstruction (Pset = 20, D = 0.4). Whatever the compliance value, $\dot{V}E$ rises toward a final plateau determined only by inspiratory time fraction and resistance. However, compliance determines rate of rise of these curves, and over the clinically relevant frequency range exerts a profound influence on $\dot{V}E$. *Bottom panel:* During simulated airflow obstruction (moderately severe), the maximum $\dot{V}E$ achievable with the same Pset and D is sharply lower and closely approached at frequencies well within clinically observable range. C = compliance, RI = inspiratory resistance, RE = expiratory resistance, D = duty cycle (Ti/Ttot). (From [82] with permission)

References

1. Marini JJ, Rodriguez RM, Lamb VJ (1986) The inspiratory workload of patient-initiated mechanical ventilation. Am Rev Respir Dis 134:902–909
2. Marini JJ, Smith TC, Lamb VJ (1988) External work output and force generation during synchronized intermittent mechanical ventilation. Effect of machine assistance on breathing effort. Am Rev Respir Dis 138:1169–1179

3. Coggeshall JW, Marini JJ, Newman JH (1985) Improved oxygenation after muscle relaxation in the adult respiratory distress syndrome. Arch Intern Med 145:1718–1720
4. Lynch JP, Mhyre JG, Dantzker DR (1979) The influence of cardiac output on intrapulmonary shunt. J Appl Physiol 46:315–321
5. Schumacker PT, Cain SM (1987) The concept of critical oxygen delivery. Intensive Care Med 13:223–229
6. Gurevitch MJ, Van Dyke J, Young ES, Jackson K (1986) Improved oxygenation and lower peak airway pressure in severe adult respiratory distress syndrome: Treatment with inverse ratio ventilation. Chest 89:211–213
7. Reynolds EOR (1971) Effect of alterations in mechanical ventilator settings on pulmonary gas exchange in hyaline membrane disease. Arch Dis Child 46:152–159
8. Westenskow DR, Pace NL (1982) Differential lung ventilation. In: Prakash O (ed) Applied physiology in clinical respiratory care. Martinus Nijhoff Boston, pp 313–324
9. Gattinoni L, Pesenti A, Mascheroni D, et al (1986) Low frequency positive pressure ventilation with extracorporeal CO_2 removal in severe acute respiratory failure. JAMA 256(7):881–886
10. Slutsky AS (1988) Nonconventional modes of ventilation. Am Rev Resp Dis 138:175–183
11. Darioli R, Perret C (1984) Mechanical controlled hypoventilation in status asthmaticus. Am Rev Respir Dis 129:385–387
12. Truwit JD, Marini JJ (1988) Evaluation of thoracic mechanics in the ventilated patient. Part 1: Primary Measurements. J Crit Care 3(2):133–150
13. Truwit JD, Marini JJ (1988) Evaluation of thoracic mechanics in the ventilated patient. Part 2: Applied Mechanics. J Crit Care 3(3):199–213
14. Cunningham DJC, Robbins PA, Wolff CB (1986) Integration of respiratory responses to changes in alveolar partial pressures of CO_2 and O_2 and in arterial pH. In: Geiger SR (ed) Handbook of Physiology, Section 3: The Respiratory System. Vol. 2. American Physiology Society Bethesda, pp 475–528
15. Prechter GC, Nelson SB, Hubmayr RD (1990) The ventilatory threshold for carbon dioxide. Am Rev Respir Dis 141:758–764
16. Veselis RA (1988) Sedation and pain management for the critically ill. Critical Care Clinics 4:167–181
17. Greenleaf JE, Kozlowski S (1982) Physiological consequences of reduced physical activity during bedrest. Exerc Sport Sci Rev 10:84–119
18. Panacek EA, Sherman B (1988) Hydrocortisone and pancuronium bromide: Acute myopathy during status asthmaticus. Crit Care Med (letter) 16:732
19. Brun-Buisson C, Gherardi R (1988) Hydrocortisone and pancuronium bromide: Acute myopathy during status asthmaticus. Crit Care Med (letter) 16:731
20. Taylor P (1985) Neuromuscular blocking agents. In: Gilman AG, Goodman LS, Rall TW, Murad F (eds) The pharmacologic basis of therapeutics, 7th Edition. MacMillan New York, pp 222–235
21. Gattinoni L, Pesenti A (1987) ARDS: the non-homogeneous lung; facts and hypothesis. Crit Care Dig 6:1–4
22. Gattinoni L, Pesenti A, Avalli L, Rossi F, Bombino M (1987) Pressure-volume curve of total respiratory system in acute respiratory failure. Computed tomographic scan study. Am Rev Respir Dis 136:730–736
23. Maunder RJ, Shuman WP, McHugh JW, Marglin SI, Butler J (1986) Preservation of normal lung regions in the adult respiratory distress syndrome. Analysis by computed tomography. JAMA 255:2463–2465
24. Albert RK, Leasa D, Sanderson M, Robertson HT, Hlastala MP (1987) The prone position improves arterial oxygenation and reduces shunt in oleic acid-induced acute lung injury. Am Rev Respir Dis 135:628–633
25. Marini JJ, Tyler ML, Hudson LD, Davis BS, Huseby JS (1984) Influence of head-dependent positions on lung volume and oxygen saturation in chronic airflow obstruction. Am Rev Respir Dis 129:101–105
26. Raine JM, Bishop JM (1963) A-a difference in O_2 tension and physiological dead space in normal man. J Appl Physiol 18:284–288

27. Refsum HE (1963) Relationship between state of consciousness and arterial hypoxemia and hypercapnia in patients with pulmonary insufficiency breathing own. Clin Sci 25:361–367
28. Schoene RB, Horbein TF (1988) High altitude adaptation. In: Murray JF, Nadel JA (eds) Textbook of respiratory medicine. W. B. Saunders, Philadelphia, pp 196–220
29. Schumacker PT, Samsel RW (1990) Oxygen supply consumption in ARDS. Clin in Chest Med 11:715–722
30. Nunn JF (1977) Applied Respiratory Physiology, Second Edition. Butterworths Boston, pp 460–470
31. Narins RG (1985) Alkali therapy of metabolic acidosis due to organic acids: The case for the judicious use of sodium bicarbonate. AKF Nephrology Letter 2:13–22
32. Arieff AI, Leach W, Park R, Lazarowitz VC (1982) Systemic effects of $NaHCO_3$ in experimental lactic acidosis in dogs. Am J Physiol 242:F586–591
33. Weil MH, Trevino RP, Rackow EC (1985) Sodium bicarbonate during CPR. Does it help or hinder? Chest (letter) 88:487
34. Fraley DS, Adler S, Bruns FJ, Zett B (1980) Stimulation of lactate production by administration of bicarbonate in a patient with a solid neoplasm and lactic acidosis. N Engl J Med (letter) 303:1100
35. Kilburn KH, Dowell AR (1971) Renal function in respiratory failure. Arch Int Med 127:754–762
36. Pesenti A (1990) Target blood gases during ARDS ventilatory management. Intensive Care Med 16:349–351
37. Dreyfuss D, Basset G, Soler P, Saumon G (1985) Intermittent positive pressure hyperventilation with high inflation pressures produces pulmonary microvascular injury in rats. Am Rev Respir Dis 132:880–884
38. Kolobow T, Moretti MP, Fumagalli R, et al (1987) Severe impairment in lung function induced by high peak airway pressure during mechanical ventilation. Am Rev Respir Dis 135:312–315
39. Gattinoni L, Pesenti A, Mascheroni D, et al (1986) Low frequency positive pressure ventilation with extracorporeal CO_2 removal in severe acute respiratory failure. JAMA 256(7):881–886
40. Morris AH, Clemmer TP, Orme JF, Wallace CJ, Suchyta MR, Dean NC (1989) Clinical trial of extracorporeal CO_2 removal (abstract). Chest 96(2):1385
41. Hickling KG, Henderson SJ, Jackson R (1990) Low mortality associated with low volume pressure limited ventilation with permissive hypercapnia in severe adult respiratory distress syndrome. Intensive Care Med 16:372–377
42. Narins RG, Bastl CP, Rudnick MR, et al (1982) Acid-base metabolism. In: Golnick HC (ed) Current Nephrology. John Wiley, New York, pp 7–9
43. Mitchell JH, Wildenthal K, Johnson RL Jr (1972) The effects of acid base disturbances on cardiovascular and pulmonary function. Kidney International 1:375–389
44. Housley E, Clarke SW, Hedworth-Whitty RB, Bishop JW (1970) Effect of acute and chronic acidemia and associated hypoxemia on the pulmonary circulation of patients with chronic bronchitis. Cardiovasc Research 4:482–489
45. Reynolds EOR (1975) Management of hyaline membrane disease. Br Med Bull 31:18–24
46. Woodring JH (1985) Pulmonary interstitial emphysema in the adult respiratory distress syndrome. Crit Care Med 13(10):786–791
47. Albelda SM, Gefter WB, Kelley MA, et al (1983) Ventilator-induced subpleural air cysts: clinical, radiographic, and pathological significance. Am Rev Respir Dis 127:360–365
48. Marini JJ, Culver BH (1989) Systemic air embolism consequent to mechanical ventilation in ARDS. Ann Intern Med 110(9):699–703
49. Chung A, Golden J, Fligiel S, Hogg JC (1983) Bronchopulmonary dysplasia in the adult. Am Rev Respir Dis 127:117–120
50. Slavin G, Nunn JF, Crow J, Core C (1982) Bronchiolectasis – a complication of artificial ventilation. Brit Med J 285:931–934
51. Pesenti A, Pelosi P, Gattinoni L (1990) Lung mechanics in ARDS. In: Vincent JL (ed) Update in intensive care and emergency medicine, vol. 10. Springer, Berlin Heidelberg New York, pp 231–238

52. Dantzker DR, Brook CJ, Dehart P, Lynch JP, Weg JG (1979) Ventilation-perfusion distributions in the adult respiratory distress syndrome. Am Rev Respir Dis 120:1039–1052
53. Gattinoni L, Mascheroni D, Basilco E, Foti G, Pesenti A, Avalli L (1987) Volume/pressure curve of total respiratory system in paralyzed patients: artefacts and correction factors. Intensive Care Med 13:19–25
54. Corbridge TC, Wood LDH, Crawford GP, Chudoba MJ, Yanos J, Sznajder JI (1990) Adverse effects of large tidal volume and low PEEP in canine acid aspiration. Am Rev Respir Dis 142:311–315
55. Matamis D, Lemaire F, Harf A, et al (1984) Total respiratory pressure volume curves in the adult respiratory distress syndrome. Chest 86:58–66
56. Benito S, Lemaire F (1990) Pulmonary pressure-volume relationship in acute respiratory distress syndrome in adults: Role of positive end-expiratory pressure. J Crit Care 5:27–34
57. Koltan M, Cattran CB, Kent G (1982) Oxygenation during high frequency-ventilation in two models of lung injury. Anesth Analg 61:323–327
58. Smith TC, Marini JJ (1988) Impact of PEEP on lung mechanics and work of breathing in severe airflow obstruction. The effect of PEEP on Auto-PEEP. J Appl Physiol 65(4):1488–1499
59. Petrof BJ, Legare M, Goldberg P, Milic-Emili J, Gottfried SB (1990) Continuous positive airway pressure reduces work of breathing and dyspnea during weaning from mechanical ventilation in severe chronic obstructive pulmonary disease. Am Rev Respir Dis 141:281–289
60. Tuxen D (1989) Detrimental effects of positive end expiratory pressure during controlled mechanical ventilation of patients with severe airflow obstruction. Am Rev Respir Dis 140(1): 5–9
61. Otis AB, Fenn WO, Rahn H (1950) Mechanics of breathing in man. J Appl Physiol 2:592–607
62. Marini JJ (1990) Lung mechanics in ARDS: Recent conceptual advances and implications for management. Clin Chest Med 11:673–690
63. Fuhrman BP, Smith-Wright DL, Venkataraman S, Orr RA, Howland DF (1989) Proximal mean airway pressure: A good estimator of mean alveolar pressure during continuous positive pressure breathing. Crit Care Med 17:666–670
64. Hyatt RE (1983) Expiratory flow limitation. J Appl Physiol, Respirat Environ Excercise Physiol 55(1):1–8
65. Boros SJ (1979) Variations in inspiratory/expiratory ratio and airway pressure waveform during mechanical ventilation. The significance of mean airway pressure. J Pediatr 94:114–117
66. Boros SJ, Matalon SV, Ewald R, Leonard AS, Hunt CE (1977) The effect of independent variations in inspiratory-expiratory ratio and end-expiratory pressure during mechanical ventilation in hyaline membrane disease: the significance of mean airway pressure. J Pediatr 91:794–798
67. Herman S, Reynolds EOR (1973) Methods for improving oxygenation in infants mechanically ventilated for severe hyaline membrane disease. Arch Dis Child 48:612–617
68. Petersen GW, Baier H (1983) Incidence of pulmonary barotrauma in a medical ICU. Crit Care Med 11:67–69
69. Cournand A, Motley HL, Werko L, Richards DW (1948) Physiologic studies of the effects of intermittent positive pressure breathing on cardiac output in man. Am J Physiol 152:162–174
70. Guyton AC, Jones CE, Coleman TC (1973) Circulatory physiology. In: Cardiac output and its regulation. W. B. Saunders, Philadelphia, p 193
71. Sladen A, Laver MB, Pontoppidan H (1968) Pulmonary complications and water retention in prolonged mechanical ventilation. N Engl J Med 279:448–453
72. Kumar A, Falke K, Geffin B, et al (1970) Continuous positive pressure ventilation in acute respiratory failure. N Engl J Med 283:1430–1436
73. Manquez JM, Douglas ME, Downs JB, et al (1979) Renal function and cardiovascular responses during positive airway pressure. Anesthesiology 50:393–398
74. Connors AF, McCaffree DR, Gray BA (1981) Effect of inspiratory flow rate on gas exchange during mechanical ventilation. Am Rev Respir Dis 124:537–543

75. Cole AGH, Weller SF, Sykes MK (1984) Inverse ratio ventilation compared with PEEP in adult respiratory failure. Intensive Care Med 10:227–232
76. Fuleihan SF, Wilson RS, Pontoppidan H (1976) Effect of mechanical ventilation with end-inspiratory pause on blood-gas exchange. Anesth Analg 55(1):122–130
77. Toben BP, Lewandowski V (1988) Nontraditional and new ventilatory techniques. Crit Care Nurs Q 11:12–28
78. Marcy TW, Marini JJ (1991) Inverse ratio ventilation in ARDS. Rationale and implementation. Chest (in press)
79. Tharatt RS, Allen RP, Albertson TE (1988) Pressure controlled inverse ratio ventilation in severe adult respiratory failure. Chest 94:755–762
80. Kacmarek RM, Hess D (1990) Pressure controlled inverse ratio ventilation. Panacea or auto-PEEP? Respir Care 35:945–948
81. Pesenti A, Marcolin R, Prato P, Borelli M, Riboni A, Gattinoni L (1985) Mean airway pressure vs. positive end-expiratory pressure during mechanical ventilation. Crit Care Med 13(1):34–37
82. Marini JJ, Crooks PS, Truwit JD (1989) Determinants and limits of pressure preset ventilation: A mathematical model of pressure control. J Appl Physiol 67(3):1081–1092
83. Marini JJ (1990) Ventilatory management of chronic obstructive pulmonary disease. In: Cherniack NS (ed) Chronic obstructive pulmonary disease. W. B. Saunders, Philadelphia, pp 495–506

Techniques of Ventilation Using Constant Flow

A.S. Slutsky

Introduction

The traditional concept of gas exchange in the lung during spontaneous breathing or conventional mechanical ventilation (MV) predicts that to achieve adequate gas exchange, the tidal volume (VT) must exceed the dead space (VD). This model is based on the concept that gas transport in the lung takes place in two distinct zones: the conducting airways where gas transport occurs by convection, and the alveolar zone where transport occurs by molecular diffusion. This concept forms the basis for the design of most mechanical ventilators that have been used very successfully over the last fifty years [1]. However, because VT must be relatively large to exceed VD, relatively large pressures are produced in the lung and this is associated with a number of complications including pulmonary barotrauma and hemodynamic compromise.

In an attempt to overcome some of these problems, a number of investigators have in recent years been examining techniques of ventilation in which the traditional concepts of gas exchange do not apply. These techniques are generally described as "non-conventional" methods of ventilation [2]. As shown in Fig. 1, these techniques can be broadly grouped into methods in which the ventilatory frequencies are substantially higher than normal, techniques termed high frequency ventilation and secondly, techniques of ventilation in which the respiratory frequencies are less than normal or even zero. The present chapter will focus on the latter ventilatory technique in which there is no VT.

Historical Perspective

The concept of ventilation using constant flows is not a new one. As long ago as 1667, Robert Hooke, the curator of the Royal Society of London, performed an elegant experiment using a technique of constant flow ventilation [3]. Hooke's interest was not in ventilation *per se*, but rather in why animals and humans breath. At the time, the accepted theory was that movement of the lungs was required to maintain adequate circulation. Hooke set out to disprove this hypothesis and in so doing had to use a technique in which it was possible to keep animals alive without cyclic lung stretch. He accomplished this by using an experimental preparation in which a catheter was placed into the trachea of a dog and a constant flow of gas was insufflated through this catheter. To provide a source by which the gas could

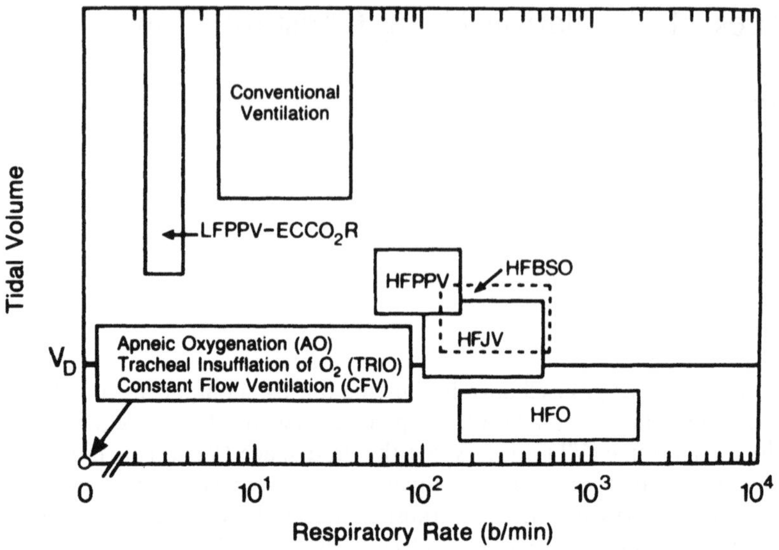

Fig. 1. Tidal volume versus respiratory rate domain for various methods of artificial ventilation. The ranges given are rough estimates. Most of the X-axis is a logarithmic scale. The methods of ventilation shown at the "origin" are the focus of this chapter and are associated with a constant flow of gas.
V_D = dead space; *LFPPV-ECCO₂R* = low frequency positive pressure ventilation with extracorporeal CO_2 removal; *HFPPV* = high frequency positive pressure ventilation; *HFJV* = high frequency jet ventilation; *HFBSO* = high frequency body surface oscillations; *HFO* = high frequency oscillations. (From [2] with permission)

leave the lungs, Hooke made multiple puncture wounds in the lungs and chest wall such that there was a constant flow of gas out via the chest wall (Fig. 2). In his description, Hooke very elegantly described the effect of starting and stopping the constant flow on the condition of the dog, and hence provided convincing evidence that cyclic lung movement was not required for an adequate circulation:

> "This (the constant flow) being continued a pretty while, the dog lay still as before, his eyes being all the time very quick, and the heart breathing very regularly; but upon ceasing this blast, and suffering the lungs to fall and lie still, the dog would immediately fall into dying convulsive fits, but he is soon revived again by renewing the fullness of the lungs ..."

In the subsequent three centuries, a number of investigators have employed techniques using constant flows in a attempt to obtain a relatively simple method of mechanical respiration. In the early 1900's, Meltzer and Auer [4, 5] developed a technique in which a catheter was placed near the carina and a constant flow of gas was insufflated. With this technique it was possible to keep dogs alive for a short period of time, but the animals died within an hour or two. In the mid 1950's, Jacoby et al. [6, 7] used a similar technique, and again were able to keep animals alive for short periods of time but they inevitably died of severe respiratory acidosis. Similar approaches were used throughout the first half of the twentieth century largely by investigators and clinicians studying subjects during anesthesia.

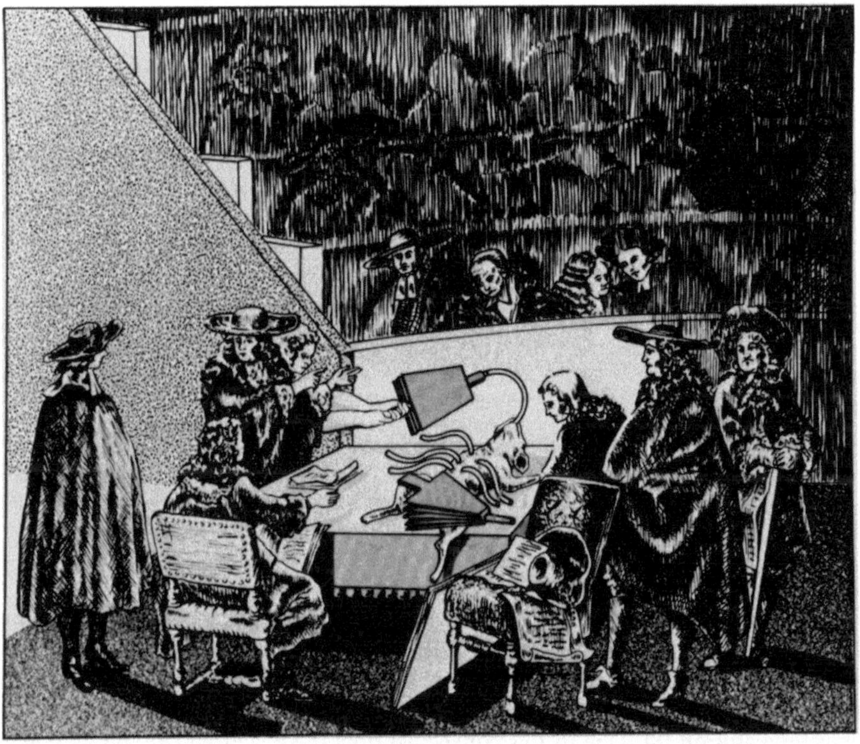

Fig. 2. Pictorial recreation of Robert Hooke's presentation to the Royal Society (London)

Apneic Oxygenation

In the mid-1940's, Draper and Whitehead [6] developed a technique which they called "diffusion respiration", which was able to maintain adequate oxygenation in apneic dogs. The term "diffusion respiration" was actually inappropriate since the primary gas transport mechanism was not diffusion, and the technique did not provide adequate respiration, since there was virtually no CO_2 removal from the lungs. This technique, however, did provide adequate oxygenation, and hence the modern term is "apneic oxygenation" [8].

The application of apneic oxygenation was relatively simple. The animal was ventilated with 100% oxygen for approximately 30–60 min to remove most of the nitrogen from the lungs. Thereafter, the dog was paralyzed while a source of 100% oxygen was placed at the airway opening. During the apnea, $PaCO_2$ rose at a rate of about 3–6 mm Hg/min [9], and PaO_2 declined from its initial value of about 500 mm Hg, at roughly the same rate at which PCO2 rose.

The mechanisms by which adequate oxygenation can take place during the prolonged apneic periods is an interesting one and is shown schematically in Fig. 3. During apnea, approximately 90% of the metabolic CO_2 production in the body is stored in tissues, with the remainder entering the lungs. By contrast, the O_2 uptake

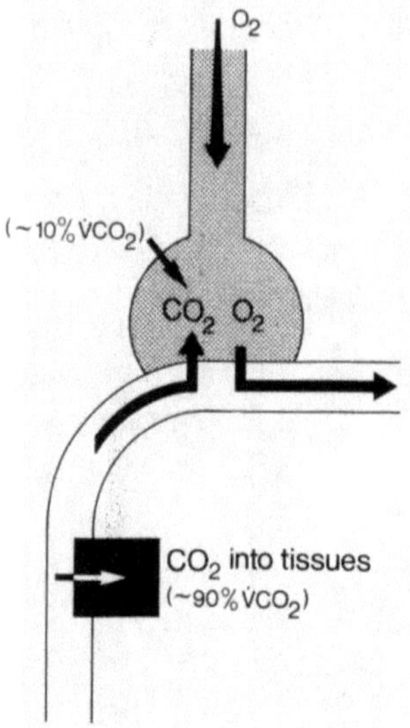

Fig. 3. Schematic respresentation of mechanism of gas transport during apneic oxygenation. During apnea, approximately 90% of the metabolic CO_2 production is stored in the tissues and only about 10% enters the lung. Since O_2 uptake from the lung remains at relatively normal levels, alveolar pressure drops below atmospheric and there is a net convective flow into the lungs

from the lungs remains relatively unchanged from non-apneic conditions and thus the net effect is movement of gas from the alveoli to the blood. This creates an alveolar pressure that is sub-atmospheric, and causes oxygen to move from the O_2 source at the airway opening into the lung by convection (bulk movement), rather than by diffusion [8]. Due to this convective flow there is essentially no CO_2 elimination from the lungs and thus, severe hypercapnic acidosis inevitably develops. Because of the severe acidosis, as well as the decreased oxygen content, partly associated with a markedly right-shifted oxyhemoglobin dissociation curve, it is possible to keep animals alive for only about 90 min [10].

The mechanisms described above should also hold true in humans, and indeed, apneic oxygenation has been applied in human subjects [7, 11, 12]. Frumin et al. [7] studied patients undergoing routing surgical procedures in whom apneic oxygenation was used for periods of time ranging from 18–55 min. In all patients, arterial oxygen saturation was greater than or equal to 98% throughout the apneic period. $PaCO_2$ ranged from 130–250 mm Hg and the lowest arterial pH ranged from 6.72–6.97. Although severe acidosis was present in all of the subjects, arrhythmias were uncommon.

Since hypercapnia is such a strong central respiratory stimulant, lack of spontaneous ventilatory efforts during apneic oxygenation has been used as a method of assessing brain death [13]. Apneic oxygenation has also been used in conjunction with extracorporeal carbon dioxide removal ($ECCO_2R$) as a means of providing oxygenation while "resting" the lungs [14]. Since cyclic lung stretch does not occur during apneic oxygenation, this technique has been used as a tool to study physiological phenomena such as control of breathing [15, 16].

Tracheal Insufflation of Oxygen

The standard management of ventilatory arrest is endotracheal intubation and controlled MV. However, under specific conditions such as respiratory arrest outside the hospital setting or in patients with upper airway abnormalities, endotracheal intubation may not be feasible. A number of approaches have been applied to manage these difficult situations. These include the insertion of a catheter percutaneously into the trachea and ventilating the patient via the catheter using conventional or high frequency ventilation, or by insufflating oxygen into the trachea. This latter approach has a number of advantages in that no special equipment is required other than the oxygen source and the catheter.

In 1985, we investigated a technique called tracheal insufflation of oxygen (TRIO) in which it was possible to obtain sufficient gas exchange to support life for prolonged periods of time in apneic dogs [17]. The experimental set-up consisted of a single catheter (approximately 2 mm ID) usually placed 1 cm proximal to the carina. A flow of oxygen of approximately 2 l/min was used and it was possible to maintain paralyzed dogs alive for 5 h. For all animals, PaO_2's were greater than 300 mm Hg, although steady state $PaCO_2$ levels were in the range of 150–250 mm Hg (Fig. 4). Flow rate was an important factor in determining the efficacy of this technique as was the catheter position. As long as the distal end of the catheter was 4 cm proximal to the carina or deeper into the lung, CO_2 elimination and the increase in oxygenation was adequate. Mackenzie et al. [18] have recently shown that O_2 flow rates as low as 91 ml/min were sufficient to maintain $PaO_2 > 55$ mm Hg for at least ½ h in apneic dogs weighing an average of 12 kg.

Mechanisms of gas exchange during TRIO are not known. It is felt that turbulence generated by the flow of gas leaving the catheter plays an important role. In addition, Burwen et al. [19] have shown that cardiogenic oscillations – the movement of gas in the lung coincident with the heart beat – plays an important role in

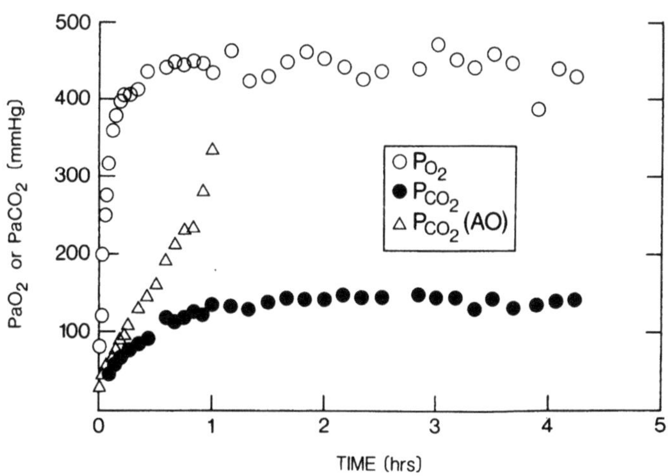

Fig. 4. $PaCO_2$ and pH during TRIO in one animal. (From [54] with permission)

augmenting gas exchange during TRIO. They studied dogs in whom the washout of nitrogen from the lungs was measured during the insufflation of oxygen. This washout was observed both under control conditions in the alive animal, and in the same animals after the dogs were killed. The time constant of the washout was approximately four times smaller in the alive compared to the dead animals, indicating that the alveolar ventilation was increased by about a factor of 4 due to the cardiogenic oscillations. The role of TRIO in clinical medicine is uncertain. This approach, applied through a simple cricothyroid puncture [20–22] could be used to ventilate patients involved in mass casualties or to increase oxygenation of patients who are difficult to intubate. The technique is not indicated in the presence of total expiratory obstruction and it is likely that patients with ventilatory failure and relatively normal lung function would probably benefit most from this technique. Stresemann et al. [23] have shown that tracheal insufflation was effective in 2 emphysematous patients.

The approach of inserting a catheter and using a constant insufflation has also been addressed in non-apneic animals with ventilatory failure [24]. The model con-

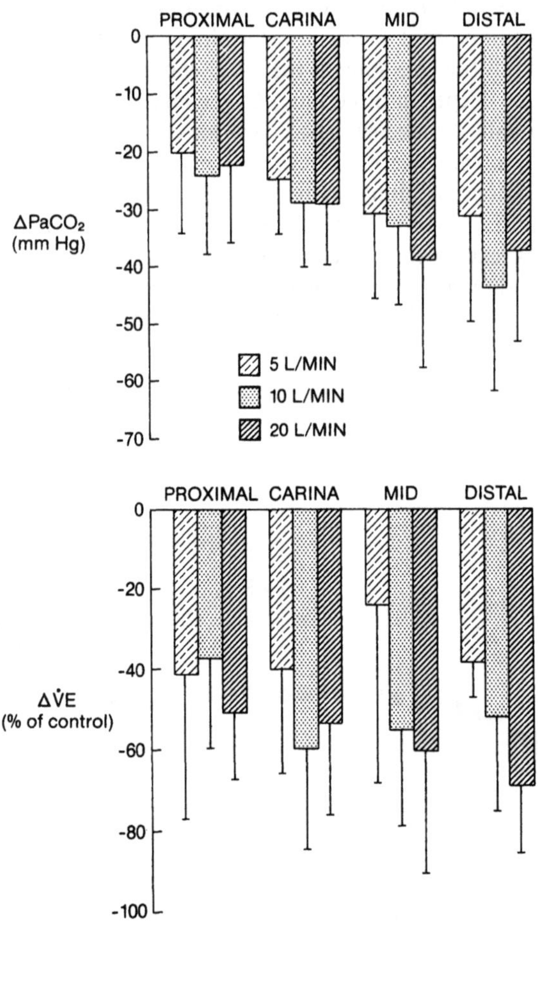

Fig. 5. Effect of constant oxygen insufflation in dogs with "ventilatory failure". The data presented are the changes in $PaCO_2$ *(top)* and minute ventilation *(bottom)* at four catheter positions and three flow rates. In the most *proximal* positions (1 cm proximal to the tracheal carina) only one catheter was used. For the other positions, there was one catheter in each lung. The bars represent standard deviations. (From [24] with permission)

sisted of anesthetized dogs that were partially paralyzed using intermittent low doses of muscle relaxant which resulted in a steady state mean $PaCO_2$ of 90±15.8 mmHg (±SD). A catheter (ID = 1.5 mm) was then inserted into each lung to the most distant position possible and then withdrawn 1–2 cm. Constant insufflation rates of oxygen ranging from 5–20 min l/min were then studied at each catheter position. The changes in $PaCO_2$ and VE due to the insufflation are presented in Fig. 5. At the most proximal position 2 cm from the carina and using a single catheter, there was a decrease in $PaCO_2$ of approximately 20 mm Hg associated with a decrease in VE of approximately 40%. The decrease in ventilation was due largely to a decrease in respiratory frequency, with little or no change in VT (Fig. 6).

There are a number of possible mechanisms by which this insufflation could have improved alveolar ventilation. The constant insufflation washes out the portion of the trachea proximal to the catheter tip, hence decreasing the VD. In addition, the jet effect created as the gas leaves the catheter would augment existing gas transport mechanisms. However, this effect is likely to be rather small in these experiments, since catheters with side holes were used. If washout of the anatomic VD is the major factor lowering $PaCO_2$, then this technique would likely be most effective in conditions of ventilatory failure with relatively normal lungs, such as

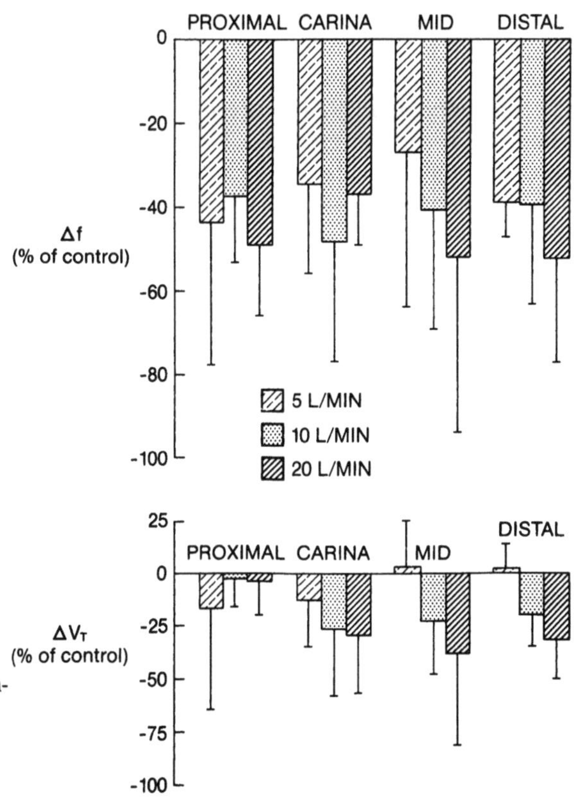

Fig. 6. Effect of constant oxygen insufflation at four catheter positions and three flow rates on changes in the respiratory frequency *(top)* and tidal volume *(bottom)*. The bars respresent standard deviations. (From [24] with permission)

neuromuscular disease, rather than conditions in which alveolar VD would be increased. In appropriate patients, tracheal insufflation might obviate the need for endotracheal intubation and conventional MV. Transtracheal catheters have been extremely well tolerated in patients who require low flow oxygen therapy for chronic hypoxemia [25]. This approach was used by Bergofsky and Hurewitz in 5 patients with COPD, scoliosis or muscular dystrophy [26]. Insufflation of room air at 5 l/min reduced VE by 18% with no change in $PaCO_2$ or PaO_2.

Constant Flow Ventilation

Although some of the techniques described above can provide a certain degree of alveolar ventilation, they cannot achieve normal level of $PaCO_2$ in apneic subjects. In 1982 [27], we described a method for maintaining normal blood gases in apneic dogs using a constant flow of gas delivered into the lungs via two catheters placed in the mainstem bronchi (Fig. 7). The technique involved the insertion of catheters which were then held against the posterior membranous sheath of the trachea using a tracheostomy tube. A constant flow of gas was then insufflated through the catheters and exited from the lungs via the tracheostomy tube. With this technique, adequate oxygenation and CO_2 removal were obtained in puppies ventilated for hours using constant flow ventilation (CFV). Subsequently, a number of investigators have confirmed these results in adult dogs and cats [28–39]. Unfortunately, the use of CFV in humans has met with only partial success. At least two groups of investigators have shown that CFV can provide from about ⅓ to ½ the normal alveolar ventilation [29, 40]. Breen et al. [40] studied CFV in 5 healthy patients in whom CFV was delivered at a total flow of 0.9–1.6 l/min. Hypoventilation was observed in all patients despite attempts to optimize flow rates and catheter positions. However, in 2 patients, $PaCO_2$ appeared to reach steady state values of approximately 50 and 70 mm Hg, indicating that alveolar ventilation was about 60–90% of baseline conditions. Similar results were obtained by Perl et al. [29] who

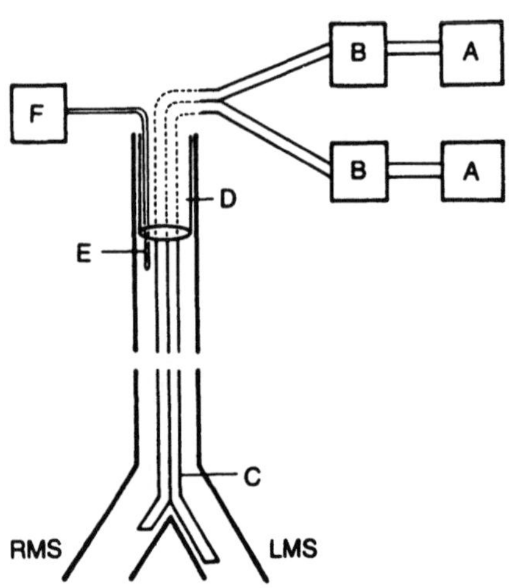

Fig. 7. Schematic diagram of the flow delivery system used during constant flow ventilation (CFV). Gas is delivered through two CFV catheters (C), from a pressurized gas source (A) through humidifiers (B). The gas leaves the animal via an endotracheal or tracheostomy tube (D) positioned such that the CFV catheters lie against the exterior membraneous sheath. (From [27] with permission)

noted that at a flow rate of 0.5 ml/kg/min, the rate of rise of Pa CO_2 was about 30% less than that observed with apneic oxygenation.

A number of investigators have examined the gas transport mechanisms by which CFV produces adequate gas exchange [37–39, 41–43]. Watson et al. [41] studied the effect of flow rate on blood gases during CFV in anesthetized, paralyzed dogs. They found that alveolar ventilation increased linearly with increasing flow over the range of 0.2–1.0 l/sec but was relatively constant at flows above 1.0 l/sec (Fig. 8). At all flow rates, there was a relatively large alveolar-arterial oxygen dif-

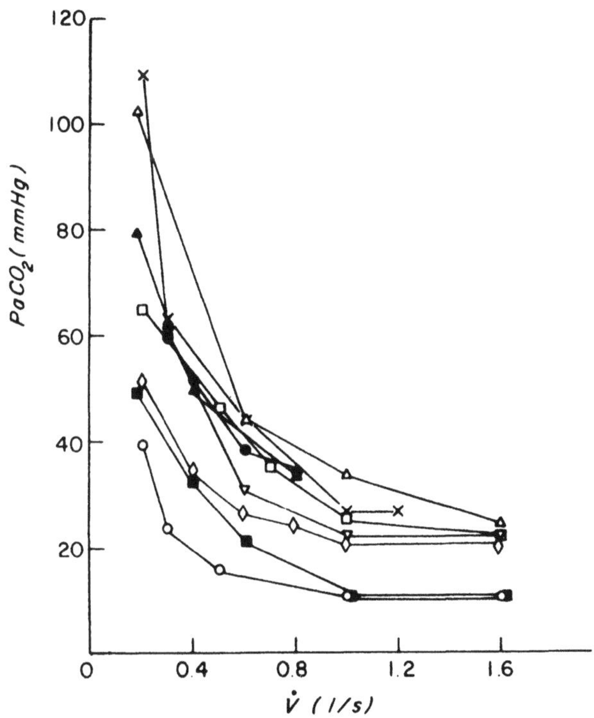

Fig. 8. $PaCO_2$ versus flow rate in 9 dogs. Note that there is a sharp decrease in $PaCO_2$ up to a flow rate of approximately 1 l/sec; thereafter, $PaCO_2$ remains relatively constant as flow rate increases. (From [41] with permission)

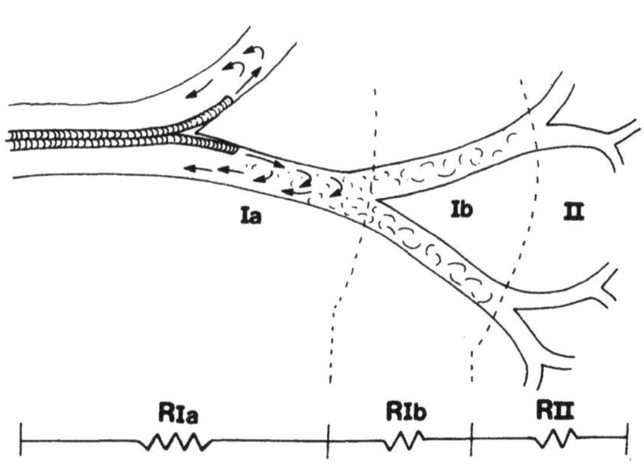

Fig. 9. *(Top)* 2-zone model of gas transport during CFV. *(Bottom)* Analogous circuit diagram for the physical model shown above, based on the concept of resistance to gas transport. Each resistor (R) represents the resistance to gas transport for the regions shown. (From [41] with permission)

ference suggesting inhomogeneities in ventilation/perfusion. To explain these results, they proposed a 2-zone serial model of the lung (Fig. 9). Zone I is the region just distal to the catheters, where turbulence generated by the jet leaving the catheters is the major gas transport mechanism. Zone II is the region distal to zone I, where molecular diffusion and cardiogenic oscillations are the primary gas transport mechanisms. This approach has been formalized into a mathematical model which predicts gas transport during CFV with reasonable accuracy [42].

A number of experimental studies have indirectly or directly tested this model. For example, Slutsky and Menon [44] showed that alveolar ventilation could be doubled when the catheter tips were simply advanced only 2–3 cm into the lungs. Recent studies have shown that alveolar ventilation is increased when a relatively dense carrier gas such as a mixture of 20% oxygen–80% sulfurhexafluoride was used as the insufflating gas rather than air [43, 45]. To examine the effect of cardiogenic oscillations, Cybulsky et al. [46] performed left heart bypass and then examined the effect on alveolar ventilation under control conditions with the heart beating, and then subsequently after the heart had been fibrillated. Ventricular fibrillation caused a decrease in the amplitude of the cardiogenic oscillations, which was associated with a decrease in alveolar ventilation in every animal. The magnitude of this decline during cardiac arrest ranged from 28–50% with a mean decrease of 37%. After the heart was defibrillated, mean alveolar ventilation increased to close to the pre-arrest values indicating that the decrease in alveolar ventilation following fibrillation was not simply due to a progressive deterioration in the experimental preparation with time (Fig. 10). These results were in accord with results that Fukuchi et al. [47] were also demonstrated that damping of cardiogenic

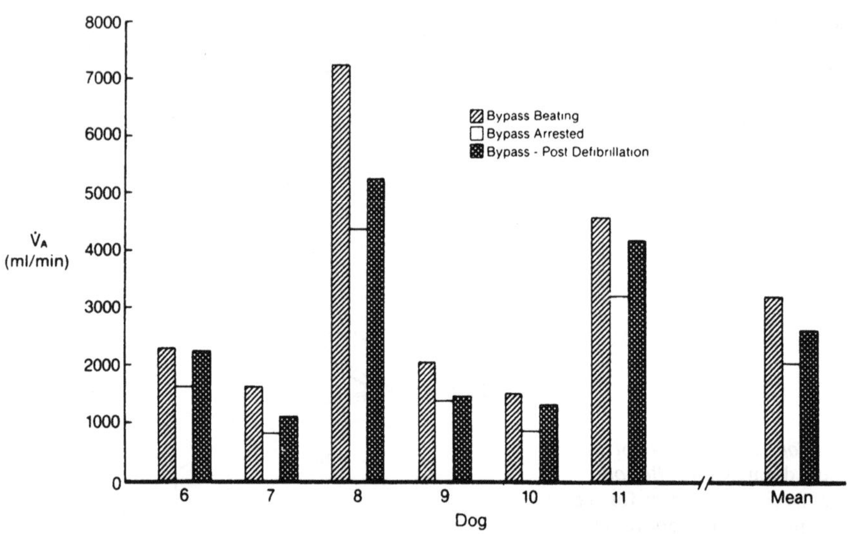

Fig. 10. Alveolar ventilation in 6 dogs studied during left heart bypass in beating, fibrillatory arrest and post-defibrillation states. Note that there was a decrease in alveolar ventilation in the arrested state and that this value returned towards the control values post-defibrillation. (From [46] with permission)

oscillations by the injection of fluid into the pericardial sac, resulted in a significant decrease in alveolar ventilation.

There are also data in the literature suggesting that other factors such as parallel inhomogeneities and collateral ventilation may play an important role during constant flow ventilation. The Chicago group showed that there are marked regional differences in alveolar pressure during CFV [37, 38] and that these inhomogeneities likely account for the large $(A\text{-}a)O_2$ differences described above. In addition, recent studies have shown that CFV is completely ineffective in pigs [48], animals known to have very high resistances to collateral ventilation [49]. It is possible that the marked differences in alveolar pressure between regions may be sufficient to cause gas flow through collateral channels thus causing a powerful convective, unidirectional flow that could produce the adequate gas exchange observed during CFV. The relative ineffectiveness of CFV in humans may be explained by this mechanism since the collateral resistance of humans is greater than that of dogs but less than of pigs [49].

Potential Application of Techniques Using Constant Flows

Tracheal insufflation of O_2 (TRIO) may find some utility as a temporizing technique for providing adequate oxygenation in patients who are difficult to intubate, since the technique of cricothyroid puncture is relatively simple [20–22]. TRIO applied through such an approach might also be helpful for ventilation of patients involved in mass casualties. Although apneic oxygenation also can maintain adequate oxygenation for short periods of time, the major advantage of TRIO is that it can improve oxygenation even when denitrogenation was not performed prior to the start of the insufflation.

The ultimate clinical application of CFV using catheters placed in each mainstem bronchus of humans is somewhat uncertain, since, to date, it has been relatively unsuccessful. However, it is possible that when the gas transport mechanism are finally elucidated, ventilation strategies will be developed that will allow for normal gas exchange in humans using CFV. The clinical appeal of CFV relates to the hypothesis that cyclic lung stretch may augment preexisting lung injury. There are a number of theoretical aspects of CFV that would suggest that it may be the ideal method of providing artificial ventilation since there are no fluctuations in airway pressure (other than those caused by the beating heart) and hence peak pressures are kept to a minimum, whereas the minimum airway pressures are kept at a maximum thus maintaining patency of airways and alveoli. It may thus serve the same purpose as LFPPV-$ECCO_2R$ but would be much less invasive and simpler to use. CFV may be also be useful for ventilating patients during surgical procedures in which no lung movement is desired [36]. However, CFV can be somewhat dangerous since relatively large flow rates have to be introduced relatively distal into the lungs. Any outflow obstruction could thus produce hyperinflation of the lungs relatively quickly, with potentially disastrous consequences.

Although the clinical utility of CFV has not been proven, and its eventual clinical utility is unknown, CFV has proven to be an excellent tool for studying a range of physiological phenomena that are influenced by the act of breathing. For example,

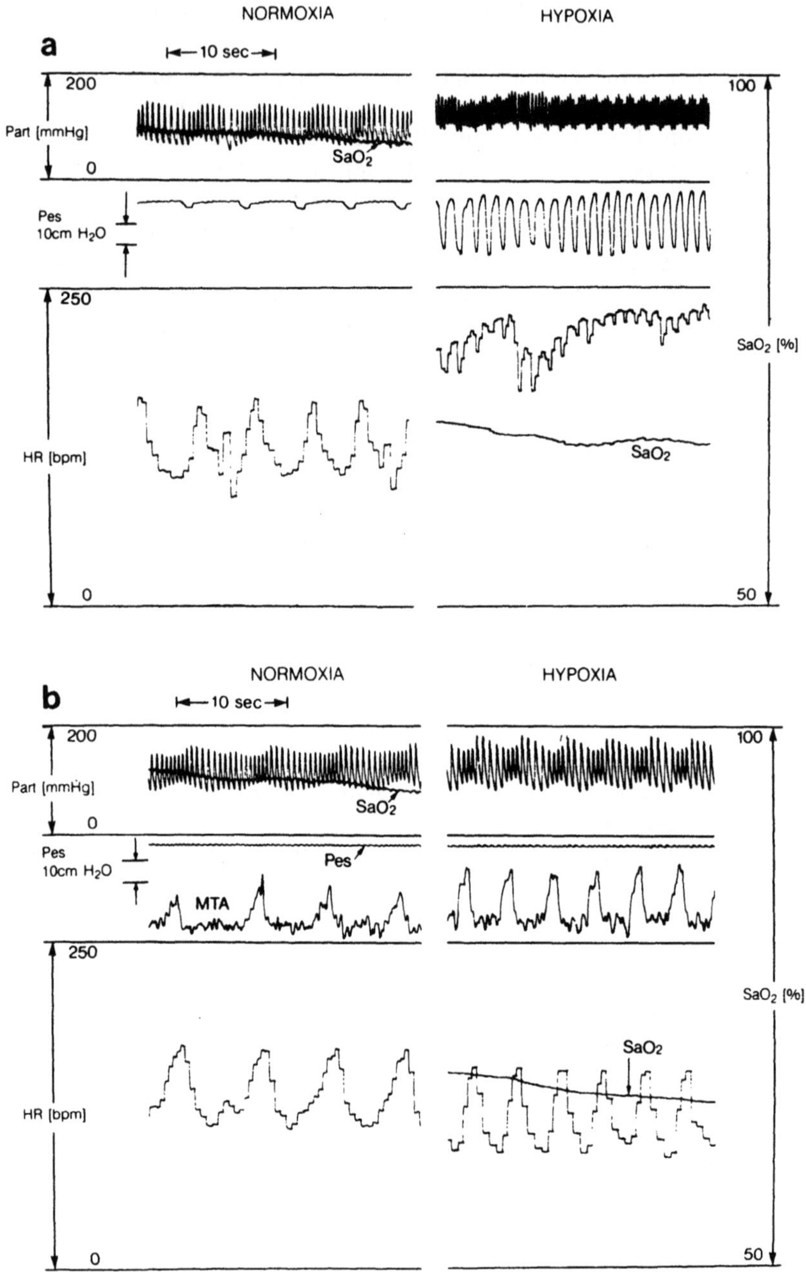

Fig. 11. Examples of experimental records showing the heart rate response to progressive hypoxemia in one dog. Heart rate (HR), arterial blood pressure *(left)* and hypoxias *(right)* in one animal breathing spontaneously
a: (upper panel) Data obtained while the animal was breathing spontaneously.
b: (bottom panel) Data obtained while the animal was being ventilated with CFV. The moving time-average (MTA) phrenic neurogram is shown for the CFV run. (From [50] with permission)

since changes in pleural pressure and changes in lung reflexes can be abolished using CFV, it has been used to investigate the mechanisms mediating the heart rate response to hypoxemia [50]. Figure 11 is an example of the heart rate response to hypoxemia during spontaneous ventilation and during CFV. While ventilated with CFV, the heart rate response to hypoxemia is bradycardia, whereas during spontaneous ventilation there is an increase in heart rate as SaO_2 decreases. Further, it is evident that respiratory sinus arrhythmia is present even in the paralyzed dog (i.e. during CFV) even though there are no changes in pleural pressure and no respiration-related changes in pulmonary reflexes. This approach has been used to show that the differences in respiratory sinus arrhythmia observed with different chemical stimuli are likely due to changes in central respiratory drive rather than any intrinsic effect of the different blood gases [51]. CFV has also been used to study control of breathing in the absence of phasic afferent information from the airways, lung and chest wall during both hypercapnia [52] and hypoxia [53].

References

1. Pontoppidan H, Wilson RS, Rie MA, et al (1977) Respiratory intensive care. Anesthesiology 47:96–116
2. Slutsky AS (1988) Nonconventional methods of ventilation. Am Rev Respir Dis 138:175–183
3. Hooke R (1667) Account of an experiment, made by R. Hooke, of preserving animals alive by blowing through their lungs with bellows. Philos Trans R Soc Lond 2:539–540
4. Meltzer SJ, Auer J (1909) Continuous respiration without respiratory movements. J Exp Med 11:622–625
5. Meltzer SJ (1911) Intratracheal insufflation. JAMA 57:521–525
6. Draper WB, Whitehead RW (1944) Diffusion respiration in the dog anesthetized by pentothal sodium. Anesthesiology 5:262–273
7. Frumin MJ, Epstein RM, Cohen G (1959) Apneic oxygenation in man. Anesthesiology 20:789–798
8. Holmdahl MH (1956) Pulmonary uptake of oxygen, acid-base metabolism and circulation during prolonged apnea. Acta Chir Scand (Suppl) 212:1–128
9. Eger EI, Severinghaus JW (1961) The rate of rise of $PaCO_2$ in the apneic anesthetized patient. Anesthesiology 22:419–425
10. Roth LW, Whitehead RW, Draper WB (1947) Studies on diffusion respiration. II. Survival of the dog following a prolonged period of respiratory arrest. Anesthesiology 8:294–302
11. Enghoff H, Holmdahl MH, Risholm L (1951) Diffusion respiration in man. Nature 168:830–835
12. Payne JP (1962) Apneic oxygenation in anesthetized man. Acta Anaesthesiol Scand 6:129–142
13. Milhaud A, Riboulot M, Gayet H (1978) Disconnecting tests and oxygen uptake in the diagnosis of total brain death. Ann NY Acad Sci 315:241–251
14. Pesenti A, Kolobow T, Buckhold DK, Pierce JE, Huang H, Chen V (1982) Prevention of hyaline membrane disease in premature lambs by apneic oxygenation and extracorporeal carbon dioxide removal. Intensive Care Med 8:11–17
15. Joels N, Samueloff M (1956) The activity of the medullary centres in diffusion respiration. J Physiol (London) 133:360–372
16. Ledlie JF, Kelson SG, Cherniack NS, Fishman AP (1981) Effect of hypercapnia and hypoxia on phrenic nerve activity and respiratory timing. J Appl Physiol 51:732–738
17. Slutsky AS, Watson J, Leith DE, Brown R (1985) Tracheal insufflation of O_2 at low flow rates sustains life for several hours. Anesthesiology 63:278–286

18. Mackenzie CF, Barnas G, Nesbitt S (1990) Tracheal insufflation of oxygen at low flow: capabilities and limitations. Anesth Analg 71:684–690
19. Burwen D, Watson J, Brown R, Josa M, Slutsky AS (1986) Effect of cardiogenic oscillations on gas mixing during tracheal insufflation of O_2. J Appl Physiol 60:965–971
20. Jacobs HB (1972) Emergency percutaneous transtracheal catheters and ventilator. J Trauma 12:50–55
21. Jacobs HB, Smyth NPD, Witorsch P (1974) Transtracheal catheter ventilation: clinical experience in 36 patients. Chest 65:36–40
22. Spoerel WE, Narayana PS, Singh NP (1971) Transtracheal ventilation. Br J Anaesth 43:932–938
23. Stresemann E, Votteri BA, Sattler FP (1969) Wash-out of anatomical dead space for alveolar hypoventilation. Respiration 26:425–434
24. Long SE, Menon AS, Kato H, Goldstein RS, Slutsky AS (1988) Constant oxygen insufflation (COI) in a ventilatory failure model. Am Rev Respir Dis 138:630–635
25. Heimlich HJ (1982) Respiratory rehabilitation with transtracheal oxygen system. Ann Otol Rhinol Laryngol 91:643–647
26. Bergosfsky EH, Hurewitz AN (1989) Airway insufflation: Physiological effects on acute and chronic gas exchange in humans. Am Rev Respir Dis 140:885–890
27. Lehnert BE, Oberdorster G, Slutsky AS (1982) Constant flow ventilation of apneic dogs. J Appl Physiol 53:483–489
28. Smith RB, Babinski M, Bunegin L, Gilbert J, Swartzman S, Dirting J (1984) Continuous flow apneic ventilation. Acta Anaesthesiol Scand 28:631–639
29. Perl A, Whitwam JG, Chakrabarti MF, Taylor VM (1986) Continuous flow ventilation without respiratory movement in cat, dog and human. Br J Anaesth 58:544–550
30. Nahum A, Sznajder I, Solway J, Wood LDH, Schumacker PT (1988) Pressure, flow, and density relationships in airway models during constant-flow ventilation. J Appl Physiol 64:2066–2073
31. Chakrabarti MK, Whitwam JG (1984) Pulmonary ventilation by continuous flow using a modified Carlen's tube. Crit Care Med 12:354–356
32. Smith RB, Sjostrand UH (1985) Apneic diffusion oxygenation and continuous flow apneic ventilation. A review. Acta Anaesthesiol Scand 29:101–105
33. Whitwam JG, Chakrabarti MK, Sapsed-Byrne S, Perl A (1986) Combined continuous-flow, normal, and high-frequency ventilation. Crit Care Med 14:202–206
34. Babinski MF, Smith RB, Bunegin L, Goldberg I (1986) Effect of nitrogen on carbon dioxide elimination during continuous flow apneic ventilation in dogs. Acta Anaesthesiol Scand 30:357–360
35. Chakrabarti MF, Whitwam JG (1984) Pulmonary ventilation by continuous flow using a modified Carlen's tube. Crit Care Med 12:354–356
36. Babinski MF, Smith RB, Bunegin L (1986) Continuous-flow apneic ventilation during thoracotomy. Anesthesiology 65:399–404
37. Sznajder I, Nahum A, Crawford G, Pollak ER, Schumacker PT, Wood LDH (1989) Alveolar pressure inhomogeneity and gas exchange during constant-flow ventilation in dogs. J Appl Physiol 67:1489–1494
38. Schumacker PT, Sznajder I, Nahum A, Wood LDH (1987) Ventilation-perfusion inequality during constant-flow ventilation. J Appl Physiol 62:1255–1263
39. Vetterman J, Brusasco V, Rehder K (1988) Gas exchange and intrapulmonary distribution of ventilation during continuous-flow ventilation. J Appl Physiol 64:1864–1869
40. Breen PH, Sznajder JI, Morrison P, Hatch D, Wood LDH, Craig DB (1986) Constant flow ventilation in anesthetized patients: efficacy and safety. Anesth Analg 65:1161–1169
41. Watson JW, Burwen DR, Kamm RD, Brown R, Slutsky AS (1986) Effect of flow rate on blood gases during constant flow ventilation in dogs. Am Rev Respir Dis 133:626–629
42. Ingenito E, Kamm RD, Watson JW, Slutsky AS (1988) Model of constant flow ventilation in a dog lung. J Appl Physiol 64:2150–2159
43. Watson JW, Kamm RD, Burwen D, Brown R, Ingenito E, Slutsky AS (1987) Gas exchange during constant flow ventilation with different gases. Am Rev Respir Dis 136:420–425
44. Slutsky AS, Menon AS (1987) Catheter position and blood gases during constant flow ventilation. J Appl Physiol 62:513–519

45. Chen FJ, Menon AS, Lichtenstein SV, Zamel N, Slutsky AS (1990) Mechanisms of gas exchange with different gases during constant-flow ventilation. J Appl Physiol 68:88–93
46. Cybulsky I, Abelo J, Menon AS, Salerno T, Lichtenstein S, Slutsky AS (1987) Contribution of cardiogenic oscillations to gas mixing during constant flow ventilation. J Appl Physiol 63:564–570
47. Fukuchi Y, Ishida K, Yano K, Kayama S, So K, Harasawa H (1984) Significance of cardiogenic gas mixing in constant flow ventilation. Am Rev Respir Dis (abstract) 129:A230
48. Webster P, Menon AS, Slutsky AS (1986) Constant flow ventilation in pigs. J Appl Physiol 61:2238–2242
49. Macklem PT (1971) Airways obstruction and collateral ventilation. Physiol Rev 51:368–436
50. Kato H, Menon AS, Slutsky AS (1988) Mechanisms mediating the heart rate response to hypoxemia. Circulation 77:407–414
51. Shykoff B, Naqvi SSJ, Menon AS, Slutsky AS (1990) Respiratory sinus arrhythmia (RSA) in dogs: effects of phasic afferents and chemostimulation. J Clin Invest (In press)
52. Menon AS, England SJ, Vallieres E, Rebuck AS, Slutsky AS (1988) Influence of phasic afferent information on phrenic neural output during hypercapnia. J Appl Physiol 65:563–569
53. Naqvi SSJ, Menon AS, Shykoff B, Rebuck AS, Slutsky AS (1990) Phrenic neural output during hypoxia in dogs: constant flow ventilation (CFV) vs spontaneous breathing. J Appl Physiol (In press)
54. Slutsky AS, Watson J, Leith DE, Brown R (1985) Tracheal insufflation of O_2 (TRIO) at low flow rates sustains life for several hours. Anesthesiology 63:278–286

Extracorporeal Carbon Dioxide Removal in ARDS

L. Gattinoni, L. Brazzi, and A. Pesenti

Introduction

The mortality rate due to acute respiratory failure (ARF) secondary to extensive inflammation of pulmonary parenchima (ARDS) varies, in different series, from 15% [1] to 90% [2] and this variability is not surprising since we are dealing with a syndrome whose etiology and subsequent outcome vary considerably.

The pathological changes in ARDS lungs are not homogeneous [3] and typically, the ARDS patients show at the CT scan a localization of radiographic densities primarily in the dependent lung regions (dorsal regions in supine patients) while the density seems rather normal in the non-dependent regions (sternal regions in supine patients) (Fig. 1). By analyzing the CT image, we were able to quantify three different parts of the lungs: normally inflated, poorly inflated and non-inflated. We

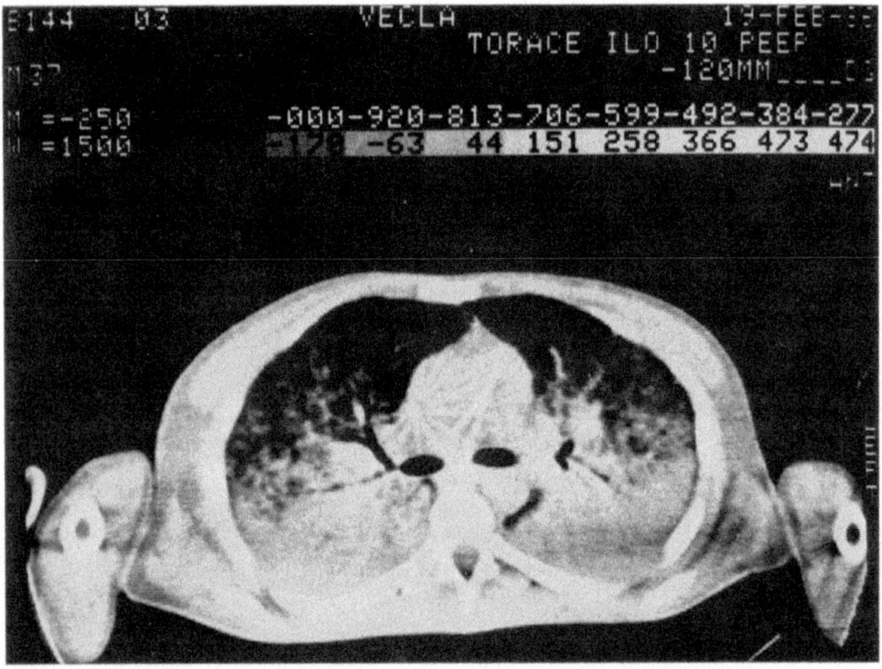

Fig. 1. Typical gravity dependent pattern of densities distribution in ARDS

found that the non-inflated parts of the lung, responsible for the shunt-related hypoxemia of ARDS patients [4], are 2–3 times heavier than normal lung tissue, and that the increased lung weight is partially responsible for the compression atelectases observed in the dependent lung areas [5]. The residual healty lung is obviously reduced, and we found that the dimensions of the relatively normal parts of the ARDS lungs are related to the value of compliance: the smaller the volume of residual normal lung tissue, the smaller the compliance (Fig. 2) [5]. When the value of compliance drops to 25–30 ml/cm H_2O, corresponding to 30–35% of normal lung volume available for ventilation, there are only few possibilities to maintain adequate gas exchange:

1. increase the inspired oxygen fraction (FiO_2);
2. increase airways pressure (peak pressure, mean airways pressure, and positive end-expiratory pressure (PEEP)); and
3. specific hyperventilation.

As regard the inspired oxygen fraction, many studies have demonstrated the effects of oxygen toxicity of normal lung [6]. Although the non-toxic FiO_2 levels in diseased lungs are unknown, there is little doubt that high FiO_2 is dangerous to the lung structure.

Looking at increased peak pressure, a number of studies on laboratory animals show the damaging effects of high peak pressure to normal lung structures independently of FiO_2 levels [7–12]. It is not clear whether the peak pressure *per se*, or the stretching of the lung structures due to volume increase, is responsible for the pulmonary injury, even if a recent study by Dreyfuss et al. [13] tends to support the concept of volotrauma instead of barotrauma. Moreover, it has been shown that specific hyperventilation decreases compliance and induces edema [9]. This may be observed independently of peak pressure elevation [14]. The possible mechanism includes local tissue alkalosis [15], due to an elevated VA/Q ratio, an increase of surfactant clearance [16], and an alteration of surfactant activity [9].

Since the lung volume available for gas exchange is reduced, an adequate gas exchange may only be obtained using high FiO_2, high peak pressure and increased

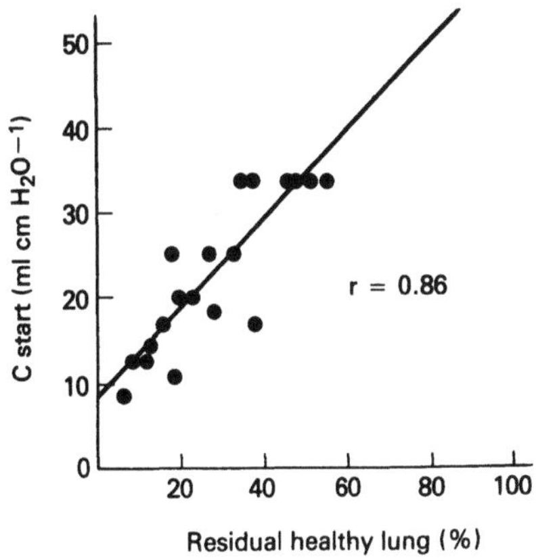

Fig. 2. Relationship between the percent of residual lung and the compliance of total respiratory system. This finding suggests the use of the compliance measurement to estimate the actual size of the residual lung open to gases

specific hyperventilation. All these factors, unfortunately, may worsen the remaining functioning lung tissue. The dimensions of the ARDS lung are reduced and we have called this condition "baby lung", since the dimensions of the relatively normal parts of the lung are comparable to the size of the lung of a baby [3]. This "baby lung" is obliged to provide an adequate gas exchange for an adult metabolism. The main goal of extracorporeal respiratory support is to avoid elevated peak pressure and FiO_2, and to abolish specific hyperventilation: the diseased lung can be treated more gently and can be ventilated in accordance with its actual dimensions.

Past Experiences with Extracorporeal Support

The first randomized study carried out to compare the efficacy of extracorporeal veno-arterial bypass plus conventional continuous positive pressure ventilation (CPPV) with CPPV by itself, was supported by the National Institute of Health (NIH) from 1974 to 1976 (ECMO study) [17]. The mortality observed was 90% [2], in a selected population with a predicted mortality of about 50%: this trial demonstrated that extracorporeal support can be provided for a prolonged period of time but it did not improve survival. Its main target was to correct hypoxemia and to "buy time" for spontaneous healing of the lungs, and this goal was generally achieved. However, the deleterious effects of CPPV on hypoperfused lung tissue were probably underestimated [18], and the perfectly acceptable concept of buying time was applied in a lung environment that was not optimal for pulmonary repair and recovery.

In 1976, the creation of a new type of artificial lung, especially designed for carbon dioxide (CO_2) removal made possible a series of laboratory tests for a possible clinical use of extracorporeal respiratory support in hypercapnic patients [19]. We found that, with extracorporeal CO_2 removal ($ECCO_2R$), it was possible to control the ventilation at will, both in spontaneously breathing [20] and in mechanically ventilated animals [21], and therefore to decrease mechanical ventilation to zero while providing a continuous oxygen flow (apneic oxygenation) equal to the consumed oxygen [22]. The progressive atelectasis formation observed during apnea could be avoided, in clinical setting, by the use of a low frequency positive pressure ventilation (LFPPV) of 3–4 breaths per minute at limited peak pressure [23]. We hypothesized that the application of $ECCO_2R$ with LFPPV could promote healing of the lungs by avoiding the potentially deleterious effects of high volume-high pressure ventilation in ARDS patients.

Techniques

A comprehensive description of the extracorporeal circulation and pulmonary support system must include:

1. the type of vascular access (veno-arterial VA; veno-venous VV). It is important to emphasize that VA bypass will also support failing heart, but it is associated

with a relative lung hypoperfusion and it was practically abandonned after the ECMO study results;
2. the ratio of the extracorporeal blood flow (ECBF) to the cardiac output. $ECCO_2R$ refers mainly to VV access with an ECBF ranging between 20–30% of the cardiac output [24] while the term $PECO_2R$ [25] indicates a very low flow VV circulation with only partial removal of the CO_2 produced (30–60%). (Recently, this technique has been applied clinically in patients with chronic lung disease [26]);
3. the respiratory support to the patient's lungs (CPPV, HFJV, LFPPV, CPAP).
   The entire circuit, which is composed by the membrane lung, roller pump, and respiratory gas tubing, is enclosed in a thermostated console (LSS6000-Kontron-Milan, Italy).

The circuit is primed with heparinized lactated Ringer's solution, which is substituted for whole blood at 37 °C immediately before $ECCO_2R$ is started. Blood from the patient is drained by gravity into a 150 ml reservoir, pumped through two membrane lungs connected in series, and then returned to the patient. The membrane lungs are ventilated in parallel by using humidified gases with an oxygen-enriched air mixture, or air alone, depending on the patient's need.

The monitoring of the extracorporeal system includes gas and blood flow meters with alarms, blood pressure transducers to follow gradients across the membrane lungs, temperature control, and venous drainage control through a flow sensor applied to the blood reservoir. A feedback system provides an automatic stop of the pump in case preset pressure limits are exceeded or venous drainage into the system decreases. We have not had any major technical problems during more than 12000 hours of $ECCO_2R$. During this extracorporeal circulation, the patient's lungs are kept inflated with PEEP, selected according to the lung volume/pressure curve, which is determined daily during static conditions using a supersyringe [27]. The lungs are normally ventilated 3–4 times per minute (LFPPV) with a pressure limit usually set at 35–45 cm H_2O. The FiO_2 is selected according to the clinical needs of the patient. During the long PEEP period, 100% oxygen is supplied via a catheter inserted through the endotracheal tube to the level of the carina, providing the oxygen consumed. Throughout the period of $ECCO_2R$, the patient is given heparin to maintain an activated clotting time (ACT) between 180 and 210 sec. ACT is measured hourly, and PT, PTT, platelets and fibrine split products (FSP) are measured at least twice a day, more frequently if indicated by the clinical conditions. Our anticoagulation monitoring and the related problems have been reviewed recently in detail elsewhere [28].

Catheters and Cannulation Sites

Main determinants in the choice of the cannulation sites are obviously the possibility of a sufficient blood drainage, a low risk of bleeding from surgical wounds and an easy management of the patient. Initially, we used a femoral-jugural bypass with two catheters (proximal and distal) surgically inserted in the femoral veins, and two (proximal and distal) in the jugular veins. This type of cannulation, much invasive, was then substituted with a special double lumen catheter with the outer lumen used for drainage and the inner for return of the blood to the patient [29]. Also, this kind of system requires cannulation of the distal femoral vein via a surgical cutdown. To further simplify the above technique, between 1986 and 1989, we developed and used the sapheno-saphenous vein technique [30]. Distal vein drainage of the legs is not required and the risk of wound bleeding is reduced, because the incisions are more superficial than with femoral vein access. Finally, we have developed the percutaneous cannulation technique [26] using the femoral-femoral or femoral-jugular approach. This technique has previously been used in dogs [31] and humans [32]. We initially utilized the percutaneous bypass only for $PECO_2R$ (ECBF 500–600 ml/min). With increased experience, we have been able to place percutaneously catheters of sizes up to 34 F, allowing total CO_2 removal. This from of cannulation is currently our first choice, since it presents considerable advantages. The catheters are easily inserted and the risk of bleeding is negligible. We have not observed any significant bleeding from the cannulation sites in the last 18 patients, who all had $ECCO_2R$ performed with this technique. The catheters are easily removed and we have not seen any vascular lesions on follow-up evaluation.

Devices for $ECCO_2R$

To our knowledge, only two types of artificial lungs have been consistently used with long-term extracorporeal circulation:

1. the Silicone Spiral Coil Membrane lung (Sci-MED) good for long-term use – up to 30 days in our experience;
2. the microporous artificial lung with heparinized surface (Carmeda) [33], which advantage is the great decrease in the need for systemic heparinization with decreased risk of bleeding.

So far, most of the long-term $ECCO_2R$ treatments in adults have been performed using a roller pump. Only occasionally a centrifugal pump has been used.

Entry Criteria

Our own inclusion criteria are based on oxygenation values as defined by the ECMO study [2]. However, we do not rely solely on gas exchange values: to undergo $ECCO_2R$ our patients must have a total static respiratory system compliance lower than 30 ml/cm H_2O, measured at 10 ml/kg inflation during anesthesia and muscle paralysis. In the past 5 years, we progressively introduced criteria based on gas exchange and CT scan response to increasing levels of PEEP (5–15 cm H_2O). Today, patients with good response to increased PEEP, as evidenced by increase PAO_2 and obvious consistent recruitment on CT scanning, are usually not treated with $ECCO_2R$. In these patients, the volume/pressure curve usually shows an inflexion point, and a great difference exists between starting compliance and inflation compliance on an adequate PEEP level. Those patients who are selected to undergo $ECCO_2R$ therapy initially respond poorly to PEEP with overinflation of ventilated lung areas rather than recruitment of new alveoli, as evidenced on CT scanning. In these patients, consolidation of the lung is a major component of the underlying pathology.

Weaning

The weaning starts as soon as the patient's gas exchange improves. First, the FiO_2 of the patient's lungs is decreased to 0.4, with PaO_2 higher than 80–90 mm Hg range. Second, we gradually decrease FiO_2 of the membrane lung, provided the PaO_2 values remain above 80 mm Hg. Third, we decrease PEEP if the PaO_2 remains above the target value. When the patient is ventilated with 40% oxygen, at 12–15 cm H_2O of PEEP, with room-air ventilating the membrane lung, and PaO_2 remaining above 80–90 mm Hg, anesthesia and paralysis are suspended and the patient is allowed to breathe spontaneously in a PSV, IMV or CPCP mode. The next step includes the withdrawal of the membrane lung ventilation, by simply clamping the gas lines. If the patient is able to maintain his/her PaO_2 target value and a PaO_2 within normal range for 4–12 h, the $ECCO_2R$ system is removed.

Complications

The main complication during $ECCO_2R$ therapy is bleeding due to systemic anticoagulation. The bleeding sites were mainly the surgical cannulation wounds, chest tube insertion sites, and, on a few occasions, other sites, such as the tracheostomy, tracheobronchial tree, gastrointestinal tract, and the arterial catheter insertion sites. The average amount of transfused blood in this patient category was approximately 1.5 liters per day.

The recent application of percutaneous cannulation technique has drastically reduced the bleeding from cannulation wound and the transfusion requests have been reduced from 1.37 ± 1.36 to 0.56 ± 1.55 per day. Also the platelets count after 72 h of bypass has been favorably affected by the reduction of transfusion requests, and the value which was 45% of the basal value with surgical approach has become 55% with the percutaneous one.

Results of $ECCO_2R$ Therapy

The most common indication for $ECCO_2R$, in our experience of 79 patients, has been pneumonia, either viral or bacterial. This was the etiology of ARDS in 45 (57%) of our patients. The survival rate was 24% in this pneumonia group, which includes 10 patients with pharmacological immunosuppression. Seventeen of our patients had post-traumatic ARDS with 6 (35%) surviving. Either pulmonary, fat, or amniotic fluid embolism was the reason for $ECCO_2R$ in 7 patients, 2 of whom

Table 1. Experience with adult respiratory extracorporeal support

	Patients	Survivors	Heparinized surface
Marburg	103	54	36
Berlin	13	8	13
Düsseldorf	4	1	—
Milan-Monza	79	36	3
Stockholm	16	6	16
Paris	19	9	—
Salt Lake City	19	8	—
Ann Arbor	11	6	—
Total	264	128 (48%)	68 (26%)

survived. Other ARDS etiologies, such as sepsis, were present in 10 patients (13%) with no less than 9 of these surviving (90%). The overall survival rate was 46% in the 79 patients.

The clinical experiences in European centers consistently using the extracorporeal support technique, are summarized in Table 1.

If we define responders as the patients who show dramatic change in gas exchange within 48 h, we had 53 (67%) in our group of 79 who improved impressively at the beginning of $ECCO_2R$. Up to 1986, survival was limited to those patients who showed a rapid response. However, in the most recent 2 years, 3 pneumonia patients have survived without such early improvement. The first sign of improvement in these patients were not noted until 2–3 weeks after initiation of $ECCO_2R$. There was no difference between survivors and nonsurvivors in the number of days they were treated with $ECCO_2R$.

As regard the causes of death, it is usually claimed that hypoxemia is not a major cause of death in ARDS [34]. However, despite the $ECCO_2R$, 21 of the 43 patients who died in our series became hypoxemic when the pulmonary shunt in some of them approached 100%. The remaining 22 of the 43 nonsurvivors in our series died with normal blood gases. Among those 22, the main causes of death were uncontrollable bleeding in 1, septic shock in 4 and multiple organ failure in 6; 8 patients were disconnected for intracranial bleeding while 3 died from pulmonary deterioration secondary to sepsis.

To improve the overal results and to increase the cost/benefit ratio of $ECCO_2R$, it would be of great importance to be able to predict survival before bypass is initiated. The presence of up to three organ failures in addition to lung failure did not prevent survival (Fig. 3). However, we have found that survival is significantly higher among patients who have had less than 1 week CPPV before extracorporeal circulation, compared to those patients who have been treated for 2 weeks or more with CPPV (Fig. 4).

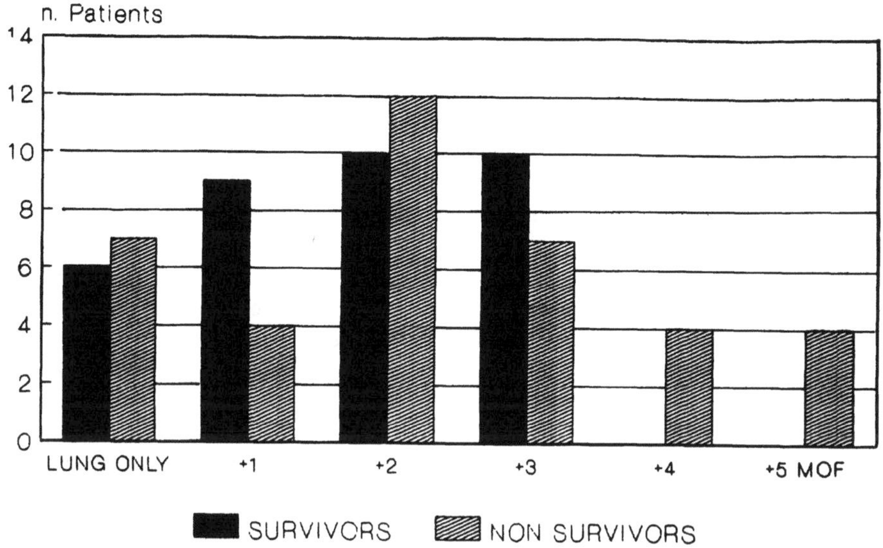

Fig. 3. MOF distribution before the bypass related to the final outcome. No patient survived with 4 or 5 organ failures other than the lung. However, surviving was not related to the number of organ failures between 0 and 3 other than the lung

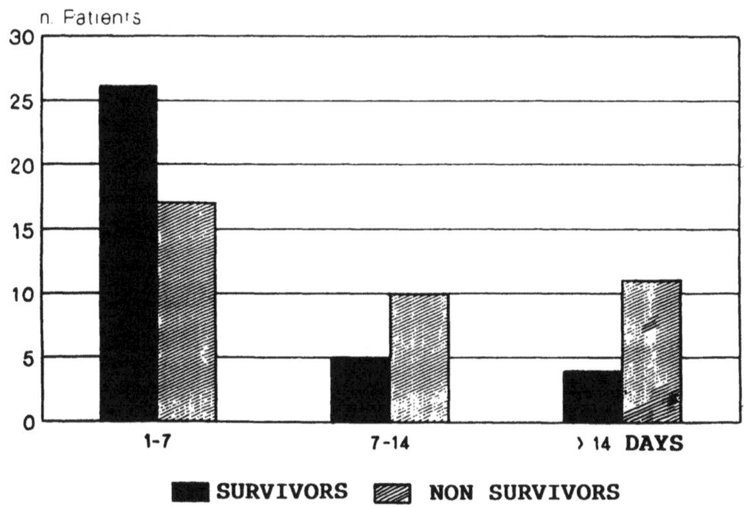

Fig. 4. Relationship between the time of conventional respiratory treatment before the bypass and the final outcome. Survival was significantly higher when the conventional respiratory treatment was limited to 1 week

Conclusions

Considering the above factors, there is little doubt in our mind that $ECCO_2R$ is a logical and rational form of therapy in severe ARDS. Still, $ECCO_2R$ is not an ideal form of treatment, since the technique carries a significant frequency of bleeding, a potentially lethal complication. We have been impressed by the finding that our survival rate is 80% among patients who do not develop severe bleeding during treatment.

It is also important to emphasize that in those cases where we were able to perform $ECCO_2R$ without bleeding complications, we observed some late responders healing after more than 4 weeks of $ECCO_2$. This observation suggests that when extracorporeal support can be performed without complications, the potential for lung recovery exists even when the lung almost completely loses its gas exchange ability.

Currently, we still consider $ECCO_2R$ an experimental technique and we do not feel it is time to recommed $ECCO_2R$ for widespread use because of the relatively high complication rate. Additional investigations are required to decrease substantially the incidence of bleeding problems. Thereafter, the effectiveness of this technique should be compared to conventional ventilatory support in a randomized study of a homogenous population of ARDS patients. Only after efficacy could be demonstrated in such a study, can this treatment be proposed for widespread utilization.

References

1. Gallagher TJ, Civetta J, Kirby RR (1978) Terminology update: optimal PEEP. Crit Care Med 6:323–325
2. Zapol WM, Snider MT, Hill JD, et al (1979) Extracorporeal membrane oxygenation in severe acute respiratory failure. JAMA 242:2193–2196
3. Gattinoni L, Pesenti A (1987) ARDS: the nonhomogenous lung. Facts and hypothesis. Intensive and Crit Care Digest 61:1–3
4. Gattinoni L, Pesenti A, Bombino M, et al (1988) Relationship between lung computed tomographic densities, gas exchange, and PEEP in acute respiratory failure. Anesthesiology 69:812–814
5. Gattinoni L, Pesenti A, Baglioni S, et al (1988) Inflammatory pulmonary edema and positive end-expiratory pressure: correlations between imaging and physiological studies. J Thorac Imaging 3:59–64
6. Deneke SM, Fanbourg BL (1982) Oxygen toxicity of the lung: an update. Br J Anaesth 54:737–749
7. Greenfield LJ, Ebert PA, Benson DW (1964) Effects of positive pressure ventilation on surface tension properties of lung extracts. Anesthesiology 25:312–316
8. Barsh J, Bibara C, Eggers GWN, et al (1970) Positive pressure as a cause of respiratory induced lung disease. Ann Intern Med 72:810–812
9. Faridy EE, Permut S, Riley RL (1966) Effect of ventilation on surface forces in excised dogs' lungs. J Appl Physiol 21:1453
10. Kolobow T, Moretti MP, Fumagalli R, et al (1987) Severe impairment in lung function induced by high peak airways pressure during mechanical ventilation. Am Rev Respir Dis 135:312–315
11. Borelli M, Kolobow T, Spatola R, et al (1988) Severe acute respiratory failure managed with CPAP and $ECCO_2R$ by artificial membrane lung. Am Rev Respir Dis 138:1480

12. Webb HH, Tierney DF (1974) Experimental pulmonary edema due to intermittent positive pressure ventilation with high inflation pressures. Protection by end-expiratory pressures. Am Rev Respir Dis 110:556–565
13. Dreyfuss D, Soler P, Basset G (1988) High inflation pressure pulmonary edema. Respective effects of high airway pressure, high tidal volume and positive end-expiratory pressure. Am Rev Respir Dis 137:1159
14. Mascheroni D, Kolobow T, Fumagalli R, et al (1988) Acute respiratory failure following pharmacologically induced hyperventilation: an experimental animal study. Intensive Care Med 15:8–12
15. Kolobow T, Spragg R, Pierce J (1981) massive pulmonary infarction during total cardiopulmonary bypass in unanesthetized spontaneously breathing lambs. Int J Artif Organs 4:76–81
16. Faridy EE (1971) Effect of food and water deprivation on surface activity of lungs of rats. J Appl Physiol 17:23–25
17. Protocol for extracorporeal support for respiratory insufficiency, collaborative program (1974). National Heart, Lung and Blood Institute, Division of Lung Disease. Bethesda, Maryland
18. Ratcliff JL, Hill JD, Fallat RL, et al (1979) Complications associated with membrane lung support by veno-arterial perfusion. Ann Thorac Surg 19:537
19. Kolobow T, Gattinoni L, Tomlinson T, et al (1977) The carbon dioxide membrane lung (CDML): a new concept. Trans Am Soc Artif Intern Organs 23:17–21
20. Kolobow T, Gattinoni L, Tomlinson T, Pierce J (1977) Control of breathing using an extracorporeal membrane lung. Anesthesiology 46:138–141
21. Gattinoni L, Kolobow T, Tomlinson T, et al (1977) Control of intermittent positive pressure breathing (IPPB) by extracorporeal carbon dioxide removal. Brit J Anaesth 50:753–758
22. Kolobow T, Gattinoni L, Tomlinson T, Pierce J (1978) An alternative to breathing. J Thorac Cardiovasc Surg 75:261–266
23. Gattinoni L, Kolobow T, Tomlinson T, et al (1978) Low frequency positive pressure ventilation with extracorporeal carbon dioxide removal (LFPPV-$ECCO_2R$): an experimental study. Anesth Analg 55:470–477
24. Gattinoni L, Pesenti A, Kolobow T, et al (1983) A new look at therapy of the adult respiratory distress syndrome: motionless lung. Int Anesthesiol Clin 21:97–117
25. Marcolin R, Mascheroni D, Pesenti A, et al (1986) Ventilatory impact of partial extracorporeal CO_2 removal ($PECO_2R$) in ARF patients. Trans Am Soc Artif Intern Organs 32:508–510
26. Pesenti A, Rossi GP, Pelosi P, et al (1990) Percutaneous extracorporeal CO_2 removal in a patient with bullous emphysema with recurrent bilateral pneumothoraces and respiratory failure. Anesthesiology 72:571–573
27. Gattinoni L, Mascheroni D, Basilico E, et al (1987) Volume/pressure curve of total respiratory system in paralyzed patients: artifacts and correction factors. Intensive Care Med 13:19–25
28. Uziel L, Cugno M, Fabrizi I, et al (1990) Physiopathology and management of coagulation during long term extracorporeal respiratory assistance. Int J Artif Organs 13:280–287
29. Artigas A (1988) Adult respiratory distress syndrome: changing concepts in clinical evolution and recovery. In: Vincent JL (ed) Update in intensive care and emergency medicine, vol 5. Springer Verlag, Berlin Heidelberg New York pp 97–114
30. Pesenti A, Romagnoli G, Fox U, et al (1983) Sapheno-saphenous cannulation for LFPPV-$ECCO_2R$ (Low Frequency Positive Pressure Ventilation with Extracorporeal CO_2 Removal). In: Tenth congress of European Society of Artificial Organs. European Society of Artificial Organs. Bologna, Italy: p 97
31. Stafford T, Wood R, Ward B (1985) Percutaneous membrane ventilation as respiratory support in acute lung injury. Anesthesiology 63S:A537
32. Jardin F, Ozier Y, Marogairez A (1984) L'épuration extracorporelle du gaz carbonique. Traitement d'appoint de certaines insuffisances respiratoires aiguës. Nouvelle Presse Med 13:743
33. Bindslev L (1987) Treatment of acute respiratory failure by extracorporeal carbon dioxide elimination performed with a surface heparinized artificial lung. Anesthesiology 67:117–120

Augmentation of Blood Gas Transfer by Means of an Intravascular Blood Gas Exchanger (IVOX)

J.D. Mortensen

Introduction

O_2 Delivery, Transport, and Utilization

Oxygen, at a concentration of about 21% of the ambient atmospheric air, enters the lung during the inspiratory phase of respiration, transits the conducting airways, and is delivered into the respiratory bronchiole-alveolar complexes of the lung. In response to the partial pressure gradient of O_2 between the alveolar air and oxygen in the blood within the pulmonary capillaries, oxygen crosses the alveolar-capillary membrane where it enters into association with the hemoglobin in the red blood cells. In this oxyhemoglobin complex, O_2 is transported with the flow of blood through the pulmonary veins into the left atrium, left ventricle, and systemic arterial system, to be delivered to the cells of the body, again crossing a systemic capillary-cellular membrane. Multiple factors, physiological and pathological, can interrupt, obtund, or impede this pathway of oxygen from the atmosphere to functioning tissue cells. If the metabolic requirements of the subject exceed the volume of oxygen delivered to the functioning cells, the oxygen content of the circulating blood decreases, hypoxemia is induced, and a state of respiratory insufficiency exists. With increasing hypoxemia, vital functions of the cells may be impaired to a life-threatening level, resulting in death if not corrected [1–4].

Methods Available for Augmenting O_2 Delivery

Simply increasing the O_2 content of inspired air by means of a face mask or nasal cannula may sufficiently increase the alveolar PO_2 to overcome hypoxemia in many clinical situations. When the added inspired O_2 cannot reach the alveoli, mechanical ventilatory assistance may be necessary. Mechanical ventilators are currently in wide use which provide sophisticated and effective means for creating gas flow, volumes, patterns, and pressures of various gas mixtures. These devices can deliver appropriate volumes of gas at desirable concentrations of O_2 to the alveoli in most patients with acute respiratory failure (ARF). Although still rather rudimentary, methods are being developed to decrease the interference of gas transfer across the edematous, thickened, inflamed alveolar-capillary membrane that exists in most patients with ARF. Adjustments in pH of the blood to permit more effective O_2-hemoglobin association/dissociation may be accomplished by the physician [5–9]. Increasing hemoglobin content of the blood and increasing flow rate of blood (cardiac output) can further aid O_2 delivery and transport. If levels of hypoxemia persist, utilization of a membrane blood gas exchanger (membrane oxygenator) may be necessary to provide temporary augmentation of O_2 delivery. Currently, this can be achieved most effectively by extracorporeal perfusion of venous blood through a cannula, pump, and external membrane blood gas exchanger, then back into the subject's circulatory system, either venous or arterial. Variously known as ECMO (Extracorporeal Membrane Oxygenation) [10–12], ECLA (Extracorporeal Lung Assist) [13], ELS (Extracorporeal Life Support) [14], or $ECCO_2R$ (Extracorporeal Carbon Dioxide Removal) [15–19], these perfusion techniques for blood gas exchange have currently reached high levels of sophistication and efficacy. A new method for adding O_2 to circulating venous blood, intracorporeally, without extracorporeal perfusion, has recently been developed. Known as IVOX [20–25], this technology is currently under clinical investigation. This new modality is discussed in depth later in this chapter.

CO_2 Production, Transport, and Removal

In the living animal, carbon dioxide produced by cellular metabolism is transported in the circulating blood to the lungs (Fig. 1). Here it is transferred across the alveolar-capillary membrane into the airways, from which it is exhausted into the atmosphere. If CO_2 production exceeds the subject's capability to remove CO_2, or if CO_2 production continues (cells remain alive) but transit of CO_2 from the living cells into the atmosphere is interrupted at any point, CO_2 accumulates in circulating blood and a state of hypercarbia exists. With increasing pCO_2 in the blood, a series of pathophysiological responses occur which may threaten the health, even the

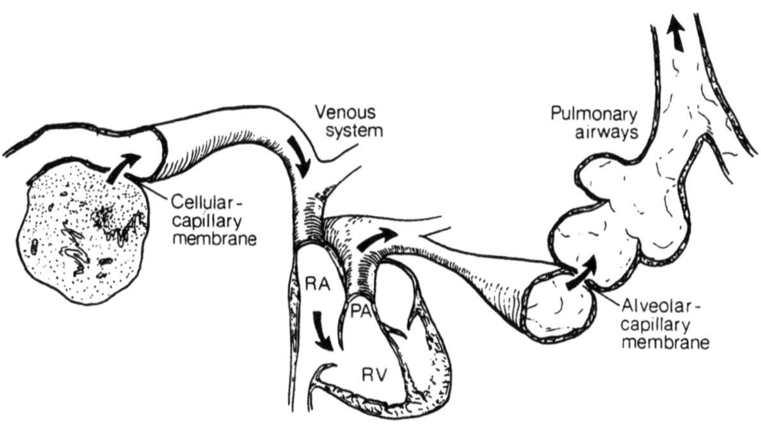

Fig. 1. Path of carbon dioxide production, transport, and elimination. From left to right: CO_2 produced in cells enters venous blood by crossing the cellular-capillary membrane, is carried in venous blood to the right heart and pulmonary arteries, crosses the capillary – alveolar membrane to enter pulmonary alveoli and respiratory bronchioles, exits the body and is exhausted into the atmosphere via pulmonary airways

life, of the subject [1–4]. In such instances, removal of excess CO_2 from venous blood may be an important, even life-saving, function.

Methods Available for Augmenting CO_2 Removal

Increased CO_2 removal from the blood can be accomplished in several ways. Physiologically, the body responds to hypercarbia by increasing gas flow through the lungs (hyperventilation), by increasing blood flow through the lungs (increased cardiac output), and/or by increasing renal excretion of the excess bicarbonate and/or carbonic acid [1–4]. The physician may augment the patient's natural responses by overcoming obstructions in the airways, by bolstering the inadequate blood flow, by stimulating renal function, and/or by administering medicine which counteracts the harmful effects on the hypercarbia/acidosis [5–9]. If these ameliorating/supportive measures are inadequate, more aggressive action may be necessary, such as increasing gas flow through the lungs by means of a mechanical ventilator [8, 9]. Augmenting CO_2 removal by dialysis has been accomplished experimentally in animals and in a few patients [26–31]. Temporarily re-routing (perfusion) of venous blood with its extra CO_2 load through an extracorporeal blood gas exchanger, then back to the body, is an extremely effective, although rather invasive method for augmenting inadequate CO_2 removal.

IVOX Utilization for Temporary Augmentation of Blood Gas Transfer

IVOX Conceptual and Design Features

IVOX is a small, elongated, gas-on-the-inside/blood-on-the-outside hollow fiber membrane oxygenator designed (Fig. 2) to lie within the vena cavae, where venous blood en route to the right heart and lungs flows over and around the hollow fibers of IVOX (Fig. 3). Gas exchange takes place between the venous blood outside the hollow fibers and the gas within the lumens of the hollow fibers. This O_2 and CO_2 transfer takes place across the gas-permeable walls of the hollow fibers. Each hollow fiber thus resembles the respiratory bronchiole-alveolus-pulmonary capillary bed complex of the natural lung, accomplishing gas transfer between venous blood and an airway, across a gas-permeable/liquid-impermeable membrane (Fig. 4). The intraluminal gas within the IVOX hollow fibers is then exhausted into the atmosphere through the gas conduits. Blood flows by natural hemodynamic forces over and around this artificial alveolar-capillary membrane interposed in the vena cavae, resulting in prepulmonary blood gas exchange which can augment or assist the gas transfer being achieved through the natural lungs. These fundamental design, materials and fundamental concepts of the IVOX device are summarized in the Table 1.

In order for the IVOX device, lying freely in the vena cavae, to transfer clinically significant quantities of O_2/CO_2 into/out of venous blood, and to remain functional for several days, significant modifications were necessary in the design and operation of this small, intracorporeal hollow fiber oxygenator. For example, a

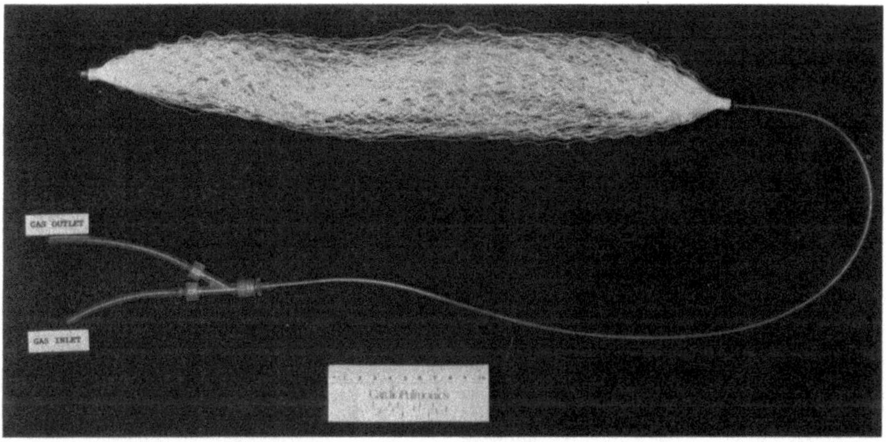

Fig. 2. Photograph of the intravascular blood gas exchanger (IVOX). The crimped hollow fibers (approximately 1.000) lie freely in the blood flowing in the SVC, IVC, and right atrium en route to the RV and lungs. Oxygen enters the inlet limb of double lumen gas conduit at atmospheric pressure. It is carried in the central gas conduit to the distal potting where it is distributed into the lumens of the hollow fibers. Gas exchange occurs with the blood outside each hollow fiber through the walls of the hollow fibers.Gas remaining in the hollow fiber lumens exits the body via the outer portion of the double lumen gas conduit, being pulled through the device by suction applied to the gas outlet limb of the double lumen gas conduit

method had to be developed for furling (compressing) the hollow fibers into a compact bundle with a cross-sectional diameter small enough to enter a peripheral access vein; then unfurling (deploying) the fibers into a configuration which would fill the cross sectional diameter of the larger vena cavae. The blood flow pattern of venous blood over and around the external surface of each hollow fiber needed to be altered to produce good mixing of the blood, rather than permitting laminar flow along the hollow fibers. Specific disadvantages of microporous hollow fibers (such as roughness of their outer surface and the filling of the mural micropores with serum) needed to be overcome if the IVOX device were to remain functional for several days in the venous blood stream. The danger of introducing gas bubbles into the blood flowing over the IVOX device (in the event hollow fibers, the gas transfer membrane, or the gas conduits were damaged and/or leaked) needed to be obviated. Finally, it was necessary to significantly reduce the thrombogenicity of the IVOX device lying in the vena cavae blood stream. The modifications of current hollow fiber oxygenator technology made by CardioPulmonics' research scientists in order to achieve these goals and to develop the IVOX device to the point that it could function safely and effectively are summarized in the Table 2.

IVOX Performance Characteristics

Following 10 years of research and development effort, including demonstration of its safety and efficacy as a blood gas exchange device in the experimental animal

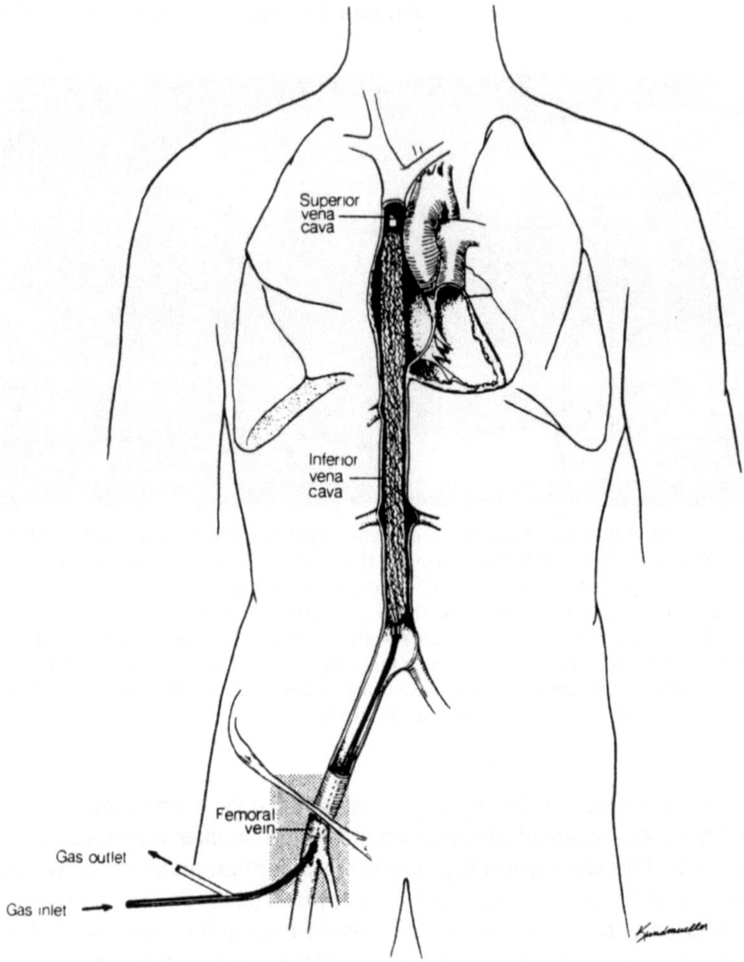

Fig. 3. Diagram of IVOX in its intravenacaval position in a human patient. In this illustration, IVOX has been introduced into the body through a venotomy in the right common femoral vein, then advanced up the iliac vein and inferior vena cava, through the lateral aspect of the right atrium, and up the superior vena cava, with its tip lying in the superior vena cava. The crimped hollow fibers lie free in the vena cavae blood stream. The double lumen gas conduit connects to the potted manifolds at the ends of the hollow fibers.The inner (inlet) gas conduit is connected to an oxygen source; the outer (outlet) gas conduit is connected to a vacuum pump which pulls the gas through the hollow fibers at controlled subatmospheric pressure. The IVOX device can remain functional in the vena cavae for up to 19 days; then (or whenever it is no longer needed) IVOX is removed and the access venotomy is repaired surgically

laboratory, IVOX is currently undergoing FDA-supervised clinical trials to assess its performance in human patients with acute, potentially reversible respiratory failure. Summary of data concerning the performance characteristics of IVOX as a means for augmenting blood gas transfer follows:

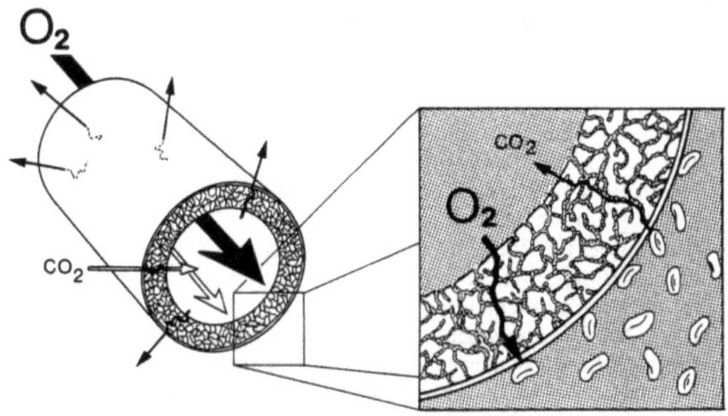

Fig. 4. Diagram of the IVOX hollow fiber gas transfer membrane. The microporous wall of the hollow fiber acts as a skeleton or framework supporting the ultra-thin siloxane gas transfer membrane and permits gas on the inside of each hollow fiber to make contact with the siloxane membrane separating the gas from the blood outside the hollow fiber. Oxygen and carbon dioxide permeate through the gas-permeable, but fluid-impermeable, siloxane membrane in response to partial pressure differences (gradient) between the gas inside the hollow fiber and blood outside the hollow fiber, as shown in the inset drawing. Composition of gas entering and flowing inside the hollow fibers of IVOX is 100% oxygen; gas flowing out of the hollow fibers and exhausted into the atmosphere contains carbon dioxide and residual oxygen. The inside diameter of each IVOX hollow fiber is 190 microns, the microporous hollow fiber wall is 30 microns thick, and the continuous siloxane gas transfer membrane is 1 micron thick. The similarities in dimensions and function between the hollow fiber component of IVOX and the natural pulmonary alveolar-capillary membrane complex is apparent

Table 1. Fundamental conceptual features of IVOX

- Fabrication of a small diameter, elongated, hollow fiber membrane oxygenator, without an external case.
- Placement of this oxygenator into the subject's vena cavae through a peripheral venotomy.
- Oxygen is introduced into the hollow fiber lumens via a small diameter gas inlet conduit which is the central limb of a double lumen gas transport tube.
- Venous blood en route to the right heart flows over and around the external surfaces of each hollow fiber.
- Blood gas exchange (O_2 into the blood and CO_2 from the blood) takes place across the walls of the hollow fibers.
- Carbon dioxide-rich gas exits the body via the outer gas outlet limb of the double lumen gas transport conduit.

Safety and efficacy testing in normal animals. The first consideration relates to the risks and hazards associated with IVOX utilization. Data from a series of standing, awake, highly instrumented by otherwise normal sheep with a functioning IVOX in the vena cavae were compared to data from similarly prepared and managed control sheep without an IVOX for up to 10 days of observation in the animal ICU. Extensive blood gas, hemodynamic, hematologic, blood chemistry, bacteriologic, and vital function testing was carried out, comparing the IVOX-implanted to the normal control animals [32]. All the animals were then euthanized and necropsy

Table 2. Cardiopulmonics' innovative design and materials modifications of the original IVOX concepts

- Coat the microporous hollow fibers with an ultra-thin, continuous, pinhole free, gas permeable siloxane coating.
- Arrange hollow fibers within the venacavae to produce a distributed blood flow pattern over and around each hollow fiber (Bellhouse principle).
- Develop a mechanism to furl the fibers into a small diameter bundle for peripheral vein entry, then unfurl the fibers to achieve optimum deployment, filling the venacaval lumen.
- Coat each hollow fiber and the entire intravascular device with an effective, covalently bonded thromboresistant coating.
- Utilizable subatmospheric pressure (vacuum) on the gas outlet to achieve optimum gas flow through the IVOX device at low (negative) intraluminal gas pressures.

findings in the two groups were compared. Results of these experiments demonstrated no significant difference between the IVOX-implanted and control animals. Utilization of the IVOX device appeared to be free from significant risks and hazards and the device was found to exchange significant quantities of O_2 and CO_2 into/out of circulating venous blood (Table 3).

Quantification of gas transfer by IVOX. The next step involved quantification of the amount of O_2 and CO_2 the IVOX device could transfer into/out of circulating venous blood [33]. This was accomplished by both *ex vivo* and *in vivo* animal experiments which indicated that the quantity of gas transferred by an IVOX device was variable, depending upon the following factors, listed roughly in order of decreasing influence on gas transfer rate:

- size of the IVOX device (surface area of gas transfer membrane exposed to blood);

Table 3. Major performance characteristics of IVOX in experimental laboratory animals

When used in compliance with established insertional and operational protocols:

- IVOX transfers clinically significant quantities of oxygen and carbon dioxide into/out of circulating venous blood (up to 170 cc/min).
- IVOX implantation in normal sheep for up to 19 days causes no mortality, morbidity, or significant gross or microscopic pathological findings at necropsy.
- IVOX in the vena cavae causes no interference with the subject's hemodynamic functions.
- IVOX implantation for up to 19 days causes no significant hematologic or blood chemistry changes, when compared to control animals without an implanted IVOX device.
- No gas leaks, bubbles, or foam have been observed in the blood of more than 150 laboratory animals with an implanted, functioning IVOX device.
- No gross or microscopic thromboemboli or pulmonary infarctions have been found in more than 150 sheep with an IVOX implanted in the vena cavae for up to 19 days.
- Neither local infection at the venous insertion site nor systemic infection in the blood stream or remote tissue have been observed during IVOX utilization for up to 19 days in awake, standing sheep.
- The IVOX device maintains its gas transfer function for up to 19 days of continuous use in moderately heparinized, awake, standing sheep.

- flow rate of blood over the IVOX hollow fibers (cardiac output/venous return of the subject with an indwelling IVOX);
- blood flow pattern around the IVOX hollow fibers (proper deployment of crimped hollow fibers, ratio of hollow fiber volume to blood volume within the vena cavae, extent of mixing of blood flowing over the IVOX device);
- PCO_2 and PO_2 in the blood exposed to IVOX (CO_2 and O_2 partial pressure gradients across the IVOX membrane);
- rate of gas flow through (in and out of) the IVOX device;
- intraluminal pressure (vacuum) of gas within IVOX hollow fibers;
- composition of gas delivered to IVOX;
- hemoglobin content of circulating blood exposed to IVOX.

These IVOX gas transfer experiments also demonstrated that quantification of CO_2 removal by the IVOX device could be accomplished accurately and easily by simply reading the flow rate of gas through the IVOX device and noting the carbon dioxide content of the exhaust gas coming out of IVOX. Placing an accurate flowmeter in the IVOX gas conduit and routing IVOX exit gas through a continuous-reading capnometer produces the necessary data to calculate the quantity of CO_2 removed from blood flowing over the IVOX. Since 100% oxygen is delivered to IVOX (CO_2 content of the IVOX inflow gas is zero), the % CO_2 in the IVOX outflow gas multiplied by the gas flow rate though IVOX (in ml/min) gives the rate of CO_2 removal from the blood by IVOX (in ml/min). This simple method of quantifying CO_2 tansfer rate can be applied whether IVOX is indwelling in the subject's vena cavae or whether blood flow passes over an extracorporeal IVOX device *in* an *ex vivo* perfusion experiment.

On the other hand, accurate assessment of the rate of O_2 transfer into blood through an IVOX device lying in the vena cavae presents formidable problems. Determination of O_2 content of gas flowing into and out of an IVOX device to the degree of accuracy necessary requires rather sophisticated techniques (such as mass spectrometry) not readily applicable or available in the operating room or the ICU. Corrections for the accumulation of nitrogen, CO_2, and water vapor in the IVOX outlet gas must also be considered. Attempts to calculate O_2 transfer rate by assessing O_2 content of blood coming to an IVOX in the vena cavae, compared to blood leaving IVOX are circumvented by inability to obtain a meaningful sample of pre-IVOX blood to compare with the readily available post-IVOX (pulmonary arterial) blood. Because of differences in O_2 content of blood entering the vena cavae from their various tributaries (femoral, lumbar, renal, hepatic, coronary sinus, azygos, subclavian, jugular veins), all of this blood being exposed to IVOX, no truly representative pre-IVOX mixed venous blood sample can be obtained.

Estimated O_2 transfer rate by means of an IVOX device indwelling in the vena cavae can be arrived at by comparing the O_2 content of pulmonary artery blood sampled with an IVOX device indwelling in the vena cavae but with no flow of gas into or out of IVOX to the O_2 content of pulmonary artery blood collected after oxygen flow through IVOX has been established for 5 min. In order to be meaningful, the IVOX-on and IVOX-off samples of PA blood must be taken with as little intervening time as possible (allowing at least 5 min for equilibration between sampling). Also, the subject's cardiac output, O_2 transfer through the natural lungs, and metabolic gas utilization/production must be stable during the IVOX-on/IVOX-off sampling time periods. Recognizing and adjusting to these variables and determining cardiac output (blood flow over the IVOX device) during the IVOX-on and IVOX-off time periods permits calculation of an estimated rate of O_2 transfer through the IVOX device. Unfortunately, as a consequence of the difficulty in maintaining physiological stability during the IVOX-on/IVOX-off time periods, this method of estimating O_2 delivery through an IVOX device in the vena cavae may produce erratic, variable, and rather inaccurate results [33].

Because of these difficulties in quantifying O_2 transfer through an IVOX device lying in the vena cavae, an *ex vivo* experimental model was utilized to accurately assess gas transfer performance of the IVOX device. In these *ex vivo* experiments, veno-venous bypass of blood from an anesthetized animal (sheep or dog) is pumped through a test chamber approximately the size and configuration of the vena cavae in which is deployed an IVOX device. In such experiments, simultaneous samples of blood entering and exiting the test chamber can be obtained for analysis of O_2 content; flow rate of blood over and around the IVOX device can be varied at will and can be accurately measured; and gas pressures, flow rates, and samples for analysis can be readily obtained. The data thus produced permits accurate, reliable quantification of both O_2 and CO_2 transfer performance of an IVOX device under conditions which simulate, but are not identical with, the *in vivo* conditions where IVOX lies in the vena cavae.

Summary of gas transfer performance of various sized IVOX devices as determined by animal *ex vivo* and animal *in vivo* experiments and in the first few human clinical trials of IVOX is recorded in the Table 4 [33].

IVOX gas transfer efficacy in experimental animals with induced acute respiratory failure. The third step in the development of IVOX was to investigate its performance in hypoxic, hypercarbic laboratory animals. Again, sheep were utilized. Acute respiratory failure was produced in anesthetized, curarized animals by hypoventilation during acute experiments; and for chronic experiments in awake, standing animals, ARF was induced by applying various methods which simulate the pathophysiology of human ARDS. IVOX performed well in all these experiments, removing significant quantities of CO_2 from hypercarbic blood and adding similar amounts of oxygen to hypoxic blood. As examples of the efficacy of IVOX in

Table 4. Quantitative gas transfer achieved by means of IVOX

IVOX	O_2 transfer cc/min		Human	CO_2 transfer cc/min		Human
Size	Animal	Animal	*in vivo*	Animal	Animal	*in vivo*
(mm OD)	*ex vivo*	*in vivo*	(ARF)	*ex vivo*	*in vivo*	(ARF)
5	15.4	18.0	—	20.5	13.8	—
6	22.8	35.5	—	33.2	24.8	—
7	28.5	66.7	52.4	44.8	39.8	48.2
8	34.9	97.5	66.3	53.2	48.6	70.5
9	45.9	115.7	73.2	66.8	60.4	72.8
10	52.9	133.0	104.7	80.7	72.2	74.3

augmenting gas transfer in laboratory animals with induced ARF, the following experiment summaries are recorded:

A normal 85 kg adult sheep was anesthetized with intravenous barbiturates, a cuffed endotracheal tube was placed, an oximetrix thermal dilution catheter was placed in the pulmonary artery via the left jugular vein, and a monitoring/sampling catheter was placed in the aortic arch via the left carotid artery. A size 10 IVOX device was placed in the vena cavae via the right external jugular vein. Baseline blood gas determinations at this time, with the animal anesthetized and breathing normally, indicated that arterial blood $PaO_2 = 92.6$ torr, $PCO_2 = 34.2$ torr, while

Table 5. Changes in blood gases in pulmonary artery blood related to turning indwelling IVOX on and off. (Sheep made mildly hypoxic and hypercarbic by hypoventilation)

	IVOX on	IVOX off
Gas flow rate into IVOX	2.640 ml/min	0
CO_2 content of IVOX exhaust gas	3.03%	0
Cardiac output	6.1 l/min	6.1 l/min
Pulmonary artery blood		
PO_2	43.9 torr	40.2 torr
PCO_2	47.3 torr	54.4 torr
pH	7.365	7.326
Hb	11.8 g/dl	11.8 g/dl
O_2 saturation	55.1%	48.4%
O_2 content	9.3 ml/dl	8.2 ml/dl

O_2 transfer by IVOX $= (9.3 - 8.2) \times 6.1 \times 10 = 67$ ml/min.

CO_2 transfer by IVOX $= 2.640 \times 0.0303 = 80$ ml/min.

Sheep # 279 (body wt = 88 kg; IVOX size = 10)

Table 6. Changes in PA blood gases with IVOX turned on and off. (Sheep made severely hypoxic and hypercarbic by hypoventilation.)

	IVOX off	IVOX On
Gas flow into IVOX	0	2.730 ml/min
CO_2 content of IVOX exhaust gas	0	4.9%
Cardiac output	4.93 l/min	4.93 l/min
PA Blood		
PO_2	20.2 torr	38.8 torr
PCO_2	97.9 torr	90.1 torr
pH	7.119	7.127
Hb	15.0 g/dl	15.0 g/dl
O_2 saturation	20.3%	32.6%
O_2 content	4.8 ml/dl	6.9 ml/dl

CO_2 transfer by IVOX $= 2.370 \times 4.9\% = 133.8$ ml/min

O_2 transfer by IVOX $= (4.93 \times 10) \times 6.9 - 4.8) = 103.5$ ml/min

Sheep # 279 (body wt = 88 kg; IVOX size = 10)

the PA blood $PO_2=51.6$ torr and $PCO_2=40.1$ torr. The animal was then paralyzed with intravenous Pavulon and hypoventilated by means of a Bennett M-I ventilator to achieve a stable condition of mild hypoxia and hypercarbia, as determined by repeated arterial and pulmonary artery blood gas determinations (Table 5). Gas flow was then instigated into/through the IVOX device. Within 1 min, the continuous-reading capnometer sampling from the IVOX exhaust gas indicated 3.03% CO_2 in the IVOX exit gas, at a flow rate of 2,640 ml of gas through IVOX. When gas flow into IVOX was turned on, the oximeter-monitored O_2 saturation in the PA rose from 48% to 55%. Cardiac output was stable at 6.1 l/min. When gas flow through IVOX was turned off, blood gases in the PA and arterial blood returned to the baseline mildly hypoxic/hypercarbic levels (Table 5). More severe respiratory insufficiency of the natural lungs was then induced by more marked hypoventilation, producing PO_2 of 35 torr and PCO_2 of 94 torr, with IVOX turned off (Table 6). PA blood under these conditions demonstrated PO_2 of 20 torr and PCO_2 of 98 torr. When gas flow through IVOX was turned on, the pulmonary artery PO_2 increased to 39 torr and the PCO_2 fell to 90 torr. PaO_2 increased to 56 torr and PCO_2 decreased to 85 torr. These changes in blood gases during IVOX utilization in the sheep made hypoxic and hypercarbic by hypoventilation are summarized in Table 5 and Table 6. The quantity of O_2/CO_2 transferred by IVOX to/from the animal's circulating blood is also shown in Table 5 and Table 6. More than 40 acute hypoventilation experiments of this type have been carried out, all demonstrating similar findings.

The following laboratory experiment is reported to illustrate utilization of the IVOX device to augment blood gas exchange in a subject with experimentally produced acute, severe, reversible respiratory failure. Acute respiratory insufficiency was induced in an otherwise normal mature 71 kg sheep by the Kolobow airway barotrauma method [34]. After 40 h of MV with peak inspiratory pressures of 50

Table 7. Effects of IVOX on arterial blood gases of a sheep with acute, severe, ventilator dependent respiratory failure (Kolobow barotrauma model)

Event	Ventilator parameter				Arterial blood gases			
	FiO_2 (torr)	Min Vol (ml)	PIP (cm H_2O)	PEEP (cm H_2O)	PaO_2 (torr)	$PaCO_2$ (torr)	O_2 Sat (%)	O_2 Content ml/dl
Baseline, pre-injury	0.21	7000	23	0	88.4	31.9	100.0	—
ARF with normal ventilatory assist	0.21	8400	23	0	24.2	58.4	30.3	—
ARF with intensive ventilatory assist	10	8400	45	13	50.7	53.0	73.4	—
Ventilatory assist & IVOX for 30 minutes	0.70	8400	45	10	55.9	38.0	85.6	18.3
Ventilatory assist & IVOX for 2 hours	0.60	8400	36	3	90.7	35.8	96.7	19.8
Ventilatory assist & IVOX for 24 hours	0.35	8400	33	0	70.1	40.3	89.6	16.6
Ventilatory assist & IVOX for 48 hours	0.30	8400	29	0	75.7	34.3	93.6	21.4

cm H_2O, and minute volume of 8.4 l/min, the PaO_2 was 50.7 torr, $PaCO_2 = 53.0$ torr, and pH = 7.179; $PAPO_2 = 42.7$ and $PCO_2 = 57.8$ torr; cardiac output was 7 l/min. These findings remained essentially unchanged during 6 h of intensive mechanical ventilator support (Table 7). At this point, a size 7 IVOX device was inserted into the vena cavae through the right jugular vein and oxygen was pulled through IVOX at 2 l/min. Within half an hour of IVOX assistance, PaO_2 had increased to 55.9 torr while the ventilator FiO_2 had been reduced to 70%. Two hours after IVOX assistance began the PaO_2 was 90 torr, and throughout the next 48 h it remained above 70 torr, while the ventilator FiO_2 was reduced to room air (Table 7). Similar, but more striking, changes were observed in $PaCO_2$. Normal ventilation in the barotraumatized animal resulted in hypercarbia, with an $PaCO_2$ of 58.4 torr and pH of 7.179. Intensive ventilator support reduced the $PaCO_2$ only slightly, to 53 torr. However, after 24 min of IVOX assistance, the $PaCO_2$ was down to 38 torr, and it remained in the normal range for 48 h, even through mechanical ventilator assistance was reduced markedly (Table 7). The relationship between FiO_2 in the ventilator to the animal's PaO_2 before and after implementation of IVOX assistance is illustrated by Fig. 5. There was a significant increase in oxygenation of the blood with IVOX assistance, even though the concentration of oxygen delivered to the injured natural lungs by the ventilator was progressively reduced. The effect of IVOX on the pulmonary arterial blood PCO_2 of the hypercarbic, ventilator supported animal was favorable, showing return to normal levels

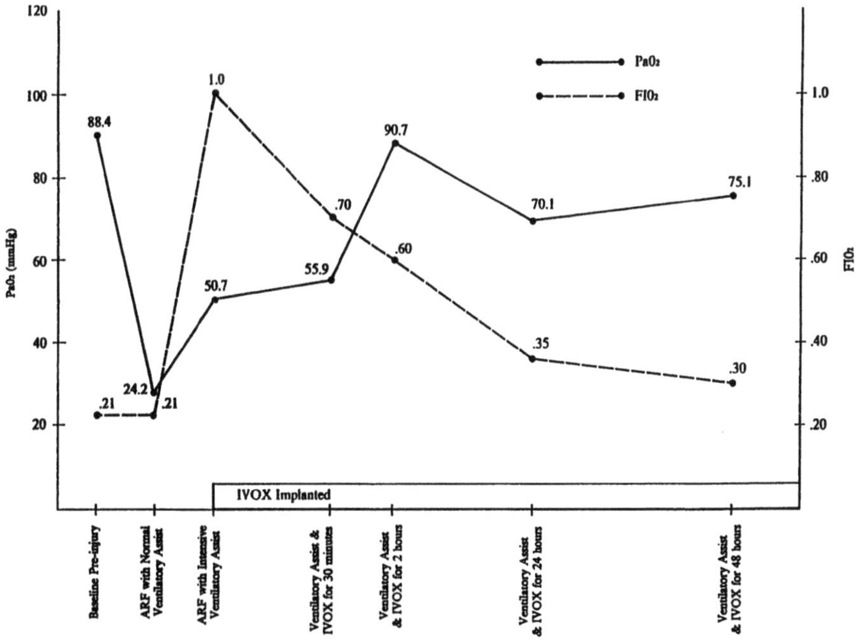

Fig. 5. Relationship between ventilator FiO_2 and PaO_2 in a ventilator-dependent ARF sheep with and without IVOX support. Note the progressive rise in arterial oxygenation when IVOX is supplied, despite the rapid reduction in FiO_2 supplied by the ventilator.

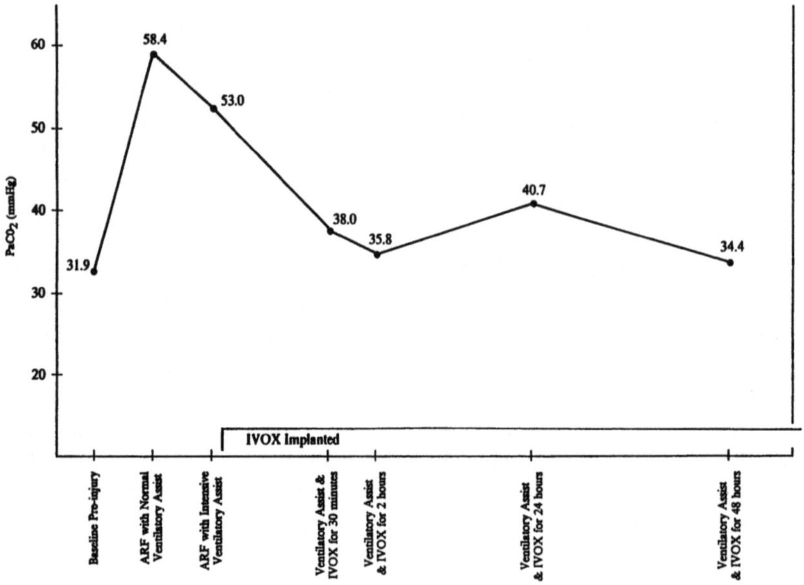

Fig. 6. Changes in $PaCO_2$ produced by IVOX in a ventilator-dependent, hypercarbic ARF sheep. Note that hypercarbia persists despite maximum ventilator support. With the additional support of IVOX the $PaCO_2$ rapidly decreases, becoming normal within 2 hours

within 2 h after IVOX support was begun (Fig. 6). The gas pressures produced in the animal's airways by the mechanical ventilator before and during IVOX utilization showed a favorable course (Fig. 7). A significant decrease in both PEEP and PIP was achieved during IVOX assistance. The quantity of oxygen delivered to the sheep's circulating blood by the IVOX device during this experiment was estimated by the difference in O_2 content of the pulmonary artery blood when the IVOX was turned off, compared to its being turned on, multiplied by the cardiac output. As shown in the Table 8; between 114 and 153 ml of O_2 were delivered by IVOX during this experiment. The amount of CO_2 transferred out of the animal's venous blood by the IVOX in its vena cavae during this experiment varied from 41 to 76 ml/min (Table 9).

Similar experiments have been carried out demonstrating the efficacy of IVOX in augmenting O_2/CO_2 transfer to/from venous blood of experimental animals with simulated ARF induced by smoke inhalation [35] and by intravenous injection of ethchlorvinyl [36].

Potential Clinical Application of IVOX

Objectives of IVOX Utilization

Based upon experience with IVOX in the experimental animal laboratory and on current human intensive care practices in respiratory ICUs, it would seem reasona-

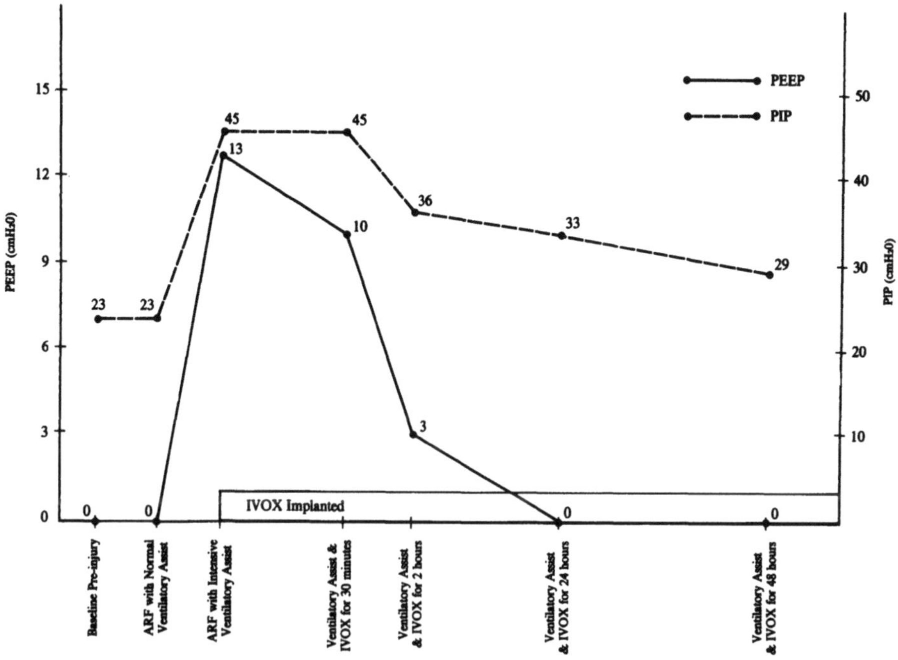

Fig. 7. Ventilator pressures in a ventilator-dependent ARF sheep with and without IVOX support. Note that with IVOX functioning, both the PEEP and peak inspiratory pressure (PIP) were decreased markedly (to normal levels), within 24 hours

Table 8. Oxygen transfer through IVOX in experimental barotrauma ARDS sheep

Time after IVOX implantation	Oxygen content of PA blood IVOX *on*	– IVOX *off*	= On-off difference	× Cardiac output l/min × 10	= O_2 transfer by IVOX (cc/min)
30 min	18.3	16.0	= 2.3	× 60	= 138
2 h	19.8	18.2	= 1.6	× 71	= 114
24 h	16.6	14.8	= 1.8	× 65	= 117
48 h	21.4	8.0	= 3.4	× 45	= 153

ble to consider the intended clinical application of IVOX to be temporary augmentation of the deficient blood gas exchange of patients with moderate to moderately severe, potentially reversible ARF in the ICU setting. With this application in mind, specific objectives for utilization of IVOX in ARF patients in different stages of lung dysfunction (severity of ARF) have been suggested in Table 10.

In patients with severe (advanced stages) ARF, including ARDS, who are hypoxic and/or hypercarbic while receiving maximum support by means of a mechanical ventilator (FiO_2 at 1.0, high airway pressures, high ventilatory minute volume),

Table 9. CO_2 transfer through IVOX in barotrauma experimental ARDS sheep

Time	% CO_2 in IVOX outlet gas (capnograph)	$PaCO_2$ (torr)	Gas flow rate through IVOX (cc/min)	CO_2 removed by IVOX (cc/min)
Immediately after IVOX turned on	3.8	53.0	2.000	76
30 min after IXOV implantation	2.3	38.0	2.000	46
2 h after IVOX implantation	2.8	35.5	1.600	44
24 h after IVOX implantation	3.4	40.3	2.000	68
48 h after IVOX implantation	3.4	34.8	1.200	41

Table 10. Objectives of IVOX utilization

In severe, reversible, ARF:
Augment inadequate mechanical ventilator support, thereby:
- Gain additional time for recovery of natural lungs
- Possibly avoid extracorporeal perfusion

Reduce the intensity of mechanical ventilator support:
- Decrase the FiO_2
- Lower the PEEP, PIP, MAP
- Decrease the MV
- Decrease danger of barotrauma/oxygen toxicity

In moderate, reversible ARF:
Decrease the time ventilator support is required
- Hasten discontinuing ventilator
- Facilitate weaning from ventilator
- Shorten stay in ICU
- Decrease danger of barotrauma/oxygen toxicity

In early, reversible ARF:
Adequately augment the deficient blood gas exchange, while at the same time:
- Avoiding endotracheal intubation
- Avoiding utilization of closed system positive pressure mechanical ventilator support

IVOX could be utilized to augment the deficient, life threatening blood gas exchange, thus supporting the patient a few days longer to permit some resolution of the natural lung dysfunction. In some cases, this "buying time" tactic of combined mechanical ventilatory and IVOX support could avoid resorting to a more invasive extracorporeal perfusion method for blood gas transfer. It can be anticipated that in some cases, with the additional gas transfer provided by IVOX, the patient's blood gases could be improved sufficiently that the intensity of mechanical ventilator support could be decreased progressively to less harmful levels. In less ill patients who are in moderate to moderately severe ARF and in whom acceptable PO_2

and/or PCO_2 can be maintained with mechanical ventilator support at rather high, potentially damaging levels (FiO_2 between 0.60 and 0.80, with PEEP >10, PIP >45, MAP >30, and/or MV >150 ml/min/kg body weight), IVOX could be utilized to permit maintenance of acceptable blood gases while the intensity of mechanical ventilator assistance is reduced to harmless levels (FiO_2 <0.50, PEEP <10, PIP <45, MAP <30, MV 150 ml/min/kg). Continued use of IVOX in this manner could shorten the time required for tracheal intubation, MV, and ICU care. The added risk of complications from prolonged MV might also be avoided. In earlier stages of ARF, when mechanical ventilator support is required at increasing levels of intensity which are at or just exceeding "safe" levels, IVOX inserted at this time could achieve and maintain satisfactory blood gases without further increases in mechanical ventilator settings, thus avoiding (preventing) the additional burden of barotrauma and/or oxygen toxicity on the existing pulmonary lesions. Finally, in certain patients in ARF, not adequately managed by O_2 administration by face mask or nasal cannula, IVOX utilization could be utilized instead of (in preference to) tracheal intubation and closed system positive pressure MV. Such patients could include any early ARF cases in whom positive airway pressure (PAP) by means of a mechanical ventilator is undesirable or contraindicated.

Perceived Indications for IVOX Utilization

With these objectives in mind for patients in various stages of ARF, currently IVOX is indicated in acute, potentially reversible respiratory insufficiency in patients with:

- Unacceptable blood gases despite maximum mechanical ventilator support;
- Borderline blood gases with mechanical ventilator settings just above maximum *SAFE* levels;
- Mandatory closed system mechanical ventilation in a patient with persistent active bronchopleural fistula and/or increasing mediastinal or subcutaneous ventilator therapy;
- Failure of the patient to tolerate the endotracheal tube, the controlled ventilation, or the sedation/muscular paralysis required for adequate mechanical ventilator therapy;
- Selected postsurgical or posttrauma patients with tracheobronchial or pulmonary tissues which cannot tolerate increased airway pressures;
- Acute, reversible, airway obstructions not amenable to mechanical ventilator therapy;
- Unsatisfactory blood gases when oxygen is administered by mask or nasal cannula and when initiation of closed system positive pressure mechanical ventilator support is undesirable, unacceptable, or particularly hazardous. (Examples: chronic asthma, emphysema, or COPD patients in respiratory insufficiency crisis).

It is readily apparent that many additional clinical scenarios present themselves in which IVOX utilization could be beneficial. The clinical trials currently underway are intended to help determine more precisely what the proper role of IVOX may be in the management of patients in ARF.

Contraindications for IVOX Utilization

As a result of experience with the IVOX device in the experimental animal laboratory coupled with observations during its early clinical trials, IVOX utilization is probably contraindicated in a number of clinical situations including:

- Likelihood that long term intensive respiratory assistance will be required (longer than 2 weeks);
- Recent major surgery or trauma in which systemic anticoagulation could cause bleeding;
- Uncontrolled sepsis (active infection, bacteremia);
- Major venous or venacaval thrombi that could embolize;
- No usable right femoral or right internal jugular access vein;
- Advanced multi-organ failure;
- Significantly depressed cardiac output, unresponsive to inotropes/fluids;
- No adequately trained personnel available for IVOX insertion and operation;
- Adequate gas transfer and anticoagulation monitoring capability not available;

In general, these contraindications have to do with preexisting conditions that could result in dislodging thrombotic material within the vena cavae or access veins, the likelihood of bleeding from the moderate systemic heparinization required during IVOX utilization, the threat of infection in or around the implanted IVOX device, the futility of temporary gas transfer augmentation in patients who are unlikely to recover, or the time limits currently imposed on IVOX utilization. As further refinements/optimization are made in the IVOX device, better understanding of its proper role as a support method is developed, and more experience is gained in its clinical application, these perceived contraindications will surely be modified considerably.

Limitations of IVOX

The small surface area of IVOX gas transfer membrane which can be inserted into the vena cavae effectively limits the quantity of O_2 and CO_2 the device can transfer into/out of circulating venous blood. Also, the relatively short time the current model of IVOX device can safely remain indwelling in the vena cavae constitutes a significant limitation to its use in ARF patients. The large venotomy, requiring an open surgical procedure for introduction and for explantation of the IVOX device, likewise limits its clinical application. The necessity for systemic anticoagulation during IVOX utilization imposes significant limitations on its application to some patients. The recognized limitations of IVOX, as it currently exists and can be used, are:

- Current models can only provide approximately 1/3 to 1/2 of the metabolic O_2 and CO_2 gas transfer requirements of most adult ARF patients (70 to 150 cc oxygen or carbon dioxide per minute).
- Time limit IVOX can safely remain indwelling in the vena cavae currently is between 7 and 19 days.
- Size of IVOX that can be inserted into vena cavae by current techniques is limited to a furled O.D. of 10 to 14 mm and with a gas transfer membrane surface area of 2,100 to 5,200 square centimeters.
- Patient must have adequate sized access right jugular or right common femoral vein and adequate vena cavae to accept the IVOX device.
- It must be feasible/possible for the patient to receive continuous mild to moderate systemic anticoagulation during utilization of current IVOX models.
- Only authorized centers and personnel who are fully trained/certified/authorized may utilize IVOX during the current clinical trials.

It may be reasonably anticipated that future modifications of the device and further optimization of its design, materials, and performance characteristics can effectively overcome or reduce these current limitations to its clinical utilization.

Current Status of IVOX

Preliminary Results of Early Human Clinical Trials of IVOX

Between February, 1990 and April, 1991 a limited number of human patients with advanced ARDS have received IVOX implantation to augment blood gas exchange, as Phase I of the IVOX clinical trials. The objective of these initial IVOX implantations was to determine the risks and hazards of IVOX utilization. Detailed protocols were followed, under FDA surveillance, to obtain data relative to the safety of IVOX utilization. By means of these clinical trials of IVOX risks and hazards, considerable preliminary data are available for consideration. Efficacy of IVOX in supporting patients in potentially reversible ARF is currently under investigation in Phase II of the ongoing clinical trials of this device.

Summary of the safety data from the first 18 patients entering the clinical trials of IVOX is recorded in Tables 11–16 and Fig. 8–10. The major safety concerns were considered to be possible IVOX-related causes of death, pulmonary thromboembolism, introduction of gas into the circulation, obstruction of venous return to the heart, and bleeding. These concerns were assessed by pathologists at necropsy of the first 10 patients dying during or after IVOX utilization. IVOX utilization did not result in necropsy evidence that any of these major concerns actually occurred (Table 12). Similarly, clinical observations by the attending physicians during IVOX utilization indicated that none of the major clinical or clinical laboratory concerns (such as febrile response, hemodynamic derangements, hematologic abnormalities, blood chemistry alterations, etc.) could be associated with utilization of IVOX (Table 12).

At necropsy, several incidental findings were recorded (Table 13), none of which the pathologists analyzing the cases considered to have clinical significance. These

Table 11. Preliminary observations from initial IVOX clinical trials

(A) Patients admitted to the trials:

- Patients receiving an IVOX implantation	18
- Cases deleted from study (user error, no data collected, insertion or utilization protocols violated)	4
- Cases with proper IVOX implantation and adequate data collection	14
- Surviving patients	4
- Patients undergoing necropsy after IVOX utilization	10

(B) IVOX insertion/utilization data

Insertion site	Number of cases
Right common femoral vein	10
Right internal jugular vein	4
IVOX size	
7	5
8	2
9	2
10	5
Time indwelling in vena cavae	
1–2 days	2
3–7 days	8
7–10 days	2
11–18 days	2

(C) Patient clinical data

Primary diagnosis producing ARDS	Number of cases	Surviving
Bacterial pneumonia	2	1
Aspiration pneumonitis	2	0
Post shock/post sepsis	3	2
Post perfusion	1	0
Viral pneumonia	3	0
Post trauma fat embolus	2	0
Post traums/pneumonectomy	1	1
	14	4

(D) Severity of ARF

		Number of cases	Surviving
+	Early ARF	0	—
+ +	Moderate ARF	0	—
+ + +	Moderately severe ARF	4	2
+ + + +	(End stage ARDS)	10	2

incidental findings were all related to the access veins utilized for IVOX insertion or to the vena cavae in which the IVOX device was indwelling. Some bleeding was noted during IVOX insertion, utilization, and removal in 5 of the first 14 clinical trials cases (Table 13). However, this problem was relatively minor in amount and

Table 12. Preliminary observations from initial IVOX clinical trials

Major IVOX safety concerns	
(A) Necropsy findings	Incidence at necropsy
IVOX-related *primary* cause of death	0/10
IVOX-related *contributing* cause of death	0/10
Grossly recognized thromboemboli in right heart/pulmonary arterial tree	0/10
Grossly recognized pulmonary infarction	0/10
Histopathologic evidence of IVOX-related thromboemboli/pulmonary infarction	0/10
Gross or microscopic gas, bubbles foam in vena cavae, right heart, or pulmonary vessels	0/10
Evidence of IVOX-related obstruction or interference to blood flow to right heart	0/10
Laceration, perforation, disruption, bleeding from vena cavae	0/10
IVOX-related sepsis, bacteremia, localized infection	0/10
(B) clinical observations relative to risks and hazards	Incidence
Clinical evidence of toxic/allergic/rejection responses to IVOX	0/14
Febrile response to IVOX	0/14
Edema/color change upstream to venotomy in:	
Right leg	3/10
Right head/neck	0/4
Infection	
Systemic	0/14
At venotomy site	0/14
Remote	0/14
Clinical evidence of pulmonary thromboembolism	0/14
Clinical evidence of pulmonary infarction	0/14

did not constitute a major risk or hazard in these patients. Hematologic changes observed during IVOX utilization were infrequent (Table 14). Platelet count decreased in 7 of 12 (58%) of the cases, but the decrease was mild and of no clinical significance, not requiring treatment. In only one case did the platelet count decrease to less than 100.000. It is possible that the transient changes in platelet counts were related to heparin administration, rather than to IVOX *per se*. White blood cell count, hemoglobin, and hematocrit were not altered by IVOX implantation. Hemolysis of red blood cells was not noted during IVOX utilization. Fibrinogen decreases noted were small in amount and appeared not to have clinical significance. Fibrin degradation products, such as D-dimer, and complement appeared not to be altered by IVOX utilization.

Hemodynamics, in general, were not depressed by IVOX indwelling in the vena cavae (Table 14). Noteworthy favorable changes included decrease in PAP in 71% of the cases, and decreased pulmonary wedge pressure and right atrial pressures in most of the patients in which signs of congestive heart failure were present before IVOX was inserted. It is particularly gratifying to note that of the 9 patients who

Table 13. Preliminary observations from initial IVOX clinical trials

Incidental IVOX-related findings at necropsy	
Finding	Incidence
Hematoma, IVOX insertion site	3/10
Thrombus in repaired vein	
Non-occlusive	2/6
Occlusive	1/6
Ligation of entry vein	
Jugular	4/4
Femoral	1/6
Thrombus on Vena Caval Intima	
Minor (1–3 patches, 0.1 cm in diameter)	4/10
Moderate (1 or more patches, >1 cm in diameter)	0/10
Extensive (non-occlusive thrombus involving 50% or more)	0/10
Occlusive (thrombotic material occluding vena cavae)	0/10
Bleeding related to IVOX utilization	
Type/location/severity	Incidence
No significant bleeding	9/14
Blood loss at insertion/explantation	
50–100 ml	2/14
>100 ml	3/14
Oozing at entry site	
Mild-no sequelae	2/14
Moderate-required non-surgical RX	2/14
Severe-requiring surgical correction	0/14
Bleeding at remote sites	
Mild-no clinical sequelae	1/14
Moderate-required transfusion but no other clinical sequelae	2/14
Severe-required transfusions, surgical intervention	0/14

needed intensive inotropic support for depressed cardiac function before IVOX was inserted, 6 (67%) experienced improvement in hemodynamics with decrease or withdrawal of inotropic medication during IVOX utilization. It is suspected that decreased airway pressures (PEEP, PIP, and MAP) required during IVOX utilization and the coincidental increase in PaO_2 were likely causes for this improved hemodynamics. Quantitative O_2 and CO_2 transfer by means of the implanted IVOX device in these first clinical trials (Table 15) indicate that the devices performed as expected, transferring significant quantities of O_2 into and CO_2 out of the circulating blood of these ARF patients.

The objective of these first clinical trials (Phase I) was to assess the risks and hazards (safety) of IVOX utilization. Most of the data collected, therefore, pertained to this subject. Nevertheless, some information was obtained relative to efficacy of the device, or to any possible benefits its utilization may have had for the patient. These observations (Table 16) indicate that 80 to 85% of the patients experienced improvement in blood gases during IVOX utilization. Similarly, in from

Table 14. Preliminary observations from initial IVOX clinical trials

Parameter	Incidence Increased >10%	Decreased >10%	No change +10% baseline
Hematologic changes			
Hb/HMCT	5/14	3/14	6/14
WBC	5/14	5/14	4/14
Platelet count	2/14	7/12 1/12*	3/12
Plasma free Hb	3/14	3/14	8/14
Fibrinogen	2/14	7/14	5/14
Fibrin degradation products (D-dimer)	4/14	4/14	6/14
Complement (C-3)	1/6	3/6	2/8
Hemodynamic effects			
Cardiac output	7/14	3/14	4/14
SVR	4/14	5/14	5/14
PVR	1/14	5/14	5/14
Cardiac support drug administration	1/9	6/9	2/9
$\overline{RAP}$ or $\overline{CVP}$	3/14	8/14	3/14
$\overline{PA}$	2/14	10/14	2/14
$\overline{CAP}$	5/14	3/14	6/14
$\overline{PWP}$	2/14	9/14	3/14

* decreased to <100000.

Table 15. Preliminary observations from initial IVOX clinical trials

Quantitative oxygen transfer through IVOX reported in the first 18 clinical trials in human ARDS patients

Size of IVOX	O_2 transfer into venous blood (cc/min) Mean	Range	Number of data points
# 7	52.4	18–128	9
# 8	66.3	42– 84	5
# 9	73.2	56– 84	4
#10	104.7	66–142	3
	CO_2 transfer into venous blood (cc/min)		
	Mean	Range	Number of data points
# 7	48.2	19– 60	9
# 8	70.5	47– 82	5
# 9	72.8	55– 90	4
#10	74.3	55–108	3

Table 16. Preliminary observations from initial IVOX clinical trials

Benefits to patients noted in first 14 IVOX implantations	
Blood gas changes	*Incidence*
Increase in PaO_2 (greater than 20%)	12/14 (85%)
Decrease in $PaCO_2$ (greater than 20%)	8/10 (80%)
Changes in ventilator settings	
Reduced FiO_2 (by more than 20%)	12/14 (85%)
Reduced FiO_2 (to <0.50)	10/14 (70%)
Reduced PEEP (by more than 20%)	9/14 (64%)
Reduced PIP (by more than 20%)	10/14 (70%)
Reduced MAP (by more than 20%)	10/14 (70%)
Reduced MV (by more than 20%)	7/9 (77%)
Changes in clinical picture	
Sealed air leak	5/8 (62%)
Reduced or discontinued cardiovascular inotropic drug support	6/9 (67%)
Decreased lung dysfunction	10/14 (70%)

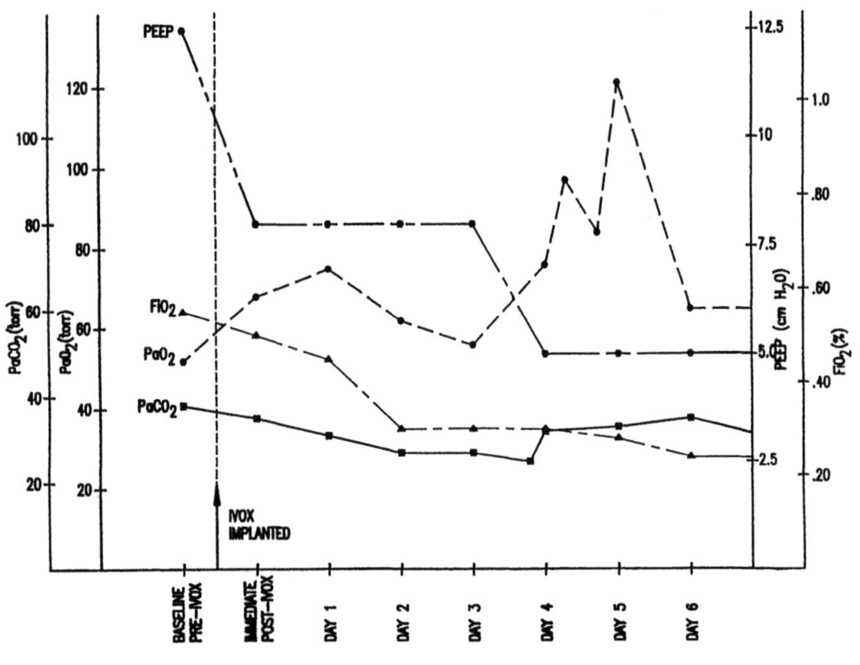

Fig. 8. Case 2. Changes in blood gases and ventilator settings following IVOX utilization in a patient with advanced ARDS. Note the rapid decrease in PEEP and FiO_2 delivered by the mechanical ventilator following insertion of IVOX. This was accompanied by recovery from the hypoxemia and hypercarbia associated with the patient's acute respiratory failure. The patient made a complete recovery

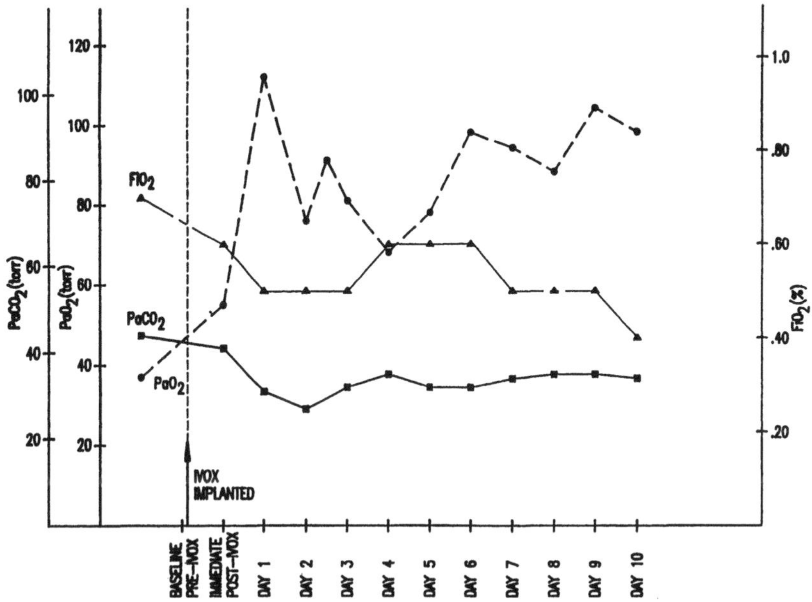

Fig. 9. Case 3. Favorable response in blood gases when IVOX was utilized in an ARDS patient who later died from non-pulmonary problems. Note the improvement in $PaCO_2$ and PaO_2, while the FiO_2 was decreased significantly; the patient's lung dysfunction being overcome nicely following augmentation of blood gas transfer by means of IVOX. However, death occurred a few days later from causes unrelated to the ARDS or to the IVOX utilization

64 to 85% of the patients it was possible to decrease the intensity of mechanical ventilator support during IVOX augmentation of blood gas transfer.

While the number of patients entering the IVOX clinical trials to date are too few in number to provide adequate data from which definitive conclusions can be made, definite safety and efficacy trends are apparent, summarized as follows:

1. No major complications, problems, or unfavorable sequelae attributed to IVOX utilization were recognized clinically or by clinical laboratory tests during or after IVOX utilization in the first 18 severely ill human ARDS patients appropriately and adequately studied in the Phase I clinical trials of IVOX.
2. No significant gross or histologic pathologic findings attributable to IVOX utilization were observed at necropsy examination of the first 10 Phase I ARDS patients who died during or after IVOX utilization.
3. Evidence of significant clinical benefit to the patient was observed in 11 of the first 14 Phase I patients (78%) in whom IVOX was utilized to augment deficient blood gas exchange. These benefits included: improved PaO_2 and $PaCO_2$ in the patient; decreased FiO_2, PEEP, PIP, mean airway pressures, and minute volume provided by the mechanical ventilator; reduced bronchopleural leak; and improved hemodynamics in certain patients, coincident with decreasing the high airway pressures delivered by the mechanical ventilator.

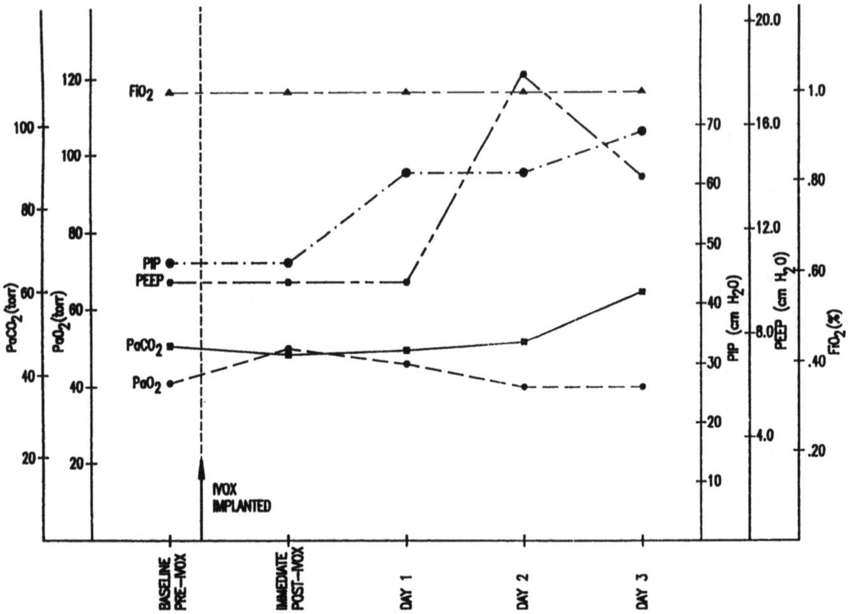

Fig. 10. Case 4. Failure of IVOX utilization and maximum ventilator support to alter the unfavorable, fatal course of a patient in end-stage ARDS. Note that the FiO_2 delivered by the mechanical ventilator remained at 1.00. Also, the airway pressures (PEEP and PIP) had to be increased significantly on the second day after IVOX was implanted. Despite all this augmentation of blood gas transfer, the hypoxemia and hypercarbia were refractory. The patient expired on the 3rd day of IVOX utilization, with complete respiratory failure, sepsis syndrome, and hemodynamic failure

4. To date, the limited data produced by the first group of human patients in severe ARDS who have received IVOX implantation/utilization appear to be consistent with the favorable safety and efficacy data previously collected from extensive experimental laboratory implantations of IVOX in normal sheep.

Selected Case Reports

The following case summaries are reported as illustrations of the effect of IVOX utilization in patients with ARF:

Case 1: This 76 year old Caucasian man underwent successful femoropoplileal bypass grafting for a severely ischemic left leg. On the 3rd postoperative day he became severely hypoxemic (PO_2 of 55 torr) and moderately hypercarbic (PCO_2 of 54 torr) despite closed system MV at an FiO_2 of 1.0 and PEEP of 10 cm H_2O. His hemodynamics were depressed, with C.I. = 3.1 l/min/m^2, wedge pressure of 12 torr while receiving an epinephrin infusion. Chest x-ray supported the clinical diagnosis of ARDS. A size 9 IVOX device was inserted through the right common femoral vein. Within 12 h, the blood gases were markedly improved with PaO_2 of 90 torr and $PaCO_2$ of 32 torr, despite significant reduction in the ventilator FiO_2 (to 0.70) and PEEP (to 6 cm H_2O). There was concomitant hemodynamic improvement, resulting in discontinuation of the inotropic support. After 6 days of IVOX augmentation of blood gas transfer the natural lungs had regained sufficient function that normal blood gases ($PaO_2 = 80$ torr; $PaCO_2 = 30$ torr) were maintained with the ventilator delivering room air at no PEEP. Two days later the endotracheal tube was removed. The patient thereafter left the ICU and has made complete recovery from his ARDS.

This case represents excellent recovery from lifethreatening ARDS when IVOX was utilized to augment blood gas transfer being achieved by intensive MV. This permitted reduction in the intensity of mechanical ventilator support, thereby possibly preventing the development of irreversible lung pathology which could have developed as a result of prolonged high intensity MV superimposed on ARDS. Four (28.6%) of the first 14 Phase I clinical trials patients with advanced ARDS followed a similar course to recovery.

Case 2: This 21 year old Caucasian man developed a viral pneumonitis which progressed rapidly so that within 2 days he was in ARF in which his PaO_2 was 51 torr and $PaCO_2$ was 38 torr despite mechanical ventilator support at an FiO_2 of 0.55, PEEP of 12.5 cm H_2O, and MV of 17 l/min. Rather than increase the intensity of the mechanical ventilatory assistance and risk adding the effects of barotrauma and oxygen toxicity to the lung dysfunction, the attending physician elected to augment the deficient blood gas exchange with IVOX. Within 1 h after IVOX insertion, the PaO_2 was 68 torr while the ventilator FiO_2 was reduced to 0.50, the MV to 11.0 l/min, and the PEEP to 8 cm H_2O (Fig. 8). Thereafter, the FiO_2 was decreased progressively to 0.30 on the 2nd day and room air on the 6th day; while the PaO_2 remained between 62 torr and 142 torr and the $PaCO_2$ between 25 torr and 35 torr. Lung dysfunction (as indicated by compliance, intrapulmonary shunt, and oxygenation index) dissipated rapidly and chest x-ray cleared completely. On the 6th day of IVOX utilization the device was removed; and 2 days later the endotracheal tube was removed (Fig. 8). The patient has remained normal, has returned to full activity and has no clinical evidence of residual sequelae from his ARF or from the 6 days of IVOX utilization.

This case represents successful utilization of IVOX to augment deficient blood gas exchange associated with potentially reversible ARF and in whom the lung dysfunction resolved quickly and the patient recovered completely without residual abnormalities. This type of course occurred in 4 (28.6%) of the first 14 ARDS patients in whom IVOX was utilized in the Phase I clinical trials.

Case 3: A 33 year old Hispanic alcoholic epileptic man aspirated vomitus during a seizure. Four days later, his aspiration pneumonitis had progressed to full-blown ARDS with hypoxia which was refractory to intensive mechanical ventilatory assistance. With a PEEP of 12.5 cm H_2O, FiO_2 of 1.00, and MV of 17.0 l/min, his PaO_2 was 38 torr (Fig. 9). When he became hemodynamically unstable on the 5th day of ARDS, a size 10 IVOX was inserted into his vena cavae via the right internal jugular vein. The device functioned well, transferring up to 95 cc O_2/min into the venous blood and removing up to 80 cc of CO_2/min. During IVOX utilization, the lung dysfunction improved so that the intensity of the mechanical ventilatory assistance could be reduced progressively until on the 7th day of IVOX support the ventilatory FiO_2 was 0.24, the PEEP was 5 cm H_2O, and the MV was 13.7 l/min; while the PaO_2 was 64 torr and $PaCO_2$ was 32 torr. Chest x-ray evidence of interstitial edema/atelectasis had cleared considerably. Two days later the IVOX device was removed and the patient's blood gases remained satisfactory with minimal support from the mechanical ventilator (Fig. 9). However, 4 days after IVOX was removed, the patient developed the sepsis syndrome, requiring inotropic hemodynamic support and increase in ventilator support, with an FiO_2 of 0.40 and PEEP of 10 cm H_2O. Blood cultures were negative. He expired suddenly the following day. Necropsy findings indicated the cause of death was acute hepatic failure with advanced liver degeneration/cirrhosis. There was no clinical or necropsy evidence of pathologic findings, injury, or harmful sequelae from the 9 days of IVOX implantation.

This case is representative of 7 (50%) of the 14 ARDS Phase I clinical trials patients in whom considerable benefit was evident from IVOX utilization, in that blood gases improved and intensity of MV decreased, but the patient did not survive hospitalization, dying from causes other than blood gas abnormalities.

Case 4: This 40 year old policeman received gunshot wounds to the right chest and right knee. Emergency resection of segments of the right upper, middle, and lower lobes was performed. Although he stabilized physiologically immediately postoperatively, 7 days later typical ARDS developed with panlobar infiltrates of the left lung and remaining portions of the right lung. He developed hypoxemia ($PaO_2 = 41$ torr) and hypercarbia ($PCO_2 = 52$ torr) which were refractory to mechanical ventilator support at 100% oxygen with PEEP of 12 cm H_2O and PIP of 48 cm H_2O (Fig. 10). Persistent air leak developed into the left pleural space, necessitating placement of 3 chest tubes connected to water seal drainage. There was no improvement after 12 days of what was considered maximum mechanical ventilator support, so a size 8 IVOX device was implanted into the vena cavae through the right common femoral vein. The device functioned well, transferring 60 to 80 cc of O_2/min into the pulmonary arterial blood and removing up to 90 cc of CO_2/min. Despite this augmented blood gas exchange by IVOX, the patient's blood gases did not improve and it was not possible to decrease the FiO_2 or PEEP supplied by the mechanical ventilator. Forty eight hours later the lung compliance decreased and the intrapulmonary shunt increased significantly, requiring considerable increases in the PEEP and PIP (Fig. 10). Thereafter, the sepsis syndrome rapidly developed and the patient required massive inotropic hemodynamic support. Finally, he became unresponsive and died 3 days after IVOX was inserted. Necropsy showed severe ARDS, multiple areas of atelectasis in both lungs, and post resectional changes in the remaining left lung tissues. There were no pathological lesions attributable to the IVOX implantation. Blood cultures were negative and there was no evidence of infection on IVOX or at the operative IVOX entry site.

This case illustrates no improvement in the patient, although IVOX appeared to be transferring significant quantities of O_2 and CO_2 into/out of the PA blood. The lung dysfunction persisted and increased to total respiratory failure, despite gas transfer augmentation by the mechanical ventilator and by IVOX. Death occurred with the patient both hypoxic and hypercarbic, the precipitating physiological derrangement being hemodynamic failure with the sepsis syndrome. Three of the first 14 Phase I clinical trials patients (21.4%) had a similar ICU course, with a persistent deterioration of clinical condition despite maximum blood gas transfer support by the mechanical ventilator plus IVOX.

Conclusions

To date, extensive experimental animal data and limited clinical trials of IVOX in human ARF patients indicate that IVOX utilization is simple and easy to carry out, is accompanied by minimal complications or adverse effects, and provides limited, but clinically significant, O_2/CO_2 transfer into/out of circulating venous blood.

The most appropriate clinical indications for IVOX utilization are to be determined by controlled clinical trials, now underway. The results will form the basis on which the physician can select the safest, most efficacious, and most cost effective modality to utilize for temporary augmentation of blood gas exchange to/from the circulating blood of specific groups of hypoxic and/or hypercarbic patients in acute, potentially reversible respiratory failure.

References

1. Levitsky MG (1986) Pulmonary physiology, 2nd ed; McGraw & Hill, New York, pp 136–156
2. Comroe JH (1974) Physiology of respiration, 2nd ed; Year Book, Chicago, pp 183–196
3. Guyton AC (1986) Text book of medical physiology, 7th edition, S. B. Saunders, Co., Philadelphia. pp 466–527
4. Selkurt EE (1984) Physiology, 5th ed. Little, Brown, and Co., Boston/Toronto, pp 336–405
5. Seaton A, Seaton D, Leitch AG (1989) Crofton and Douglas's respiratory diseases, 4th ed. Blackwell Scientific Publications, London, pp 526–538
6. Zapol WM, Folke KJ (1985) Acute respiratory failure, Marcel Dekker, Inc., New York, pp 1-21
7. Gordon BL, Carlton RA, Faber LP (1969) Clinical cardiopulmonary physiology - 3rd edition. Grune and Stratton, New York, pp 327–403 and 702–728
8. Shapiro BA, Harrison RA, Trout CA (1979) Clinical application of respiratory care, Yearbook Medical Publishers, Chicago, Chap. 7, pp 133–152
9. Spearman CB, Sheldon RL (1982) Egan's fundamentals of respiratory therapy. C.V. Mosby Co., St. Louis, Chap 12, 13:422-562
10. Bartlett RH, Gazzaniga AB, Wetmore NE, Rucker R, Huxtable RF (1980) Extracorporeal membrane oxygenation (ECMO) in the treatment of cardiac and respiratory failure in children. Trans Am Soc Artif Int Org 26:578
11. Bartlett RH, Andrews AF, Toomasian J, et al (1982) Extracorporeal membrane oxygenation for newborn respiratory failure: Forty five cases. Surgery 92:425–433
12. Hirschl RB, Bartlett RH (1987) Extracorporeal membrane oxygenation support in cardiorespiratory failure. Adv Surg 21:189–212
13. Funakubo A, Fukui Y, Kawamura R (1987) A compact extracorporeal oxygenator (ECMO) system using a single lumen catheter. Trans ASAIO 33:429–433
14. Sinard JM, Bartlett RH (1990) Extracorporeal membrane oxygenation (ECMO): Prolonged bedside cardiopulmonary by-pass. Perfusion 5:239–249
15. Gattinoni L, Kolobow T, Damia G, Agostoni A, Pesenti A (1979) Extracorporeal carbon dioxide removal ($ECCO_2R$): A new form of respiratory assistance. Intern J of Artif Organs 2:183
16. Gattinoni L, Agostoni A, Pesenti A, et al (1980) Treatment of acute respiratory failure with low-frequency positive-pressure ventilation and extracorporeal removal of CO_2. The Lancet:292–294
17. Kolobow T, Gattinoni L, Fumagalli R, et al (1982) Carbon dioxide and the membrane artificial lung: Their roles in the prevention and treatment of respiratory failure. Trans Am Soc Artif Int Org 28:20
18. Porrington KL, McRae K, Bellhouse BJ (1987) Extracorporeal CO_2 removal ($ECCO_2R$) improves oxygenation in a lung lavage model of acute respiratory failure. Trans ASAIO 33:574–578
19. Gattinoni L, Pesenti A, Mascheroni D, et al (1986) Low frequency positive-pressure ventilation with extracorporeal CO_2 removal in severe acute respiratory failure. JAMA 256:881–886
20. Mortensen JD (1987) An intravenacaval blood gas exchange (IVCBGE) device. Trans Am Soc Artif Intern Organs 33:570–573
21. Mortensen JD, Berry G (1989) Conceptual and design features of a practical, clinically effective, intravenous, mechanical blood oxygen/carbon dioxide exchange device (IVOX). Internat Journ Artif Org 12:384–389
22. Mortensen JD, Berry G, Winters S (1990) IVOX: An intracorporeal device for temporary augmentation of blood gas transfer in subjects with acute respiratory insufficiency. Cardiac Chronicle 4:1–6
23. Mortensen JD, Schaap RN, Henrie JN (1991) IVOX: An intravenous oxygenator. Hospimedica 9:32-36
24. Morioka, Tohru (1990) A method for intravenous blood gas exchange. Clinical Anesthesia (Japan) 14:1149–1156

25. Kallis P, Al-Saady NM, Bennett D, Treasure R (1991) Clinical use of intravascular oxygenation, The Lancet (letter), Vol 337, no 8740, p 549
26. Matsunobe S, Isobe J, Mitsuno H, Shimizu Y (1987) Extracorporeal CO_2 removal by hemodialysis in patients with chronic respiratory failure. Trans Am Soc Artif Int Org 33:441–445
27. Stuart J, Updike J, Shults AM (1973) Excretion of carbon dioxide using an artificial kidney. J Appl Physiol 34:274–276
28. Zborowski M, Kmiotek W, Slwinsku J, Ciszecki J, Werynski A (1983) Carbon dioxide removal by a hemodialyzer with dialysate channel coupled to a bubble oxygenator. Artif Organs 7:481
29. Gille JP, Sauneir C, Baluais C, Battistella P (1984) Extracorporeal CO_2 removal by hemodialysis. ASAIO Journal 7:80–84
30. Gille JP, Bauer P, Bollaert PE, Tousseul B, Kachani-Nasour R, Munsch L (1989) CO_2 removal with hemodialysis and control of plasma aortic pressure. Trans Am Soc Artif Int Org 35:654–657
31. Nolte SH, Jonitz WJ, Grau J, Roth H, Assenbaum ER (1989) Hemodialysis for extracorporeal bicarbonate/CO_2 removal (EC-BIC CO_2R) and apneic oxygenation for respiratory failure in animal experiments. Trans Am Soc Artif Int Org 35:30–34
32. Mortensen JD (1989) Laboratory studies relative to IVOX safety and efficacy. Report to FDA. CardioPulmonics Inc., Salt Lake City
33. Bagley B, Bagley A, Froerer C, Brohamer J, Henrie J, Burkart J, Mortensen JD (1991) Quantification of blood gas transfer by means of IVOX. Trans Am Soc Artif Int Org (in press)
34. Mascheroni D, Kolobow T, Fumagalli R, et al (1985) Respiratory failure following induced hyperventilation: An experimental study. Critical Care Med 13:330
35. Cox CS, Zwischenberger JR (1991) Use of an intravascular membrane oxygenator (IVOX) in an ovine model. ASAIO (Abstracts) 20:63
36. Mortensen JD. CardioPulmonics, Inc., (unpublished data)

Weaning Assessment

M.J. Tobin

Introduction

Although mechanical ventilation (MV) can be lifesaving, it is associated with numerous complications, and thus, it should be discontinued as soon as possible. However, determination of the optimal time to discontinue ventilator support can be very difficult. While an experienced physician can frequently judge the likely outcome of a weaning trial, it is desirable to have objective measurements that decrease the dependence on the wisdom and skill of a physician [1–3]. By identifying patients who are likely to fail a weaning trial, such indices can prevent a premature weaning attempt and the development of severe cardiorespiratory and/or psychological decompensation. On the other hand, by identifying the earliest time that a patient is able to resume and sustain spontaneous ventilation, indices help to avoid unnecessary prolongation of the period of ventilator support. Finally, since these indices assess many different physiological functions, they may provide insight into the reasons for ventilator dependency in an individual patient and suggest alterations in management.

An ideal weaning index should include the following features:

1. It should assess the true pathophysiological determinants of weaning outcome;
2. It should provide precise quantitation of a physiological function, being proportional to the magnitude of an abnormality;
3. It should be easy to measure;
4. It should require minimal patient cooperation;
5. The index should have good reproducibility, and the underlying function being assessed should have limited natural variability; and
6. It should have high positive and negative predictive values.

The first of these points is especially critical: assessment of the true determinants of weaning outcome. These can be grouped into three major categories: psychological

Table 1. Indices used to predict weaning outcome

Oxygenation indices	Maximum voluntary ventilation
Vital capacity	Airway occlusion pressure
Maximum inspiratory pressure	Breathing pattern
Respiratory system compliance	Work of breathing
Minute ventilation	

problems, for which we have no simple objective indices, and abnormalities of pulmonary gas exchange and respiratory muscle pump function, for which we have a number of indices [4]. The physiological functions that are commonly assessed are listed in Table 1, and their rationale and predictive power are discussed below.

Pulmonary Gas Exchange

No single index of oxygenation is universally accepted to prohibit weaning, and a number of different criteria derived from arterial blood gas (ABG) measurements have been proposed [5].

Alveolar-arterial O_2 tension difference ($AaPO_2$) is calculated as $PAO_2 - PaO_2$, where PAO_2 (alveolar O_2 tension) can be estimated according to the modified alveolar gas equation

$$PAO_2 = (PB\text{-}PH20) \times FiO_2 - PaCO_2/R,$$

where PB = barometric pressure, PH20 = water vapor pressure (usually 47 torr), FiO_2 = fractional inspired O_2 concentration, $PaCO_2$ = arterial carbon dioxide tension, and R = respiratory exchange ratio (assumed to be 0.8), respectively. It remains normal when hypoxemia is solely due to hypoventilation, but any other factor making gas exchange less efficient will increase the $AaPO_2$ gradient. A major limitation of this index is that it changes unpredictably (depending on the ventilation/perfusion distribution) with changes in FiO_2. An $AaPO_2$ of less than 350 torr while inhaling an FiO_2 of 1.0 has been proposed as a predictor of a successful weaning outcome [6].

The *arterial/alveolar O_2 tension ratio* (PaO_2/PAO_2) remains more stable with changing levels of FiO_2 than $AaPO_2$ [7]. Thus, it is preferred as an index of gas exchange, although a value considered predictive of weaning outcome has not been proposed.

The *arterial/inspired O_2 ratio* (PaO_2/FiO_2) is the easiest index to calculate since it does not require solving the alveolar gas equation. However, unlike the PaO_2/PAO_2 ratio, it fails to adjust for fluctuations in $PaCO_2$ although this has little influence on calculations at high levels of FiO_2. Krieger et al. [8] recently examined the accuracy of a PaO_2/FiO_2 ratio of 238, which equivalent to a PO_2 of 50 torr with an FiO_2 of 0.21. In a retrospective study of 269 patients, the positve predictive value was 90%, indicating that 90% of the patients who had a PaO_2/FiO_2 ratio of 238 or more were successfully weaned. However, the negative predictive value was only 10%, indicating that only 10% of the patients with a PaO_2/FiO_2 ratio of less than 238 failed the weaning trial.

Vital Capacity

Vital capacity (VC) is the greatest volume of gas that a subject is able to exhale after taking a maximum inspiration. The normal VC is usually between 65 and 75 ml/kg; a VC of 10 ml/kg [9] or more [10] has been suggested as being essential to sustain spontaneous ventilation. This value is approximately twice the predicted tidal volume (VT) [11]. A VC of more than 10 or 15 ml/kg has been suggested as a standard predictor of weaning outcome [5, 10]. However, Tahvanainen et al. [12] found that a VC of 10 ml/kg was falsely positive in 18% of patients (predicted success but actual failure) and falsely negative in 50% (predicted failure but actual success). Similarly, in a prospective study of 33 postoperative patients, where weaning success was defined as sustained spontaneous respiration with a pH greater than 7.35, Milbern et al. [13] found that a VC of 15 ml/kg was falsely positive in 15% of patients and falsely negative in 63%.

Maximal Inspiratory Pressure

One of the major determinants of weaning outcome is the capacity of the respiratory muscles to meet ventilatory demands. The overall strength of the respiratory muscles is usually assessed by measurement of maximum inspiratory pressure (PI max) [14]. In patients being considered for a weaning trial, this is measured with a manometer attached to the opening of an endotracheal tube, and the best of three efforts is usually selected [7]. PImax is greatest following a complete expiration to residual volume. In healthy men, PImax is approximately 111 ± 34 cm H_2O, while values in women are approximately 25% lower. Considering the critical importance of respiratory muscle capacity in determining weaning outcome, one would expect PImax to be a good predictor. Indeed, Sahn and Lakshminarayan [15] found that all patients who generated PImax values of -30 cm H_2O or lower could be extubated successfully, while all patients with a PImax higher (i.e. less negative) than -20 cm H_2O required continued ventilator support. In a subsequent prospective study, Tahvanainen et al. [12] found that a threshold value of -30 cm H_2O was falsely negative in 100% of patients (predicted failure but actual success) and falsely positive in 26% (predicted success but actual failure). Other investigators have also found that PImax has limited power in predicting weaning outcome, especially in patients receiving prolonged MV [16, 17]. These disapointing results may have arisen because PImax does not take into account thoracic compliance or the position on the pressure-volume curve at which tidal breathing is occurring. Hyperinflation causes the patient to breathe on the upper, less compliant portion of the pulmonary pressure-volume curve and, also, causes shortening of the inspiratory muscles, which, respectively, lead to an increased work of breathing and the generation of less effective inspiratory pressure swings [18]. Another factor that may account for the poor predictive power of PImax is its dependence on respiratory muscle strength rather than endurance, since the latter may be a more important determinant of weaning outcome.

Respiratory System Compliance

To achieve adequate ventilation, it is necessary to generate sufficient muscular force to overcome the frictional resistance to airflow throughout the tracheobronchial tree, the frictional resistance during movement of the tissues of the lungs and chest wall, and the elasticity of the lungs and the chest wall. Elasticity is the reciprocal of compliance, which is the change in volume for a given change in distending pressure (the static pressure difference between the airway opening and the atmosphere for the respiratory system or between the airway opening and the pleural space for the lung). In patients receiving MV, respiratory system compliance (Crs) is calculated by dividing the delivered volume by the pressure registered on the ventilator gauge [7]. "Dialing in" an inspiratory pause will achieve conditions of zero gas flow at end-inspiration and airway pressure will fall to a plateau. If the patient is receiving positive end-expiratory pressure (PEEP), this must be substracted from the pressure reading before calculating Crs, i.e. Crs = volume delivered/(Plateau pressure - PEEP). The normal range is 60–100 ml/cm H_2O. Another index termed "dynamic characteristic" or "dynamic compliance" (Cdyn) can be calculated in a similar manner, i.e. tidal volume/peak inflationary pressure [7]. As in the case of Crs, Cdyn values are lower in the presence of disorders that decrease lung or chest wall elasticity, but Cdyn is also decreased in the presence of increased airway resistance. These indices are attractive because of their sound physiological basis, independence of patient effort, and relative independence of patient cooperation. However, a rigorous prospective examination of their accuracy in predicting weaning outcome has never been untertaken, although a Crs of less than 25 ml/cm H_2O is commonly considered predictive of an unsuccessful weaning outcome [4], because the associated work of breathing makes it difficult to sustain a level of ventilation necessary to achieve satisfactory gas exchange.

Minute Ventilation and Maximum Voluntary Ventilation

The relationship between minute ventilation (VE) and $PaCO_2$ provides a good indication of the demands being placed on the respiratory system [7]. Normal VE is about 6 l/min and a value of less than 10 l/min is desirable in a patient being considered for a weaning trial. Maximum voluntary ventilation (MVV), i.e. the volume of air that can be inhaled and exhaled with maximum effort over one minute, is normally 50 to 250 l/min. The relationship between VE and MVV provides a measure of ventilatory reserve [7]. A patient who is being considered for a weaning trial should be able to at least double his/her VE during a MVV maneuver. A problem with the MVV maneuver is its major dependence on motivation and the patient's ability to cooperate. Sahn and Lakshiminarayan [15] found that the combination of a VE of less than 10 l/min and the ability to double this value during a MVV maneuver was able to predict 100% of the weaning successes and 71% of the failures. However, Tahvanainen et al. [12] found that the VE criterion was falsely positive in 11% of patients (predicted success but actual failure) and falsely negative in 75% of patients (predicted failure but actual success), and the MVV criterion was falsely positive in 14% and falsely negative in 76% of patients.

Airway Occlusion Pressure

While a decreased respiratory drive [19] can lead to hypoventilation and hypercapnia, an inappropriately elevated respiratory drive places considerable stress on the

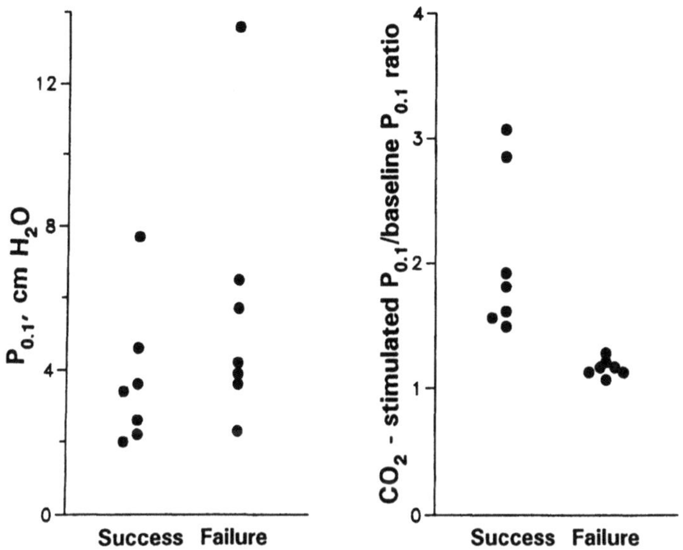

Fig. 1. Airway occlusion pressure (P0.1) responses in patients being weaned from mechanical ventilation (*left*). Note overlap in values between the patients who were successfully weaned and those who failed the weaning trial. The ratio of CO_2-stimulated P0.1 to baseline P0.1 in the same patients (*right*). Note that all of the successful patients have ratios of ≥ 1.49, whereas all of the failure group have ratios of ≤ 1.28. (From [40] with permission based on data from [23])

respiratory system. The airway pressure generated at 0.1 sec after initiating an inspiratory effort against an occluded airway (P0.1) is an index of respiratory drive [19]. Three groups of investigators [20–22] have recently reported that a high P0.1 value predicts weaning failure. The threshold value of P0.1 separating weaning success from weaning failure varied among the studies but appears to be approximately 4–6 cm H_2O (normal < 2 cm H_2O). In contrast to these studies, Montgomery et al. [23] found no difference in P0.1 values between patients with a successful and unsuccessful weaning outcome (Fig. 1). They also observed no difference between the patient groups in P0.1 measurements made during a hypercapnic challenge (inhaling 3% CO_2). However, hypercapnic augmentation of P0.1 expressed as the ratio of the CO_2-stimulated P0.1 to the baseline P0.1 was greater in the patients who were successfully weaned than those who failed the weaning trial. Further prospective studies are needed to document the accuracy of airway occlusion pressure (stimulated or unstimulated) as a predictor of weaning outcome.

Breathing Pattern

Attention has been recently focused on the pattern of breathing as a guide to weaning outcome, i.e. respiratory frequency (f), VT and rib cage-abdominal motion. This largely stems from a study by Cohen et al. [24] which suggested that respiratory muscle fatigue might be a primary cause of failure to wean from MV, and also that a bedside diagnosis of respiratory muscle fatigue could be made by detecting paradoxical motion of the abdomen (inward displacement during inspiration) and respiratory alternans (alteration in the contribution of the rib cage and abdomen to VT). This conclusion was based on a study of 12 patients exhibiting difficulty during weaning, 7 of whom developed a power spectral shift in their diaphragmatic electromyogram (EMG), which the investigators interpreted as indicating respiratory muscle fatigue. Abnormal rib cage-abdominal motion was observed in 6 of these 7 patients, but in none of the 5 patients without EMG changes. However, certain features of this study need to be noted. Ventilator support was reinstituted in all 12 patients within 40 min, thus limiting the clinical significance of these findings. Also, power-spectral shift of the EMG is not directly related to low-frequency fatigue, the form that is physiologically important [25]. Finally, no distinction was made between work of breathing and fatigue.

If detection of abdominal paradox truly indicates the presence of respiratory muscle fatigue, one would expect that all patients who display abdominal paradox should fail a trial of weaning. However, in a recent prospective study, Tobin et al. [26] found no difference in the amount of abdominal paradox between patients who were successfully weaned and those who failed a weaning trial (Fig. 2). Two other abnormalities of rib cage-abdominal motion did discriminate between the weaning success and weaning failure patients. The first of these indices was maximum compartmental amplitude to VT ratio (MCA/VT) (see derivation in Fig. 3), which quantitates *both* asynchronous and paradoxical motion of *both* the rib cage and abdomen. The superiority of this index over other indices of asynchronous and

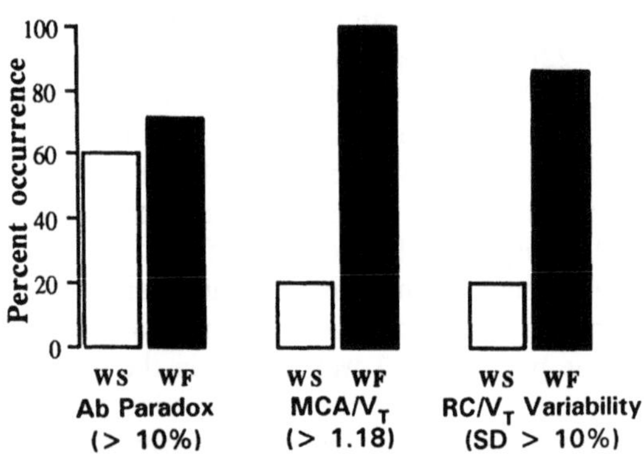

Fig. 2. The frequency of significant abnormalities of rib cage-abdominal motion in patients who were successfully weaned (WS) and in patients who failed a weaning trial (WF). Significant abdominal (Ab) paradox was considered present when paradoxic volume was >10% of the total Ab volume excursion (both in and out of phase). The maximum compartmental amplitude to tidal volume ratio (MCA/VT) (see derivation in Fig. 3) was considered significantly increased when it exceeded 1.18. A significant increase in the breath-to-breath variability in the relative contribution of the rib cage (RC) and Ab to tidal volume (VT) was considered present when the standard deviation (SD) of the RC/VT ratio exceeded 10%. Significant differences were observed between the two groups of patients in the occurrence of an increased MCA/VT ratio ($p < 0.001$) and increased variability of the RC/VT ratio ($p < 0.05$), but not for increased Ab paradox. (From [26] with permission)

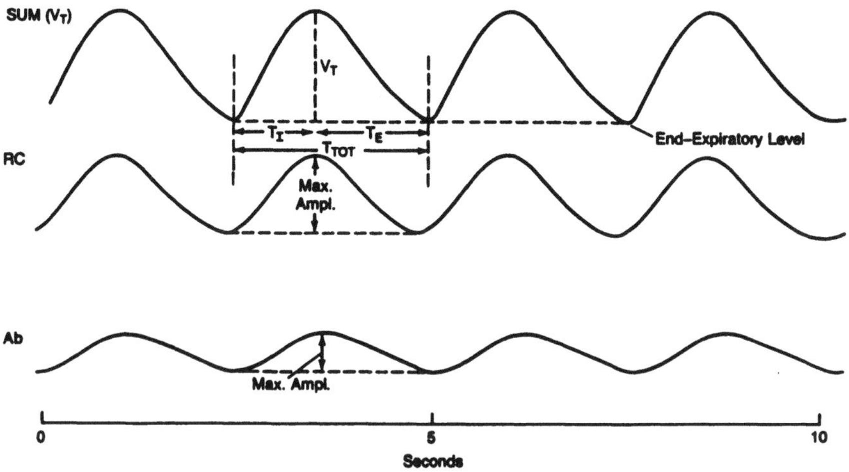

Fig. 3. Schematic recording of the respiratory cycle that depicts the points of reference for computation of the various breathing pattern parameters. The signals have been obtained with a respiratory inductive plethysmograph; thus SUM (VT) indicates tidal volume, which has been calibrated to spirometry and represents the algebraic sum of the rib cage (RC) and abdominal (Ab) excursions. TI represents inspiratory time; TE, expiratory time; Ttot, time of a total breath; and VT/TI, mean inspiratory flow. Alterations in the end-expiratory level represents changes in functional residual capacity, provided movement artifact is absent. Maximum amplitude is the trough-to-peak amplitude of the rib cage and abdominal excursions, irrespective to their phase relationship to the SUM signal; their arithmetic sum, designated maximum compartmental amplitude (MCA), is equivalent to the algebracic SUM signal when the rib cage and abdomen move in phase. (From [7] with permission)

paradoxical motion as predictors of weaning outcome was probably related to the fact that the patients who failed a weaning trial displayed considerable breath-to-breath fluctuation in the relative contribution of the rib cage and abdomen to VT, and the extent of abnormal motion tended to be divided between the two compartments [26]. The second discriminating index quantitated the breath-to-breath variability in the relative contribution of the rib cage and abdomen to VT in terms of the standard deviation of the rib cage/VT ratio (RC/VT). Patients who failed a weaning trial showed considerable breath-to-breath variation in the relative contribution of the rib cage and abdomen to VT, whereas the contribution was more constant in the successfully weaned patients [26]. Breath-by-breath plots of the MCA/VT ratio and RC/VT ratio in representative patients with unsuccessful and successful weaning outcomes are shown in Fig. 4 and 5, respectively. Of interest was the immediate onset of abnormal rib cage-abdominal motion following discontinuation of ventilator support in the patient who failed the weaning trial. Conceptually, it is difficult to reconcile this pattern of immediate alteration in breathing pattern (without subsequent progression) with the development of respiratory muscle fatigue. Indeed, further studies in healthy volunteers indicate that fatigue is neither a sufficient nor a necessary condition for the development of abnormal motion [27]; instead, abnormal motion is primarily related to increased respiratory load.

More simple indices of the breathing pattern also appear to be very useful. Res-

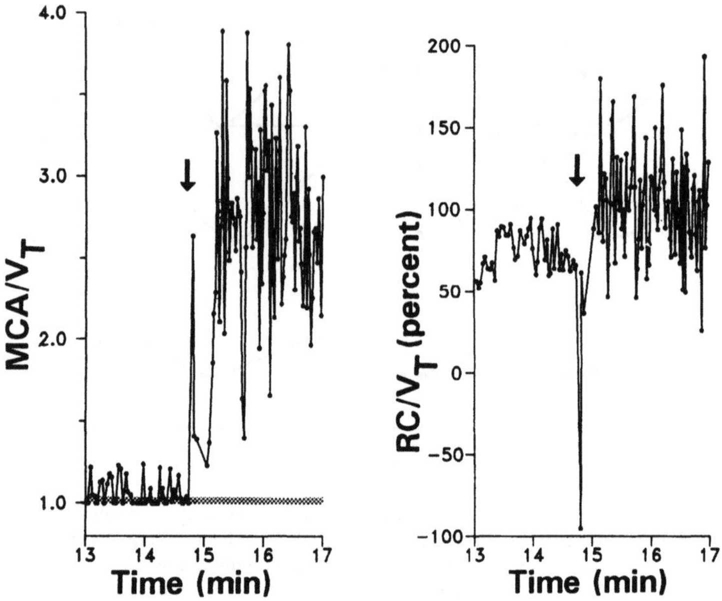

Fig. 4. A breath-to-breath plot of maximum compartmental amplitude/tidal volume (MCA/VT) ratio (*left*) and rib cage contribution to tidal volume ratio (RC/VT) (*right*) in a patient who failed a weaning trial. The arrow indicates the point of resuming spontaneous breathing following discontinuation of ventilator support. The shaded area represents the 95% confidence limits of the mean value of MCA/VT in healthy subjects. Note that discontinuation of ventilator support resulted in an almost immediate increase in MCA/VT, an index of rib cage-abdominal asynchrony and paradox (see Fig. 3 for its derivation), and in the breath-to-breath variability of the RC/VT ratio. (From [41] with permission)

piratory frequency is normally 17 breaths/min, and a value of 25 breaths/min or higher suggests that a weaning trial is likely to result in an unsuccessful outcome (Fig. 6 and 7) [28, 29]. VT is normally about 400 ml, and a value of less than 300 ml is also suggestive of an unsuccessful weaning outcome [28]. These two indices can be combined into an index of rapid shallow breathing by dividing f by VT (f/VT ratio) and a value of greater than 100 breaths/min/liter suggests an unsuccessful outcome [4].

Work of Breathing

Several investigators have examined the relationship between work of breathing and weaning outcome. Assessments have been based on both the work per minute (obtained by multiplying work per breath by f) and work per liter (obtained by dividing work rate per minute by VE). Proctor and Woolson [30] found that a work per minute value of 1.34 kg.m/min provided the best separation between ventilator-independent and ventilator-dependent patients; however, it was associated with a false-positive rate of 14% and false-negative rate of 14%. From the

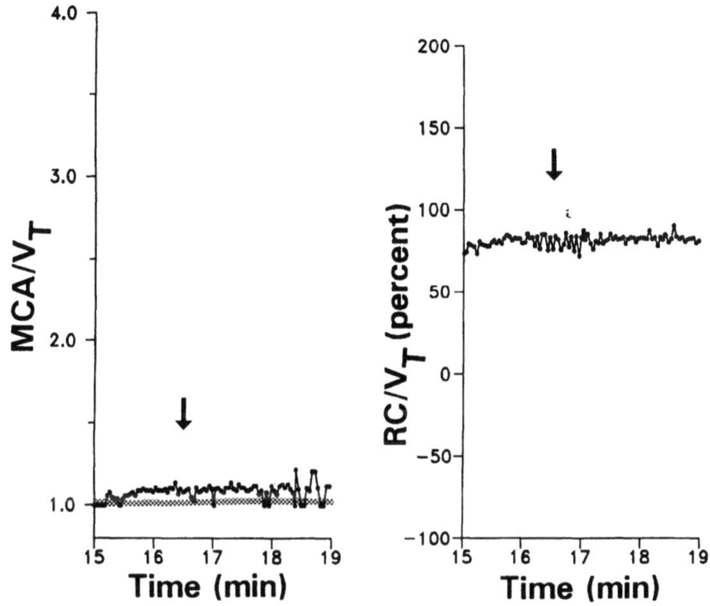

Fig. 5. A breath-by-breath plot of maximum compartmental amplitude/tidal volume (MCA/VT ratio) (*left*) and rib cage contribution to tidal volume ratio (RC/VT) (*right*) in a patient who was successfully weaned from mechanical ventilation. The arrow indicates the point of dicontinuing ventilator support, and the shaded area represents the 95% confidence limits of the mean value of MCA/VT in healthy subjects. In contrast to Fig. 4, note that the resumption of spontaneous breathing caused minimal alteration in the MCA/VT ratio. (From [41] with permission)

data of Peters et al. [31], it appears that a work per liter value of approximately 0.10 kg.m/l and a work per minute value of approximately 1.0 kg.m/min provided the best separation between ventilator-dependent and ventilator-independent patients, but there was considerable overlap between the two groups (precise extent is impossible to judge). Fiastro et al. [16] found that all of their ventilator-independent patients had both work per liter values of ≤ 0.14 kg.m/l and work per minute values of ≤ 1.6 kg.m/min, whereas all of their ventilator-dependent patients had work per minute values of > 1.6 kg.m/min and 66% of the patients had work per liter values of > 0.14 kg.m/l.

Another way of assessing respiratory work is to measure the O_2 cost of breathing. This is usually taken as the differences in the total O_2 consumption between a period when the patient is relaxed and receiving MV, and a period when he/she is breathing spontaneously [32]. In normal subjects, the O_2 cost of breathing is less than 5% of total O_2 consumption, whereas it may exceed 50% in patients being weaned from VE [32]. Conflicting findings exist as to whether the O_2 cost of breathing is higher in patients who fail a weaning trial compared with those who are successfully weaned [33–36].

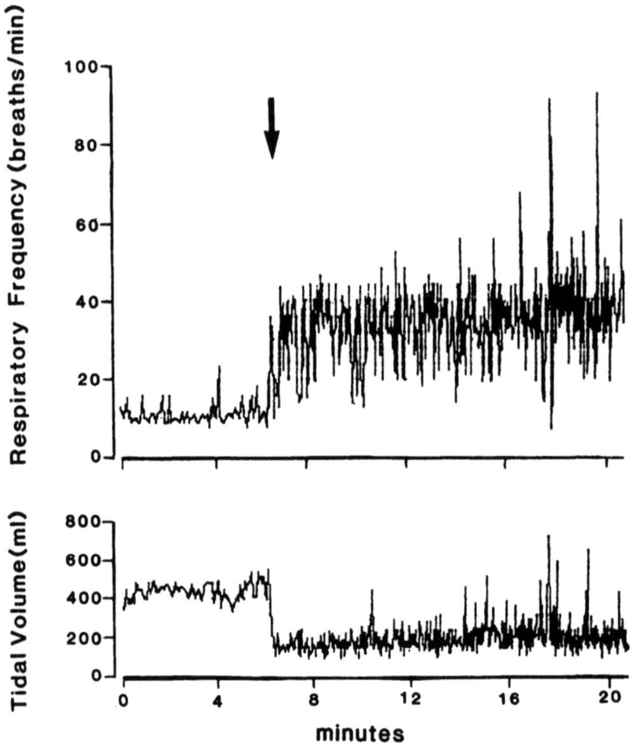

Fig. 6. A time-series, breath-by-breath plot of respiratory frequency and tidal volume in a patient who failed a weaning trial. The arrow indicates the point of resuming spontaneous breathing following discontinuation of ventilator support. Rapid, shallow breathing developed almost immediately, which suggests the prompt establishment of a new steady state. Although it has been considered that rapid, shallow breathing may reflect the presence of respiratory muscle fatigue, its almost instantaneous development without subsequent progression is difficult to reconcile with the development of respiratory muscle fatigue. (From [28] with permission)

Physical Examination

Probably one of the most helpful methods of judging the likelihood of successful weaning is to conduct a careful physical examination at a time when the patient is breathing spontaneously (Fig. 8). The patient should be checked for the presence of cyanosis, although this is not a very accurate physical sign [7]. When carefully counted over a one minute period, an elevated respiratory rate is a very sensitive sign of respiratory distress [37]. In contrast, bedside estimation of VT is very inaccurate. It is important to form a clinical impression of the patient's work of breathing, especially in relation to $PaCO_2$. Evidence of increased patient effort is signalled by nasal flaring, accessory muscle recruitment, recession of the suprasternal and intercostal spaces, and paradoxical motion of the rib cage and abdomen [18, 27, 38]. The chest should be ausculated to detect the development of wheezing or

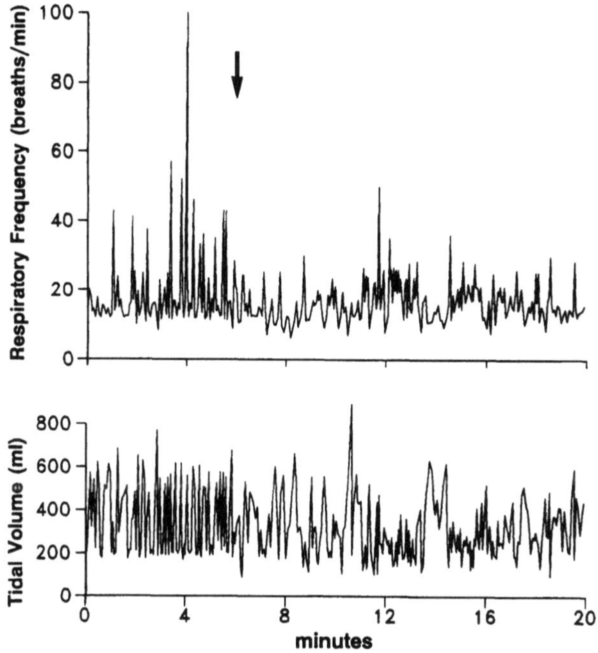

Fig. 7. A time-series, breath-by-breath plot of respiratory frequency and tidal volume in a patient who was successfully weaned. The arrow indicates the point of resuming spontaneous breathing following the discontinuation of ventilator support. In contrast with the patient in Fig. 6, note the lack of change in breathing pattern.

crackles. In addition, one needs to assess the patient's level of dyspnea, mental status, blood pressure, and heart rate and rhythm.

What Accounts for Varied Performance of Weaning Predictors?

From the above discussion it is clear that a number of the indices that were initially proposed to accurately predict weaning outcome were found to be considerably less accurate in subsequent studies. Several reasons may account for the discrepancies between studies.

The type of patient in an original study may differ from that in subsequent studies. For example, 60% of the patients of Sahn and Lakshminaryan [15] were postoperative, a group renowned for the ease with which ventilator support can be discontinued, whereas Tahvanainen et al. [12] excluded surgical patients. Also, the duration of ventilator support differs between studies; for example, the patients of Sahn and Lakshminarayan [14] required ventilator support for only about 37 h, whereas other investigators examined patients who were ventilated for 30 days or more [16, 17].

There may be differences in the methods of making the measurements. In contrast to measurements of pulmonary function in ambulatory patients which have been well standardized to ensure quality assurance, the methods of assessing pulmonary function in ICU patients have never been standardized [7].

The threshold value that is selected may not achieve the best discrimination between the patient groups. While a maximum inspiratory pressure of 30 cm H_2O is

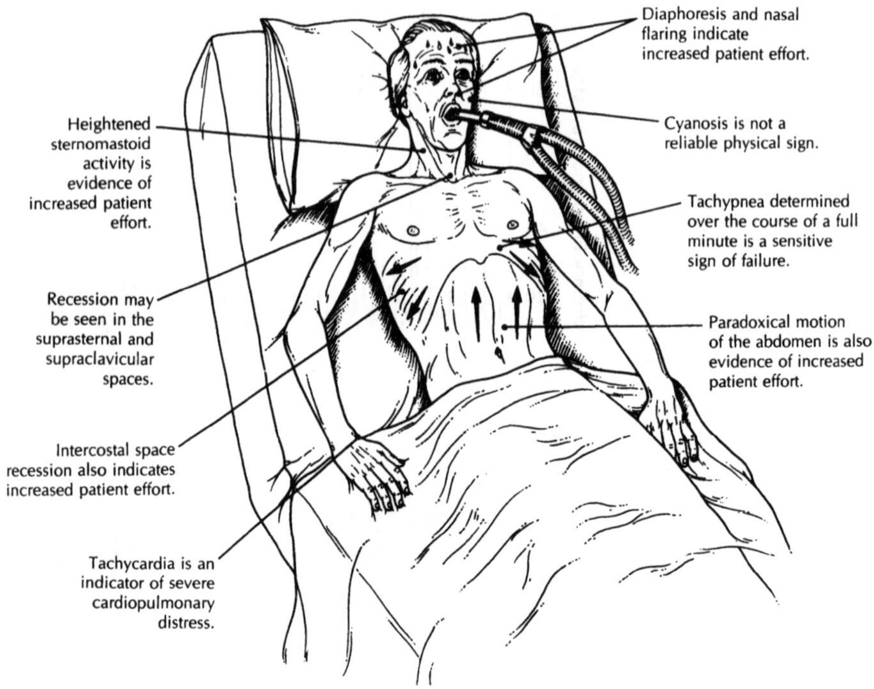

Fig. 8. Physical signs that may be evident in a patient who is failing a trial of weaning from mechanical ventilation. (From [42] with permission)

obviously easier to remember than a value of 27 cm H_2O, it does not follow that the "rounded-off" value will provide better discrimination between patients. Few, if any, of the recent studies reporting the poor performance of the standard predictors have addressed the possibility that prediction might be enhanced by the selection of a different threshold value.

The end points of different studies have been poorly defined. While the definition of weaning success is fairly straightforward (usually defined as successful spontaneous ventilation for at least 24 h following extubation), the definition of weaning failure is more difficult. While a number of investigators indicate some arterial blood gas criteria to indicate weaning failure, almost all investigators state that weaning failure was defined by arterial blood gases changes *or* clinical deterioration. This absence of standardized objective criteria of weaning failure makes it difficult to compare the performance of predictive indices in different studies, because patients judged to have failed a weaning trial in one study might have been successfully weaned by a physician who managed the patient in a more aggressive manner.

Finally, the index being measured may not be an accurate reflection of the true determinants of weaning outcome. Indeed, since weaning failure is commonly multifactorial in origin, an index that assesses only a single function is not likely to be a very accurate predictor. Instead, an alogrithm of several indices or an index that integrates the major determinants of weaning outcome are likely to be more successful. In a recent preliminary study of patients being weaned from MV, Yang and Tobin [39] examined accuracy of an index that integrates respiratory load (Cdyn·respiratory rate), respiratory muscle strength (PImax) and gas-exchange function (PaO_2/PAO_2 ratio). The index equals (Cdyn·PImax·PaO_2/PAO_2)/respiratory rate, and it has been dubbed the CROP index, an acronym for *C*ompliance, *r*ate, *o*xygenation and *p*ressure. In their preliminary study of 41 patients, a high CROP value was associated with an 87% likelihood of successful weaning outcome, compared with likelihoods of only 55% for VE $\leq$10 l/min and 61% for a PImax $\geq$30 cm H_2O.

In conclusion, physiological indices that predict weaning outcome are useful in that they decrease dependence on the clinical judgement of an individual physician and they provide clues to the cause of ventilator dependency. Investigations conducted over the last 10 years have given us a better understanding of the true determinants of ventilator dependency, and an index that assesses a single physiological function is likely to have limited predictive power, and an assessment of the balance between respiratory load and respiratory capacity is likely to be more accurate.

References

1. Editorial (1987) Predictors of successful weaning in ventilated patients. Lancet 1:1245–1246
2. Milic-Emili J (1986) Is weaning an art or science? Am Rev Respir Dis 134:1107–1108
3. Tobin MJ (1988) Predicting weaning outcome. Chest 94:227–228
4. Tobin MJ (1990) Weaning from mechanical ventilation. In: Simmons DH (ed) Current Pulmonology. Volume 11. Year Book Medical Publishers, Chicago pp 47–105
5. Pierson DJ (1983) Weaning from mechanical ventilation in acute respiratory failure: Concepts, indications, and techniques. Respir Care 28:646–662
6. Pontoppidan H, Laver MB, Geffin B (1970) Acute respiratory failure in the surgical patient. In: Welch CE (ed) Advances in Surgery. Chicago, Year Book Medical Publishers, pp 163–254
7. Tobin MJ (1988) State of the art: Respiratory monitoring in the intensive care unit. Am Rev Respir Dis 138:1625–1642
8. Krieger BP, Ershowsky PF, Becker DA, Gazeroglu HB (1989) Evaluation of conventional criteria for predicting successful weaning from mechanical ventilatory support in the elderly. Crit Care Med 9:858–861
9. Bendixin HH, Egbert LD, Hedley-White J, et al (1965) Respiratory Care. St. Louis, CV Mosby, p 149
10. Feeley TW, Hedley-White J (1975) Weaning from controlled ventilation and supplemental oxygen. N Engl J Med 292:903–906
11. Radford EP (1975) Ventilation standards for use in artifical respiration. J Appl Physiol 7:451–460
12. Tahvanainen J, Salenpera M, Nikki P (1983) Extubation criteria after weaning from intermittent mandatory ventilatory and continous positive airway pressure. Crit Care Med 11:702–707
13. Milbern SM, Downs JB, Jumper LC, et al (1978) Evaluation of criteria for discontinuing mechanical ventilation support. Arch Surg 113:1441–1443
14. Moxham J (1990) Tests of respiratory muscle function, In: Tobin MJ (ed) The respiratory muscles. JB Lippincott Co., Philadelphia pp 312–328
15. Sahn SA, Lakshminarayan S (1973) Bedside criteria for discontinuation of mechanical ventilation. Chest 63:1002–1005
16. Fiastro JF, Habib MP, Shon BY, et al (1988) Comparison of standard weaning parameters and mechanical work of breathing in mechanically ventilated patients. Chest 94:232–238

17. Morganroth ML, Morganroth J, Nett LM, Petty TL (1984) Criteria for weaning from prolonged mechanical ventilation. Arch Intern Med 144:1012–1016
18. Tobin MJ (1988) Respiratory muscles in disease. Clinics Chest Med 9:263–286
19. Whitelaw WA, Derenne JP, Milic-Emili J (1975) Occlusion pressure as a measure of respiratory center in conscious man. Respir Physiol 23:181–189
20. Herrera M, Blasco J, Venegas J, Barba R, Doblas A, Marquez E (1985) Mouth occlusion pressure: P0.1 in acute respiratory failure. Intensive Care Med 11 (3):134–139
21. Sassoon CSH, Te TT, Mahutte CK, Light RW (1987) Airway occlussion pressure: An important indicator for successful weaning in patients with chronic obstructive pulmonary disease. Am Rev Respir Dis 135:107–113
22. Murciano D, Boczkowski J, Lecocguic Y, et al (1988) Tracheal occlusion pressure: A simple index to monitor respiratory muscle fatigue during acute respiratory failure in patients with chronic obstructive pulmonary disease. Ann Intern Med 108:800–805
23. Montgomery AB, Holle RHO, Neagley SR, et al (1987) Prediction of successful ventilator weaning using airway occlusion pressure and hypercapnic challenge. Chest 91:496–499
24. Cohen C, Zagelbaum G, Gross D, et al (1982) Clinical manifestations of inspiratory muscle fatigue. Am J Med 73:308–316
25. Moxham J, Edwards RHT, Aubier M, et al (1982) Changes in the EMG power spectrum (high-to-low) with force fatigue in humans. J Appl Physiol 53:1094–1099
26. Tobin MJ, Guenther SM, Perez W, et al (1987) Konno-Mead analysis of ribcage-abdominal motion during successful and unsuccessful trials of weaning from mechanical ventilation. Am Rev Respir Dis 135:1320–1328
27. Tobin MJ, Perez W, Guenther SM, et al (1987) Does ribcage abdominal paradox signify respiratory muscle fatigue? J Appl Physiol 63:851–860
28. Tobin MJ, Perez W, Guenther SM, et al (1986) The pattern of breathing during successful and unsuccessful trials of weaning from mechanical ventilation. Am Rev Respir Dis 134:1111–1118
29. Krieger BP, Ershowsky P (1988) Noninvasive detection of respiratory failure in the intensive care unit. Chest 94:254–261
30. Proctor HJ, Woolson R (1973) Prediction of respiratory muscle fatigue by measurements of the work of breathing. Surg Gynecol Obstet 136:367–370
31. Peters RM, Hilberman M, Hogan JS, et al (1972) Objective indications for respiratory therapy in posttrauma and postoperative patients. Am J Surg 124:262–269
32. Field S, Kelly SM, Macklem PT (1982) The oxygen cost of breathing in patients with cardiorespiratory disease. Am Rev Respir Dis 126:9–13
33. Lewis WD, Chwals W, Benott PN, et al (1988) Bedside assessment of the work of breathing. Crit Care Med 16:117–122
34. Kemper M, Weissman C, Askanazi J, et al (1987) Metabolic and respiratory changes during weaning from mechanical ventilation. Chest 92:979–983
35. Hubmayr RD, Loosbrock LM, Gillespie DJ, et al (1988) Oxygen uptake during weaning from mechanical ventilation. Chest 94:1148–1155
36. Shikora SA, Bistrian BR, Borlase BC, et al (1990) Work of breathing: reliable predictor of weaning and extubation. Crit Care Med 18:157–162
37. Browning IB, D'Alonzo GE, Tobin MJ (1990) Importance of respiratory rate as an indicator of respiratory dysfunction in patients with cystic fibrosis. Chest 97:1317–1321
38. Tobin MJ, Jenouri GA, Watson H, et al (1983) Noninvasive measurement of pleural pressure by surface inductive plethysmography. J Appl Physiol 55:267–275
39. Yang KL, Tobin MJ (1989) Decision analysis of parameters used to predict outcome of a trial of weaning mechanical ventilation. Am Rev Respir Dis (abstract) 139:A98
40. Tobin MJ, Yang KL (1990) Weaning from mechanical ventilation. In: Tobin MJ (ed) Critical care clinics: mechanical ventilation. WB Saunders, Philadelphia p 735
41. Tobin MJ, Yang KL (1990) Respiratory muscle dysfunction in patients being weaned from mechanical ventilation. In: Tobin MJ (ed) The respiratory muscles. JB Lippincott, Philadelphia p 429
42. Tobin MJ (1990) Respiratory parameters for successful weaning. J Crit Illness 5:819–837

Proportional Assist Ventilation and Pressure Support Ventilation: Similarities and Differences

M. Younes

Introduction

Proportional assist ventilation (PAV) [1, 2] and pressure support ventilation (PSV) [3, 4] are two recently introduced methods of partial ventilatory support. They are intended for patients whose respiratory drive is normal or high but who have difficulty sustaining an adequate level of ventilation on their own. In the absence of ventilatory support, respiratory distress develops.

The patient who is a candidate for partial support is one who must exert a greater effort (defined here as percent of maximum available inspiratory pressure, MIP) than a normal person in order to attain the same tidal volume (VT) or ventilation. This is brought about by respiratory muscle weakness, abnormal respiratory mechanics, or both. In the case where the problem is in the muscles, MIP is decreased so that a greater effort is required to generate the same pressure. In the case of abnormal respiratory mechanics, a greater pressure (and hence a greater % MIP) is required to generate the same ventilation. In either case, there is an abnormal relation between effort and ventilatory consequences (neuro-ventilatory coupling) and this is an important cause of respiratory distress [5–7]. Furthermore, when the pressure required to maintain adequate ventilation is a large fraction of MIP (i.e. when effort is high), respiratory muscle fatigue may develop [8, 9] with potentially catastrophic consequences (acute respiratory failure, ARF).

A fundamental feature that distinguishes these two methods (PAV and PSV) from other methods of partial support is that in both cases the objective is to assist each inspiration; each inspiratory effort that succeeds in decreasing airway pressure below a critical value causes the ventilator to raise airway pressure (Paw). With each inspiration the patient therefore receives more air than he would on his own. The relation between effort and ventilatory consequences (flow and/or VT) is improved with each breath. This is expected to result in greater comfort than with the other two methods of partial support, airway pressure release ventilation (APRV) and synchronized intermittend mandatory ventilation (SIMV). With the two latter methods the ventilator also contributes a fraction of total ventilation. However, this contribution is sporadic or intermittent.

With SIMV only, some of the spontaneous efforts are assisted and the assist is in the form of a predetermined VT delivered with a predetermined flow pattern [10]. Since the setting of the IMV breaths are determined by the physician or therapist, and not by the patient, the VT and flow need not agree with the patient's own demand, and conflict may arise. Furthermore, efforts made by the patient to adjust flow or volume to suit his needs during the IMV breaths are futile; the ventilator simply readjusts its own pressure output such that the programmed flow and volume are delivered [1, 2]. The remaining breaths are not assisted. Since in these patients the relation between effort and ventilatory consequences is abnormal, with SIMV the patient alternates between breaths in which effort is futile (IMV breaths) and breaths in which the ventilatory return is too low relative to effort (spontaneous breaths).

With APRV [11], airway pressure is maintained at a positive level for the majority of the time. Machine contribution to ventilation is accomplished by periodically reducing pressure to a lower level, thereby causing lung emptying, and then raising it again to return lung volume to the baseline value. The spontaneous efforts between the transient pressure release maneuvers are again not assisted and are therefore subject to the poor relation between effort and ventilatory return. In fact, the relation may be even worsened since these efforts are superimposed on a already elevated volume (relative to functional residual capacity FRC); it is well known that the ability of inspiratory muscle to generate pressure decreases as lung volume increases [12–14].

As indicated earlier with both PSV and PAV, positive airway pressure is delivered with each inspiratory effort that succeeds in triggering the ventilator. The fundamental difference between the two methods is in the function that governs airway pressure behavior once the machine is triggered (Fig. 1). With PSV, Paw follows a predetermined function of time, usually a nearly square pattern. Differences in level of effort beyond the trigger point should, ideally, not influence the level of Paw. (In practice many ventilators are not capable of maintaining Paw at the prescribed level in the face of increasing patient effort; Paw generally falls with increased effort.) Thus, Paw will rise to the same level, set by the physician, whether the effort is large or small (Fig. 1, left). Paw is maintained at the set level until a cycling off condition is met. The condition that resets the pressure varies from one ventilator to another [4] and is most commonly a decrease in flow rate below a critical value. This point (cycling off) is not inherently linked to the termination of patient effort.

With PAV airway pressure changes as a function of patient effort [1]; the more

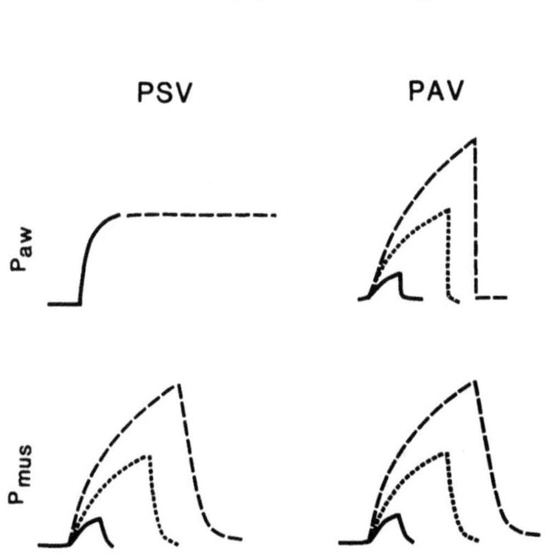

Fig. 1. Schematic respresentation of ideal response of airway pressure (Paw) to different intensities of patient effort (Pmus) with pressure support ventilation (PSV) and proportional assist ventilation (PAV). With PSV, neither the pattern nor the magnitude of Paw is affected by intensity of patient effort beyond the trigger point. With PAV, both the pattern and magnitude of Paw reflect the pattern and magnitude of patient effort.

the patient pulls, the more Paw rises. This relation not only applies as level of effort changes from breath to breath but the pattern of Paw within each inspiration also reflects the pattern of pressure generated by the patient (Pmus, Fig. 1, right). Neither the level of pressure nor flow or volume are set. Rather, what is set is the proportionality between instantaneous Paw and instantaneous patient effort (Pmus). The operation of PAV is analogous to power steering, or to the patient acquiring an extra set of muscles which remain entirely under the control of respiratory centers, much as the patient's own muscles. If, for example, the proportionality is set at 1/1 (1 cm H_2O of Paw/cm H_2O of Pmus), ventilator and patient share the work equally at all times regardless of level of ventilation, breathing pattern or flow pattern. If the proportionality is set at 3/1, the ventilator assumes three quarters of the work, and so on. With all settings, however, all attributes of breathing are determined by the patient through changes in his own effort.

How Does a Ventilator Sense Instantaneous Effort

Theoretically, it is possible to record the activity from a respiratory muscle (EMG) or nerve and use the signal to drive the ventilator. Systems of this kind have been developed and used to produce a "normal" breathing pattern in experimental animals subjected to thoracotomy or paralysis [15, 16]. Such an approach is not practicable in clinical practice; it is clearly not reasonable to entertain recording from the phrenic nerve in order to drive the ventilator, and the current technology for non-invasive, or minimally invasive recording from inspiratory muscles is not adequate to permit the acquisition of reliable, stable signals.

The amount of pressure generated by the respiratory muscles at any instant can however be inferred or estimated from the equation of motion [17]. This approach is based on the classical mechanical concept that the pressure applied to a system (Pappl) is dissipated against the elastic, resistive and inertial properties of the system. For the respiratory system, inertial properties are negligible [17] so that the equation simplifies to:

$$\text{Pappl} = \text{Pel} + \text{Pres} \quad (1)$$

where P01 is pressure dissipated against the elastic elements and Pres is pressure dissipated against the resistance.

Since it is possible to calculate P01 from volume (V) and respiratory elastance (Ers), and Pres from flow ($\dot{V}$), and resistance (Rrs), it is also possible to calculate the time course of Pappl from V and $\dot{V}$ if one knows the elastic and resistive properties of the respiratory system (both properties can be, and are routinely, measured in ventilated patients). In the event elastance and resistance are constant (i.e. linear P-V and P-$\dot{V}$ relations):

$$\text{Pappl} = \text{V} \cdot \text{Ers} + \dot{\text{V}} \cdot \text{Rrs} \quad (2)$$

In spontaneously breathing subjects, where Paw = 0, the pressure generated by the respiratory muscles (Pmus) is the sole force applied to the respiratory system

(Pappl = Pmus). Computation of Pappl according to equation 2, therefore, directly results in Pmus [17]. Where Paw is not zero, Pappl is the sum of Pmus and the pressure applied by the device to the airway (Pappl = Pmus + Paw). Thus,

$$\mathrm{Pmus} + \mathrm{Paw} = \mathrm{V} \cdot \mathrm{Ers} + \dot{\mathrm{V}} \cdot \mathrm{Rrs} \tag{3}$$

Rearranging:

$$\mathrm{Pmus} = \mathrm{V} \cdot \mathrm{Ers} + \dot{\mathrm{V}} \cdot \mathrm{Rrs} - \mathrm{Paw} \tag{4}$$

Since V, $\dot{\mathrm{V}}$ and Paw can be continuously monitored, and Ers and Rrs can be measured or estimated, the time course of Pmus can be computed continuously.

This approach for estimating the time course of Pmus has been extensively used in the past to identify the response of subjects and patients to various experimental manipulations of airway pressure [18–21] or ventilator settings [22, 23]. It is also the approach used, with some modifications [1] to control the ventilator in PAV.

The concept of PAV, along with methods of implementation, the various advantages and potential drawbacks, and the results of initial clinical testing are described in detail elsewhere [1, 2].

Ability to Modulate Breathing with PAV and PSV

Both PSV and PAV are capable of unloading the inspiratory muscles [1, 2, 24–27]. In addition, with either method, the extent of pressure expenditure, or work of breathing (WOB), that is assumed by the ventilator can be varied from trivial to near total. In this respect, however, these two methods are not different from other methods of ventilatory support where ventilator cycle is synchronized with patient's inspiration, for example assist/control or SIMV [22, 23].

The main alleged advantage of PSV and PAV is the freedom retained by the patient to modulate breathing while being assisted. It is in this respect that the two methods need to be contrasted. In the remainder of this chapter, the effect of the different airway pressure behavior (independent of Pmus in PSV and positively related to Pmus in PAV) on patient ability to modulate breathing will be explored. The practical implications of differences in this respect will also be outlined. Apart from meeting its main objective (how free is the patient really?), such analysis should provide a framework for the correct interpretation of changes in breathing pattern that may be observed in patients during PSV and PAV.

Because of the large number of variables involved, and the difficulty of changing any of them in a controlled fashion in real patients, this kind of assessment is best done by modeling. The validity of model predictions necessarily depends on how good the model is. In this case, the variables at issue are well defined and there is sufficient information to permit their correct representation in a model. The model to be used here is one that was used extensively earlier to estimate the ventilatory consequences of different patterns of respiratory motor output in spontaneously breathing subjects under a variety of physiological and pathological conditions [28–30]. The model has been modified from time to time to suit the particular application. The version that most closely resembles the one used here was described in detail in a recent publication [29]. This has been further modified to permit the addition of PSV and PAV. A brief description is provided in the appendix.

In general, the effect of a given inspiratory effort on breathing will depend on how much pressure this effort generates (a function of muscle strength), the pattern and duration of the effort, respiratory mechanics both during inspiration and expiration, and on the level of assist (preset pressure with PSV and proportionality with PAV). Because each of these variables may span a very wide range, the number of possible combinations that can be modeled is nearly infinite. It is, therefore, necessary to select specific conditions for illustration. Although the qualitative conclusions apply in general, the quantitative relations are specific to the conditions selected. In the following account the conditions outlined below were utilized unless otherwise specified.

Patient physical characteristics: Muscle strength: Maximum inspiratory pressure at FRC = 30 cm H_2O (30% of normal). Resistive properties: A resistance of 12 cm H_2O/l/sec is assumed. Elastic properties: Vital capacity (VC) is 2.0 l, representing 40% of normal, and the pressure-volume relation retains its sigmoid nature within this restricted range. Near FRC, the elastance is 25 cm H_2O/l.

Characteristics of motor output: Inspiratory activity rises from 0 to a peak value in a ramp manner with the ramp being somewhat convex to the time axis (Pmus, Fig. 3). The peak value is altered from near 0 (virtually no effort, just enough to trigger the ventilator) to 60% of maximum effort, corresponding in this case to 18 cm H_2O. Peak pressure levels in excess of 60% MIP are associated with a tension-time index [9] greater than 15% max, and are not sustainable [8, 9]. Beyond peak level, inspiratory pressure declines to zero rapidly (Fig. 3) and there is no expiratory effort. Unless otherwise specified, neural inspiration is 35% of total cycle duration (Ti/Ttot = 35%).

Machine characteristics: For PSV, the machine was triggered as soon as inspiratory effort succeeded in generating inspiratory flow or in reducing Paw below the CPAP level (here assumed to be zero). Once triggered, pressure increased to the set level (range = 0–30 cm H_2O) at a fast rate (time constant = 0.1 sec). The effect of slower rise in pressure is examined separately. Pressure was cycled off when inspiratory flow decreased to 0.08 l/sec (5 l/min) unless otherwise indicated. For PAV, pressure began increasing once inspiratory effort succeeded in generating inspiratory flow. Proportionalities ranging from 1 (Paw/Pmus = 1) to 8 (Paw/Pmus = 8) were modeled (see appendix).

Effect of changes in peak inspiratory effort on tidal volume (VT) and inspiratory duration (Ti): With PSV, the effect of a given patient effort on Ti and VT depends critically on the Ti and VT that would occur as a result of the pressure support alone; that is in the absence of patient effort. The events following the triggering of pressure in the absence of patient effort (pressure control) have been detailed by Marini et al. [31]. Soon after the pressure is introduced, volume, and hence elastic recoil pressure (P01) is small. Much of the pressure is applied against the resistance (see equation 1) resulting in a high initial flow (Fig. 2). As volume rises, P01 also rises. Since the total pressure is unchanged, less pressure is available for flow (Pres). Flow accordingly declines with time (Fig. 2). In a system where resistance and elastance can be represented by constants (linear P–V and P–$\dot{V}$ relations) and the applied pressure is square, volume rises and flow declines along an exponential function with a time constant given by R/E, where R is resistance and E is elastance. With pressure control ventilation (PCV) pressure is cycled off at a preset time. Ti is therefore predetermined, and volume at the end of inspiration is that which is determined by the exponential volume function and the preset Ti (Fig. 2) [31].

With PSV, taking the case of a patient who makes just enough effort to trigger the ventilation but ceases his effort thereafter, the time course of flow and volume after triggering would be identical to the case with the machine triggered breath in PCV. The difference is in the cycling-off criterion. Rather than a set Ti (this would defeat the purpose of PSV responsiveness to patient), the pressure is cycled off when flow declines to a preset level ($\dot{V}$th, Fig. 2). The latter is machine specific [4]. With PSV, volume (and hence P01) will rise until Pres (i.e. PS – P01, Fig. 2)

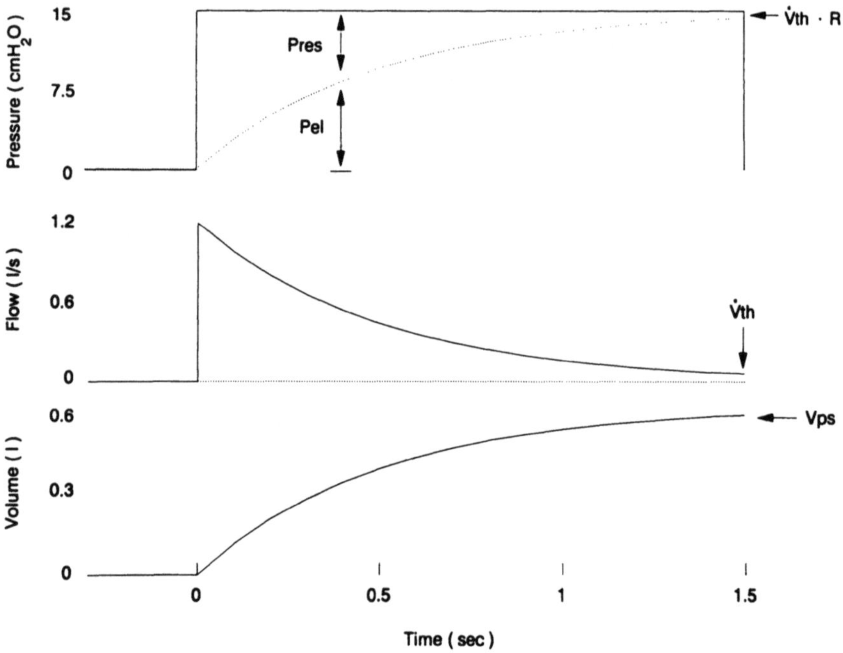

Fig. 2. Schematic representation of time course of flow and volume following onset of pressure support in the absence of significant patient effort (triggering effort only). Volume rises and flow falls along an exponential function until flow declines to the level at which PS is cycled off. This expiratory triggering flow level is $\dot{V}$th. A progressively increasing fraction of PS is applied against elastic recoil of the respiratory system (P01). The balance (Pres) is applied against resistance (R) to generate flow. The maximum volume that can be sustained by PS alone (VPS) is that which leaves just enough Pres to generate $\dot{V}$th, and is given by $\dot{V}$th·R. (See text)

declines to just below the level required to generate $\dot{V}th$ (i.e. $\dot{V}th \cdot R$). At this point, flow declines below $\dot{V}th$ and pressure is cycled off. There is, therefore, a maximum P01, and hence volume, that can be sustained by PS alone. Since at the end of the breath:

$$PS - P01 = \dot{V}th \cdot R$$

the highest P01 that can be achieved in the absence of patient effort (P01max) is given by:

$$P01max = PS - \dot{V}th \cdot R$$

and the highest volume that can be sustained by PS alone (VPS) is:

$$VPS = P01max/E = (PS - \dot{V}th \cdot R)/E$$

It can be seen that the volume that can be sustained by PS alone is a function of PS level, mechanical properties of the system and $\dot{V}th$.

Inspiratory duration, on the other hand, is determined by the time taken for the exponentially declining flow to reach $\dot{V}th$. Where the time constant (R/E) of the exponential decline is long, small differences in $\dot{V}th$ can have an important effect on Ti. For example, with a time constant of 0.6 sec (e.g. R = 15, E = 25), Ti with a $\dot{V}th$ of 0.05 l/sec (3 l/min) is 0.4 sec longer than if $\dot{V}th$ were 0.1 l/sec (6 l/min).

We now examine the effect of progressively increasing patient effort on Ti and VF (Fig. 3). a low $\dot{V}th$ (0.05 l/sec) was deliberately chosen to enhance the phenomenon being illustrated. PS level is 15 cm H_2O. All other mechanical parameters are as outlined at the beginning of this section. With only a triggering effort (solid line) Ti is 1.65 sec. The maximum volume that can be sustained by PS alone (VPS) is 560 ml, and this is indicated by the horizontal arrows in the volume panel.

With the next effort level, the patient makes an inspiratory effort that lasts 0.7 sec beyond the trigger. Pmus increases to a peak level of 3 cm H_2O (10% maximum effort) and then decreases to zero. In the first 0.7 sec, the combined action of Pmus and PS results in a greater flow, and hence greater rate of increase in volume. At the end of inspiratory effort however, volume is still lower than VPS. When inspiratory effort ceases, flow will therefore remain higher than $\dot{V}th$, albeit lower than at the same time in the absence of effort (see flow panel). Inspiration continues beyond patient effort although Ti will be shorter than in the case without effort (because flow is closer to $\dot{V}th$). In this case, therefore, patient effort resulted in reduction in Ti with no effect on VT.

At the next higher level of effort, peak Pmus reaches 6 cm H_2O (20% max) in the same neural Ti (0.7 sec). Flow is initially higher but VT just barely reaches VPS at the end of the effort. Cessation of patient effort, leaving PS alone, results in earlier termination of inspiration (shorter Ti) but still the same VT. Termination of PS now nearly coincides with termination of patient effort. From this point on, further increases in peak patient effort will result in greater volume with little change in Ti.

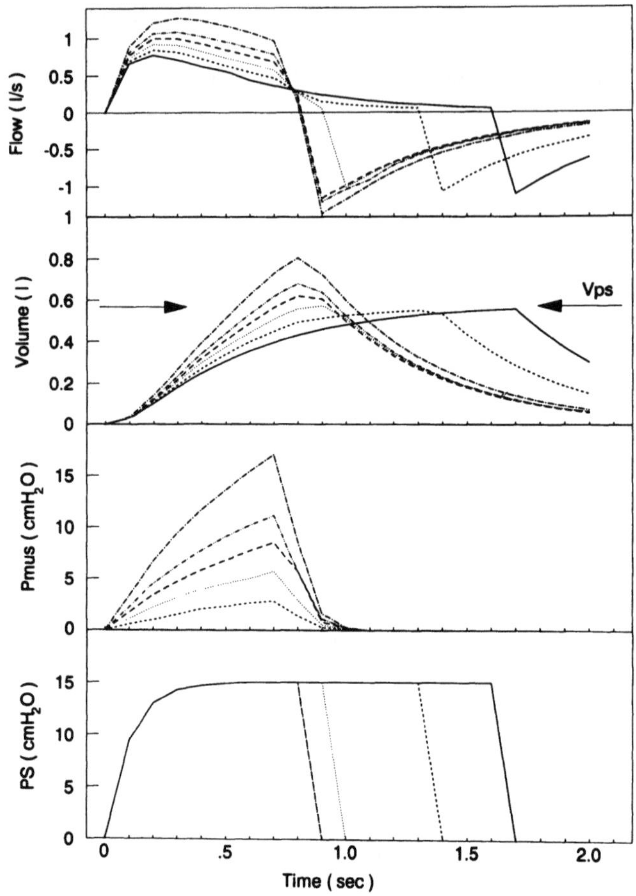

Fig. 3. Effect of progressively increasing peak inspiratory effort (Pmus) on time course of flow and volume during PSV. The rising phase of Pmus is 0.7 sec in all cases. Solid lines represent pattern with triggering effort only. Note that increasing peak effort results in greater flow and volume during the period of inspiratory effort. Termination of pressure support (PS) and inspiratory flow coincide with termination of patient effort only with higher levels of effort. At lower levels, patient effort has little effect on VT and only succeeds in reducing the duration of inspiratory flow. VPS is maximum volume that can be sustained by PS in the absence of patient effort (see Fig 2).

It follows that, in the case of PSV, when neural Ti is less than the Ti that would be obtained with PS alone, progressive increases in peak effort at the same Ti will elicit reduction in mechanical Ti with no change in VT. Only when the effort is sufficiently intense to cause synchronous termination of machine and patient inspiration, will VT become sensitive to patient effort. During PSV, duration and peak value of inspiratory flow should be more sensitive than VT, as indicators of changes in intensity of patient effort.

It also follows that synchrony between termination of PS and termination of patient inspiratory effort is not assured with PSV. A critical level of effort must be reached first before the two events are synchronized. Below this level, PS may continue during the patients's neural expiration. This may cause discomfort, or insufficient time for expiration before the next spontaneous breath is initiated. Alternatively, patient may establish synchrony through activation of expiratory muscles or through prolongation of his own inspiratory effort. Since neither of these options may exist spontaneously, the patient may have to resort to deliberate manipulation of his output to establish synchrony, a strategy that is only available during wakefulness and, because it is not natural, may not be well tolerated.

With proportional assist (PAV), Paw rises and falls with patient effort. As effort decreases at the end of neural inspiration, Paw will also decrease. Unlike PSV, there is therefore little possibility of non-synchrony between end of neural and mechanical inspirations. For the same mechanical properties, changes in VT and Ti reflect corresponding changes in neural output. On the other hand, because with PAV the increase in Paw during inspiration cannot appreciably outlast the end of neural inspiration, the duration of pressure assist may be too brief in patients with very short inspiratory times. It remains to be seen whether patients with rapid rates and short neural Ti will slow their rate with use of PAV [1].

Figure 4 illustrates the relation between peak inspiratory effort (% max) and VT and different levels of PSV (left) and PAV (right) in the typical patient described earlier. The corresponding changes in mechanical Ti are also shown (bottom). Neural Ti was 0.7 sec and, to avoid the confounding influence of auto-PEEP, neural Ti was sufficiently long to permit lung volume to return to passive FRC before the onset of the next inspiration. Cycling off in the case of PSV occurred at a flow threshold of 0.08 l/sec (5 l/min).

The relation between peak inspiratory effort and VT in a normal subject (VC = 5.0 l, Rrs = 4.0 cm H_2O/l/sec and maximum inspiratory pressure (MIP) = 100 cm H_2O) is given by the line marked N. For our example patient (VC = 2.0 l, Rrs = 12.0 cm H_2O/l/sec and MIP = 30 cm H_2O) the relation in the absence of any support is given by the line marked "O". The slope of any line in this plot is a reflection of the patient's ability to modulate VT through changes in peak inspiratory effort. The patient's slope, without support, is 7 ml/1% max. This is one ninth the normal slope (63 ml/1%/max). This difference is in part related to weaker muscles (a given effort results in less pressure) and in part due to abnormal mechanics (a given pressure change results in a smaller VT).

With PSV, a maximum VT is delivered even in the absence of any significant effort (Y intercepts). As indicated earlier, this point is followed by a range in which VT is insensitive to patient effort (i.e. slope is nearly 0); changes in effort simply result in reduced Ti (bottom panel). As a result of patient effort total work is increased because the same VT is reached sooner (higher flow rate). But there are no benefits in terms of VT or ventilation. The flat range is followed by an effort responsive range. However, the slope in this range is no higher than in the absence of assist (7 ml/1% effort, or less). It follows that with PSV, patient's ability to modulate VT remains curtailed by the disease process which resulted in the institution of ventilatory support. In the example illustrated, the patient's control over VT is much closer to assist/control (slope = 0) than it is to the normal state (63 ml/1% effort). Clearly, if the disease process does not impair the patient's ability to control VT, the slope of the relation between effort and VT during PSV will also be higher than in the illustrated example. Thus, in the extreme, a normal subject retains normal control over VT during PSV. However, if the underlying relation between peak effort and VT is close to normal, the need for ventilatory assist no longer exist.

The implications of this state of affairs deserve consideration. In a given patient, a PSV level is selected because, at the moment, it is associated with apparent comfort, and reasonable VT and PCO_2. The patient's respiratory drive increases. This may occur because of a change in the gas exchanging or mechanical properties of the respiratory system, due for example to change in position or disease progression. Under these conditions, PCO_2 will tend to rise and PO_2 may fall. Alternatively, respiratory drive may increase because of an increase in metabolic rate brought about by a change in level of consciousness (sleep state), movement, shivering or an increase in temperature. With the exception of temperature, changes in blood gas tensions or metabolic rate elicit primarily changes in demand (and are expressed as an increased peak inspiratory effort) [32]. Significant changes in frequency occur with much higher levels of increased drive [32]. In this patient, at the original PS level, such increase in VT demand will result in little increase in actual VT, and hence ventilation. If the patient is awake, anxiety may develop and this will aggravate the situation. If asleep or unconscious, PCO_2 will rise, ultimately causing respiratory efforts to be visibly labored or frequency to increase. The PS level is adjusted upwards until a new comfortable level is reached. As the initial cause of increased drive disappears, the new PS level represents overassist. If the PS level is adjusted down again because PCO_2 is low, a new episode of increased drive will cause distress. The tendency will therefore be to keep PS at the level that is appropriate for the highest level of drive encountered during the moment to moment, or day to day variations.

The relations described in Fig. 4, which show that the patient's ability to alter VT is as impaired as it is without PS, represent in fact a best case scenario. Several factors may cause the relation between peak effort and VT during PSV to be even worse than it is without PSV. First, we assumed that trigger sensitivity is very high. This is not always the case. When trigger sensitivity is substantially less than zero (e.g. -2 or -3cm H_2O), triggering is delayed relative to onset of inspiratory effort. This reduces the time during which patient effort is contributing to flow and volume (i.e. balance of neural Ti). Second, because PS by itself results in a finite flow and this is usually highest early in inspiration when patient effort is operative, patient effort will cause flow to increase from a high to an even higher level (Fig. 3), as opposed to increasing from zero as in the case with no PS. Because the flow resistance of ET tubes increases with flow [33], patient effort is expended against a higher resistance than would be the case in the absence of PS. Likewise, because PS, *per* se, results in a finite VT, any increase in VT produced by patient effort will have to be in a higher volume range (relative to FRC) than would otherwise be the case (i.e. in the absence of PS). Since elastance is generally higher at higher volumes, patient effort is expended against a higher elastance. It follows that the impedance facing patient effort during PSV may be substantially higher than the impedance without PSV. The slope of the relation between peak effort and VT would accordingly be even lower during PSV than otherwise. Third, in many commercial ventilators PS is not sustained at the set level when flow increases as a result of

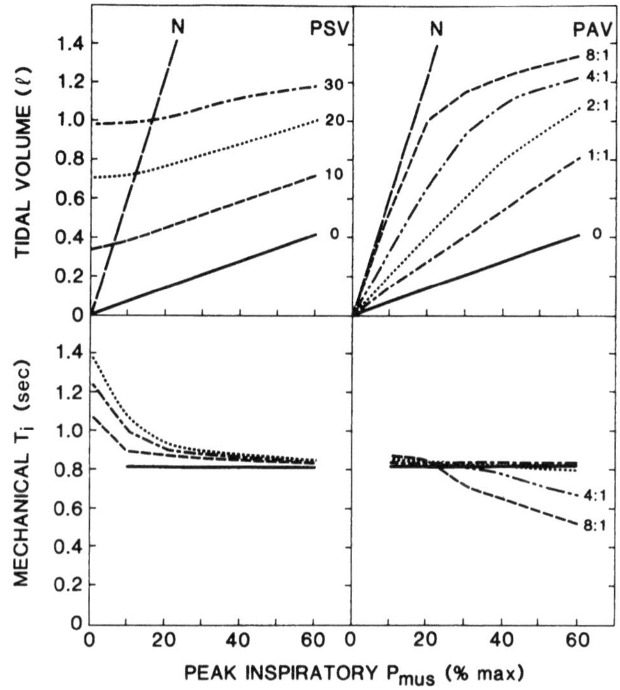

Fig. 4. Effect of increasing peak inspiratory effort on VT and mechanical Ti at different levels of pressure support (isopleths, units in cm H_2O) and PAV (isopleths represent different proportionalities). The line marked N pertains to a normal subject. Other lines pertain to a patient with low maximum inspiratory pressure (30 cm H_2O), high resistance (12 cm H_2O/l/sec) and high elastance (2.5 times normal). The slope of any line in the VT panel reflects the ability of the patient to alter VT as a result of changing his own effort. Note that with PSV the slopes remain substantially abnormal relative to the normal line. In all cases, the duration of neural inspiration was 0.7 sec. (See text)

incrased patient effort. The total applied pressure (Paw + Pmus), therefore, increase less than would otherwise occur as a result of the increase in effort. The ventilatory consequences (increased volume and/or flow) are accordingly reduced. Fourth, with some PSV delivery systems, the increase in pressure is rather slow. For a given PS level, the time taken to reach $\dot{V}$th, and hence Ti in the absence of effort, is increased. More effort is, therefore, required before end of PS and end of spontaneous inspiration are synchronized. Furthermore, if patient Ti is less than the time required for Paw to reach the set PS level, such synchrony for the end of inspiration will cause end-inspiration to occur prior to Paw reaching the set PS level. The greater the reduction in Ti the less pressure assist the patient receives. The effect of a change in the rise time constant from 0.1 sec (as used in Fig. 4) to 0.4 sec (as is the case in some commercial ventilators) on the relation between increased effort on one hand and VT and Ti on the other hand is illustrated, for one PS level, in Fig. 5. The 0.1 sec line is similar to the line in Fig. 4 at PSV of 20 cm H_2O. It can be seen that the effort insensitive range of VT extends over a much wider effort range.

In summary, in the patient with severe impairment of neuroventilatory coupling (as in most patients that require partial ventilatory support) the patient's ability to modulate VT through changes in his own effort remains substantially abnormal with PSV and may in fact be little different from patient triggered volume cycled ventilation (assist/control). Rather than appropriately altering VT, changes in peak inspiratory effort are more likely to be reflected in changes in peak inspiratory flow or in the duration of mechanical inspiration. The latter two indices (on the product VT/Ti are more appropriate for monitoring changes in intensity of patient effort than VT is.

With PAV, the patient's ability to alter VT through changes in this own effort (slope of effort vs VT, neuroventilatory coupling) progressively improves as the proportionality of the assist (Paw/Pmus) is increased (Fig. 4, right). In our typical patient, where the slope is one ninth normal, a proportional assist of 8/1 returns neuroventilatory coupling to normal. The substantial deviation from normal at volumes in excess of 1 liter is due to the progressive stiffening of the respiratory system

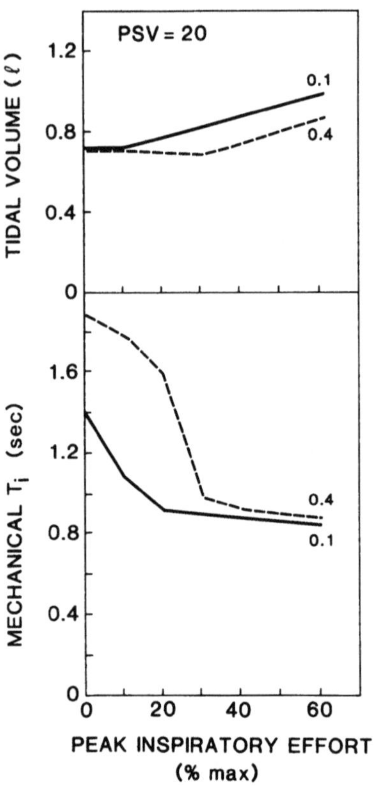

Fig. 5. Effect of rise time of pressure support on relation between peak inspiratory effort and VG and mechanical Ti. A pressure support of 20 cm H_2O was modeled. 0.1 and 0.4 reflect the time constant of the rising phase of PS in seconds. Mechanical Ti is mechanical duration of inspiratory flow. The rising phase of inspiratory Pmus (neural Ti) was 0.7 sec in duration. Note that with the slower rising phase mechanical Ti is longer and the range over which VT is insensitive to patient effort is wider.

near total lung capacity (TLC) which in this patient (VC = 2.0 l) is at a VT of 1.3 l. In the model used here, the proportionality is set based on the mechanical properties of the respiratory system near FRC (see appendix). Thus, if elastance (E) near FRC is 25 cm H_2O/l and resistance (R) is 12 cm H_2O/l/min, and 8/1 assist is obtained by setting the volume-proportional component to 8/9 of 25 and the flow proportional component of 8/9 of 12. So long as Ers and Rrs do not deviate substantially from these values, proportionality remains near 8/1. However, since elastance increases progressively near TLC, the actual proportionality decreases as volume approaches TLC. It is possible to eliminate this problem by designing PAV delivery systems with which the volume related assist is non-linear, reflecting the non-linear behavior of the pressure-volume (P-V) curve. It is questionable whether this would be advantageous since it would then be possible for volume to exceed the value associated with flattening of the P-V relation (physiologic ceiling). It is almost certain that venturing in this range would be associated with a much greater risk of barotrauma. Setting the degree of proportional assist according to elastance near FRC, therefore, insures that the physiologic ceiling will not be exceeded. Should it become necessary to exceed this ceiling to obtain adequate ventilation (ceiling is too close to FRC), other modalities of ventilatory support would be preferable.

The implication of improved neuro-ventilatory coupling with PAV is that the patient can respond to changes in respiratory mechanics, gas exchange or metabolic rate through relatively small changes in his effort (cfr PSF). Once the level of PAV is set to a comfortable range (i.e. near normal relation), there is a lesser chance for respiratory distress to develop as demand increases. There is also little chance of overventilation as demand decreases. The price of this enhanced control by patient is, however, that there is no minimum VT (cfr PSV). With PAV, breathing can be very shallow if peak inspiratory effort is very small. This may occur with central depression (peak inspiratory effort fails to increase as PCO_2 rises) or where rapid shallow breathing is not related to poor neuroventilatory coupling but to reflexes originating in the lung. Where shallow breathing is not due to poor neuroventilatory coupling, increasing coupling (with PAV) may not increase (VT); effort may be down-regulated to sustain the desired (by the respiratory centers) shallow pattern.

As indicated earlier, with PAV there is no likelihood for mechanical inspiration to appreciably outlast the end of neural inspiration. This is shown in the bottom right panel of figure 4. Mechanical Ti is close to neural Ti except when volume encroaches on TLC. At this point inspiratory flow may terminate before end of neural inspiration due to incomplete assist (see above).

Effect of changes in spontaneous respiratory rate on observed rate: In the preceding analysis we have assumed that lung volume always returns to passive FRC before the onset of the next spontaneous inspiratory effort. Under these conditions, minimal inspiratory effort should cause respiratory flow to begin, or Paw to decrease, in such a way that the assist is initiated. Every inspiratory effort would then be assisted and patient and machine rates would be identical. In actuality however, a return to passive FRC before the onset of the next effort is not assured (auto-PEEP) [34–36]. Under these conditions, the patient must first generate enough pressure to counteract the elastic recoil of the respiratory system before airway pressure can be decreased below baseline level [34–36]. To this must be added the reduction in Paw required to trigger the ventilator. As pointed out by Marini [37], auto-PEEP blunts effective triggering sensitivity.

With PSV or PAV, if peak patient effort is less than the sum of auto-PEEP and the set trigger sensitivity, triggering will not take place and a spontaneous breath will go unassisted. Because there is little or no inflation during this breath, lung volume continues to decline in the ensuing expiration so that the patient is in a better position to trigger the ventilator on the next spontaneous cycle. With PSV and PAV therefore, there exists the potential for machine rate (number of triggered breaths per minute) to underestimate the spontaneous rate. Furthermore, lung volume at the beginning of spontaneous inspiration may vary substantially from breath to breath. Although failure to "trigger" is recognized by most clinicians who use PSV, there has been, to my knowledge, no systematic examination of the circumstances leading to this phenomenom or the implications of this occurrence to the ongoing assessment of patients while receiving PSV.

As applicable to other situations [31, 34–37] the extent of "auto-PEEP" at the onset of spontaneous inspiration is increased when VT is large, when time available for expiration is reduced, and when the rate of lung emptying is decreased due to high expiratory resistance or flow limitation. Furthermore, for a given amount of auto-PEEP at the beginning of inspiration, "non-triggering" is more likely to occur when the pressure generated by the patient is small. When applied to the specific case of PSV, non-triggering is more likely to happen with higher PS levels (larger VT), higher spontaneous respiratory rate (shorter expiratory time), high expiratory resistance, and when patient generates little pressure during inspiration. In addition, PSV provides an additional feature that would tend to promote non-triggering of some breaths, namely the potential for mechanical Ti (duration of inspiratory flow) to substantially outlast the end of neural inspiration (see above). Much of the spontaneous expiratory duration may be encroached upon by mechanical inspiration leaving little time for emptying. For the same respiratory rate, therefore, non-triggering is more likely to occur with PSV than with assist/control, where the duration of the inflation phase is predetermined, and hence less likely to be excessive.

Figure 6 (top) shows the relation between spontaneous rate and the rate of machine-assisted breaths in our typical patient, at different levels of PSV (left to right) and different levels of peak inspiratory effort (isopleths). At PS of 10 cm H_2O, there is good agreement between spontaneous and machine rates at all levels of effort and at respiratory rates of 35 or less. For the 10% effort level however, as patient rate increases from 35 to 40 min^{-1}, machine rate decreases from 35 to 30 min^{-1}. One in every four breaths fails to trigger the ventilator. In this example, lung volume at the onset of spontaneous inspiration progressively increases over 3 breaths but it is not sufficiently high to preclude triggering. By the fourth breath, auto-PEEP is higher than patient generated Pmus and no triggering occurs. This permits lung volume to return back towards passive FRC and the four breath cycle is repeated. At higher PS levels, the same phenomenon is observed except that discrepancies occur at higher levels of effort and may be more pronounced, with machine rate falling to half the spontaneous rate. The implications of these discrepancies should be evident. A patient on PSV of 20 whose spontaneous rate is 30 is

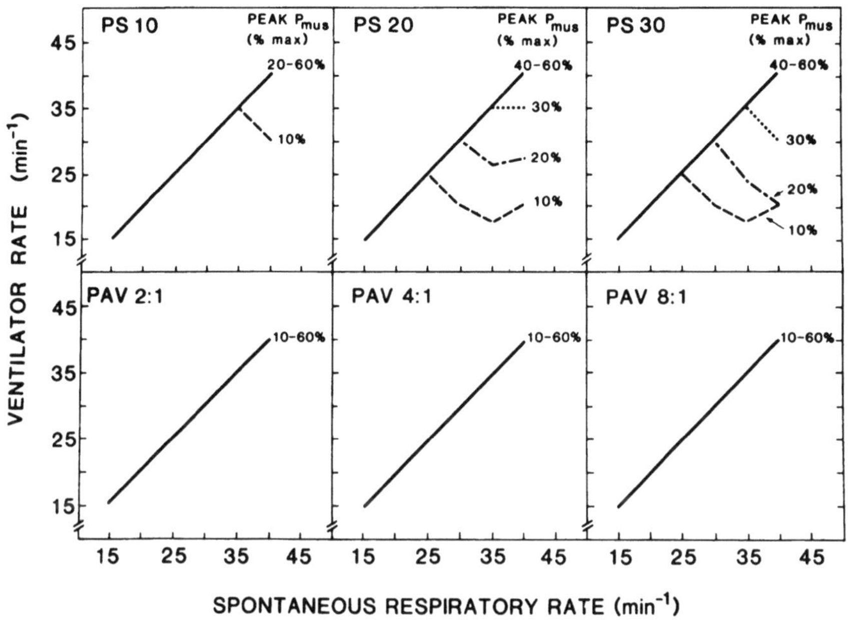

Fig. 6. Relation between spontaneous respiratory rate and ventilator rate at different levels of pressure support *(top)* and PAV. The relations were determined for different levels of peak inspiratory effort (peak Pmus, % max). Note that with PSV discrepancies between ventilator rate and spontaneous rate occur, particularly at low levels of patient effort and high levels of PS.

"triggering" only two out of every three breaths because his peak inspiratory effort is 10% max (i.e. middle panel, 10% effort). The patient increases his peak effort to 20% max (i.e. twice the VT demand) with no change in frequency. He now triggers the machine with every breath. The change in apparent breathing pattern (as judged from machine output) is an increase in rate (from 20 to 30^{-1}) with little change in VT (Fig. 4). This is exactly the opposite of what actually happened (doubling of VT demand with no change in frequency). Likewise, machine frequency may increase while patient's frequency decreases, and *vice versa*. An extreme example is provided in Fig. 6 with PS = 30 where a decrease in patient rate from 40 to 30 min^{-1} (20% effort line) is associated with an increase in machine rate from 20 to 30 min^{-1}. By prolonging Ti, the slowing of spontaneous frequency permitted the patient to trigger the ventilator every breath, as opposed to every other breath. The flow, volume and Paw tracings associated with this example are shown in Fig. 7.

Figure 7 illustrates several additional points. First, note that pressure support continues well beyond the end of neural inspiration. There is thus no synchrony at the end of inspiration. Second, with the 1/1 triggering pattern (bottom) there is an increase in end-expiratory volume (i.e. more auto-PEEP). Third, with the 1/2 rhythm (Fig. 7, top) the expiratory flow displays a biphasic pattern with the nadir being coincident with the "missing" inspiratory effort. The inspiratory effort, while failing to reduce Paw to the trigger level, nonetheless acts to retard expiratory flow.

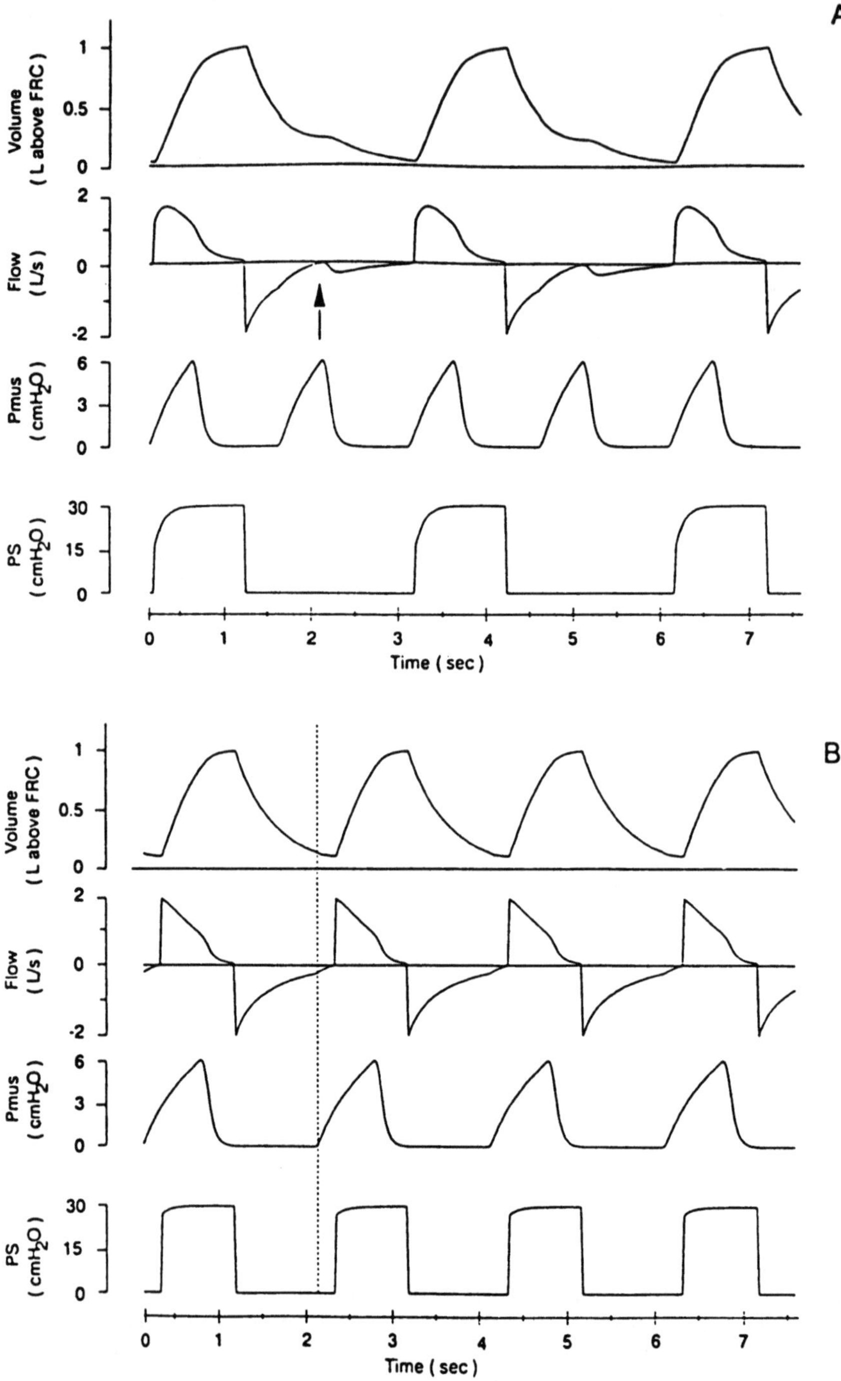

Fig. 7. *Top:* Example of 1/2 rhythm where pressure support (PS) is triggered every other spontaneous inspiratory effort. The intervening spontaneous breaths fail to trigger PS because volume, and hence elastic recoil, is greater than can be overcome by the inspiratory effort. The latter

This suggests that with PSV, monitoring expiratory flow (or Paw during expiration) should provide a more accurate assessment of the patient's spontaneous rate than simply monitoring the rate of machine cycles.

The results for similar analysis with PAV at three levels of proportionality (2/1, 4/1, 8/1) are shown in the bottom panels of figure 6. There was no discrepancy between patient and machine rates at any frequency or inspiratory effort level. In fact, this analysis was extendend up to a rate of 60 min^{-1} and the resistance was increased from 12 to 20 cm H_2O/l/sec to promote even slower emptying. No discrepancies were observed. This is not to say that non-triggering would never occur with PAV. Thus, a breath with a large inspiratory effort will be associated with a large VT and a tendency for lung volume to be higher at the onset of the next inspiration (see above). If the next inspiratory effort happens to be feeble (i.e. inconsistent inspiratory efforts), non-triggering may occur. Other situations may also be envisaged where non-triggering may occasionally occur. Nonetheless, this analysis seems to indicate that, all else being the same, the tendency for discrepancies between patient and machine rates should be less with PAV.

The reduced likelihood for non-triggering with PAV is related to two factors. First, with PAV, the time available for expiratory flow cannot be compromised because of non-concordance between end of inspiratory flow and end of inspiratory effort (see above). The entire duration of neural expiratory is therefore available for expiratory flow under all circumstances. Second, one of the most important factors that promote auto-PEEP, and hence, non-triggering, is a large VT (see above). With PAV, large VT are more likely to occur when inspiratory effort is high. Higher inspiratory efforts are, however, associated with a reduced likelihood of non-triggering. With PSV on the other hand, large VT are generally the result of the set PS level. VT may be large even when inspiratory effort, and hence the ability to counteract the resulting auto-PEEP, is not high.

In summary, with PSV, the patient receives a mandatory amount of support (pressure) but his ability to modulate ventilatory pattern through changes in his own motor output remains impaired, and there is a potential for significant discrepancies to occur between the respiratory rates of patient and machine. In the patient with severe impairment of neuroventilatory coupling (weak muscles and/or poor respiratory mechanics) PSV is much closer to assist/control than it is to the normal situation where subject is in total control of all aspects of breathing. With PAV, the ability of the patient to modulate ventilatory pattern is enhanced and the potential for discrepancies between patient and machine rates is much reduced. The ventilator essentially becomes an extension of the patient's own muscles. The consequence of this improved control by patient is that the responsibility for determining ventilation and breathing pattern is shifted from the physician to the patient's own control mechanisms. Since the optimal pattern of breathing in various disease

simply causes a momentary hesitation in expiratory flow (arrow) due to braking. Note that PS and inspiratory flow continue well past the end of inspiratory effort in the triggered breaths. This is in part responsible for failure of volume to reach FRC before the onset of the next spontaneous effort. *Bottom:* Same conditions except that patient's rate decreases from 40/min (as in A) to 30/min allowing more time for expiration. Each effort now triggers PS. Machine rate increases while patient rate has actually decreased.

states is not known, and the behavioral, chemical and reflex control in patients requiring ventilatory support is little understood, much experimental work is required before one can identify the situations in which delegating this responsibility to patient's control mechanisms is in the patient's best interest.

Appendix:

The model calculates the time course of flow and volume by iteration at finite intervals (generally 5 msec intervals). At each iteration, the direction and magnitude of flow ($\dot{V}$) is computed from the balance between instantaneous applied pressure (Pappl), opposing elastic recoil pressure (P01), and respiratory resistance:

$$\dot{V} = [\text{Pappl} - \text{P01}]/\text{Rrs}$$

Flow is inspiratory when Pappl exceeds the elastic recoil at the moment. It is expiratory when the bracketed term is negative. Flow is integrated over the iteration period to provide volume at the next iteration (Vi). The latter is then used to calculate P01 for the next iteration, resistance or maximal flow (in the event of volume dependence of these parameters), and for the conversion of patient effort to pressure output (Pmus) which is also volume dependent [29].

Applied pressure at any instant (Pappl) is made up of the sum of patient generated pressure (Pmus) and ventilator pressure (pressure support or PAV).

$$\text{Pappl} = \text{Pmus} + \text{Paw}$$

Instantaneous Pmus is a function of the pattern of neural activation of muscle and several factors that affect the conversion of neural activation to pressure [29, 38]. These include muscle reaction time, muscle strength (expressed by maximum inspiratory pressure) (Pimax) at FRC, instantaneous volume (through the dependence of Pimax on volume) and instantaneous flow (through the force-velocity relation). The latter two factors are not very important in the present simulation since Pimax is not significantly volume dependent in the volume range of FRC to FRC + 1 l (the volume encompassed in the present simulation) and flow is small relative to maximum inspiratory flow [1].

Patient inspiratory effort is represented as rising from a minimal value at the beginning of neural inspiration (a value of zero was used in the present simulation) to a peak value at the end of neural inspiration. It then declines to the minimal value and remains there for the balance of the duration of expiration. The durations of the rising and declining phases, as well as the duration of neural expiration, are variable. The shape of the rising and declining phases can also be adjusted. Expiratory activity can be included (not used in the present simulation).

Patient contribution is expressed as % of max inspiratory effort. This has the advantage (i.e. over use of pressure units) of accounting for muscle weakness which is often present in ventilator dependent patients. Thus, a pressure output of 10 cm H_2O may represent 10% effort in a normal subject while being 50% effort in a patient with much reduced muscle strength. This has obvious implications to respiratory distress.

Airway pressure (Paw) was modeled after PSV or PAV. For PSV, pressure is triggered whenever inspiratory pressure (Pmus) exceeds P01. The ventilator, therefore, is assumed to be very sensitive (triggering occurs whenever Paw decreases below zero). Following triggering, PS rises in an exponential fashion to a present level (variable). The time constant of the rising phase is adjustable, permitting nearly square to very slowly rising functions. PS remains in effect until flow decreases below a set threshold level ($\dot{V}$th). The latter could be varied to examine the effect of this parameter (which differs from machine to machine [4]) on the results.

For PAV, Paw was calculated according to the following function beginning with the first iteration showing [Pmus > P01]:

$$\text{Paw} = K_1 \cdot \dot{V}_1 + K_2 \cdot \text{Vi}$$

where $\dot{V}_1$ is instantaneous flow at the last iteration and Vi is volume at the last iteration, referenced to volume at the beginning of the breath. K_1 is a fraction of respiratory resistance and K_2 is the same fraction of respiratory elastance [1]. The fractions used were 1/2, 2/3, 4/5 and 8/9 to produce proportionalities (PAW/Pmus) of 1/1, 2/1, 4/1 and 8/1, respectively. The elastance value used was the slope of the P-V relation near FRC. This treatment results in degradation of the proportionality as volume encroaches on the flat part of the P-V curve near TLC (see text).

Elastic recoil at any instant (P01) is a function of the pressure-volume relation of the respiratory system. The latter was represented as a sigmoid function; the system is most compliant near FRC while becoming progressively less compliant near the extremes of VC [29]. To simulate restriction, VC was simply reduced. This has the effect of decreasing compliance at all volumes, while the P-V relation retains its sigmoid nature.

While the model permits the use of non-linear pressure-flow relations, as well as flow limitation during expiration, linear pressure-flow relation was used in this simulation. The slope (Rrs) was the same for inspiration and expiration.

Iterations began at the beginning of neural inspiration and continued for a whole cycle. If lung volume at the end of the cycle was not the same as at the beginning, iterations continued for another cycle using the volume at the end of the preceding cycle as the starting volume. Iterations continued until end-expiratory volume stabilized, thereby providing the steady state solution.

Acknowledgments. The author thanks Z. Bshouty and J. Freedman for modifying the software to include pressure support and PAV and K. Harlos for secretarial assistance. The analogy of PAV to power steering was provided by Dr. W. Sanborn. This work was supported by the Respiratory Health Network of Centres of Excellence.

References

1. Younes M (1991) Proportional assist ventilation, A new approach to ventilatory support: Theory. Amer Rev Resp Dis (in press)
2. Younes M, Puddy A, Roberts D, et al (1991) Proportional assist ventilation: Results of an initial clinical trial. Amer Rev Resp Dis (in press)
3. MacIntrye NR (1986) Respiratory function during pressure support ventilation. Chest 89:677–683
4. Kacmarek MR (1988) The role of pressure support ventilation in reducing work of breathing. Respir Care 33:99–120
5. Killian KJ, Campbell EJM (1985) Dyspnea. In: Roussos C, Macklem PT (eds) The thorax. Lung biology in health and disease. Dekker, New York, vol 29, chapt 26, pp 787–928
6. Altose MD (1986) Dyspnea. In: Simmons DH (ed) Current pulmonology. Year Book Medical Publishers. Chicago, vol. 7, pp 199–226
7. Zechman FW, Wiley RL (1986) Afferent inputs to breathing: respiratory sensation. In: Handbook of physiology. The respiratory system. Control of breathing. Bethesda, MD. Am Physiol Soc, vol II, pp 449–474
8. Roussos C, Fixley M, Gross D, Macklem PT (1979) Fatigue of inspiratory muscles and their synergic behavior. J Appl Physiol 46:897–904
9. Bellemare F, Grassino A (1982) Effect of pressure and timing of contraction on human diaphragm fatigue. J Appl Physiol 53:1190–1195
10. Downs JB, Klein EF, Desautels D, et al. (1973) Intermittent mandatory ventilation: A new approach to weaning patients from mechanical ventilators. Chest 64:331–335
11. Downs JB, Stock MC (1987) Airway pressure release ventilation: A new concept in ventilatory support. Critical Care Med 15:459–461
12. Marshall R (1962) Relationships between stimulus and work of breathing at different lung volumes. J Appl Physiol 17:917–921
13. Grassino A, Goldman MD, Mead J, Sears TS (1978) Mechanics of the human diaphragm during voluntary contraction: statics. J Appl Physiol 44:829–839

14. Eldridge FL, Vaughn KZ (1977) Relationship of thoracic volume and airway occlusion pressure: muscular effects. J Appl Physiol 43:312–321
15. Remmers JE, Gautier H (1976) Servorespirator constructed from a positive pressure ventilator. J Appl Physiol 41:252–256
16. Daubenspeck JA, Pichon D, Knuth KV, Bartlett D Jr, St John WM (1988) An inexpensive servorespirator based upon regulation of a shunt resistance. Respir Physiol 73:87–96
17. Mead J, Agostoni E (1964) Dynamics of breathing. In: Handbook of physiology. Respiration. Am Physiol Soc, Washington DC, vol. 1, pp 411–427
18. Im Hof V, West P, Younes M (1986) Steady state response of normal subjects to inspiratory resistance load. J Appl Physiol 60:1471–1481
19. Im Hof V, Daniels V, Dubo H, Younes M (1986) Steady state response of quadriplegic subjects to inspiratory resistive load. J Appl Physiol 60:1482–1492
20. Gallagher CG, Younes M (1989) Effect of pressure assist on ventilation and respiratory mechanics in heavy exercise. J Appl Physiol 66:1824–1837
21. Gallagher CG, Sanii R, Younes M (1989) Response of normal subjects to inspiratory resistive unloading. J Appl Physiol 66:1113–1119
22. Marini JJ, Rodriguez RM, Lamb V (1986) The inspiratory workload of patient-initiated mechanical ventilation. Am Rev Resp Dis 134:902–909
23. Marini JJ, Smith TC, Lamb VJ (1988) External work output and force generation during synchronized intermittent mechanical ventilation. Effect of machine assistance on breathing pattern. Am Rev Resp Dis 138:1169–1179
24. Brochard L, Pluskwa F, Lemaire F (1987) Improved efficacy of spontaneous breathing with inspiratory pressure support. Am Rev Respir Dis 136:411–415
25. Brochard L, Harf A, Lorino H, Lemaire F (1989) Inspiratory pressure support prevents diaphragmatic fatigue during weaning from mechanical ventilation. Am Rev Respir Dis 139:513–521
26. Brochard L, Isabey D, Piquet J, et al (1990) Reversal of acute exacerbations of chronic obstructive lung disease by inspiratory assistance with a face mask. N Eng J Med 323:1523–1530
27. MayIntyre NR, Leatherman NE (1990) Ventilatory muscle loads and the frequency-tidal volume pattern during inspiratory pressure-assisted (pressure-supported) ventilation. Am Rev Resp Dis 141:327–331
28. Younes M, Riddle W (1984) Relation between respiratory neural output and tidal volume. J Appl Physiol 56:1110–1119
29. Younes M (1991) Determinants of thoracic excursions during exercise. In: Whipp BJ, Wasserman K (eds) Pulmonary physiology and pathophysiology of exercise. Vol. 52: Lung biology in health and disease series. Dekker, New York, pp 1–65
30. Younes M (1990) Load responses, dyspnea and respiratory failure. Chest 97:59S–68S
31. Marini JJ, Crooke PS, Truwit JD (1989) Determinants and limits of pressure-preset ventilation: a mathematical model of pressure control. J Appl Physiol 67:1081–1092
32. Hey ENB, Lloyd BB, Cunningham DJC, Jukes MGM, Bolton DPG (1966) Effect of various respiratory stimuli on the depth and frequency of breathing in man. Respir Physiol 1:193–205
33. Tobin MJ (1990) Weaning from mechanical ventilation. Current Pulmonology 11:47–105
34. Pepe PE, Marini JJ (1982) Occult positive end-expiratory pressure in mechanically ventilated patients with airflow obstruction: the auto-PEEP effect. Am Rev Resp Dis 26:166–170
35. Gottfried SB, Rossi A, Higgs BD, et al (1985) Noninvasive determination of respiratory system mechanics during mechanical ventilation for acute respiratory failure. Am Rev Resp Dis 131:414–420
36. Rossi A, Gottfried SB, Zocchi, et al (1985) Measurement of static compliance of the total respiratory system in patients with acute respiratory failure during mechanical ventilation. The effect of intrinsic positive end-expiratory pressure. Am Rev Resp Dis 131:672–677
37. Marini JJ (1990) Lung mechanics determination at the bedside: Instrumentation and clinical application. Respir Care 35:669–696
38. Younes M (1981) A model for the relation between respiratory neural and mechanical outputs. I Theory. J Appl Physiol 51:963–978

Pressure Support Ventilation

L. Brochard

Introduction

Pressure support ventilation (PSV) is a mode of partial ventilatory support which can be used in spontaneously breathing patients, both in the early phase of acute respiratory failure (ARF) and during weaning from mechanical ventilation (MV) [1]. It offers numerous advantages among which the fact that it is generally easily accepted by the patients, but has also some limitations which must be well known before proposing an extensive use of this mode in Intensive Care Units (ICU). Some data probably suggest it is one of the most interesting method to be used in difficult-to-wean patients but more information is needed about its role as a full ventilatory support.

Principles

During PSV, each spontaneous breath is assisted by a more or less constant positive pressure applied in the ventilator circuit during the duration of inspiration. Expiration is free of assistance and a positive end-expiratory pressure (PEEP), lower than the inspiratory plateau pressure, can be applied. Breathing frequency is determined by the patient since no controlled cycle is delivered. Tidal volume (VT) depends mainly upon the effort of the patient and no preset VT is delivered.

Three phases can be distinguished:

1. recognition of the beginning of inspiration;
2. pressurization;
3. recognition of the end of inspiration.

These three phases constitute the working principles of PSV and can vary from one ventilator to another. As discussed below, these variations may induce important differences in the effect of PSV for similar levels of pressurization. A schematic representation of PSV is illustrated in Fig. 1.

Recognition of Inspiration

Triggering of inspiration is initiated by the inspiratory effort of the patient and is usually detected by a pressure sensor. The trigger sensitivity is usually adjustable.

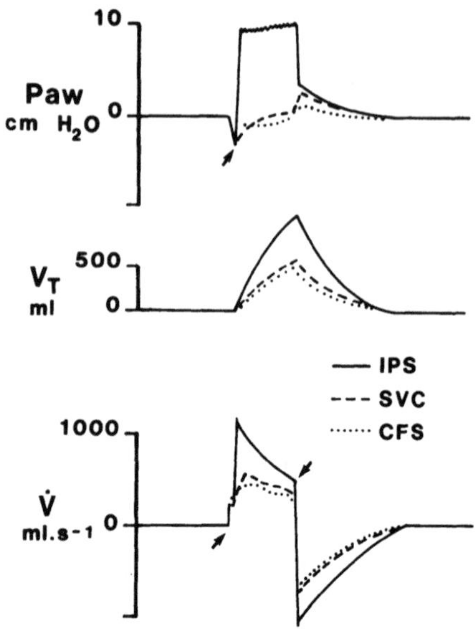

Fig. 1. Diagram of airway pressure (Paw), tidal volume (VT) and flow (V) during inspiratory pressure support (IPS), and two modes of spontaneous breathing without assistance (spontaneous circuit of a Servo 900 C ventilator, SVC, and a continuous flow system, CFS). The beginning and end of IPS are indicated with arrows on the flow trace, while opening of the demand valve is indicated on the pressure trace. (From [13] with permission)

This mechanism requires an effort from the patient; however, modern demand valves have been much improved and have a short time response. A few ventilators (Erica, Elvira) trigger inspiration on flow demand instead of pressure. The opening time delay varies between 50 and 150 msec depending upon the ventilator, and published data are available in the literature [2–3]. Although studies specifically concerning PSV are lacking, there is general agreement that, whenever respiratory cycles are patient-initiated, a high sensitivity of the trigger, together with a fast time response of the ventilator, allows a reduction of work of breathing (WOB) [2, 3] and make the patient more comfortable. Obviously, sensitivity must not be so high as to cause self-cycling.

Pressurization

Once inspiration has been initiated, the ventilator delivers a high inspiratory flow which rapidly decreases throughout the whole of inspiration. The servo regulatory mechanism maintains the proper flow necessary to reach the appropriate preset pressure support level and maintains it broadly constant until expiration occurs. The flow regulation varies between the different ventilators, determining the exact pressure wave form.

Pressure increases according to a rate that is system-specific and generally non-adjustable. A high pressurization rate results in a square pressure wave, while a low pressurization rate results in a more progressive achievement of the preset pressure support level. Only a few ventilators (Siemens Servoventilator 900C, Dräger EV-A and EVITA) allow the setting of this parameter.

Pressurization rate has been shown to influence the ventilatory pattern [4]. A low pressurization rate is disadvantageous since it may excessively increase Ti/Ttot.

This is true at least for ventilators whose expiratory trigger sensitivity is dependent on the inspiratory peak flow (see below). On the other hand, a high pressurization rate induces lower values of Ti/Ttot. The resulting square wave should be also more efficacious from the standpoint of assistance to the patient, although it can be associated with a reduction of VT in the extreme situations. It was recently shown that the "fast" pressure wave had a greater efficacy than the "slow" one to reduce WOB [5]; this was mainly explained by the higher mean airway pressure found with a fast pressure wave form. Intermediate pressure wave can also be advantageous for other patients [6].

For any inspiratory effort, the addition of pressure support augments the pressure difference between the circuit and the alveoli, leading to a higher inspiratory flow rate and a higher VT than during spontaneous breathing. Thus, whatever the IPS level, this mode always increases the inspiratory flow rate of the patient in a way which remains under patient regulation. This is the main characteristic which individualizes PSV from all other ventilatory modes. For example, during the assist-control mode, the inspiratory effort of the patient leads only to a reduction in the ventilator work but does not modify either flow or volume; if the required flow becomes greater than the flow supplied by the ventilator, the patient will exhaust his inspiratory effort without any resulting increase in VT.

Recognition of the End of Inspiration

During PSV, the cycling to exhalation is triggered by a decrease of the inspiratory flow from the peak to a system-specific threshold value. This critical decrease of the inspiratory flow is a signal that the inspiratory muscles have begun to relax. The threshold value for cycling, that represents the sensitivity of the expiratory trigger, is non-adjustable. According to the ventilator, expiration is triggered when either an absolute level of flow (between 2 and 6 l/min), or a fixed percentage of the peak (25 or 12%) is reached.

The effects of different expiratory trigger sensitivities have been investigated by means of a modified ventilator, provided with a high pressurization rate and a selection of different percentages of sensitivity [7]. From this study, it has been concluded that the optimal sensitivity for a ventilator is a function of the pressurization rate. A combination of high pressurization rate and low sensitivity of the expiratory trigger could be the most advantageous setting.

The detection of a small degree of over pressure (1–3 cm H_2O) above the fixed IPS level, which necessitates a sudden expiratory effort from the patient, can also be used, either alone, either in association with the flow criteria, to stop assistance. Lastly, as a part of the control of PSV, a time limit for inspiration is usually added. This works as a safety mechanism when a leak is present in the circuit and the two previous systems become inoperative. Hazards have been reported in the absence of this device when constant insufflation at PSV level have created high CPAP levels [8].

Set Up

For regular use, the following parameters must be adjusted:

- The trigger level, in cm H_2O below PEEP; keeping in mind that the aim of PSV is to reduce the effort done by the patient, this should be set at its maximal sensitivity.
- The pressure support level, usually adjustable from 0 to 30 or 60 cm H_2O. The degree of assistance given to the patient depends on this pressure level.

Adjustment of this level needs a different approach that in any mode of volume-controlled ventilation. The effects of PSV depend on both respiratory mechanics of the patient and its respiratory drive which result in part from its ventilatory needs. Since these parameters cannot be quantified easily and routinely, the clinician has to adjust the pressure level at the bedside after examining the effects of an arbitrarily chosen level. The two parameters which well reflect the effects of PSV and can be easily monitored, are VT and respiratory rate. Upon initiation, PSV can be adjusted to obtain a predetermined VT of 10 ml/kg. However, it is probably easier to look only at the respiratory rate, and to set the PSV level necessary to obtain the desired respiratory rate, usually between 15 and 25 breaths per minute. Adaptation of the breathing pattern to the new loading conditions is very rapid [9] and this can be observed in a minute or two. It is essential to monitor clinical status of the patient at the same time, verifying the absence of signs of respiratory distress such as recruitment of the sternocleidomastoid muscles during inspiration [10].

It must be stressed that excessive levels of PSV may be detrimental by inducing hyperinflation, generally followed by periods of apnea [11]. These deleterious high levels are dependent on respiratory mechanics of the patient. It is likely that 15 cm H_2O of PSV can induce hyperventilation on a normal lung, while 40 cm H_2O may not be sufficient in a patient with ARDS.

Because of the principles upon which PSV works, neither volume nor frequency settings can be used. In modern ventilators, a back-up ventilation is present in case of prolonged apnea.

Servocontrolled pressure support level is an interesting way to resolve the question of the adequate level of pressure and its modification over time. This is proposed by several ventilators and the controlled parameter is either minute ventilation (VE) or the breathing frequency (f) of the patient. This last modality seems to be an interesting and promising mode of partial ventilatory support [12].

Monitoring

Monitoring is an important aspect of ventilation with PSV. Indeed, the volume delivered to the patient at each breath can vary if any worsening of respiratory mechanics occurs, and the patient can feel discomfort if his respiratory drive is altered without any adaptation of the pressure delivered. Respiratory rate is a key feature of this monitoring, suggesting, when normal, the adequacy between the patient's need and the level of support [10]. An alarm of high respiratory rate is often proposed by modern ventilators.

Effects of PSV on Respiratory Muscle Activity

Breathing Pattern

As discussed above, addition of PSV modifies the spontaneous breathing pattern. By comparison to spontaneous breathing, VT increases and respiratory rate decreases suggesting an adaptation to the decreased workload [10, 13, 14]. With increasing levels of pressure support, gradual increase in VT and reduction in respiratory rate are observed. Some data suggest that this reduced respiratory rate may reduce auto-PEEP because of expiratory time lengthening [10, 15]. VE can either be increased or either remain at the same level [10, 13, 16, 17].

In patients with deteriorating gas exchange during spontaneous breathing, i.e. hypoxemia and hypercapnia, alveolar ventilation and arterial blood gas tensions are improved by the addition of pressure support allowing the patient to breathe with a normalized $PaCO_2$ [10].

Respiratory Muscle Work

A recent study examined the effects of PSV on the mechanical WOB, the oxygen cost of breathing and diaphragmatic activity [10]. In eight patients with difficulty in tolerating discontinuation from MV despite adequate therapy several levels of PSV were compared, from 0 (i.e. spontaneous breathing without assistance) to 20 cm H_2O of pressure support. During PS = 0 the patients exhibited a characteristic pattern of breathing, with small VT at a high rate. This has been found to be associated with unsuccessful weaning [9]. This particular breathing pattern was ac-

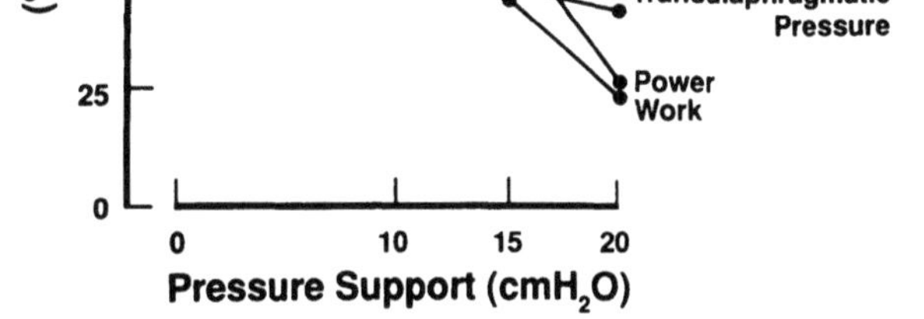

Fig. 2. Mean values of respiratory muscle function parameters obtained in eight patients with difficulties to tolerate discontinuation from mechanical ventilation. Values are expressed in percentage of the highest values which were found during spontaneous breathing without pressure support. Addition of successive levels of pressure induced a gradual decrease in power of breathing, in work per liter of ventilation, in transdiaphragmatic pressure as well as in total oxygen consumption by reducing the oxygen cost of breathing

companied by a decrease in PaO_2 and a significant increase in $PaCO_2$. All patients exhibited intense activity of the sternocleidomastoid muscles. In the same period, patients performed high levels of WOB and the oxygen cost of breathing was estimated to be as high as 25% of total oxygen consumption. Diaphragmatic electromyogram (EMG) studies were recorded and the ratio of high frequency to low frequency components of the diaphragmatic EMG (H/L), an index indicative of excessive workload and impending fatigue, were measured. During PS = 0, 7 of the 8 patients exhibited electrical signs of impending diaphragmatic fatigue, a finding concomittant with their inability to be weaned from the ventilator. Pressure support was then delivered at 10, 15 and 20 cm H_2O. With increasing levels of PSV, alterations in breathing pattern and arterial blood gases were observed, as described above. A dramatic reduction in the WOB performed by the patients, the oxygen cost of breathing [18] and diaphragmatic activity was also demonstrated. The magnitude of the work was inversely correlated with the level of pressure support delivered. Diaphragmatic activity, although always present, was progressively reduced. All these data are summarized in Fig. 2. In addition, the EMG signs of diaphragmatic fatigue were suppressed at 10 cm H_2O in 4 patients and at 20 cm H_2O in 3 patients. Interestingly at this "optimal level", activity of the sternocleidomastoid muscles was minimized or no longer present. In addition, respiratory rate was markedly decreased. These findings are illustrated in Fig. 3. In another study performed in post-operative patients without preexisting pulmonary disease, 15 cm H_2O PSV was shown to take over the major part of the WOB assessed by the oxygen cost of breathing [19]. In patients with COPD, similar findings have been demonstrated [20]. In these patients, 15 cm H_2O of PSV decreased markedly both the oxygen cost of breathing and the diaphragmatic pressure time index by comparison to CPAP. Thus by setting the pressure level adequately, the physician may regulate WOB and find an optimal workload for the respiratory muscles.

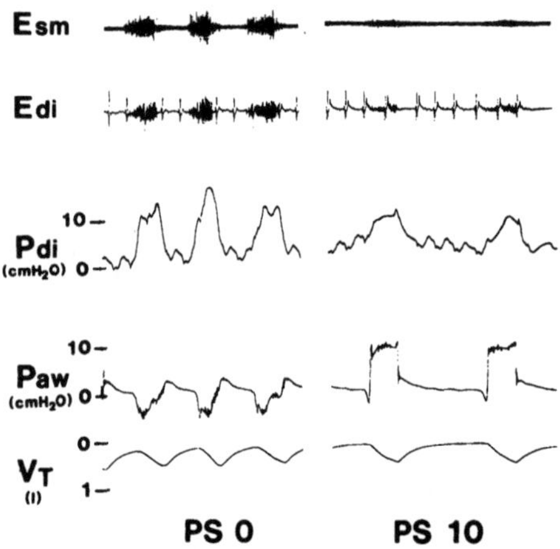

Fig. 3. Recordings of electrical activity of the sternocleidomastoid muscle (Esm) and of the diaphragm (Edi), transdiaphragmatic pressure (Pdi), airway pressure (Paw) and tidal volume (VT) for one representative patient during PS = 0 and PS = 10. Diaphragmatic activity, assessed by Pdi, is reduced during PS = 10 but is still present. Sternocleidomastoid activity is no longer present during PS = 10 and respiratory rate is markedly decreased. (From [9] with permission).

Compensation of the Additional Work Induced by the Endotracheal Tube and the Demand Valve

It has been proposed that PSV could be used to compensate the extrawork of breathing induced by the presence of an endotracheal tube [21, 22]. In addition, the presence of a demand valve and the ventilator circuitry imposes a supplemental load which can be overcome by a certain amount of PSV. Breathing through the endotracheal tube has been found to induce a significant extra-workload [22]. This additional work was much higher in patients with chronic lung disease (nearly 40% of the work measured after extubation) than in patients free of lung disease in whom the additional work was virtually negligible (13% of the work measured after extubation). The pressure support level necessary to compensate this additionnal work in patients with lung disease was always above 8 to 10 cm H_2O. Thus, intubated patients with chronic lung disease (who represent most of the patients with difficulties to be weaned) who have an adequate breathing pattern at a pressure support level of 8 cm H_2O for several hours, can probably be extubated without risks of excessive respiratory muscle work. In patients free of lung disease however, much lower levels of pressure support are able to suppress the extrawork induced by the tube.

Clinical Applications

Inspiratory pressure support increases markedly the efficacy of spontaneous breathing in patients intubated for respiratory failure while reducing the activity of the inspiratory muscles. The ventilator-to-patient synchronization is optimized since the respiratory rate is determined by the patient and as each breath is efficiently assisted, the patient can breathe spontaneously for sustained periods. Sophisticated monitoring of ventilation is performed by ventilators offering the pressure support mode. There is no evidence to date, however, that PSV can reduce complications related to MV.

Full Ventilatory Support

PSV can be used early in the course of respiratory failure. Its potential advantages are a lesser need for sedation and a better comfort for the patient. PSV has been compared to other modes of ventilation in short term studies. It has been used to lower the peak airway pressure and decrease spontaneous respiratory rate of patients ventilated with assist-control ventilation [23]. Other studies have focused on patients ventilated with PSV instead of conventional controlled MV [24, 25]. In patients with moderate acute respiratory insufficiency and in whom extravascular lung water was measured as almost normal, improvement in oxygenation has been observed with PSV by comparison to continuous positive pressure ventilation [25]. It is possible that this improvement resulted at least partly from a lesser use of sedation in patients with PSV. Since a significant amount of work can be performed during assist-control ventilation [26, 27], comparison of this mode with PSV was interesting. A mode of pressure assisted ventilation similar to PSV has been shown to have a greater efficacy than assist-control ventilation to decrease WOB in patients with normal respiratory drive [28]. It has also a greater efficacy than the classical intermittent positive pressure breathing [29].

Several factors also favor the use of PSV in certain circumstances: the hemodynamic status seems to be similar during PSV and other modes of ventilatory support [24, 30], while several authors have reported that patients felt more comfortable during PSV than during CPAP or assisted MV (AMV) [13]. Another study in post-operative patients has shown that the arterial blood gases were improved in PSV compared with AMV despite a lower VE and that these patients required less sedation [30].

All these data are not conclusive enough to demonstrate the superiority of PSV over other ventilatory support but show that

1. it can be used early in the course of MV for ARF, and
2. it is likely that some advantages can result form the use of PSV in some patients such as a lesser need for sedation and a better comfort for the patients.

It must be emphasized that, by definition, no preset VT or VE is present. Efficacy of a certain level of pressure therefore depends upon mechanics of the respiratory system. Any change in compliance or resistance may induce a modification of the efficacy of PSV, requiring, at best, an adjustment of the level of pressure support. In unstable and/or severely injured patients, precise monitoring is mandatory since rapid deterioration of the patient may result from inadequate assistance. Thus, in some patients, it may be uneasy to use PSV as a "full support" and its potential advantages, mainly comfort and lesser use for sedation, must be counterbalanced with the need of adequate monitoring. The use of PSV requires an adequate ventilatory drive, and heavily sedated patients or with depressed ventilatory command are not candidates for this technique.

Weaning form Mechanical Ventilation

PSV seems to be a very promising alternative for use during the weaning phase. During this phase, the critical problem is no longer oxygenation but the ability of respiratory muscle function to face the supplemental workload imposed by weaning. Most patients recovering from ARF can be easily weaned from MV, and in this case the choice of weaning method is not critical. However there are difficult-to-wean patients, ranging from 10 to 40% of the ventilated patients, who should benefit from an optimal method [9, 31–33]. Decreasing the workload imposed on their muscles and assessing their ability to be extubated should be the two goals of the weaning strategy. PSV has the ability of both decreasing respiratory muscle work and evaluating respiratory adaptation to the imposed workload. Indeed, the level of pressure support needed by the patient to achieve a satisfactory breathing pattern is an important tool to estimate his ability to be weaned [22]. Preliminary data from a multicenter trial comparing PSV, synchronized intermittent mandatory ventilation (SIMV) and T-piece trials in difficult-to-wean patients suggest that the use of PSV results in significantly less weaning failure and a shorter duration of successful weaning [34]. In this study, no pressure support was applied during the spontaneous cycles of SIMV and the T-piece trials. Although there is no data to support it, it is likely that SIMV should be best applied with some pressure support to help overcome circuit and endotracheal tube resistance.

Non Invasive Ventilation

Since both endotracheal intubation and MV have numerous complications, there is a need for methods of ventilatory assistance that could obviate the need for intubation in patients with ARF. Several approaches have been proposed, all presenting difficulties in their clinical use [35, 36]. PSV delivered with a face mask by the means of a special device has recently been used in patients admitted for acute exacerbations of chronic obstructive lung disease [37]. The short term effects of this mode of ventilation were similar to what is observed in intubated patients.

Figure 4 provides an example of the effects of this inspiratory assistance delivered via a face mask. A decrease in respiratory muscle activity was obtained while hypoxemia was corrected. In addition, respiratory acidosis was partially or totally corrected. Therefore, the two goals of MV, i.e. correction of gas exchange abnormalities and decrease of respiratory workload, were achieved. Also application of the method was not easy, requiring to use well fitted face mask and especially de-

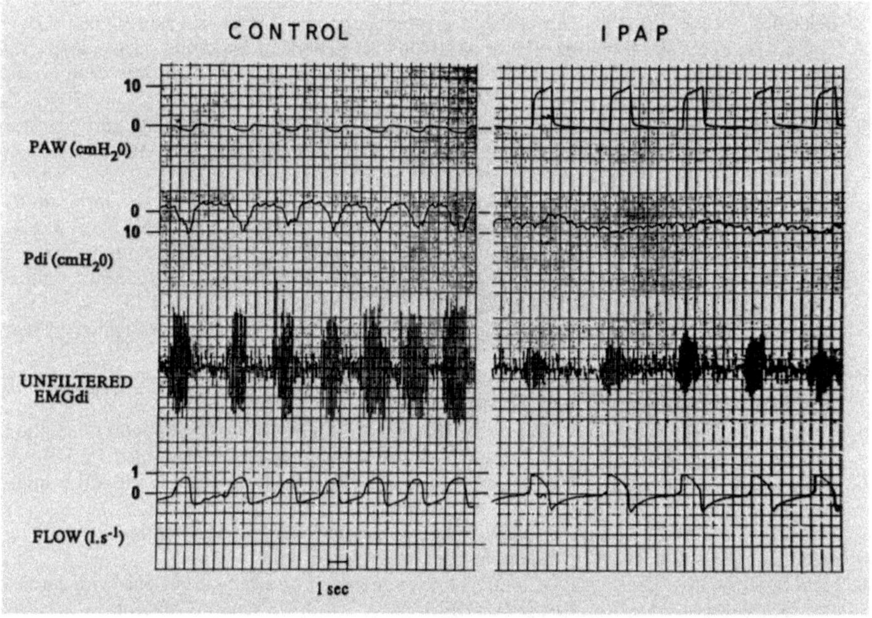

Fig. 4. Recordings for a representative patient during the control period and after 45 min of treatment with inspiratory positive airway pressure. From top to bottom, recordings of airway pressure, transdiaphragmatic pressure, unfiltered diaphragmatic electromyographic activity and flow. Note the decrease in muscular activity and in respiratory rate during treatment. (From [30] with permission)

signed device, most patients with acute exacerbation of their disease could be treated with this method. Most patients receiving PSV avoided tracheal intubation, resulting in a shorter stay in ICU than control patients treated conventionally whose tracheas were intubated in most of the cases.

References

1. Kacmarek RM (1988) The role of pressure support ventilation in reducing work of breathing. Respir Care 33:99–120
2. Cox D, Tinloi SF, Farrimond JG (1988) Investigation of the spontaneous modes of breathing of different ventilators. Intensive Care Med 14:532–537
3. Samodelov LF, Falke KJ (1988) Total inspiratory work with modern demand valve devices compared to continuous flow CPAP. Intensive Care Med 14:632–639
4. Braschi A, Rodi G, Sala Gallini G, Iotti G, Chiaranda M (1989) Relationships between pressurization rate and breathing pattern during pressure support ventilation. Am Rev Respir Dis (Abstract) 139:A155
5. Messadi AA, Ben Ayed M, Brochard L, Iotti G, Harf A, Lemaire F (1990) Comparison of the efficacy of two waveforms of inspiratory pressure support: Slow versus fast pressure wave. Am Rev Respir Dis (Abstract) 141:A519
6. MacIntyre NR, Ho Li (1991) Effects of initial flow rate and breath termination criteria on pressure support ventilation. Chest 99:134–138
7. Braschi A, Sala Gallini G, Rodi G, Iotti G, Chiaranda M, Villa S (1989) Relationships between sensitivity of the expiratory trigger and breathing pattern during pressure support ventilation. Am Rev Respir Dis (Abstract) 139:A361
8. Black JW, Grover BS (1988) A hazard of pressure support ventilation. Chest 93:333–335
9. Tobin MJ, Perez W, Guenther SH, et al (1986) The pattern of breathing during successful and unsuccessful trials of weaning from mechanical ventilation. Am Rev Respir Dis 134:1111–1118
10. Brochard L, Harf A, Lorino H, Lemaire F (1989) Inspiratory pressure support prevents diaphragmatic fatigue during weaning from mechanical ventilation. Am Rev Respir Dis 139:513–521
11. Ben Ayed M, Axler O, Lemaire F (1986) Un accident de la ventilation avec aide inspiratoire: bradypnée avec hyperinsufflation thoracique. Réan Soins Intens Med Urg (Abstract) 3:262
12. Boyer F, Bruneau B, Gaussorgues P, Jay-Lassonnery S, Robert D (1989) Aide inspiratoire avec asservissement du niveau de pression: volume ventilé minute versus fréquence ventilatoire. Réan Soins Intens Med Urg 5:227–232
13. MacIntyre NR (1986) Respiratory function during pressure support ventilation. Chest 89:677–683
14. Brochard L, Pluskwa F, Lemaire F (1987) Improved efficacy of spontaneous breathing with inspiratory pressure support. Am Rev Respir Dis 32:1011–1016
15. Conti G, Bufi M, Antonelli M, Rocco M, Gasparetto A (1989) Pressure support ventilation reverses hyperinflation induced isorythmic A-V dissociation. Intensive Care Med 15:319–321
16. Ershowsky P, Krieger B (1987) Changes in breathing pattern during pressure support ventilation. Resp Care 32:1011–1016
17. Tokioka H, Saito S, Kosaka F (1989) Effect of pressure support ventilation on breathing patterns and respiratory work. Intensive Care Med 15:491–494
18. Field S, Kelly SM, Macklem PT (1982) The oxygen cost of breathing in patients with cardiorespiratory disease. Am Rev Respir Dis 126:9–13
19. Viale JP, Annat GJ, Bouffard YM, Delafosse BX, Bertrand OH, Motin JP (1988) Oxygen cost of breathing in post-operative patients. Chest 93:506–509
20. Annat GJ, Viale JP, Dereymez CP, Bouffard YM, Delafosse BX, Motin JP (1990) Oxygen cost of breathing and diaphragmatic pressure time-index. Measurement in patients with COPD during weaning with pressure support ventilation. Chest 98:411–414

21. Fiastro JF, Habib MP, Quan SF (1988) Pressure support compensation for inspiratory work due to endotracheal tubes and demand continuous positive airway pressure. Chest 93:499–505
22. Brochard L, Rua F, Lorino H, Lemaire F, Harf A (1988) Suppression of the extrawork of breathing due to the endotracheal tube with inspiratory pressure support. Am Rev Respir Dis (Abstract) 137:A64
23. Tokioka H, Saito S, Kosaka F (1989) Comparison of pressure support ventilation and assist control ventilation in patients with acute respiratory failure. Intensive Care Med 15:364–367
24. Prakash O, Meij S (1985) Cardiopulmonary response to inspiratory pressure support during spontaneous ventilation vs conventional ventilation. Chest 88:403–408
25. Zeravik J, Borg U, Pfeiffer UJ (1990) Efficacy of pressure support ventilation dependent on extravascular lung water. Chest 97:1412–1419
26. Marini JJ, Capps JS, Culver BM (1985) The inspiratory work of breathing during assisted mechanical ventilation. Chest 87:612–618
27. Marini JJ, Rodriguez RM, Lamb VI (1986) The inspiratory workload of patient-initiated mechanical ventilation. Am Rev Respir Dis 134:902–909
28. Cinnella G, Barboni E, Conti G, et al (1990) Comparison of assist-control ventilation and assist pressure controlled ventilation. Intensive Care Med (Abstract) 16:S70
29. Mancebo J, Brochard L, Amaro P, Mollo JL, Harf A, Lemaire F (1988) Is inspiratory pressure support similar to intermittent positive breathing? Intensive Care Med 14:A326
30. Fargier JJ, Robert D, Boyer F, et al (1987) Positive pressure inspiratory aid vs assisted mechanical ventilation after esophageal surgery. J Crit Care 2:101–108
31. Schachter EN, Tucker D, Beck GJ (1981) Does intermittent mandatory ventilation accelerate weaning? JAMA 246:1210–1214
32. Sassoon CSH, Te TT, Mahutte CK, Light RW (1987) Airway occlusion pressure. An important indicator for successful weaning in patients with chronic obstructive pulmonary disease. Am Rev Respir Dis 135:107–113
33. Murciano D, Boczkowski J, Lecocguic Y, Milic-Emili J, Pariente R, Aubier M (1988) Tracheal occlusion pressure: A simple index to monitor respiratory muscle fatigue during acute respiratory failure in patients with chronic obstructive pulmonary disease. Ann Intern Med 108:800–805
34. Brochard L, Rauss A, Benito S, et al (1991) Comparison of three techniques of weaning from mechanical ventilation. Results of an european multicenter trial. Am Rev Respir Dis (Abstract) 143:A602
35. Meduri GU, Conoscenti CC, Menashe P, Nair S (1989) Non invasive face mask ventilation in patients with acute respiratory failure. Chest 95:865–870
36. Carrey Z, Gottfried SB, Levy RD (1990) Ventilatory muscle support in respiratory failure with nasal positive pressure ventilation. Chest 97:150–158
37. Brochard L, Isabey D, Piquet J, et al (1990) Reversal of acute exacerbations of chronic obstructive lung disease by inspiratory assistance with a face mask. N Engl J Med 323:1523–1530

The Role of PEEP in the Mechanically Ventilated COPD Patient

S.B. Gottfried

Introduction

The approach to mechanical ventilation (MV) of the critically ill patient will vary according to the pathophysiological events underlying the development of acute respiratory failure. In this regard, it is clinically useful to classify acute respiratory failure into two major categories - "type 1" or hypoxemic respiratory failure and "type 2" or hypercapnic ventilatory failure [1]. The former category is best exemplified by the adult respiratory distress syndrome (ARDS). The underlying pathophysiology in this condition is one of diffuse alveolar injury characterized by extensive alveolar edema and collapse, a reduction in lung volume, and marked hypoxemia relatively refractory to high inspired concentrations of oxygen [2]. MV with the addition of positive end-expiratory pressure (PEEP) is the treatment modality most commonly employed to improve oxygenation in such patients. PEEP is considered to act through its ability to re-expand flooded and atelectatic alveolar units, increase functional residual capacity, and thereby reduce the magnitude of venous admixture [2].

In contrast, hypercapnic ventilatory failure is identified by the inability of the "failing respiratory pump" to provide a level of alveolar ventilation sufficient to meet the required metabolic demands [3]. While this may be due to central depression of respiratory drive, neuromuscular disorders, or chest wall abnormalities, perhaps the most common etiology in the ICU setting is an acute exacerbation of severe underlying chronic obstructive pulmonary disease (COPD). MV is instituted in this instance in order to provide an appropriate level of alveolar ventilation while allowing for improvement in pulmonary function and recovery from presumed respiratory muscle fatigue to occur [3]. In this setting, PEEP has been considered unhelpful and in fact contraindicated for several reasons [1, 2, 4, 5]. First, the level of hypoxemia observed in such patients is generally mild and responds readily to low levels of supplemental oxygen. Second, severe COPD is characterized by substantial elevations in lung volume; a further increase in lung volume induced by PEEP would not only impair respiratory muscle efficiency but also enhance the risk of hemodynamic depression and barotrauma.

The rationale against the use of PEEP in mechanically ventilated COPD patients appears to be quite logical and sound. However, it is of interest to bear in mind that PEEP (or more appropriately "continuous positive pressure breathing") was originally introduced in the U.S. by Barach specifically for its proposed benefit in patients with severe airway obstruction [6]. In addition, more recent work indicates that PEEP can play a significant and important role in the management of the mechanically ventilated patient with severe COPD [7, 8]. Accordingly, the aims of the following chapter will be to 1) review the physiological background supporting the use of PEEP, 2) examine the role of PEEP (or continuous positive airway pressure, CPAP) during assisted modes of MV and particularly when discontinuation of ventilatory support is being attempted, and 3) present a number of recommendations concerning the administration and monitoring of PEEP (or CPAP) therapy in the COPD patient with acute respiratory failure.

Dynamic Hyperinflation and Intrinsic PEEP: Implications for the Inspiratory Muscles

An appreciation of the indications for and use of PEEP in the mechanically ventilated patient with severe COPD requires a firm grasp of the unique pathophysiological events occurring. This topic has been presented elsewhere in this volume and in a number of previous publications [8, 9, 10]. It will nevertheless be of benefit to briefly review a number of specific points in the context of the discussion to follow.

It is now commonly accepted that dynamic hyperinflation is a cardinal feature recognized in nearly all mechanically ventilated patients with severe COPD, particularly at the time of initial presentation [11-15]. Because the rate of lung emptying is unduly prolonged relative to the available expiratory duration, expiration is interrupted by the subsequent breath before the relaxation volume of the respiratory system can be reached. The presence of dynamic hyperinflation implies that alveolar pressure remains positive throughout expiration, in contrast to the normal circumstance. This positive pressure now present at end-expiration is commonly referred to as *auto* or *intrinsic PEEP* (PEEPi) [12, 16].

Dynamic hyperinflation has a number of adverse effects on inspiratory muscle function and energetics. The dynamic increase in lung volume places the inspiratory muscles on a disadvantageous position of their force-length relationship as well as reducing force-generating capacity because of alterations in thoracic geometry and other considerations [17, 18]. It should be noted that this is in addition to any increase in *static* lung volume which may have occurred due to pulmonary emphysema and reduced elastic recoil. While recent evidence indicates that adaptation to chronic changes in resting muscle length are possible [19, 20], it is unlikely that this would be of benefit for the acute changes in muscle length expected with dynamic hyperinflation.

In addition to alterations in efficiency, dynamic hyperinflation also directly increases the mechanical load imposed on the disadvantages inspiratory muscles (Fig. 1). This is due to the extensive degree of overall hyperinflation which places the patient on the flat, relatively stiff portion of the volume-pressure relationship of the total respiratory system [18]. The decreased compliance against which the inspiratory muscles must act will contribute to increase the work and oxygen cost of breathing. Moreover, the presence of intrinsic PEEP also requires that the inspiratory muscles must generate sufficient force to overcome the opposing recoil pressure before inspiratory flow will begin [9, 13]. In this respect, PEEPi acts as an inspiratory threshold load and represents an additional impedence with which the disad-

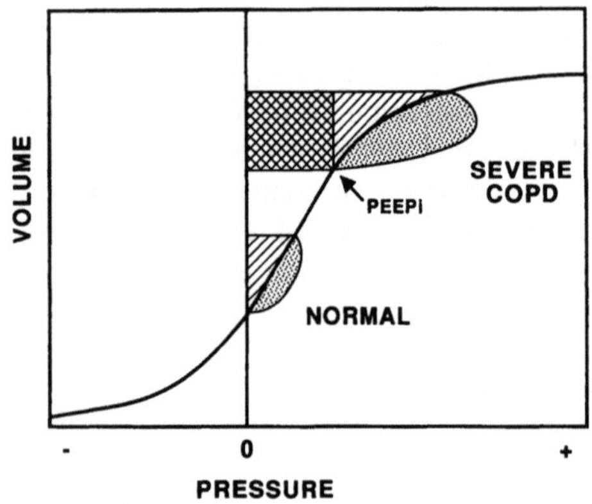

Fig. 1. Schematic representation of the volume-pressure relationship of the respiratory system demonstrating the manner in which the mechanical work of breathing is increased in a patient with severe COPD and acute respiratory failure. Compared to a normal subject, the inspiratory resistive work of breathing *(stippled area)* is significantly increased. In addition, the extensive degree of hyperinflation forces the COPD patient to breathe on the relatively flattened portion of the volume-pressure relationship, considerably increasing the elastic work of breathing *(diagonally striped area)*. Inspiratory effort is also required to overcome the positive recoil pressure present at end-expiration, or intrinsic PEEP (PEEPi), further adding to the increased elastic *(cross-hatched area)* and total work of breathing which must be performed. (Adapted from [22, 23])

vantaged muscles are faced [13]. As will be discussed shortly, this has important clinical consequences during assisted modes of mechanical ventilation as well as when discontinuation of ventilatory support is being attempted.

Management of Dynamic Hyperinflation and Intrinsic PEEP

It has been clearly demonstrated that dynamic hyperinflation has significant adverse effect on cardiovascular as well as respiratory function in the mechanically ventilated patient [11, 12, 21]. Reducing the degree of dynamic hyperinflation, and consequently the magnitude of PEEPi, is therefore an important clinical objective in such patients. Obviously, management should be directed toward those factors contributing to the level of dynamic hyperinflation present. As a general approximation, this will be proportional to tidal volume and inversely related to expiratory duration and the rate of expiratory flow which can be achieved [11, 12, 16]. Attempts at decreasing PEEPi will therefore include measures to reduce the severity of airway obstruction and minimize ventilatory requirements [9, 11, 12]. Ventilator settings should also be adjusted in order to provide as much time as possible for complete exhalation to occur while still being consistent with patient comfort and satisfactory gas exchange [12, 16]. The severity of clinical illness and airway obstruction, however, are often such that the success of these approaches are limited and clinically important levels of intrinsic PEEP persist. Under these circumstances, other alternative therapeutic modalities are needed.

Importance of Dynamic Airway Compression and Flow Limitation

Expiratory flow limitation occurring as a consequence of dynamic airway compression is nearly always present in mechanically ventilated COPD patients in whom PEEPi can be found [11, 13, 24–27]. Under these circumstances, it had been reasoned that increases in downstream impedance (e.g. PEEP) relative to the site of flow limitation would have little effect on expiratory flow-volume events until the existing level of PEEPi was approached [9, 13, 25]. Thus, PEEP applied through the external ventilator circuit could serve to counterbalance the positive recoil pressure present at end-expiration. In effect, PEEP would replace PEEPi and in this fashion eliminate the threshold load imposed [9, 16, 24].

This assumption has been examined by several investigators during controlled MV in which errors in interpretation due to variability in breathing pattern, patient effort, or the nature of respiratory muscle recruitment could be avoided [24, 25, 28]. Briefly, low levels of PEEP much less than the amount of PEEPi present generally had no effect on expiratory flow and lung volume remained unchanged. However, as the amount of PEEP applied increased relative to the existing level of PEEPi, a value of PEEP could be identified above which expiratory flow was reduced and lung volume increased. Of importance, this occurred at a level of PEEP somewhat less than the value of PEEPi. This level of applied pressure has been referred to as Pcrit (or Pmax), analogous to the use of that term to describe the transpulmonary pressure at which expiratory flow limitation occurs during forced expiration [11, 28–30].

These findings are in fact entirely consistent with the physiological principles originally described to explain the transpulmonary pressure, flow, and volume interrelationships observed during forced expiratory maneuvers in both health and disease [29, 30]. Under these circumstances, the transpulmonary pressure at which expiratory flow limitation occurs must be somewhat less than the total elastic recoil pressure available, due to resistive pressure losses across the upstream segment proximal to the point of dynamic airway collapse. In terms of the mechanically ventilated COPD patient, this implies that the critical value of PEEP (Pcrit) above which changes in flow-volume events and end-expiratory lung volume will first occur must be somewhat less than the existing level of PEEPi. Available data indicates that in general Pcrit amounts to about 75% of PEEPi, the actual value presumably varying with the upstream resistance and maximum flow achieved [24, 25, 28].

This analysis can be best understood considering the lung as a simple one-compartment model, not unlike that used to describe flow through a Starling resistor or across a vascular "waterfall" (Fig. 2) [29–31]. The results obtained, however, are also consistent with a more complex system with marked heterogeneity of regional mechanical properties [7, 24, 32]. McNamara et al. [33] have demonstrated through direct measurements of regional alveolar pressure in experimental animals that significant heterogeneity in the presence and magnitude of expiratory flow limitation amongst regional lung units may occur and not be evident from examination of flow-volume events at the airway opening. Of interest, they described a number of physical mechanisms which tended to limit the degree of variability in flow limitation which could occur. Whether these principles apply in pathological

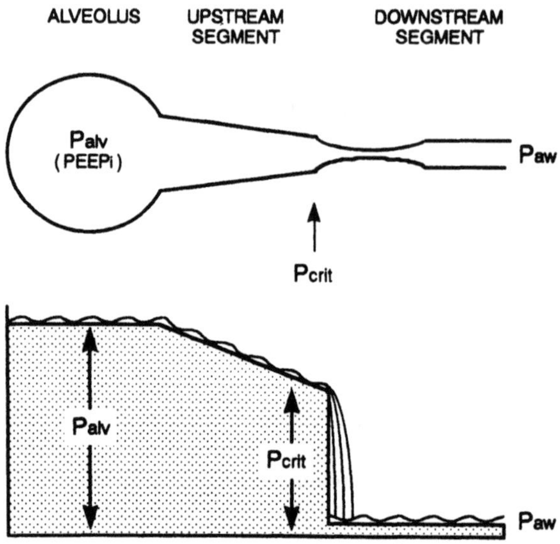

Fig. 2. Schematic representation depicting expiratory flow limitation within the lung. In the *upper figure,* the lung is modeled as a single alveolus and conducting airway divided into upstream and downstream segments. Alveolar pressure (Palv) exceeds the critical pressure (Pcrit) at which dynamic airway compression occurs, the difference due to resistive pressure losses across the upstream segment. Palv at the end of passive expiration in a dynamically hyperinflated patient is equivalent to intrinsic PEEP (PEEPi). Expiratory flow limitation will persist as long as the positive pressure applied at the airway (Paw) does not exceed Pcrit, rather than PEEPi. The *lower figure* displays analogous circumstances governing flow across a waterfall. The amount of flow over the waterfall remains constant until the level of water in the stream below (Paw) reaches the height of the waterfall (Pcrit) and not the stream above (Palv)

conditions in man remains to be determined. The clinical importance of this is that such considerations will influence the therapeutic use of PEEP, indicating that the absence of changes in flow-volume events and end-expiratory lung volume may not entirely exclude the presence of significant regional hyperinflation and the risk of barotrauma in COPD patients (see below).

Dynamic Hyperinflation in Acute Asthma

As recently demonstrated by Tuxen [34, 35], dynamic hyperinflation is also a common occurrence in patients mechanically ventilated for treatment of acute asthma. In contrast with the prior observations in COPD patients however, PEEP appeared to uniformly increase lung volume and worsen hyperinflation [35]. Expectedly, this was associated with often marked increases in airway pressure and circulatory impairment. Though not examined in further detail, these results would indicate that expiratory flow limitation is not a characteristic feature of acute life-threatening asthma.

Considering the basic pathophysiology of asthma, it is not surprising that the results obtained may differ substantially from previously reported findings in patients with well-documented and longstanding, severe airway obstruction due to COPD. Increased airway collapsibility has been recognized in patients with advanced COPD [36]. This has been attributed to destruction of lung parenchyma with loss of lung elastic recoil (and the ability to tether open conducting airways) as well as structural changes within the airway wall itself. In contrast, the increases in airway smooth muscle, bronchomotor tone, and inflammatory infiltration characteristic of severe asthma may actually serve to stiffen the airway wall and decrease collapsibility despite the considerable reduction in airway caliber [37–39]. Alternatively, differences between asthmatic and COPD patients in the heterogeneity and distribution of airway obstruction with flow limitation amongst lung units may also explain these results [7, 24].

Anecdotal reports have described the ability of PEEP (often at remarkably high levels) to directly improve airway function, relieving refractory bronchoconstriction in acute life-threatening asthma [40–42]. These reports appear to be exceptional and isolated circumstances, however. Considering the limited nature of these clinical observations, the importance of other confounding factors cannot be entirely excluded. With this in mind, the general dictum against the use of PEEP in acute asthma (in contrast to mechanically ventilated COPD patients) remains justified at the present time [7].

Role of PEEP During Assist-Control Ventilation

It had been generally considered that patient effort was minimal during assisted MV, and as a result the work of breathing was largely assumed by the ventilator. However, a number of recent studies have shown that the work actually performed by a patient during assisted ventilation is considerable and often a significant fraction of values observed during unsupported spontaneous breathing [43–45]. One of the major determinants of patient work during ventilator-assisted breaths is in fact the trigger sensitivity set on the machine [43]. In normal individuals subjected to assisted MV, a modest reduction in triggering sensitivity increased the work of breathing performed by as much as 50% [43]. This is particularly relevant in the mechanically ventilated COPD patient where PEEPi reduces the "effective" trigger sensitivity, requiring the patient to generate a negative inspiratory force equivalent in magnitude to the opposing positive recoil pressure present at end-expiration (i.e. PEEPi) plus the triggering pressure set on the ventilator before an assisted breath can be initiated (Fig. 3) [9, 24]. Considering the relative magnitude of PEEPi encountered clinically in these patients (about 10 cm H_2O) compared to the customary trigger sensitivity set on the ventilator (1–2 cm H_2O), the manner in which PEEPi would act to increase patient effort during assisted ventilation can be readily appreciated.

The importance of these concepts has been supported by direct quantitative measurements of the inspiratory work of breathing in COPD patients with acute respiratory failure. The work of breathing was shown to be considerably increased during spontaneous breathing, averaging 15.2 joules/min, but was only reduced to

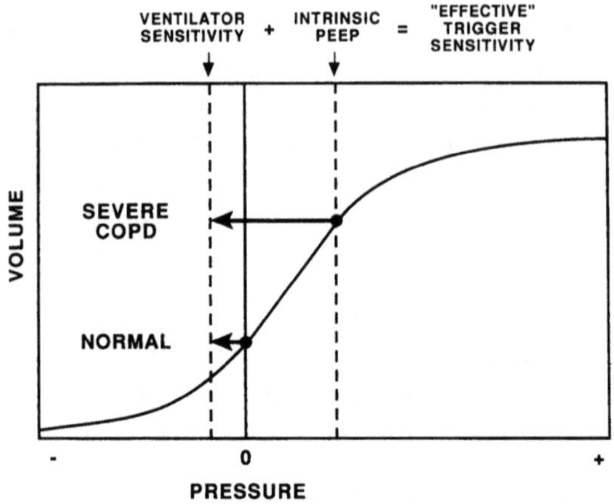

Fig. 3. The end-expiratory position *(filled circle)* during assist-control ventilation in a normal subject and a patient with severe COPD and intrinsic PEEP is depicted on the static volume-pressure relationship of the respiratory system. To trigger a machine-assisted breath, the normal subject must produce an inspiratory force *(horizontal arrow)* slightly more negative than the sensitivity set on the ventilator *(left vertical dashed line)*. Intrinsic PEEP *(right vertical dashed line)* increases the "effective" trigger sensitivity *(horizontal arrow)* in the patient with severe COPD, requiring that inspiratory effort exceeds ventilator sensitivity *plus* the opposing recoil pressure present at end-expiration (i.e. intrinsic PEEP) in order to initiate a ventilator-assisted breath

10.6 joules/min when assist-control ventilation was provided [24]. Thus, the capacity of assist-control ventilation to reduce patient effort, and thereby relieve dyspnea and promote recovery from respiratory muscle fatigue, was severely limited in such patients. Accordingly, Smith and Marini [24] investigated the consequences of externally applied PEEP on the existing level of PEEPi and its ability to alter the excessive workload experienced during assist-control ventilation in these patients. As anticipated, the addition of PEEP did decrease the level of PEEPi present. While end-expiratory lung volume was not directly measured, failure of PEEP to appreciably increase peak airway pressure was considered as evidence that lung volume was unaltered. This was associated with a significant reduction in the total inspiratory work of breathing, which averaged approximately 50% of the baseline value when 10 cm H_2O PEEP was applied. Although partitioning work into its resistive and elastic components during assisted ventilation was not possible, inspiratory resistance and compliance did not change indicating that the observed improvement was due to removal of the inspiratory threshold load imposed by PEEPi. Although applied for relatively brief periods, no complications due to the use of PEEP were reported. Similar findings have been obtained more recently by other investigators [26].

PEEP and Synchronized Intermittent Mandatory Ventilation

Intermittent mandatory ventilation (IMV) was introduced by Downs et al. [46] in 1973 as an alternative mode of ventilatory support with a number of proposed advantages over the conventional forms of MV then available. This included improvement in patient work, comfort, and coordination with the mechanical ventilator. At the time of a recent survey by Venus et al. [47], IMV appeared to be the most common form of MV used in ICUs in the United States. Currently, this ventilator mode is generally provided in its synchronized form, SIMV, taking advantage of the internal demand valve system of current generation ventilators to provide inspiratory airflow during both spontaneous and positive-pressure ventilator breaths.

Despite its widespread use, the efficacy of SIMV in patients with severe COPD and PEEPi has not been examined. This issue is of importance for a number of reasons. Not unlike assist-control ventilation, the presence of PEEPi will increase the inspiratory effort required to produce flow for both ventilator and spontaneous breaths (see below). In addition, the pattern of breathing during SIMV is inherently heterogeneous and variable due to the combination of both spontaneous and posi-

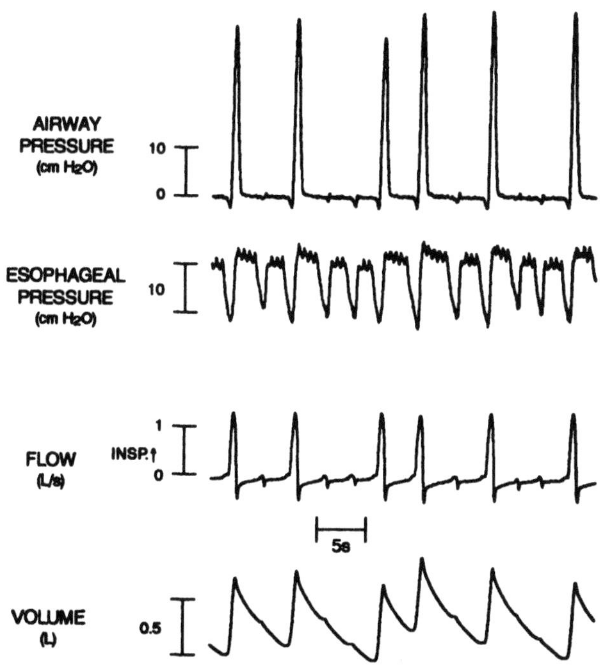

Fig. 4. Experimental record demonstrating marked variability in lung volume and inability to trigger the machine during assisted ventilation in a patient with severe COPD and intrinsic PEEP. Note the progressive increase in inspiratory effort (indicated by negative deflections in esophageal pressure) for several consecutive breaths before a sufficient reduction in airway pressure capable of opening the ventilator demand valve occurs. (In this patient, a sine wave rather than a constant inspiratory flow pattern was being used with a Puritan-Bennett 7200 ventilator).

tive-pressure breaths. In the patient with severe COPD, small temporal changes in tidal volume or respiratory rate can result in significant increases in the degree of dynamic hyperinflation and thus the level of PEEPi present [48]. This will reduce inspiratory muscle efficiency and unnecessarily increase the effort required for the subsequent spontaneous or machine-assisted breath. In the extreme, inspiratory force generating capacity will be insufficient to trigger inspiratory flow through the ventilator demand valve (Fig. 4) [49]. This is one instance where SIMV would not be beneficial, worsening patient-ventilator asynchrony and dyspnea while increasing the work of breathing.

With this in mind, Ranieri et al. [26] examined the effect of PEEP on inspiratory effort during SIMV. In 7 COPD patients, PEEP (0–10 cm H_2O) was applied at 5 SIMV rates, varying from fully assisted ventilation (100% SIMV, assist-control ventilation) to completely unsupported spontaneous breathing through the ventilator circuit (0% SIMV). Reducing SIMV rate produced graded increases in inspiratory effort, as previously described in patients with acute respiratory failure of varied etiology [50]. However, the addition of PEEP significantly reduced inspiratory effort at all levels of ventilator support, i.e. 0 to 100% SIMV. For the intermediate SIMV rates, PEEP was equally effective in reducing patient effort during both spontaneous and ventilator-assisted breaths. This was true when estimating inspiratory effort by graphical analysis of the work of breathing or the pressure-time integral of esophageal and transdiaphragmatic pressure. The magnitude of this effect increased with the level of PEEP (within the range of applied pressure examined) and occurred with little change in breathing pattern or end-expiratory lung volume.

PEEP and Pressure Support Ventilation

Pressure support is a new and unique mode of partial ventilatory support. As discussed in greater detail elsewhere in this volume, it offers a number of potential advantages over the previously available modes of assisted ventilation, i.e. assist-control and IMV [51–53]. First, it allows the patient to adjust the level and pattern of inspiratory flow as well as tidal volume and respiratory rate while machine assistance is provided with each spontaneous effort [52, 53]. Second, minute ventilation generally increases with the level of pressure support while providing graded reductions in the work and oxygen cost of breathing [53]. In fact, it has been suggested that an optimal level of pressure support can be individually determined which would sufficiently support ventilation, avoiding both excessive respiratory muscle effort as well as the potential complications of excessive positive pressure ventilation and lung inflation [53]. In this respect, pressure support would appear to be well-suited to the problematic COPD patient in whom a gradual and cautious transition from assisted ventilation to spontaneous breathing may be required.

Is pressure support equally effective in COPD patients with acute respiratory failure? While much emphasis has been placed on the ability of pressure support to minimize patient effort while improving ventilation and gas exchange, little attention has been focused on the interaction between pressure support and PEEPi. It must be stressed that pressure support is another form of patient-triggered assisted ventilation which requires that airway pressure falls below the triggering pressure set on the ventilator before the demand valve will open and inspiratory airflow can begin. Moreover, pressure support requires sufficient inspiratory effort not only to initiate but in addition to maintain airflow throughout the course of each pressure-assisted breath. It would appear that the presence of significant levels of PEEPi would limit the ability of pressure support to assist ventilation in such patients. In this regard, Calderini et al. [27] recently examined the ability of PEEP to improve the efficacy of pressure support in mechanically ventilated COPD patients. Pressure support alone did increase minute ventilation and improve breathing pattern, providing a larger tidal volume with a lower breathing frequency. While measures of inspiratory effort fell with increasing levels of pressure support, the values obtained were less than might be expected considering the magnitude of pressure support applied. However, the addition of PEEP markedly decreased patient effort, as measured by both work of breathing and the pressure-time integral of esophageal

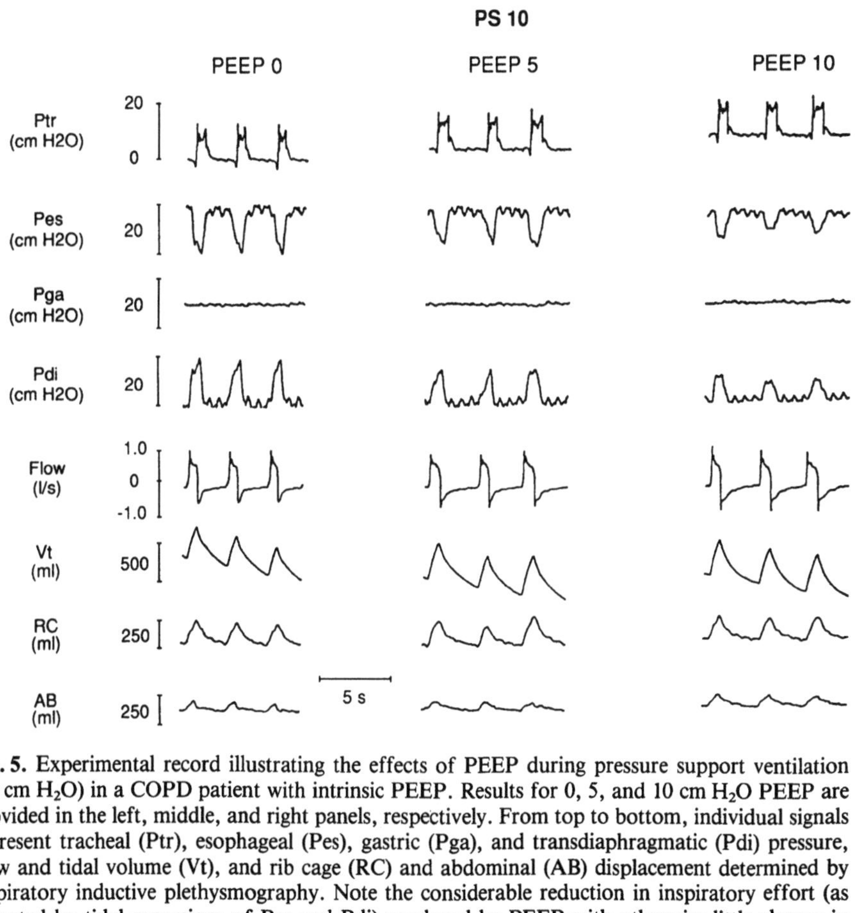

Fig. 5. Experimental record illustrating the effects of PEEP during pressure support ventilation (10 cm H_2O) in a COPD patient with intrinsic PEEP. Results for 0, 5, and 10 cm H_2O PEEP are provided in the left, middle, and right panels, respectively. From top to bottom, individual signals represent tracheal (Ptr), esophageal (Pes), gastric (Pga), and transdiaphragmatic (Pdi) pressure, flow and tidal volume (Vt), and rib cage (RC) and abdominal (AB) displacement determined by respiratory inductive plethysmography. Note the considerable reduction in inspiratory effort (as reflected by tidal excursions of Pes and Pdi) produced by PEEP with otherwise little change in breathing pattern or end-expiratory lung volume. Evidence of expiratory muscle recruitment with PEEP is not apparent.

pressure and transdiaphragmatic pressure, at all levels of pressure support evaluated (Fig. 5) [27]. The reduction in inspiratory effort increased with the amount of PEEP applied and occurred with no change in breathing pattern. As seen previously, PEEP had little or no effect on end-expiratory lung volume in these flow-limited patients [24–26].

Effect of PEEP on Hemodynamics and Gas Exchange

As noted above, the primary indication for PEEP in the mechanically ventilated COPD patient is to reduce the increased cardiac index, heart rate, stroke volume, and right ventricular ejection fraction determined by the thermodilution technique [55]. Arterial PO_2 and PCO_2 were also unaltered. It was not until higher levels of PEEP sufficient to increase lung volume (reflected by increases in total PEEP and reduced compliance) were applied that some alteration in these hemodynamic parameters was apparent. These effects were small which is perhaps not surprising, considering that the effective level of PEEP applied (as indicated by the increase in total end-expiratory recoil pressure, i.e. total PEEP) was about half of the nominal value set on the ventilator. Of note, there was no change in alveolar ventilation or dead space, as indicated by the stable arterial PCO_2 at a fixed minute ventilation and breathing pattern with a presumably constant CO_2 production. There was improvement in arterial PO_2 and venous admixture at the highest level of applied PEEP, perhaps explained in part by the decrease in cardiac output. These results suggest that the appropriate use of PEEP to decrease inspiratory effort during assisted ventilation need not be complicated by adverse effects on hemodynamics and gas exchange.

CPAP During Weaning from Mechanical Ventilation

While PEEP is a useful means of reducing patient effort during assisted modes of MV, this principle is also of particular importance when complete discontinuation of MV is being attempted. COPD patients recovering from acute respiratory failure at some point in time are required to inspiratory muscle effort attributable to PEEPi during assisted forms of ventilatory support. While PEEP should not be provided as a means of improving oxygenation (at least in the absence of other complicating medical illness), its potential effects on both hemodynamics and gas exchange should not be overlooked. Considering the reasons for the longstanding admonition against the use of PEEP in severe COPD, one might expect previous studies to have demonstrated significant hemodynamic depression, worsened oxygenation, and increased dead space ventilation with PEEP therapy in these patients. Remarkably, the effect of PEEP on hemodynamics and gas exchange has not been systematically examined in severe COPD patients. The influence of PEEPi in this context has also never been considered. In order to address these issues, routine hemodynamic parameters, indices of gas exchange, and respiratory mechanics were determined in 10 intubated COPD patients during controlled MV with 4 levels of PEEP ranging from 0 to 15 cm H_2O [54]. Patients were selected for evaluation on the basis of significant levels of PEEPi during routine MV. The presence of expiratory flow limitation was also confirmed in all patients [13, 28]. These results are summarized in Table 1.

As previously shown, low levels of PEEP approaching the recorded level of PEEPi had no significant effect on respiratory compliance, total PEEP, or end-expiratory lung volume. In these circumstances, there was no change in the hemodynamic parameters examined, including systemic and pulmonary arterial pressures, breathe spontaneously without the help of conventional positive pressure ventilation. The presence of PEEPi in the spontaneously breathing patient implies that the inspiratory muscles must now generate sufficient force to overcome this opposing positive recoil pressure not only to initiate but in addition to maintain airflow throughout the course of every inspiratory effort [9, 13, 32]. As noted earlier, in effect PEEPi functions as an inspiratory threshold load [56]. This represents a significant additional workload for the difficult to wean COPD patient, whose inspiratory muscles are already operating under disadvantageous conditions caused by force-length considerations, abnormal thoracic geometry, and a number of other factors [17, 18].

Analogous to the use of PEEP during assisted modes of MV, Petrof et al. [32] reasoned that CPAP should prove equally effective when used during spontaneous breathing trials in COPD patients being weaned from MV. This concept was examined in a group of 7 patients with well-documented severe COPD in whom some

Table 1. Effects of PEEP on hemodynamics and gas exchange in mechanically ventilated COPD patients

	PEEP 0	PEEP 5	PEEP 10	PEEP 15
SAPs (mm Hg)	121±9	122±8	121±9	110±9
SAPd (mm Hg)	56±3	59±4	58±4	60±5
PAPs (mm Hg)	39±6	40±5	40±5	40±4
PAPd (mm Hg)	21±3	21±3	22±3	23±2
PCWP (mm Hg)	11±2	11±2	12±2	14±2*
CI (l/min/M2)	3.0 ±0.2	3.0 ±0.2	2.9 ±0.2	2.5 ±0.2*
HR (b/min)	85±4	83±5	85±5	88±6
SVI (ml/M2)	36±3	36±3	34±2	29±2*
RVEF (%)	38±3	37±3	36±3	32±2**
PaO_2 (mm Hg)	97±10	98±10	99±10	129±14**
$PaCO_2$ (mm Hg)	40±2	40±3	39±3	39±2
pH	7.46±0.02	7.46±0.02	7.46±0.02	7.46±0.02
Qs/Qt (%)	17±1	16±1	15±1	12±1**
PEEPt (cm H_2O)	8.6 ±0.6	9.0 ±0.4	10.6 ±0.3	15.6 ±0.2**
Cst, rs (ml/cm H_2O)	63±8	63±9	63±8	56±7*

Values are means ± SEM. * $p<0.05$; ** $p<0.01$: PEEP 0 vs PEEP 5, 10, and 15 (two-way ANOVA and Dunnet modification of paired t-test).

SAPs, SAPd = systolic and diastolic systemic arterial pressure; *PAPs, PAPd* = systolic and diastolic pulmonary arterial pressure; *PCWP* = pulmonary capillary wedge pressure; *CI* = cardiac index; *HR* = heart rate; *SVI* = stroke volume index; *RVEF* = right ventricular ejection fraction; PaO_2 = arterial partial pressure of oxygen; PCO_2 = arterial partial pressure of carbon dioxide; *Qs/Qt* = shunt fraction; *PEEPt* = total PEEP; *Cst, rs* = static compliance of the total respiratory system

difficulty in discontinuing MV had been experienced. As anticipated, CPAP decreased the total inspiratory work of breathing in all patients. This was accounted for by a reduction in PEEPi and elastic work performed, while pulmonary resistance and the resistive work of breathing remained unchanged. For the group as a whole, the reduction in inspiratory effort increased with the amount of CPAP applied. These patients were able to assess changes in their subjective sense of dyspnea. All reported a decrease in breathlessness with the use of CPAP, consistent with the reduction in inspiratory effort observed. In addition, work by O'Donnell et al. [57] suggest that dynamic airway compression *per se* may heighten the sense of dyspnea. To the extent that the application of CPAP reduced the degree of dynamic airway collapse in the downstream flow-limited segment, this may have also contributed to the decrease in dyspnea observed.

These initial observations were extended in a subsequent study by Reissmann et al. [58] in a second group of patients in whom CPAP ($\simeq$7.5 cm H_2O) was randomly applied to one of two consecutive weaning trials which lasted a maximum of 30 min. Only 2 of 7 patients (29%) were able to tolerate weaning for the prescribed 30 min period during the control condition compared to 6 patients (86%) with CPAP ($P < 0.05$) (Fig. 6). Weaning duration improved in all 5 patients who failed to complete the control trial. The duration of spontaneous breathing tolerated increased significantly with CPAP for the group as a whole, averaging 28.0 ± 2.0 min compared to 15.7 ± 3.9 min when CPAP was not applied ($P < 0.05$). With the somewhat longer period of CPAP administration compared to the previously cited study, breathing pattern also improved (becoming less rapid and shallow in nature) with no change in minute ventilation. This was associated with enhanced alveolar ventilation and a fall in arterial PCO_2. While more detailed assessment of inspiratory muscle effort was not performed, both P100 and visual analog scale assessments of dyspnea did improve. In the absence of a well-designed large scale clinical trial, taken together these studies strongly support the judicious use of CPAP in severe COPD patients requiring weaning from MV.

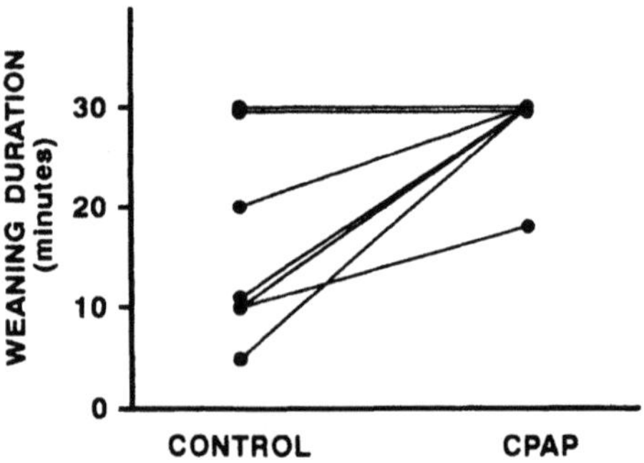

Fig. 6. Individual values for weaning duration in COPD patients breathing spontaneously (control) or with the addition of CPAP. CPAP significantly increased the time which spontaneous breathing could be tolerated ($P < 0.05$).

Importance of CPAP Circuit Design

Of considerable practical importance is the fact that the operating characteristics of the CPAP system play a critical role in determining the ability of CPAP to reduce the inspiratory work of breathing. To be effective, the level of airway pressure must be maintained as constant as possible throughout the respiratory cycle. This can best be accomplished with a CPAP circuit containing a high flow gas source sufficient to meet patient demands, a reservoir, and a PEEP valve whose function is unaffected by the flow passing through it [59]. Reductions in inspiratory airway pressure, particularly below atmospheric pressure, will not only decrease the efficacy of CPAP but will itself considerably increase the work of breathing. In addition, the demand valve systems by which many of the newly designed ventilators provide CPAP can themselves substantially increase the work of breathing [60]. This can be attributed to the decrease in airway pressure required to open the demand valve as well as delivery of an insufficient level of flow once inspiration has begun. While using the ventilator to administer CPAP offers the advantage of ease of application and the alarm systems which the ventilator provides, it may in fact hamper rather than facilitate discontinuation of MV.

Pursed Lip Breathing

The use of PEEP or CPAP has been likened to the act of pursed lip breathing often adopted spontaneously by severely dyspneic COPD patients with apparent symptomatic improvement [61]. While it has been generally accepted that pursed lip breathing can relieve dyspnea in such patients, the exact mechanism(s) by which this may occur have not been fully elucidated. Evidence from previous physiological investigations suggest that a number of factors may be responsible [62–64]. These include an altered pattern of breathing, improved gas exchange, and differences in the pattern of inspiratory muscle recruitment [62–65]. As noted earlier, dynamic airway compression itself may produce afferent sensory information which contributes to the sense of dyspnea experienced [57]. A reduction in the degree of dynamic airway compression during pursed lip breathing could therefore also contribute to the alleviation of breathlessness in these patients. It is relevant to point out that dynamic hyperinflation and PEEPi have been described in spontaneously breathing COPD patients in the absence of acute respiratory failure [66]. To the extent that dynamic hyperinflation is present in severely dyspneic COPD patients, assumption of a slower, deeper breathing pattern during pursed lip breathing may reduce PEEPi and thereby the inspiratory work of breathing. This could certainly play a role in relieving dyspnea, though its relative importance to the other mechanisms discussed is difficult to estimate. It should be noted, however, that the positive airway pressure produced during expiration by pursed lip breathing cannot act to counterbalance the threshold load imposed by PEEPi during inspiration. Pursed lip breathing is an expiratory phenomenon. While dynamic hyperinflation and PEEPi develop as a result of events occurring during expiration, the mechanical consequences of this are most evident during inspiration for the respiratory muscles.

CPAP and Non-Invasive Forms of Ventilatory Support

The mortality occurring in patients requiring MV for management of acute respiratory failure will obviously vary with the nature and severity of the underlying disease. However, both the morbidity and mortality related to the complications of intubation and conventional positive pressure ventilation (CPPV) are not insignificant [67]. This is of some importance for patients with severe COPD in whom extended periods of ventilatory support may be required. The monetary expenditure and medical resources required to mechanically ventilate such patients for prolonged periods of time must also be kept in mind [68].

Such considerations have led a number of physicians to examine the role of alternative, non-invasive forms of ventilatory support in the treatment of hypercapnic respiratory failure in patients with severe COPD [69–72]. Along these lines, a preliminary report by Goldberg et al. [71] demonstrated the feasibility of administering CPAP through a facemask or mouthpiece device to severely dyspneic, hypercapnic patients experiencing an acute exacerbation of their underlying severe airway obstruction. CPAP breathing for 15–20 min produced significant reductions in indices of inspiratory muscle effort in all the patients evaluated. While minute ventilation was generally unchanged or increased slightly, breathing pattern improved becoming less rapid and shallow in nature. This was associated with some reduction in arterial PCO_2. These results were similar in many respects to those obtained in intubated patients examined after a number of days of CPPV [32, 58]. In contrast to the initial report by Petrof et al. [32], however, breathing pattern improved in these later two studies. This may be explained by the relatively brief period of CPAP administration used by Petrof and coworkers (3–5 min compared with up to 30 min).

Brochard et al. [72] demonstrated the ability to satisfactorily assist ventilation and reduce inspiratory effort in a non-invasive fashion by administering a form of pressure support ventilation through a tightly fitting facemask. Moreover, this was associated with a decreased need for endotracheal intubation and CPPV when compared to an historical control group. A significant reduction in the average number of days of ventilatory support as well as the duration of ICU stay was also noted. In light of the earlier discussion demonstrating the utility of PEEP during pressure support as well as other forms of assisted ventilation, the addition of PEEP in this setting would be expected to further improve the efficacy of such forms of non-invasive support. Conceivably, the addition of PEEP would allow non-invasive ventilatory support to be provided successfully to patients in whom either CPAP or assisted ventilation alone were insufficient to avoid the need for intubation and conventional MV.

Use of Negative Extrathoracic Pressure

Implicit in the use of the term PEEP or CPAP is that increases in transthoracic pressure are accomplished by the application of positive pressure to the airway opening. However, a number of studies in both experimental animals and patients with ARDS have demonstrated that comparable effects on respiratory function can be achieved when applying negative pressure at the body surface [73, 74]. Patient acceptance of negative pressure devices is variable and may be limited by musculoskeletal complaints, bulk and inconvenience of use, and poor physical access for medical and nursing care [75]. However, there are a number of potential advantages when compared with the use of PEEP or CPAP, particularly in the non-intubated patient. This is particularly true for those individuals in whom satisfactory levels of positive airway pressure cannot be applied because of patient comfort or a poorly fitting commercial mask. In addition, the upper airway remains unencumbered, facilitating expectoration and clearance of secretions without the need to temporarily discontinue use. The increased risk of gastric distention and aspiration of gastric contents should also be reduced. Negative pressure ventilation has been associated with functionally significant upper airway obstruction, particularly during sleep [75, 76]. This should not be the case with continuous negative extrathoracic pressure (CNEP, analogous to CPAP) used to reduce PEEPi in COPD patients, where the development of increased negative transmural upper airway pressures would not be expected to occur. CNEP has been shown to be effective in reducing inspiratory muscle effort without adversely effecting minute ventilation, breathing pattern, or end-expiratory lung volume in less acutely ill COPD patients [77]. The negative pressure device was generally well tolerated and evidence of upper airway obstruction was not apparent. These results were in fact not different than those obtained using equivalent levels of CPAP in the same subjects [78].

Several commercially available CPAP devices can be easily modified to provide a constant level of negative extrathoracic pressure throughout the respiratory cycle. In addition, a currently available Emerson ventilator (model # 33-CR) allows for continuous negative pressure ventilation (CNPV, analogous to CPPV with PEEP), providing different levels of negative pressure during the inspiratory and expiratory phases of the respiratory cycle. Through the use of nasal cannulae or prongs to sense patient effort, an assisted mode of negative pressure ventilation can also be obtained with this machine. To the extent that PEEP is effective with various forms of assisted ventilation in intubated COPD patients, negative end-expiratory pressure (NEEP) should be also beneficial when providing non-invasive support with negative pressure ventilation.

Indications and Guidelines for the Use of PEEP or CPAP

Comprehensive instructions concerning the indications for and proper use of PEEP or CPAP in mechanically ventilated COPD patients remains to be defined on the basis of more extensive clinical experience. However, a number of practical and important recommendations can be made with the information available at this time. In view of the previous discussion, these points should be apparent and are outlined in Table 2.

It is important to recognize that PEEP will have no salutary effect on the degree of dynamic hyperinflation already present or those adverse effects not directly related to PEEPi, i.e. reduced inspiratory muscle efficiency due to altered force-length and geometric considerations, hemodynamic depression, or risk of barotrauma. Its beneficial effect relates only to the ability to reduce the inspiratory thres-

Table 2. Criteria for use of PEEP or CPAP in mechanically ventilated patients with intrinsic PEEP

Relative Indications	*Relative Contraindications*
1. Severe COPD	Airway obstruction not severe Other causes of airway obstruction - acute asthma Dynamic hyperinflation without airway obstruction - high minute ventilation - rapid, shallow breathing - small or kinked endotracheal tube - high expiratory circuit resistance
2. PEEPi > 5 cm H_2O	PEEPi < 5 cm H_2O
3. Flow limitation present Peak airway pressure, total PEEP, and lung volume stable when small amounts of PEEP or CPAP applied Expiratory muscle recruitment does not occur in response to PEEP or CPAP	Flow limitation absent Peak airway pressure, total PEEP, and lung volume increase with small amounts of PEEP or CPAP Expiratory muscles actively recruited when PEEP or CPAP is applied
4. Assisted mechanical ventilation - assist-control ventilation - intermittent mandatory ventilation - pressure support ventilation Spontanous breathing	Controlled mechanical ventilation
5. Excessive patient effort - ineffective triggering - extreme dyspnea - marked asynchrony with machine - prominent accessory muscle use	Patient comfortable - triggers ventilator easily - no noticeable dyspnea - well coordinated with ventilator - no inspiratory accessory muscle use

hold load imposed by PEEPi and the associated increase in work and oxygen cost of breathing. Accordingly, externally applied PEEP is not indicated for the patient receiving controlled MV whose respiratory muscles are being intentionally rested. Similarly, little benefit would be anticipated in those less severely ill COPD patients with modest levels of PEEPi in whom discontinuation of MV and successful extubation is anticipated shortly.

As a general rule, PEEP or CPAP should not be used in patients with PEEPi without evidence of significant airway obstruction for several important reasons. First, while PEEPi is not uncommon in MV patients, occurring in up to 25% of such individuals without known airflow obstruction, the levels are generally low and usually do not exceed 5 cm H_2O except in very particular circumstances [9, 16, 79, 80]. Second, in the absence of expiratory flow limitation, active recruitment of expiratory muscle activity would be required in order to defend lung volume and prevent further hyperinflation [81]. The potential benefit of such a strategy would be to allow part of the total work of breathing to be assumed by the expiratory muscles, thus providing some relief for the taxed inspiratory muscles [81]. While conceptually appealing, this approach has not been critically examined and its efficacy demonstrated on a more widespread clinical basis. Previous work has demonstrated that recruitment of expiratory abdominal muscles can themselves contribute significantly to the overall oxygen cost of breathing and, even in the presence of reductions in inspiratory muscle activation, heighten the sense of dyspnea [82, 83]. In addition, there are a number of factors frequently encountered in critically ill ICU patients which would interfere with effective expiratory muscle recruitment, including abdominal distention or recent surgery, recumbency, sleep, sedation, and reduced consciousness for other reasons [84–86]. In these circumstances, further hyperinflation would ensue and no clinical benefit would be realized.

Optimal Level of PEEP or CPAP

The optimal level of PEEP or CPAP is difficult to define but it should take into consideration the beneficial effects of a reduction in the inspiratory work of breathing as well as potential adverse consequences related to increases in lung volume that may be induced by positive airway pressure. The response to PEEP or CPAP in a given patient will vary depending on the pre-existing level of PEEPi and severity of airway obstruction. Provided expiratory flow limitation is present and end-expiratory lung volume remains stable in the absence of expiratory muscle activity, applying PEEP (or CPAP) approaching the level of PEEPi should be of benefit without adverse effects in terms of inspiratory muscle function and work. Continued decreases in the work of breathing with increasing PEEP beyond the level at which hyperinflation first occurs (i.e. PEEP >Pcrit) are also theoretically possible if one considers the implications of a lung that exhibits regional inhomogeneity of its mechanical properties [32]. In this regard, time constant inequalities should lead to varying levels of PEEPi within the lung, with the highest regional PEEPi values present in the slowest-emptying units. Under these circumstances, increasing the level of PEEP would be expected to produce further decreases in work as PEEPi was progressively reduced in those units with the highest regional PEEPi. This would only be true, however, provided that any hyperinflation occurring in faster-emptying lung units (with lower levels of PEEPi) did not increase overall pulmonary elastance with attendant increases in elastic work, thus tending to negate the beneficial effects obtained by eliminating PEEPi in the slower-emptying units.

Although further reductions in inspiratory work may occur despite increases in lung volume with the use of higher levels of PEEP (i.e. PEEP >Pcrit), a cautionary note is warranted. While external work may decrease, further increases in lung volume will predictably reduce inspiratory muscle efficiency (due to force-length and other considerations), so that no overall improvement in metabolic demands placed on the respiratory muscles would actually be achieved. In addition, heterogeneity of mechanical properties within the lung may lead to excessive regional hyperinflation, and an increased risk of barotrauma, even through the absolute increase in overall lung volume is small. With this in mind, PEEP or CPAP approaching the existing level of PEEPi and without a measurable increase in lung volume should be of benefit and without undue risk. Levels of applied pressure much in excess of PEEPi and accompanied by significant increases in lung volume should not be encouraged, and if employed only with extreme caution. Such an approach should be justified by firm evidence of clinically important reductions in patient effort and dyspnea while close monitoring would necessarily be required.

Monitoring Intrinsic PEEP and the Response to PEEP or CPAP

It has been suggested by several authors that PEEPi should be routinely monitored in all mechanically ventilated patients [9, 16, 79, 80, 87]. Such recommendations are justified considering the diagnostic and therapeutic implications of PEEPi in a number of clinical settings [9, 15, 16, 80, 88, 89]. Monitoring PEEPi and the response to PEEP or CPAP is of particular importance in the mechanically ventilated COPD patient. Ideally, this would include the ability to separately and reliably assess both the beneficial and adverse effects of PEEP or CPAP in an individual patient. Unfortunately, quantitative measurements of inspiratory muscle function, work, and oxygen cost or breathing cannot be considered part of routine clinical practice at the present time. Clinical assessment of inspiratory accessory muscle activation and dyspnea is worthwhile, however, and should not be overlooked [32, 53].

In the absence of being able to more conveniently and precisely quantify changes in inspiratory muscle function and work, interest has naturally focused on minimizing potential adverse effects by closely monitoring changes in lung volume or alveolar pressure. Measurement of changes in peak airway pressure, total PEEP, and end-expiratory lung volume determined by respiratory inductive plethysmography have all been utilized for this purpose. Each of these approaches will be reviewed and the relative advantages and limitations discussed.

Measurement of Peak Airway Pressure

Peak airway pressure can be continuously monitored during assist-control ventilation with the addition of PEEP, and will remain stable provided that the level of PEEP applied is not excessive and further hyperinflation does not occur [24, 25]. Peak airway pressure reflects the positive pressure applied by the ventilator to overcome PEEPi as well as the resistive and elastic impedance of the respiratory system. Considering the absolute magnitude of PEEPi relative to the peak airway pressure observed in mechanically ventilated COPD patients, which frequently exceeds 30–40 cm H_2O, this may not prove to be as sensitive a method as would be hoped for [21, 22]. The significant breath-to-breath variability in airway pressure frequently seen during assist-control ventilation is another complicating feature, although this may be offset by the continuous and precise pressure monitoring capabilities available on the newer microprocessor-based ventilators [90]. Measurement of peak airway pressure will obviously not be useful during pressure support and other related pressure-assisted forms of ventilation in which the peak airway pressure achieved is an independent variable set on the ventilator and continuously controlled throughout the course of inspiration. This is also true for the use of CPAP during unassisted spontaneous breathing or for spontaneous breaths occurring with SIMV.

Measurement of Total PEEP

Some of these limitations can be overcome by utilizing direct measurements of end-expiratory recoil pressure both before and after the application of PEEP or CPAP. Again provided that PEEP replaces PEEPi without altering lung volume, the *total* recoil pressure at end-expiration, or total PEEP (i.e. the sum of applied PEEP and remaining PEEPi), should be unchanged. Such measurements can be obtained, during both assisted and spontaneous breathing, by occluding the airway at end-expiration and recording the plateau in airway pressure developed between the subsequent occluded inspiratory efforts (Fig. 7 and 8) [26, 27, 32, 54]. The end-expiratory hold function, first introduced on the Siemens 900C and now available on a number of machines, facilitates such measurements by providing prolonged periods of airway occlusion accurately timed to the end of the ventilator or spontaneous respiratory cycle [90].

A modification of the manual exhalation port occlusion method popularized by Pepe and Marini [12, 24] can be used during assisted ventilation with other ventilators, but difficulty in ensuring accurate timing and duration of airway occlusion is problematic. This is particularly relevant during assisted or spontaneous breathing modes where an increased variability in the pattern of breathing would necessarily be expected. Limited access to the exhalation port in certain newer generation ventilators (e.g. Puritan-Bennett 7200) can make rapid and complete manual airway occlusion difficult to perform [79]. An alternative approach utilizing a 3-way valve placed in the inspiratory limb of the external ventilator circuit has been described which overcomes these drawbacks, enabling prolonged and accurately timed end-expiratory occlusions to be performed with all currently available ventilators [91].

These methods of end-expiratory occlusion apply as well to spontaneously breathing patients when a demand valve CPAP system is being used. However, an external continuous flow CPAP circuit will require an additional valve to enable airway occlusions to be performed [14, 32]. Determination of intrinsic or total PEEP from occluded airway pressure measurements does assume that significant expiratory muscle activation does not occur during uninterrupted breathing or in response to airway occlusion. While this may be inferred from a stable and reproducible plateau in occluded airway pressure, more detailed and invasive methodology beyond the scope of routine clinical practice would be required to confirm this point.

Use of Respiratory Inductive Plethysmography

Changes in end-expiratory lung volume determined by respiratory inductive plethysmography can also be used to indirectly estimate PEEPi and monitor the response to PEEP or CPAP [25–27, 32, 92]. For the reasons discussed earlier, the amount of positive airway pressure applied at which end-expiratory lung volume begins to increase will be somewhat less than the actual magnitude of PEEPi present (i.e. PEEPi will be greater than Pcrit). As a result, PEEPi and its related adverse effects (i.e. reduced force-generating capacity, excessive work of breathing and dyspnea, hemodynamic depression, and risk of barotrauma) will all be under-

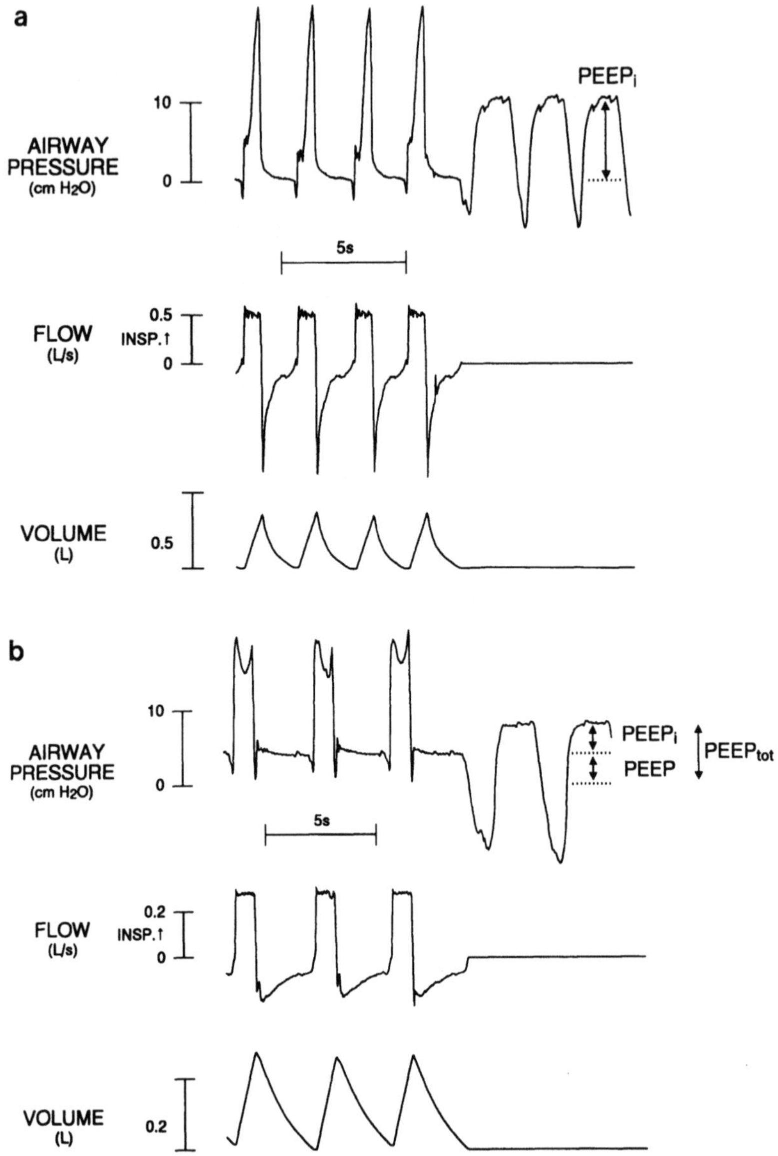

Fig. 7. The top record illustrates measurement of intrinsic PEEP (PEEPi) during assist-control ventilation. The airway was occluded at end-expiration and maintained for several consecutive respiratory efforts using the end-expiratory hold function on a Siemens 900C ventilator. The plateau in airway pressure between inspiratory efforts represents the magnitude of PEEPi. In a second patient with severe COPD (bottom record), end-expiratory occlusion was performed during assist-control ventilation with externally applied PEEP. The plateau in occluded airway pressure relative to the PEEP applied indicates the amount of PEEPi present. The total positive recoil pressure at end-expiration, or total PEEP (PEEPtot), is equal to the sum of these two values

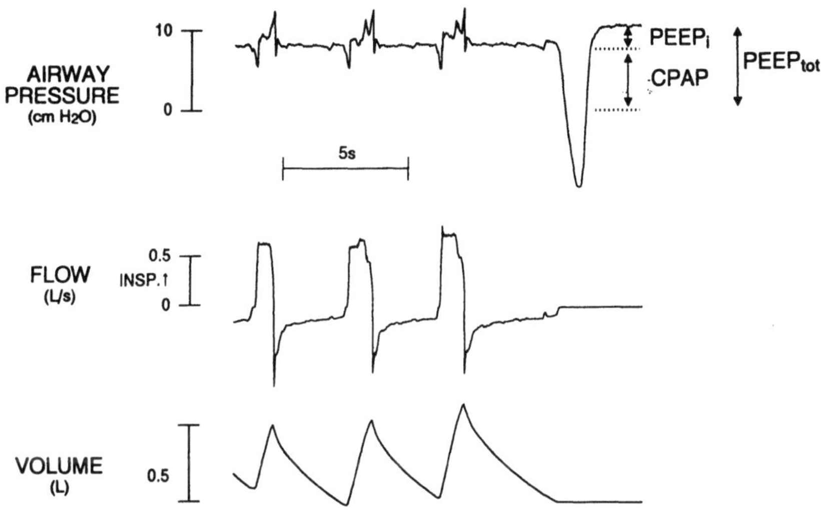

Fig. 8. Experimental record illustrating measurement of intrinsic (PEEPi) and total PEEP (PEEPtot) during spontaneous breathing with continuous positive airway pressure (CPAP) applied through a Siemens 900C ventilator in a patient with severe COPD. The end-expiratory hold function allows airway occlusion to begin at the end of a spontaneous breath. PEEPtot is indicated by the plateau in airway pressure relative to atmosphere. The difference between PEEPtot and the CPAP applied represents PEEPi

estimated to some extent. It should be noted that this approach is most suitable for COPD patients with dynamic airway compression and confirmed flow limitation. In the dynamically hyperinflated patient in whom expiratory flow limitation is absent, any level of external positive airway pressure should in theory reduce expiratory flow, increase lung volume, and preclude accurate determination of PEEPi. In either instance, expiratory muscle recruitment in response to excessive amounts of PEEP or CPAP may prevent noticeable changes in lung volume from occurring. This would then provide misleading information as to the level of PEEPi present as well as the indication for and amount of positive pressure which may be safely applied.

Stable calibration factors for the respiratory inductive plethysmograph can be difficult to maintain for prolonged periods of time in the critically ICU patient, where the need for repeated calibration may be considered burdensome and time consuming to busy medical or nursing ICU staff. This is particularly true for those devices which do not have an automated calibration procedure. This issue is of lesser importance in the present context, where detection of an immediate increase in lung volume is being sought. While the exact magnitude of the degree of hyperinflation induced is of interest, this is of less concern if the level of PEEP or CPAP to be used clinically will be limited to amounts below the value at which hyperinflation occurs.

A number of other methods for measurement of PEEPi have been described [16, 32, 87]. However, the need for expensive or sophisticated equipment, measurement of esophageal pressure, or controlled ventilation limits their widespread clinical application in general as well as for monitoring the response to PEEP or CPAP during assisted or spontaneous breathing modes.

In addition to such measurements, the usefulness of clinical examination should again be kept in mind. Worsening dyspnea or increased use of inspiratory accessory muscles are signs that either the level of applied pressure is excessive or respiratory function has deteriorated for other reasons (e.g. increased bronchospasm, tracheobronchial secretions, etc.). Alternatively, a previously acceptable amount of PEEP or CPAP may become inappropriately high if improvement in respiratory function or breathing pattern occurs and, as a result, the baseline level of PEEPi falls. Lastly, excessive levels of PEEP or CPAP may also be recognized by the development of expiratory muscle activation in an attempt to defend end-expiratory lung volume. While expiratory muscle recruitment may not occur for a number of reasons, as noted earlier, its presence in response to the addition of PEEP or CPAP should be a signal for a more thorough evaluation of the indications for and amount of positive pressure which should be applied.

Conclusions

Management of the mechanically ventilated patient with severe COPD remains a difficult and challenging clinical problem. This chapter has attempted to illustrate the fundamental importance of PEEPi and the mechanisms by which externally applied PEEP or CPAP can be useful in such patients. Like any therapeutic modality, it should be used judiciously and the value of any benefit to be realized weighed against the possible adverse effects which may occur in an individual patient. This will require careful consideration with respect to the indications for PEEP or CPAP use, the amount of positive pressure to be applied, and the need for continued monitoring to ensure patient benefit and avoid unnecessary complications. With this in mind, current evidence indicates that PEEP and CPAP can be important therapeutic modalities to help improve the care and hopefully the ultimate outcome of the severe COPD patient with acute respiratory failure.

Acknowledgements. This work was supported in part by the Medical Research Council of Canada, the Canadian Cystic Fibrosis Foundation, and the EL/JTC Memorial Fund. The author is a Medical Research Scholar of the Fonds de la Recherche en Santé du Québec.

References

1. Balk R, Bone RC (1983) Classification of acute respiratory failure. Med Clin NA 76:551–556
2. Johanson WG, Peters JI (1988) Respiratory failure: pathophysiology and treatment. In: Murray JF, Nadel JA (eds) Textbook of respiratory medicine, 1st ed. W.B. Saunders, Philadelphia, pp 2017–2034
3. Roussos C (1982) The failing ventilatory pump. Lung 160:59–84
4. Ashbaugh DG, Petty TL (1973) Positive end-expiratory pressure. Clinical indications and contraindications. J Thorac Cardiovasc Surg 65:165–170

5. Gong H Jr (1982) Positive-pressure ventilation in the adult respiratory distress syndrome. Clin Chest Med 3:69–88
6. Kacmarek RM, Petty TL (1988) Historical development of positive end-expiratory pressure. Respir Care 33:422–433
7. Marini JJ (1989) Should PEEP be used in airflow obstruction? Am Rev Respir Dis 140:1–3
8. Rossi A, Brandolese R, Milic-Emili J, Gottfried SB (1990) The role of PEEP in patients with chronic obstructive pulmonary disease during assisted ventilation. Eur Respir J 3:818–822
9. Gottfried SB, Rossi A, Milic-Emili J (1986) Dynamic hyperinflation, intrinsic PEEP, and the mechanically ventilated patient. Intensive Crit Care Digest 5:30–33
10. Derenne JP, Fleury B, Pariente R (1988) Acute respiratory failure of chronic obstructive pulmonary disease. Am Rev Respir Dis 138:1006–1033
11. Kimball WR, Leith DE, Robins AG (1982) Dynamic hyperinflation and ventilator dependence in chronic obstructive pulmonary disease. Am Rev Respir Dis 126:991–995
12. Pepe PE, Marini JJ (1982) Occult positive end-expiratory pressure in mechanically ventilated patients with airflow obstruction. The auto-PEEP effect. Am Rev Respir Dis 126:166–170
13. Gottfried SB, Rossi A, Higgs BD, et al (1985) Non-invasive determination of respiratory system mechanics during mechanical ventilation for acute respiratory failure. Am Rev Respir Dis 131:414–420
14. Fleury B, Murciano C, Talamo C, Aubier M, Pariente R, Milic-Emili J (1985) Work of breathing in patients with chronic obstructive pulmonary disease in acute respiratory failure. Am Rev Respir Dis 131:822–827
15. Broseghini C, Brandolese R, Poggi R, et al (1988) Respiratory mechanics during the first day of mechanical ventilation in patients with pulmonary edema and chronic airway obstruction. Am Rev Respir Dis 138:355–361
16. Rossi A, Gottfried SB, Zocchi L, et al (1985) Measurement of static compliance of the total respiratory system in patients with acute respiratory failure during mechanical ventilation: the effect of intrinsic PEEP. Am Rev Respir Dis 131:672–677
17. Macklem PT (1984) Hyperinflation. Am Rev Respir Dis 129:1–2
18. Tobin MJ (1988) Respiratory muscles in disease. Clin Chest Med 9:263–286
19. Farkas GA, Roussos C (1983) Diaphragm in emphysematous hamsters: sarcomere adaptability. J Appl Physiol 54:1635–1640
20. Similowski T, Yan S, Gauthier AP, Macklem PT, Bellemare F (1990) Contractile properties of the human diaphragm during chronic hyperinflation. Am Rev Respir Dis 141:A166
21. Conti G, Bufi M, Antonelli M, Rocco M, Gasparetto A (1989) Pressure support ventilation reverses hyperinflation induced isorhythmic A-V dissociation. Intensive Care Medicine 15:319–321
22. Marini JJ (1991) Ventilatory management of COPD. In: Cherniack NS (ed) Chronic obstructive pulmonary disease, W.B. Saunders Company, Philadelphia, pp 495–519
23. Roussos C (1985) Energetics. In: Roussos C, Macklem PT (eds) The Thorax. Marcel Dekker, New York, pp 437–492
24. Smith TC, Marini JJ (1988) Impact of PEEP on lung mechanics and work of breathing in severe airflow obstruction. J Appl Physiol 65:1488–1499
25. Simkovitz P, Brown K, Goldberg P, Milic-Emili J, Gottfried SB (1987) Interaction between intrinsic and externally applied PEEP during mechanical ventilation. Am Rev Respir Dis 135:A202
26. Ranieri M, Calderini E, Eissa T, Petrof B, Gottfried SB (1990) PEEP reduces inspiratory effort during synchronized intermittent mandatory ventilation (SIMV) in COPD. Am Rev Respir Dis 141:A572
27. Calderini E, Petrof B, Gottfried SB (1989) Continuous positive airway pressure improves efficacy of pressure support ventilation in severe COPD. Am Rev Respir Dis 139:A155
28. Gay CG, Rodarte JR, Hubmayr RD (1989) The effects of positive expiratory pressure on isovolume flow and dynamic hyperinflation in patients receiving mechanical ventilation. Am Rev Respir Dis 139:621–626
29. Mead J, Turner JM, Macklem PT, Little JB (1967) Significance of the relationship between lung recoil and maximum expiratory flow. J Appl Physiol 22:95–108

30. Pride NB, Permutt S, Riley RL, Bromberger-Barnea (1967) Determinants of maximal expiratory flow from the lungs. J Appl Physiol 23:646–662
31. Permutt S, Riley RL (1963) Hemodynamics of collapsible vessels with tone: the vascular waterfall. J Appl Physiol 18:924–932
32. Petrof BJ, Légaré M, Goldberg P, Milic-Emili J, Gottfried SB (1990) Continuous positive airway pressure reduces work of breathing and dyspnea during weaning from mechanical ventilation in severe chronic obstructive pulmonary disease. Am Rev Respir Dis 141:281–289
33. McNamara JJ, Castile RG, Glass GM, Fredberg JJ (1987) Heterogeneous lung emptying during forced expiration. J Appl Physiol 63:1648–1657
34. Tuxen DV, Lane S (1987) The effects of ventilatory pattern on hyperinflation, airway pressures, and circulation in mechanical ventilation of patients with severe air-flow obstruction. Am Rev Respir Dis 136:872–879
35. Tuxen DV (1989) Detrimental effects of positive end-expiratory pressure during controlled mechanical ventilation of patients with severe airflow obstruction. Am Rev Respir Dis 140:5–9
36. Pride NB, Macklem PT (1986) Lung mechanics in disease. In: Fishman AP (ed) Handbook of physiology, section 3: The respiratory system, volume 3, Mechanics of breathing. Americam Physiological Society, Bethesda, pp 659–692
37. James AJ, Paré PD, Hogg JC (1989) The mechanics of airway narrowing in asthma. Am Rev Respir Dis 139:242–246
38. Ebina M, Yaegashi H, Chiby R et al (1990) Hyperreactive site in the airway tree of asthmatic patients revealed by thickening of bronchial muscles. Am Rev Respir Dis 141:1327–1332
39. Djukanovic R, Roche WR, Wilson JW et al (1990) Mucosal inflammation in asthma. Am Rev Respir Dis 142:434–457
40. Qvist J, Anderson JB, Pemberton M, Bennike KA (1982) High level PEEP in severe asthma. N Engl J Med 307:1347–1348
41. Weng JT, Smith DE, Graybar GB, Kirby RR (1984) Hypotension secondary to air trapping treated with expiratory flow retard. Anesthesiology 60:350–353
42. Tenaillon A, Salmona JP, Burdon M (1983) Continuous positive airway pressure in asthma. Am Rev Respir Dis 127:658
43. Marini JJ, Capps JS, Culver BH (1985) The inspiratory work of breathing during assisted mechanical ventilation. Chest 87:612–618
44. Marini JJ, Rodriguez RM, Lamb V (1986) The inspiratory workload of patient-initiated mechanical ventilation. Am Rev Respir Dis 134:902–909
45. Ward ME, Corbeil C, Gibbons W, Newman S, Macklem PT (1988) Optimization of respiratory muscle relaxation during mechanical ventilation. Anesthesiology 69:26–35
46. Downs JB, Klein EF, Desautels D, Modell JH, Kirgy RR (1973) IMV: a new approach to weaning patients from mechanical ventilation. Chest 64:331–335
47. Venus B, Smith RA, Mathru M (1987) National survey of methods and criteria used for weaning from mechanical ventilation. Crit Care Med 15:530–533
48. Braschi A, Iotti G, Rodi G, Emmi V, Sala Gallini G (1988) Dynamic pulmonary hyperinflation during intermittent mandatory ventilation. Intensive Care Med 14:284
49. Fernandez R, Benito S, Blanch LL, Net A (1988) Intrinsic PEEP: a cause of inspiratory muscle ineffectivity. Intensive Care Med 15:51–52
50. Marini JJ, Smith TC, Lamb VJ (1988) External work output and force generation during synchronized intermittent mechanical ventilation: effect of machine assistance on breathing effort. Am Rev Respir Dis 138:1169–1179
51. Kacmarek RM (1988) The role of pressure support ventilation in reducing imposed work of breathing. Respir Care 33:99–120
52. MacIntyre NR (1986) Respiratory function during pressure support ventilation. Chest 89:677-683
53. Brochard L, Harf A, Lorino H, Lemaire F (1989) Inspiratory pressure support prevents diaphragmatic fatigue during weaning from mechanical ventilation. Am Rev Respir Dis 139:513–521
54. Ranieri VM, Giuliani R, Gottfried SB, et al (1991) Effects of PEEP on hemodynamics and gas exchange in mechanically ventilated COPD patients (in press)

55. Dhainaut JF, Brunet F, Monsallier JF, et al (1987) Bedside evaluation of right ventricular performance using a rapid computerized thermodilution method. Crit Care Med 15:148–152
56. Campbell EJM, Dikinson CJ, Dinnick OP, Howell JBL (1964) The immediate effects of threshold loads on the breathing of men and dogs. Clin Sci 172:321–331
57. O'Donnell DE, Sanii R, Anthonisen NR, Younes M (1987) Effect of dynamic airway compression on breathing pattern and respiratory sensation in severe chronic obstructive pulmonary disease. Am Rev Respir Dis 135:912–918
58. Reissmann H, Ranieri M, Goldberg P, Gottfried SB (1990) CPAP improves breathing pattern and gas exchange during weaning in COPD. Chest 98:76S
59. Hillman DR, Finucane KE (1985) Continuous positive airway pressure: a breathing system to minimize respiratory work. Crit Care Med 13:38–43
60. Gibney RIN, Wilson RS, Pontoppidan H (1982) Comparison of work of breathing on high gas flow and demand-valve continuous positive airway pressure systems. Chest 82:692–695
61. Barach AL (1973) Physiologic advantages of grunting, groaning, and pursed-lip breathing: the development of continuous positive pressure breathing. Bull NY Acad Med 49:666–673
62. Thoman RL, Stroker GL, Ross JC (1966) The efficacy of pursed lip breathing in patients with chronic obstructive pulmonary disease. Am Rev Respir Dis 93:100–106
63. Ingram RH Jr, Schilder DP (1967) Effect of pursed lip breathing on the pulmonary pressure-flow relationship in obstructive lung disease. Am Rev Resp Dis 96:381–388
64. Mueller RE, Petty TL, Filley GF (1970) Ventilation and arterial blood gases induced by pursed lip breathing. J Appl Physiol 28:784–789
65. Fitting JW, Chartrand DA, Bradley TD, Killian KJ, Grassino A (1987) Effect of thoracoabdominal breathing patterns on inspiratory effort sensation. J Appl Physiol 62:1665–1670
66. Haluszka J, Chartrand DA, Grassino AC, Milic-Emili J (1990) Intrinsic PEEP and arterial PCO_2 in stable patients with chronic obstructive pulmonary disease. Am Rev Respir Dis 141:1194–1197
67. Pierson DJ (1990) Complications associated with mechanical ventilation. Crit Care Clin 6:711–724
68. Rosen RL, Bone RC (1988) Economics of mechanical ventilation Clin Chest Med 9:163–170
69. Meduri GU, Conoscenti CC, Menashe P, Nair S (1989) Noninvasive face mask ventilation in patients with acute respiratory failure. Chest 95:865–870
70. Carrey Z, Gottfried SB, Levy RD (1990) Ventilatory muscle support in respiratory failure with nasal positive pressure ventilation. Chest 97:150–158
71. Goldberg P, Reissmann H, Ranieri M, Gottfried SB (1990) CPAP reduces inspiratory effort during acute respiratory failure. Chest 98:76S
72. Brochard L, Isabey D, Piquet J, et al (1990) Reversal of acute exacerbations of chronic obstructive lung disease by inspiratory assistance with a face mask. New Engl J Med 323:1523–1530
73. Skaburskis M, Helal R, Zidulka A (1987) Effects of external continuous negative pressure ventilation (CNPV) compared to continuous positive pressure ventilation (CPPV) in dogs with acute lung injury. Am Rev Respir Dis 136:886–891
74. Morris AH, Elliott G (1985) Adult respiratory distress syndrome: successful support with continuous negative extrathoracic pressure. Crit Care Med 13:989–990
75. Hill NS (1986) Clinical application of body ventilators. Chest 90:897–905
76. Scharf SM, Feldman NT, Goldman MD, Haut HZ, Bruce E, Ingram RHM (1978) Vocal cord closure: a cause of upper airway obstruction during controlled ventilation. Am Rev Respir Dis 117:391–397
77. Gottfried SB, Simkovitz P, Skaburskis M (1987) Effect of constant negative extrathoracic pressure on breathing pattern and respiratory muscle function in severe COPD. Am Rev Respir Dis 135:A202
78. Gottfried SB, Simkovitz P, Skaburskis M (1987) Effect of constant positive airway pressure on breathing pattern and respiratory muscle function in chronic obstructive pulmonary disease. Chest 92:127
79. Brown DG, Pierson DJ (1986) Auto-PEEP is common in mechanically ventilated patients: a study of incidence, severity, and detection. Respir Care 31:1069–1074

80. Benson MS, Pierson DJ (1988) Auto-PEEP during mechanical ventilation of adults. Respir Care 33:557–565
81. Martin JG, Shore S, Engel LA (1982) Effect of continuous positive airway pressure on respiratory mechanics and pattern of breathing in induced asthma. Am Rev Respir Dis 126:812–817
82. Paton JY, Swaminathan S, Sargent CW, Keens TG (1989) Expiratory muscle endurance and the oxygen cost of expiration in normal adults. Am Rev Respir Dis 139:A345
83. Petrof BJ, Calderini E, Gottfried SB (1990) Effect of CPAP on respiratory effort and dyspnea during exercise in severe COPD. J Appl Physiol 69:179–188
84. Druz WS, Sharp JT (1981) The activity of respiratory muscles in upright and recumbent man. J Appl Physiol 51:1552–1561
85. Begle RL, Skatrud JB, Dempsey JA (1987) Ventilatory compensation for changes in functional residual capacity during sleep. J Appl Physiol 62:1299–1306
86. DiMarco AF, DiMarco MS, Strohl KP, Altose MD (1984) Effects of expiratory threshold loading on thoracoabdominal motion in cats. Respir Physiol 57:247–257
87. Gottfried SB, Milic-Emili J (1986) Non-invasive monitoring of respiratory system mechanics. In: Cherniack NS, Nochomovitz M (eds) Non-invasive respiratory monitoring. Churchill Livingston, New York, pp 59–82
88. Duncan SR, Rizk NW, Raffin TA (1987) Inverse ratio ventilation, PEEP in disguise? Chest (letter) 92:390–392
89. Solway J, Rossing T, Saari A, et al (1986) Expiratory flow limitation and dynamic pulmonary hyperinflation during high frequency ventilation. J Appl Physiol 60:2071–2076
90. Kacmarek RM, Meklaus MD (1990) The new generation of mechanical ventilators. Crit Care Clin 6:551–578
91. Reissmann H, Ranieri VM, Gottfried SB (1991) A simple method for the measurement of intrinsic PEEP during controlled and assisted modes of mechanical ventilation. (in press)
92. Hoffman RA, Ershowsky P, Kreiger BP (1989) Determination of auto-PEEP during spontaneous and controlled ventilation by monitoring changes in end-expiratory thoracic gas volume. Chest 96:613–616

Which Patients Need a Weaning Technique?

S. Benito, I. Vallverdu, and J. Mancebo

Introduction

One of the aims of artificial substitution of ventilation is to recuperate spontaneous ventilation as early as possible and in the most optimal conditions. Withdrawal from artificial ventilation may appear simple, but is sometimes more difficult than maintaining mechanical ventilation (MV) itself according to the different options proposed in the literature [1–3]. The process of withdrawal from ventilation, or taking the decision to begin this process, is empirical in most cases [4].

To recover spontaneous ventilation, the patient must have the capacity to carry out the work of breathing, but the level of consciousness, the synergy of the respiratory muscles and the nutritional state should also be maintained. The patient should either have recovered from or be recovering from the illness causing the acute respiratory failure (ARF) before artificial ventilation is withdrawn. It would be unwise to attempt to reinstate spontaneous ventilation in patients with hemodynamic instability, psychomotor agitation or pyrexia. In spite of the weaning unpredictability, in most cases the changeover is a short and successful process.

Weaning: Magnitude of the Problem

Few words in medical technology have been so strongly accepted as "weaning", possibly due to the significant symbolism and sound of this term. It refers to the transition period between artificial ventilation and spontaneous respiration, and it expresses the concept of a progressive process. Weaning is therefore defined as the gradual withdrawal from the artificial substitution of ventilation. When patients have not fully recovered from acute respiratory failure, or when their requirements cannot be spontaneously supplied, partial substitution techniques during the process of weaning should be used.

Although special care should be taken regarding the moment to interrupt MV in those patients who have presented ARF only a minority actually require a gradual transition to spontaneous ventilation (Table 1). In the now classical study by Sahn and Lakshminarayan [5] in which the clinical parameters to interrupt MV were described, only 17% of patients required a weaning technique. Hilberman et al. [6] found a similar percentage (18%) of patients requiring weaning in their series of postoperative heart surgery patients. Although the series of patients in Tahvanainen et al. study was smaller [7], a similar percentage of patients required weaning. In a series of patients with ARF due to different etiologies, Tomlinson et al. [8]

Table 1. Incidence of patients requiring weaning. This table shows the overall incidence of patients requiring weaning according to different series. In general, about 20% of intubated patients need a weaning technique. However, and according to their recruitment, the majority of COPD patients (80%) need weaning from artificial ventilation

Reference	Patients	% Weaning	Recruitment
Sahn et al., 1973 [5]	100	17%	Med-Surg
Hilberman et al., 1976 [6]	124	18%	Postop. CC
Tahvanainen et al., 1983 [7]	47	19%	Med
Tomlinson et al., 1989 [8]	165	18%	Med-Surg
Menzies et al., 1989 [9]	95	80%	COPD
Krieger et al., 1989 [10]	269	10%	CPE-Elderly

also found that 18% of their 165 patients needed progressive withdrawal from artificial ventilation.

The incidence of patients requiring weaning from artificial respiration varies according to the etiology of respiratory failure. It is obviously very different if patients are ventilated due to respiratory complications during surgery for example, or due to decompensation of chronic obstructive pulmonary disease (COPD). Menzier et al. [9] found that more than half of the COPD patients with ARF needed a prolonged period of weaning, although successful extubation was obtained in 76% of cases. This prolonged weaning of these patients was explained by severe limitation of basal FEV_1, which is a strong predictive index of the capacity of recuperating spontaneous respiration. This was not the case however in Krieger et al. series [10] in which only 10% of 259 patients required weaning from artificial ventilation even though they were elderly. The clinical characteristics of the patients also influenced the results in Krieger et al. series [10]: the cause of the ARF was cardiogenic pulmonary edema following abdominal surgery in 75% of patients, and the percentage who required a weaning technique was particularly low.

In our experience, in a group of 169 patients with ARF due to different causes, and in whom we used a strict protocol of exploration of spontaneous ventilatory capacity before initiating weaning, 28% of patients required progressive withdrawal from MV. Therefore, although recuperation of spontaneous breathing may be difficult and not immediate, weaning is only necessary in a determined proportion of mechanically ventilated patients.

Total or Partial Substitution of Ventilation

The ventilatory mode that should be used during the initial phase of ARF is controversial, although we suggest a mode that provides total substitution for ventilation. By this, we understand the assist mode ventilation (AMV), meaning that the respiratory cycle may be patient-initiated. The control mode ventilation (CMV) should be reserved for those cases in which the driving of the respiratory center should be eliminated, by heavy sedation and paralysis if necessary, due to the high inspiratory effort of the patient to trigger the ventilator [11]. It seems, however, that the use of these modes (AMV and CMV) is very common in the initial phase of ARF, as was clearly shown in the survey by Venus et al. [3] which demonstrated that the vast majority of patients were ventilated with intermittent mandatory ventilation (IMV) from the onset of ARF.

The use of AMV is also controversial because, as shown by Marini et al. [12], it may increase the inspiratory work of breathing if the sensitivity of the trigger of the machine or the inspiratory flow are not adequate for the patient's ventilatory requirements, producing fatigue and dyspnea.

When discussing weaning, it is of interest to analyze the mode of ventilation to be used during the initial phase of ARF. According to "non-use muscular atrophy", it is recommended to maintain a certain degree of contraction of the respiratory muscles. This may lead to a better starting point at the moment of recuperating spontaneous ventilation. Furthermore, continual muscular contraction during fatigue may produce "use-atrophy". It is presently agreed that the functional reserve of respiratory muscles is high and that rest improves muscular contraction in fatigued patients [13]. It appears that adequate selection of the ventilatory mode to be used should be individualized. In one patient, a determined ventilatory mode may contribute to fatigue and be harmful, while in another, it may be beneficial by preventing atrophy.

Although there may be some controversy over the use of total substitution of ventilation during the initial phase of ARF, it is generally accepted that patients who do not tolerate interruption of MV, require progressive recuperation of spontaneous respiration for a greater or lesser period. During this period of weaning, ventilatory modes which provide partial substitution of ventilation are used. The most common ventilatory modes included in this group are the T-tube, IMV, and pressure support. With their specific differences, these modes permit a gradual and progressive recuperation of ventilation according to clinical tolerance. Furthermore, for some patients, several authors have suggested the use of systems which allow the inspiratory muscles to train during weaning in order to improve their strength and endurance and help to achieve withdrawal from artificial ventilation [14].

Criteria for Discontinuing Mechanical Ventilation

One subject of constant interest in MV is to determine useful parameters to define the moment at which to interrupt artificial ventilation. The classically recommended criteria are related to ventilatory capabilities. Thus, when vital capacity (VC) is less than 10 ml/kg [15] or inferior to 1l [16] or when minute volume (VE) is superior to 10 l/min and patients are unable to double VE during maximum minute ventilation (MMV) [17], patients are considered unable to maintain spontaneous breathing.

Sahn and Lakshminarayan [5] showed that although MMV and VE were not useful parameters to predict the success of the interruption of MV, all those patients capable of generating maximal inspiratory pressures (PImax) superior to 30 cm H_2O could breathe spontaneously. Other authors [7, 8, 18, 19] however, have not found these parameters useful criteria to predict spontaneous respiratory capacity.

Gaseous exchange is not a limiting factor in carrying out the weaning process, although it is usually included in the concept of improving the ARF prior to interrupting MV. An A-a O_2 gradient <350 mm Hg with FiO_2 1 is required, or in other words, a PaO_2 >60 mm Hg with FiO_2 0.4. Adequate alveolar ventilation expressed by the quotient VD/VT is another classical gaseous exchange parameter [1, 20] although it is currently only occasionally used. VD/VT values superior to 0.6 are believed to oblige the patient to carry out a high VT to maintain adequate alveolar ventilation and a high VE although this situation may be difficult to maintain if fatigue ensues. These parameters related to gaseous exchange were described by Sahn et al. [1] as "more sophisticated" measures, and as well as the A-a O_2 and the VD/VT which we have mentioned, they included a functional residual capacity (FRC) >50% of the predicted value and a VE <180 ml/kg/min for a PaO_2 of 40 mm Hg.

The low predictive value of these parameters for some patients, especially those who have required a prolonged period of MV, has led to investigation of other variables. Morganroth et al. [21] proposed an Adverse Factor Score (AFS) and a Ventilator Score (VS) which correlated well with the weaning ability. The AFS is composed of a series of variables which are stratified with corresponding scores, and refer to cardiocirculatory variables, quantity and type of respiratory secretions, level of consciousness, and the need for drug therapy. The VS refers to pulmonary mechanics and the parameters used in the ventilator. Menzier et al. [9] considered that the prediction of weaning in COPD patients was directly related to the plasma levels of albumin, and the previous quality of life, and proposed a formula which allowed the estimation of weaning possibilities.

One interesting approach to the problem is the utilization of the oxygen cost of breathing as a predictor of weaning capacity. McDonald et al. [22] found a good correlation between the oxygen cost of breathing and the duration of weaning. Shikora et al. [23] found the difference in VO_2 between spontaneous and MV to be of greater predictive value than traditional criteria. These aspects were not confirmed in Kemper et al. [24] study which also analyzed VO_2. When the work of breathing (WOB) is measured not as VO_2 of the respiratory muscles, but from its mechanical point of view, we are analyzing the VE, the VT, and the lung compliance and resistance. Fiastro et al. [25] proposed that the WOB could be of greater utility than the standard parameters, specially in patients who had undergone a prolonged period of MV.

Another totally different approach has been to use the central respiratory drive, assessed by the tracheal occlusion pressure at 0.1 sec after onset of inspiration (P0.1). It has been shown that P0.1 is a good predictor for successful weaning in COPD patients [26], either as an isolated parameter or expressed as the ratio of P0.1 during CO_2-stimulated to baseline value [27]. Additionally, P0.1 is a valid and simple index to assess respiratory muscle fatigue in COPD patients on weaning from MV [28]. In an attempt to relate demands expressed as P0.1, and ventilatory capacity, expressed as PImax, we proposed an index [29] which increases the reliability of P0.1 in detecting the need for MV.

The apparent difficulty in defining useful parameters for predicting weaning capacity in a concrete patient contrasts with the evident clinical signs presented by patients who do not tolerate spontaneous respiration. In their excellent work with non-invasive methods, Tobin et al. [30] demonstrated the evolution of the ventilatory pattern in ventilated patients a short time after initiating spontaneous respiration. Those who did not tolerate spontaneous breathing presented a well-maintained VI, a low VT, a high respiratory frequency and a high and progressive increase in VT/TI. When from the evolution of ARF, it is considered that MV may be interrupted, spontaneous respiration may be attempted. If the patient then develops rapid and shallow breathing [30], spontaneous respiration should be interrupted and a partial substitution technique for ventilation should be initiated allowing progressive recuperation from MV.

We participated in a cooperative study [31] in which we analyzed patients in whom MV could be interrupted by means of a previously defined protocol which was followed by the attending physician. If three of four criteria were met (PaO_2 60 mm Hg with FiO_2 0.4, PImax 20 cm H_2O; RR 35 breath/min; VC 10 ml/kg) patients were allowed to breathe spontaneously. If this pause was well tolerated for 2 hours, patients were extubated. For one year in our unit, 169 patients were included in the above mentioned protocol (Fig. 1). Of these, 122 tolerated the 2-hour spontaneous breathing trial. Extubation was unsuccessful in 13 of these 122 cases and patients were reintubated. If extubation had been performed when 3 of the 4 above mentioned criteria were met, the percentage of successful extubation would have been 65%. However, it rose to 89% when this 2-hour T-tube pause was added. It therefore appears that adding a spontaneous respiration capacity test may make it easier to differentiate those patients who need a technique of progressive withdrawal from ventilation, from those who do not.

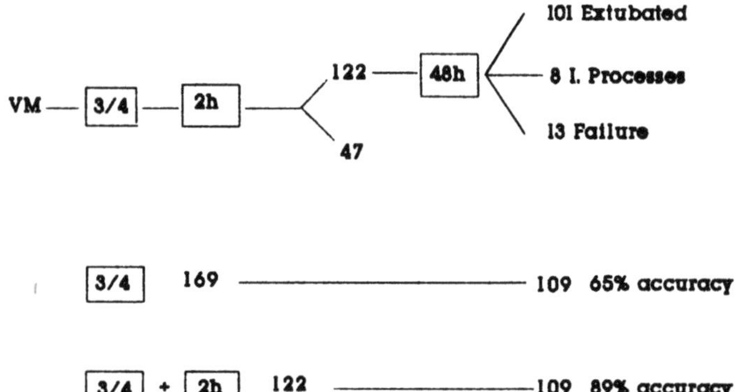

Fig. 1. In one year, 169 patients were included in a weaning protocol: 122 tolerated a 2-hour spontaneous breathing and were extubated, and of these 13 were reintubated. This means that if extubation had been performed when 3 of the 4 criteria for extubation were met, the percentage of success would have been 65%. However, when a 2-hour T-piece trial pause was added, the percentage of successfully extubated patients rose to 89%

Clinical Profile of Patients Requiring a Weaning Technique

It is important to identify those patients needing a weaning period to interrupt MV. As these patients require a longer control, early clinical identification is important. From the point of view of clinical investigation, it is interesting to know the group of patients who may require a weaning technique to interrupt MV. Some works for example have compared weaning techniques and found no differences [8, 32]. This was because they analyzed patients who did not require progressive recuperation of spontaneous ventilation as shown by the fact that extubation time was only hours.

It seems therefore that differences between one weaning technique and another could be more clearly appreciated if only patients with difficult weaning were included. In our previously mentioned study carried out over a one-year period, we analyzed the clinical and functional characteristics of these intubated patients on MV. These patients were grouped according to tolerance to spontaneous respiration into successfully extubated (group 1), reintubated due to failure of extubation (group 2), reintubated due to an intercurrent process not related to an extubation failure (group 3) and patients who required some weaning technique (group 4) (Fig. 2, Table 2).

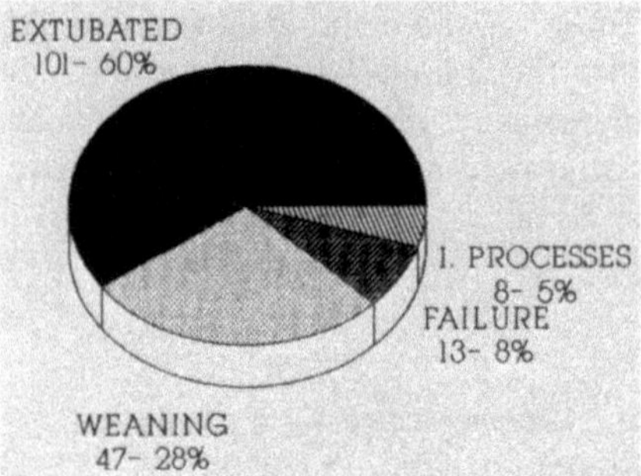

Fig. 2. This pie shows the distribution of patients in our series according to their evolution. Of the 169 patients included, 101 (60%) were successfully extubated, 13 (8%) were extubated and then reintubated because of failure of the decision to extubate, 8 (5%) were extubated and then reintubated because of a problem not related to the decision to extubate, and finally 47 (28%) required a weaning technique

Table 2. Functional characteristics of patients at the onset of weaning according to the clinical evolution

Group	DVM	VT	f	VE	$P0_1$	MIP	VVC	MEP
1	6.4±0.9	432±13	25±0.6	11.5±1	3.7±0.1	64±0.9	1.223±98	54±3.1
2	10.3±2.8	451±33	26±2.6	10.4±1	4.8±0.8	61±4.9	1.170±215	36±3.8
3	8.7±2.7	425±45	26±1	11±1	4.4±0.3	66±8.9	1.775±825	32±5.2
4	14.2±2.1	334±16	32±1.3	10±0.3	5±0.3	53±2.3	953±62	41±2.9
p	0.001	0.001	0.001	0.7 (NS)	0.002	0.01	0.03	0.005

Group 1: extubated; Group 2: failure of extubation; Group 3: intercurrent process; Group 4: weaning technique.

DVM: days of mechanical ventilation; *VT:* tidal volume (ml); *f:* frequency (resp/min); *VE:* expired minute volume (ml); *$P0_1$:* occlusion pressure (cm H_2O); *MIP:* maximal inspiratory pressure (cm H_2O); *VVC:* Voluntary vital capacity (l); *MEP:* maximal expiratory pressure (cm H_2O)

Furthermore, in order to determine the evolutive differences during withdrawal from MV regarding the basal disease, 3 categories of patients were established: COPD (Fig. 3), neurologic (Fig. 4), and acute patients (Fig. 5) (Table 3).

From these results, it could be concluded that patients requiring weaning techniques presented a longer period of MV as well as a pattern of rapid and shallow

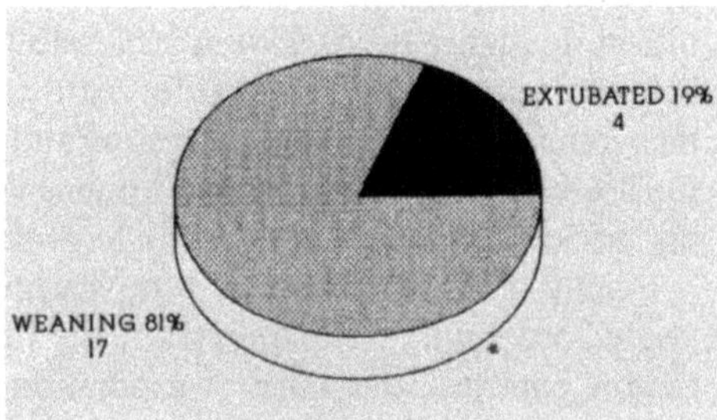

Fig. 3. According to the etiology, 21 patients had a COPD. Of these, 17 (81%) required a weaning technique, and 4 (19%) were extubated without needing weaning

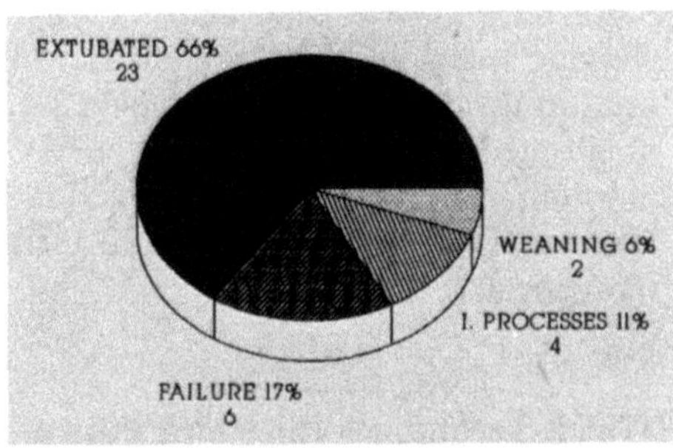

Fig. 4. According to the etiology of IRF, 35 patients had a neurological disease. Of these only 2 (6%) required weaning, 6 (17%) were an extubation failure, 4 (11%) were reintubated because of an intercurrent process, and 23 (66%) were extubated without needing weaning

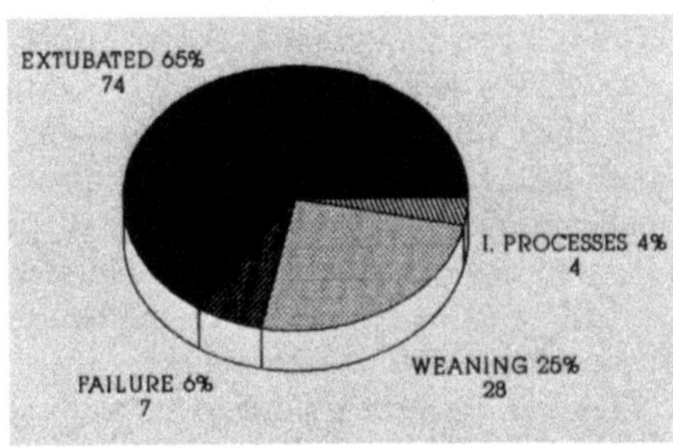

Fig. 5. According to the etiology, 113 patients had an acute respiratory failure. Of these, 28 (25%) required a weaning technique, 7 (6%) were an extubation failure, 4 (4%) were reintubated because of an intercurrent process, and 74 (65%) were extubated without needing weaning

Table 3. Evolutive differences during withdrawal from mechanical ventilation regarding the basal disease

		COPD (n = 21)	NEURO-LOGIC (n = 35)	ACUTE (n = 113)	P
Extubated	(Group 1)	4 (19%)	23 (65%)	74 (65%)	0.0002
Failure	(Group 2)	0	6 (17%)	7 (6%)	0.038
Intercurrent process	(Group 3)	0	4 (11%)	4 (3%)	0.08
Weaning	(Group 4)	17 (80%)	2 (6%)	28 (25%)	0.0001

respiration with high RR and low VT, characteristics already described in this type of patients [30].

Sassoon et al. [26] confirmed the utility of P0.1 in patients with weaning difficulties, and her findings coincide with our data in which the P0.1 was significantly higher ($p = 0.002$) in the group of patients who did not tolerate spontaneous respiration. Additionally, the indexes of muscular strength such as PIM and PEM were lower in patients who did not tolerate extubation. Furthermore, the PEM was significantly higher ($p = 0.005$) in successfully extubated patients, and this index may help to determine the moment for extubation. An example would be those patients recovering from neurologic illnessess and absence of lung complications, in whom the need for adequate bronchial hygiene would retard extubation because of coughing difficulties, which in turn would prolong weaning.

Finally, and in agreement with the literature [9], 80% of our COPD patients needed a weaning technique, while the figure was only 6% in neurologic patients. On the contrary, the index of extubation failures was nihil in COPD patients and the majority of those in whom extubation failed had a neurologic disease.

All these clinical characteristics may help to define those patients needing a weaning technique. Nevertheless, as Milic-Emili stated [4], the non-scientific aspects in the process of weaning have yet to be considered. This is particularly demonstrated in the case of patients on MV who deliberately extubate themselves and in whom reintubation is only required in 11% of cases [33]. We are therefore still a long way from being able to define the totality of problems regarding weaning in our patients.

Which Techniques for which Patient?

This is a very important question. However, there is not yet sufficient information available to be able to reply fully. As explained previously, we are generally able to recognize which patients need a weaning technique. Additionally, it seems to have been demonstrated that the period of weaning is shortened when difficult-to-wean patients are ventilated with pressure support (PS). Besides, it is logical to think that PS may not be a universal weaning technique for all patients. Most important would be to determine which mechanism is responsible for recuperating spontaneous respiration in each patient.

Several excellent reports have analyzed the weaning process [34–36] and also dealt with aspects for making decisions regarding withdrawal from artificial ventilation, aspects indicating the correct evolution and also the weaning modalities we can use.

Nevertheless, it may be clinically difficult to separate the determinants which make a patient dependent on a ventilator. In a review by Marini [38] the most important causes of this ventilation dependence and the eventual therapeutic approaches are described. Although hypoxemia is a clearly recognized situation, the hemodynamic instability caused by the extra-effort due to spontaneous inspiration may require invasive exploratory maneuvers in some cases. The most frequent cause of failure in patients unable to tolerate spontaneous respiration is the unbalance between capabilities and demands.

Careful examination of functional parameters which explore ventilatory necessities, strength, endurance, ventilatory reserve and adequacy of ventilatory drive may provide sufficient information about the clinical status of a patient who cannot breathe spontaneously, and may help in knowing the reason for the mismatch between demands and capabilities. From a clinical point of view the most frequent causes are slightly increased demands coupled with decreased muscular reserves, which in turn make it difficult to reach the necessities or limit the ventilatory reserve [39].

We do not know of any report analyzing in detail which mode is the most adequate for each clinical situation. However, there is detailed information available which can help in specific situations. For example, PS disminishes the WOB and increases the sense of comfort [40] as PS helps in decreasing duration and intensity of contraction of the inspiratory muscles [41], thus preventing diaphragmatic fatigue [42]. These characteristics probably make PS a very effective technique in patients with prolonged starvation and loss of muscular mass, and also in patients with COPD and weak and/or fatigued muscles. Another group of patients which may benefit from PS are patients with mitral valve disease or with congestive heart failure because these patients present associated alterations in respiratory muscles [43, 44].

It is unlikely that PS will be useful in patients who, after suffering an ARDS, present a restrictive respiratory pattern and low pulmonary compliance. These patients will probably benefit from weaning with the T-tube. Furthermore, those anxious patients who fight against the ventilator will possibly benefit from the T-tube weaning technique.

Although it has been demonstrated that the progressive decrease of frequency of SIMV breaths augments the WOB of both spontaneous and mandatory breaths [45], those patients with low WOB requiring low ventilatory demands and with an irregular respiratory pattern, such as those with central nervous system abnormalities (i.e. cranial trauma), may perhaps benefit from SIMV weaning. In post cardiac surgery patients with low ventilatory reserves and with chest wall instability SIMV may probably be a beneficial weaning technique.

Such comments about possible indications of one technique versus another in certain diseases only aim to point out that these are differential aspects among techniques which may be beneficial in concrete clinical situations if these techniques are judiciously employed. Additionally, we should keep in mind that in the majority of patients, the transition between MV and spontaneous respiration is only extubation, and in those patients who require weaning, viewed as a whole group, the most useful weaning technique among PS, SIMV and T-tube, is PS because it shortens the weaning time.

References

1. Sahn SA, Lakshminarayan S, Petty TL (1976) Weaning from mechanical ventilation. JAMA 235:2208–2212
2. Skillman JJ, Malhotra JV, Palotta JA, Bushnell LS (1971) Determinants of weaning from controlled ventilation. Surgical Forum 22:198–200

3. Venus B, Smith RA, Mathru M (1987) National surgery of methods and criteria used for weaning from mechanical ventilation. Crit Care Med 15:530–533
4. Milic-Emili J (1986) Is weaning an art or a science? Am Rev Respir Dis 134:1107–1108
5. Sahn SA, Lakshminarayan S (1973) Bedside criteria for discontinuation of mechanical ventilation. Chest 63:1002–1005
6. Hilberman M, Kamm B, Lamy M, et al (1976) An analysis of potential predictors of respiratory adequacy following cardiac surgery. J Thorac Cardiovasc Surg 71:711–720
7. Tahvanainen J, Salmenpera M, Nikki P (1983) Extubation criteria after weaning from intermittent mandatory ventilation and continuous positive airway pressure. Crit Care Med 11:702–707
8. Tomlinson JR, Miller KS, Lorch DG, Smith L, Reines HD, Sahn SA (1989) A prospective comparison of IMV and T-piece weaning from mechanical ventilation. Chest 96:348–352
9. Menzies R, Gibbons W, Goldberg P (1989) Determinants of weaning and survival among patients with COPD who require mechanical ventilation for acute respiratory failure. Chest 95:398–405
10. Krieger BP, Ersowsky PF, Becker DA, Gazeroglu HB (1989) Evaluation of conventional criteria for predicting successful weaning from mechanical ventilatory support in elderly patients. Crit Care Med 17:858–861
11. Fernández R, Benito S, Sanchis J, Milic-Emili J, Net A (1988) Inspiratory effort and occlusion pressure in triggered mechanical ventilation. Intensive Care Med 14:650–653
12. Marini JJ, Copps JS, Culver BH (1985) The inspiratory work of breathing during assisted mechanical ventilation. Chest 87:612–618
13. Braun NM, Faulkner J, Hughes RL, Roussos C, Sahgal V (1983) When should respiratory muscles be exercised? Chest 84:76–84
14. Aldrich TK, Karpel JP, Uhrlass RM, Sparapani MA, Erano D, Ferranti R (1989) Weaning from mechanical ventilation: adjuntive use of inspiratory muscle resistive training. Crit Care Med 17:143–147
15. Bendixen HH, Egbert LD, Hedley-Whyte J, et al (1965) Management of patients undergoing prolonged artificial ventilation. In: C. V. Mosly (ed) Respiratory care. St. Louis, p 149
16. Safar P, Kunkel HG (1965) Prolonged artificial ventilation. In: Safar P (ed) Respiratory Therapy. Philadelphia FA Davis, p 126
17. Stetson JB (1970) Introductory essay in prolonged tracheal intubation. Int Anesthesiol Clin 8:774–775
18. Millbern SM, Downs JB, Jumper LC, et al (1978) Evaluation of criteria for discontinuing mechanical ventilation support. Arch Surg 113:1441–1444
19. DeHaven GB, Hurst JM, Branson RD (1986) Evaluation of two different extubation criteria: Attributes contributing to success. Crit Care Med 14:92–94
20. Pontoppidan H, Laver MB, Geffin B (1970) Acute respiratory failure in the surgical patient. In: Welch CE (ed) Advances in surgery. Chicago. Year Book Medical Publishers 4:163–254
21. Morganroth ML, Morganroth JL, Nett LM, Petty TL (1984) Criteria for weaning from prolonged mechanical ventilation. Arch Intern Med 144:1012–1016
22. McDonald NJ, Lavelle P, Gallacher WN, Harpin RP (1988) Use of the oxygen cost of breathing as an idex of weaning ability from mechanical ventilation. Intensive Care Med 14:50–54
23. Shikora SA, Bistrian BR, Borlase BC, Blackburn GL, Stone MD, Benotti PN (1990) Work of breathing: reliable predictor of weaning and extubation. Crit Care Med 18:157–162
24. Kemper M, Weissman C, Askanazi J, Hyman AI, Kinney JM (1987) Metabolic and respiratory changes during weaning from mechanical ventilation. Chest 92:979–983
25. Fiastro JF, Habib MP, Shon BY, Campbell SC (1988) Comparison of standard weaning parameters and the mechanical work of breathing in mechanically ventilated patients. Chest 94:232–238
26. Sassoon CSH, Te TT, Mahutte CK, Light R (1987) Airway occlusion pressure. An important indicator for successful weaning in patients with chronic obstructive pulmonary disease. Am Rev Respir Dis 135:107–113
27. Montgomery BA, Holle RHO, Neagley SR, Pierson DJ, Schoene RB (1987) Prediction of successful ventilator weaning using airway occlusion pressure and hypercapnic challenge. Chest 91:496–499

28. Murciano D, Boczkowski J, Lecocguic Y, Milic-Emili J, Pariente R, Aubier M (1988) Tracheal occlusion pressure: a simple index to monitor respiratory failure in patients with chronic obstructive pulmonary disease. Ann Intern Med 108:800–805
29. Fernández R, Cabrera J, Calaf N, Benito S (1990) P0.1/PImax: an index assessing respiratory capacity in acute respiratory failure. Intensive Care Med 16:175–179
30. Tobin MJ, Pérez W, Guenther SM, et al (1986) The pattern of breathing during successful and unsuccessful trials of weaning from mechanical ventilation. Am Rev Respir Dis 134:1111–1118
31. Brochard L, Rauss A, Benito S, et al (1990) Comparaison de trois modalités de sevrage de la ventilation artificielle. Résultats d'un essai multicentrique européen. Réan Soins Intens Méd Urg 6:517
32. Prakash O, Meij S, Van Der Borden B (1982) Spontaneous ventilation test vs intermittent mandatory ventilation. Chest 81:403–406
33. Coppolo DP, May JJ (1990) Self-extubation. Chest 98:165–169
34. Pierson DJ (1983) Weaning from mechanical ventilation in acute respiratory failure: concepts, indications, and techniques. Respir Care 28:646–662
35. Hall JB, Wood LDH (1987) Liberation of the patient from mechanical ventilation. JAMA 257:1621–1628
36. Morganroth ML, Grum CM (1988) Weaning from mechanical ventilation. J Intensive Care Med 3:109–120
37. Schuster DP (1990) A physiologic approach to initiating, maintaining and withdrawing mechanical ventilatory support during acute respiratory failure. Am J Med 88:268–278
38. Marini JJ (1986) The physiologic determinants of ventilator dependence. Respir Care 31:271–282
39. Boysen PG (1987) Respiratory muscle function and weaning from mechanical ventilation. Respir Care 32:572–583
40. MacIntyre NR (1986) Respiratory function during pressure support ventilation. Chest 89:677–683
41. Brochard L, Pluskwa F, Lemaire F (1987) Improved efficacy of spontaneous breathing with inspiratory pressure supprt. Am Rev Respir Dis 136:411–415
42. Brochard L, Harf A, Lorino H, Lemaire F (1989) Inspiratory pressure support prevents diaphragmatic fatigue during weaning from mechanical ventilation. Am Rev Respir Dis 139:513–521
43. De Troyer A, Estenne M, Yernault JC (1980) Disturbance of respiratory muscle function in patients with mitral valve disease. Am J Med 69:867–873
44. Hammond MD, Bauer KA, Sharp JT, Rocha RD (1990) Respiratory muscle strength in congestive heart failure. Chest 98:1091–1094
45. Marini JJ, Smith TC, Lamb VJ (1988) External work output and force generation during synchronized intermittent mechanical ventilation. Am Rev Respir Dis 138:1169–1179

Ventilatory Failure: Innovative Support Techniques

M.A. Branthwaite, M.W. Elliott, and A.K. Simonds

Introduction

Ventilatory failure is usually defined in terms of measured abnormalities of arterial blood gas tensions. This implies an absolute distinction between its presence or absence but makes no allowance for chronicity, variability, changes between sleeping and wakefulness, or the coincident presence of other abnormalities which influence tissue oxygen delivery or demand.

An alternative approach is to consider the respiratory system as a balance (Table 1) between demand (respiratory work) and capacity (the strength and endurance of the respiratory muscles). Under normal circumstances, this system is polarised in favor of the respiratory muscles. There are reserves of strength and endurance which permit considerable increases in demand, e.g. on exercise, without the onset of either respiratory muscle fatigue or ventilatory failure. Pathology which interferes with the efficiency of gas exchange, which impairs the capacity of the respiratory muscles or which increases metabolic demand, can erode these reserves so that eventually arterial blood gas status deteriorates and/or respiratory muscle fatigue supervenes. Presented in these terms, it is easy to envisage that respiratory failure is

Table 1. Concept of a balance between the work of breathing and the capacity of the respiratory muscles

Respiratory muscles – supply and demand

Work	Muscles
Factors increasing respiratory work	Factors decreasing strength/endurance
Lung pathology	Myopathic/neurogenic weakness
	Disadvantageous configuration
Rigidity/deformity	Malnutrition
	Fatigue
Metabolic demand	– Overload
	– ↓Perfusion
	– ↑PCO_2
	– ↓PO_2

not necessarily absolute but that conditions can fluctuate when demand and capacity are finely balanced.

Bellemare and Grassino [1] present a similar concept in their plot of transdiaphragmatic pressure as a proportion of the maximum that can be generated, against the duration of inspiration as a proportion of the total respiratory cycle. Using these two variables, they indicate the extremes where respiratory muscle fatigue is either absent or inevitable, and include an intermediate 'risk zone' where the ability to sustain adequate gas exchange without fatigue is uncertain. Several consequences follow from this analysis. First, is that there are many potential causes for patients to fail a trial of weaning and highly likely that the manifestations of each will differ. For example, the development of pulmonary congestion as a consequence of venoconstriction in a patient with left ventricular dysfunction will differ clinically from weaning failure caused by sputum retention. This challenges the concept that any test is likely to predict reliably whether or not a weaning trial will be successful. Furthermore, the dynamic nature of the balance between respiratory work and resources means that whichever test is chosen will only be representative for a brief period. The ideal test for predicting successful weaning would address the most severely compromised and most rapidly changing factor contributing to the unstable equilibrium.

The therapeutic consequences of considering ventilatory capacity in terms of this balance are more encouraging. Small and individually insignificant improvements in several variables will contribute to the return of spontaneous ventilation, even when respiratory reserves are very limited. More importantly, the need for mechanical assistance is likely to vary with time. Techniques used intermittently should be as unobtrusive as posssible and, above all, avoid introducing additional problems. Endotracheal intubation and tracheostomy provide a first class airway but can augment respiratory work, promote the secretion of bronchial mucus, predispose to infection, interfere with nutrition and possibly necessitate sedation. It is these concepts which have led to renewed enthusiasm for non-invasive methods of controlling or assisting ventilation mechanically, and it is the indications, techniques and results of this approach which are reviewed here.

Indications for Non-Invasive Ventilatory Support

There are three clinical circumstances where the balance between respiratory demand and capacity is likely to be finely poised.

First is the patient with an acute exacerbation of chronic lung disease in whom some intercurrent event, often a respiratory tract infection, precipitates the onset or unacceptable worsening of ventilatory failure. Factors which disturb the equilibrium of the respiratory balance in these circumstances are illustrated in Table 2.

Similar abnormalities are likely during recovery from severe acute respiratory failure (ARF) requiring prolonged and often continuous mechanical ventilation (MV), particularly if there is a background of chronic respiratory, cardiac or neuromuscular disease. This is the familiar situation in the intensive care unit (ICU) when patients are 'slow to wean'.

Finally, and numerically an important group, are patients in whom the onset of

Table 2. Factors adversely and acutely affecting the balance between respiratory work and capacity in exacerbations of chronic obstructive pulmonary disease (COPD)

Acute changes in COPD

Work	Muscles
Factors increasing respiratory work	Factors decreasing strength/endurance
● Lung pathology	Myopathic/neurogenic weakness
	Disadvantageous configuration
Rigidity/deformity	Malnutrition
● Metabolic demand	Fatigue
	– Overload ●
	– $\downarrow$Perfusion (●)
	– $\uparrow PCO_2$ ●
	– $\downarrow PO_2$ ●

The size of the solid circles represents the relative importance of each factor.

sleep precludes the maintenance of adequate alveolar ventilation so that episodes of desaturation and hypercapnia occur, either in all sleep stages or, more commonly, during periods of rapid eye movement sleep. Sleep diminishes central chemosensitivity, abolishes or makedly decreases the contribution of accessory respiratory muscles and reduces intercostal activity to such an extent that ventilation depends almost exclusively on diaphragmatic contraction during rapid eye movement sleep. Repeated episodes of hypoventilation occurring every night during sleep lead eventually to day-time hypoxemia and hypercapnia as well, and hence pulmonary hypertension, cor pulmonale and death (Fig. 1). This is the characteristic pattern of cardio-respiratory failure in patients with central sleep apnea or severe extra-pulmonary restrictive disorders such as chest wall rigidity, deformity or weakness [2, 3]. It also occurs when pulmonary and extra-pulmonary disease co-exist, a good example being healed pulmonary tuberculosis treated surgically by measures such as thoracoplasty which create restriction [4]. Intermittent sleep-related hypoventilation is a prominent feature of patients with advanced chronic obstructive pulmonary disease (COPD) [5] and here too may contribute to the genesis of cor pulmonale. Mild to moderate nocturnal hypoventilation can be controlled by suppressing rapid eye movement sleep using protriptyline, 5–10 mg nocte, a regime which is effective and well-tolerated by many patients with restrictive chest wall disease [6]. Similar albeit more modest benefit can be demonstrated in those with COPD (Fig. 2) but symptomatic improvement is usually only slight and the anticholinergic side-effects are often poorly tolerated by patients who are generally in the older age groups [7]. Assisting ventilation by mechanical means during sleep is the only rational alternative when drug therapy is either ineffective or cannot be tolerated.

It is apparent from this analysis that non-invasive methods of ventilatory support have a potential role in the management of acute on chronic respiratory insufficien-

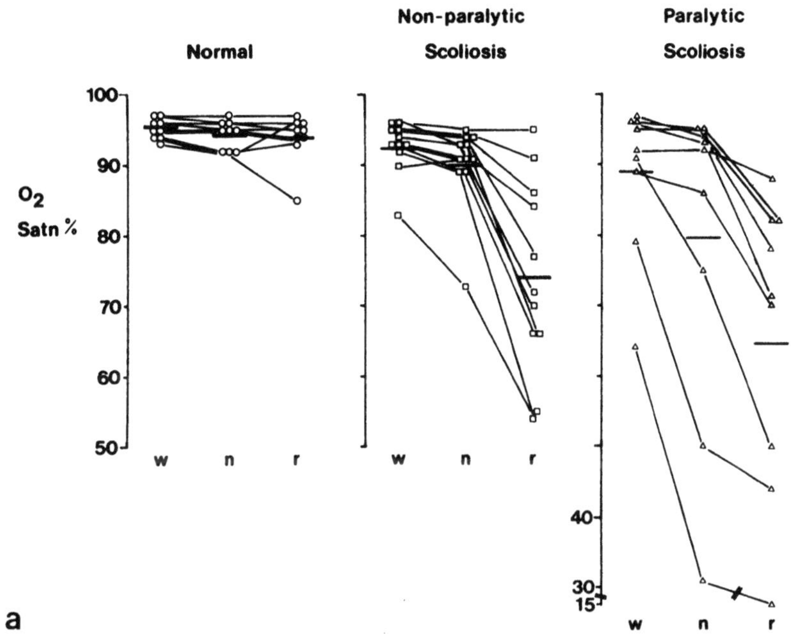

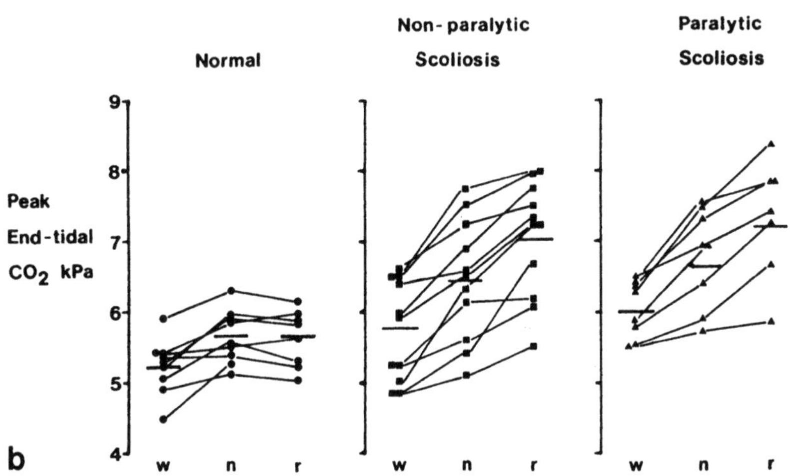

Fig. 1. a Minimum oxygen saturation during wakefulness (w), non-rapid eye movement (n) and rapid eye movement (r) sleep in patients with scoliosis compared to a control group matched for age and sex. **b** Highest values for end-tidal carbon dioxide tension under similar circumstances in the three groups. (5.3 kPa = 40 mm Hg)

cy, during prolonged weaning from conventional MV, and for long-term use in a domiciliary environment when the primary abnormality is sleep-related hypoventilation.

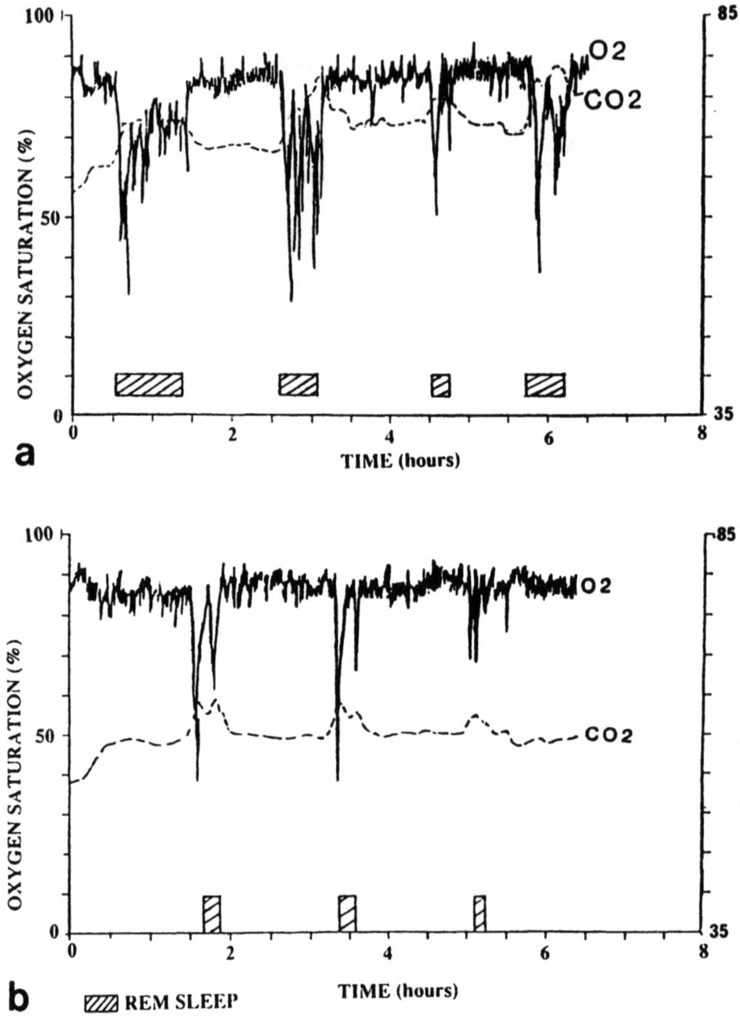

Fig. 2. Control of sleep-related hypoventilation using protriptyline in a patient with chronic obstructive pulmonary disease. Oxygen saturation and transcutaneous carbon dioxide tension during sleep while on no treatment (upper panel) and when taking protriptyline 10 mg nocte (lower panel). Cross-hatched areas = periods of rapid eye movement sleep. (From [7] with permission)

Techniques of Non-Invasive Ventilation or Ventilatory Support

MV can be provided intermittently and non-invasively using either negative pressure applied to the chest wall or positive pressure applied to the upper airway.

Negative pressure devices [8, 9]. The original tank ventilators were designed to maintain gas exchange in subjects with respiratory muscle paralysis but in whom lung function was usually unimpaired. In these circumstances, their bulk, relative inefficiency and the need for an assistant to manipulate the sealing mechanism were of no concern. The current resurgence of interest in their use centers not only on augmenting gas exchange but also on their ability to rest the respiratory muscles, usually in patients in whom muscle function is otherwise unimpaired but who have severe respiratory disease. Then the clumsy, cumbersome tank and loss of independence associated with its use are far less appropriate or acceptable. An even more important constraint is that application of negative pressure to the thoraco-abdominal wall accentuates any tendency to upper airway obstruction during sleep in the recumbent and supine patient.

Simpler derivatives of the original tank ventilator include those which are patient operated, smaller and more easily disassembled, but portability remains a problem and an uninterrupted power supply is essential for most models.

The cuirass or body shell, and jacket, pneumosuit or pneumowrap are less efficient than the tank ventilator but can operate from a smaller and more mobile pump. A few patients are well suited to these devices, particularly those who are thin and have extensive weakness, but many find them uncomfortable, clumsy and difficult to operate so that compliance with recommended treatment programs is poor.

Non-invasive positive pressure ventilation. Anaesthetized, paralyzed patients are usually easy to ventilate using positive pressure delivered through a face-mask. It is the inconvenience of maintaining a secure seal between the face and the mask which prompts intubation when ventilation is to be continued for any length of time. An alternative approach is to accept a variable leak and use exceptionally high volumes and/or flow rates, aiming to compensate for the leak to such an extent that alveolar ventilation can be sustained.

Only a minority of conscious patients find a close-fitting face-mask acceptable for long, although Brochard et al. [10] have achieved notable success using pressure support ventilation (PSV) by face-mask. Alba et al. [11] advocate a mouth-piece held between the teeth, but the most popular variant is a nasal mask [12] which most patients find more acceptable than a full face-mask and with which it is usually possible to secure a better seal. The most recent innovation consists of soft plastic plugs inserted in the nares [13], shaped so that delivery of positive pressure through the lumen helps seal the wall of the plug against the inner surface of the nasal vestibule. The device and its associated circuit were designed for continuous positive airway pressure (CPAP) during sleep but it can be modified for intermittent positive pressure ventilation (IPPV) and has been used successfully with inflation pressures of up to 30 cm H_2O [14].

All the positive pressure techniques have the advantage of helping to preserve patency of the upper airway and indeed, nasal IPPV is a derivative of nasal CPAP introduced by Sullivan et al. [15] for the relief of obstructive sleep apnea. Several small, simple positive pressure ventilators have been designed with this application in mind, and their suitability for use outside the hospital environment has been an important requirement [16]. Many incorporate a trigger function so that conscious patients, capable of taking or initiating at least a small breath, can dictate respiratory frequency when necessary. The sensitivity and response time of the trigger are important determinants of comfort and acceptability, but the inspiratory effort of patients with COPD may do no more than merely lower the persistently raised intra-thoracic pressure (the auto-PEEP phenomenon) so that the trigger threshold is never reached and thus their own efforts fail to coincide with the imposed respiratory cycle [17]. These considerations mean that the ventilator must be capable of controlling ventilation, as distinct from assisting spontaneous breathing, and requisite safeguards to warn of disconnection or mechanical failure must be incorporated. Major and often variable leaks are an almost inevitable feature of non-invasive positive pressure ventilation and a number of patients remain asleep even though respiratory excursion and gas exchange have been markedly reduced and a loud alarm is ringing close by. An innovative technique which aims to compensate for even quite major leaks is incorporated in the Respironics BiPAP [18] which is a pressure preset device with a variable flow capable of increasing automatically to compensate for losses from the circuit. The limiting factor on its performance is that it is pressure and not volume preset so that patients with high airway resistance or poor compliance may be ventilated inadequately, especially during sleep [19].

Results of Non-Invasive Ventilatory Support

Negative pressure methods. The early role of negative pressure ventilation in the management of respiratory failure caused by acute, potentially reversible paralysing illnesses such as poliomyelitis is too well known to be reiterated here. The reports discussed below all derive from the last decade or so.

Spencer [20] was one of the first to report a large series of patients, most with marginal respiratory function caused by chest wall deformity, weakness or both, in whom negative pressure ventilation was used electively. He has employed the tank ventilator to treat acute exacerbations of respiratory failure, often caused by infective episodes, and to facilitate extubation when conventional positive pressure ventilation had been used during and after major surgery. He is also an advocate of negative pressure techniques in the domiciliary environment. A number of other authors have used negative pressure equipment successfully both for acute, in-hospital treatment and at home, most series reporting patients with extra-pulmonary restrictive disorders [8, 9, 21–23].

Simonds et al. [24] described the use of the tank ventilator to secure the return of unassisted spontaneous breathing in patients previously identified as 'weaning failures'. The technique is not a universal panacea for the chronically ventilator dependent in the ICU but is most appropriate for those with severe but stable respiratory disability in whom other pathology has been fully treated as far as possible. There is an obvious hazard of aspiration of gastric contents into the lungs if gastro-intestinal function is impaired or glottic reflexes are sluggish, a risk which is accentuated by physical constraint of the patient who can virtually only lie supine in the tank. The risk of upper airway obstruction is also accentuated by the supine posture, and another troublesome side-effect is gaseous distension of the abdomen. Last but by no means least, the management of back-ache and skin soreness over pressure points demands skilful nursing.

Samuels and Southall [25] have extended the use of negative pressure techniques to neonates and infants and treated various types of respiratory insufficiency, including respiratory distress syndrome of the newborn. They advocate the application of either constant negative pressure of varying magnitude, or intermittent negative pressure ventilation with a sustained but lower negative pressure during the expiratory phase. The physiological rationale is analogous to that intended with CPAP in adults with acute respiratory insufficiency, or IPPV with PEEP. Apart from the advantages of avoiding intubation in the very young, they claim a lower incidence of adverse cardiovascular consequences and, possibly, a lower incidence of intra-ventricular hemorrhage by comparison with conventional techniques, but these postulated benefits await confirmation.

Most interest in negative pressure techniques in the recent past has focused on their possible role in the management of COPD [26, 27]. Both subjective and objective benefit has been reported from periods of assisted ventilation using negative pressure ventilators in patients with COPD treated in hospital [28, 29] but attempts to continue treatment at home, particularly overnight, have met with only limited success [30, 31], either because patients are poorly compliant or because upper airway obstruction during sleep precludes overnight use. A reduction in diaphragmatic EMG activity can be demonstrated during negative pressure ventilation in patients with COPD [32, 33], and even in normal subjects during sleep [34, 35]. Sustained improvement in arterial blood gas tensions during spontaneous ventilation and higher values for maximum inspiratory and expiratory mouth pressures have also been reported [29, 36]. Relief of chronic respiratory muscle fatigue has been postulated as the mechanism for achieving benefit [37–39], and it has been suggested that patients with COPD can be selected for treatment on the basis of a low maximum inspiratory mouth pressure [40].

Positive Pressure Methods. Nasal positive pressure ventilation has found immediate popularity and, unlike negative pressure techniques, has been adopted in many centers. This difference probably reflects its greater efficiency, acceptability, and comparability to other equipment used currently to assist ventilation mechanically.

Although described initially as a means of providing long-term support, Elliott et al. [41] described the relief of severe, acute on chronic respiratory failure in six patients who would otherwise have been expected to die or to require endotracheal intubation and conventional ventilation. Included in this series was one patient with cystic fibrosis awaiting heart-lung transplantation. This effective but non-invasive technique of ventilatory support (Fig. 3) has since proved invaluable in the management of other patients in the same predicament and, in a number, has provided a bridge to subsequent successful transplantation. The advantages of using nasal positive pressure ventilation in these circumstances are that there is little or no erosion of the quality of life in the terminal stages of an illness which can only be salvaged by transplantation, there is far less need for scarce resources because the technique can be continued in a well-supervised general ward and, perhaps most importantly, the avoidance of tracheal intubation provides a better chance of a successful outcome if donor organs do become available.

Similar concepts are expressed in two recent abstracts reporting the value of NIPPV in the management of acute on chronic respiratory failure, primarily in patients with COPD [42] and in elderly subjects (mean age 79 years) where intuba-

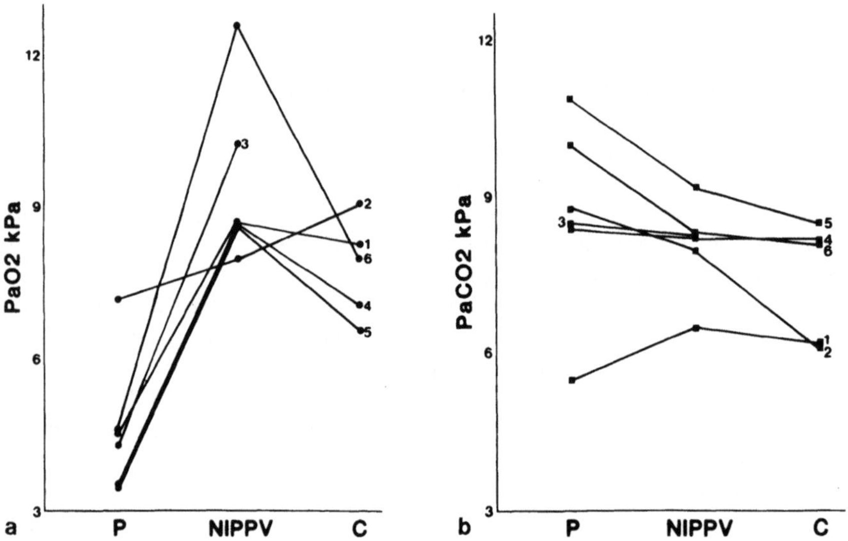

Fig. 3. Changes in arterial oxygen tension (PaO_2) and carbon dioxide tension ($PaCO_2$) in six patients with life-threatening, acute on chronic respiratory failure. Patients 2 and 5 (suffering from chronic obstructive pulmonary disease and cystic fibrosis respectively) were breathing 24 or 28% oxygen at presentation.
P at presentation, breathing spontaneously; *NIPPV* values recorded approximately two hours later during NIPPV, with added oxygen (1 litre) in all patients; *C* during convalescence, 7–10 days later, breathing spontaneously (patient 5 still using oxygen). (5.3 kPa = 40 mm Hg)

tion and conventional ventilation were considered questionable [43]. A comparable philosophy has been followed by Brochard et al. [10] who demonstrated improved gas exchange and reduced respiratory work in patients with an acute exacerbation of COPD treated with inspiratory pressure support by face-mask. Patients using this technique required ventilatory assistance for a shorter time and were discharged from ICU sooner than a historical control group, most of whom required intubation and conventional ventilation.

The ability to offer effective ventilatory assistance, continued at home if necessary, but without imposing all the disadvantages and complications of tracheostomy, has also re-opened a dialogue on the role of MV in the management of progressive neuromuscular disease [44], and it is important to note in this context that the technique of nasal IPPV has even been mastered and tolerated by relatively young children [45, 46].

Given that nasal IPPV can be used to avoid intubation and conventional MV, it is hardly surprising that it has also been used to assist the return of spontaneous ventilation and secure extubation. It is now the technique of choice at this hospital for achieving extubation or closure of a tracheostomy in otherwise stable patients who are only able to breathe for limited periods, for example after cardiac surgery complicated by bilateral diaphragm paresis or paralysis, and when ARF occurring against a background of chronic respiratory disability has been treated by conventional mechanical measures but the patient 'fails to wean' [47]. Presence of a well-established tracheostomy is no barrier to using nasal IPPV provided the stoma is either occluded completely, or the trachestomy tube is fenestrated and perfectly aligned. Surgical emphysema is a potential complication if there is a tracheal opening but is unlikely if there is a well-formed track to the skin. Continued presence of the tube, or at least a mini-tracheostomy, provides a route for endotracheal suction in patients with profuse secretions, but unacceptable leaks are common in these circumstances so that non-invasive ventilation is most likely to succeed in those who either have few secretions or can clear them spontaneously.

The most notable role for nasal IPPV to date has been in the provision of home care, particularly for patients who only require ventilation overnight [12, 48–52]. Considerable success has been reported (Table 3), primarily in patients with restrictive disease, but even some of the early series included patients with primary lung disease [51]. Practical problems which complicate management include unacceptable leaks through the open mouth, abrasion or even ulceration of the skin of the nasal bridge, and gaseous distension of the abdomen, particularly when high inflation pressures are necessary. Careful attention to the detail of mask selection and adjustment of the ventilator controls usually circumvents these difficulties, and most patients can handle the system at home without assistance. Wider use of this life-saving technique on a domiciliary basis underlines the need for an effective home-care program providing not only support for patient and family, but also prompt response to mechanical breakdowns and reliable arrangements for readmission if emergencies supervene [53].

The incidence of home care ventilation will undoubtedly increase enormously if sustained benefit can be demonstrated in patients with COPD. The results of long-term IPPV by tracheostomy in COPD have been disappointing [54] with survival figures little different from those achieved by more conservative means. Nasal IPPV has yet to be fully evaluated in these cirumstances but Elliott et al. [55] reported improved daytime blood gas status in 10 of 12 patients with stable hypercapnic COPD treated by night-time NIPPV for four weeks [55]. Nocturnal hypo-

Table 3. Outcome of home mechanical ventilation using nasal IPPV over approximately 5 years

Domiciliary ventilation c̄ NIPPV (mortality: August 1986–January 1991)

	8.86–1.88	1.88–1.89	1.89–1.90	1.90–1.91
8.86–1.88 (n = 41)	74F (R) 27F (N – R)		64F (R)	52M (R)
1.88–1.89 (n = 29)		34F (N – R)	63M (N – R)	59F (N – R)
1.89–1.90 (n = 38)			63F (R) 17F (R/N – R)	57F (N – R)
1.90–1.91 (n = 24)				

The number of patients (n) recruited over each time period is shown on the left and individual deaths (M male; F female) are shown, with age at death, in the columns.
N – R indicates death caused by non-respiratory disease and R denotes patients in whom death was attributed to respiratory insufficiency. Both respiratory and non-respiratory disease contributed to one death. All other patients were alive and well in January 1991.

ventilation was considerably improved such that without oxygen enrichment, the median percentage of the night spent with an oxygen saturation greater than 80% increased from 52% (range 0–100%) to 94% (range 16–100%), and there were corresponding falls in transcutaneous carbon dioxide tension. Subjective reports of improved sleep quality in the majority have since been confirmed by formal assessment [56] and, after a year, 7 patients have elected to continue treatment. Contrary results were reported by Strumpf et al. [57] in whose series of 23 patients, 4 were excluded because of coincident obstructive sleep apnea, 7 withdrew with intercurrent illness and 6 because of intolerance to the nasal mask. The 6 patients who completed the three month study and control periods showed neurospychiatric improvement but no significant change in daytime blood gas status or pulmonary function.

Technical considerations may explain some of the discrepancies between these conflicting reports but, even if successful control of ventilation can be secured overnight in patients with COPD, the technique can only be advocated for widespread use if it prolongs life or enhances its quality. The results of long term domiciliary oxygen [58] and of MV through a tracheostomy [54] are disappointing and more information is needed on the mechanisms by which lung damage and destruction progress and how these detrimental effects might be alleviated. The putative importance of respiratory muscle fatigue and the therapeutic potential of rest continue to receive emphasis [59] but a reduction in respiratory load, correction of alveolar hypoventilation, particularly during sleep, and enhancement of central drive may be of equal or greater importance [60].

Conclusion

It is perhaps worth considering the possible basis for the remarkable success achieved with nasal IPPV in the few years it has been available. It uses the natural airway and so has the benefit of filtering, warming and humidifying the inspired air. It can assist or control ventilation during unsedated wakefulness or sleep and, provided the characteristics of the trigger are chosen with care, it can reduce respiratory muscle work in both the control and the assist modes. Finally it can, when necessary, be combined with a sustained positive pressure during the expiratory phase. Thus, unlike a number of other innovative ventilatory support techniques introduced during the last decade, nasal IPPV is based firmly on the principles of normal physiology. It has considerable potential for both hospital and home use and, particularly in the management of the later stages of COPD, warrants wider exploitation and evaluation.

References

1. Bellemare F, Grassino A (1982) Evaluation of human diaphragm fatigue. J Appl Physiol 53:1196–1206
2. Sawicka EH, Branthwaite MA (1987) Respiration during sleep in kyphoscoliosis. Thorax 42:801–808

3. Midren B, Petersson K, Hansson L, Eriksson L, Airikkala P, Elmqvist D (1988) Nocturnal hypoxaemia in severe scoliosis. Br J Dis Chest 82:226–236
4. Phillips MS, Miller MR, Kinnear WJM, Gough SE, Schneerson JM (1987) Importance of airflow obstruction after thoracoplasty. Thorax 42:348-352
5. Catterall JR, Douglas NJ, Calverley PMA, et al (1983) Transient hypoxemia during sleep in chronic obstructive pulmonary disease is not a sleep apnea syndrome. Am Rev Respir Dis 128:24–29
6. Simonds AK, Parker RA, Sawicka EH, Branthwaite MA (1986) Effects of protriptyline on sleep related disturbances of breathing in restrictive chest wall disease. Thorax 41:586–590
7. Carroll N, Parker RA, Branthwaite MA (1990) Effects of protriptyline on respiratory failure in patients with chronic airflow limitation. Europ Respir J 3:746–751
8. Hill NS (1986) Clinical applications of body ventilators. Chest 90:897-905
9. Kinnear W, Petch M, Taylor G, Schneerson JM (1988) Assisted ventilation using cuirass respirators. Eur Respir J 1:198–203
10. Brochard L, Isabey D, Piquet J, et al (1990) Reversal of acute exacerbations of chronic obstructive lung disease by inspiratory assistance with a face mask. New Eng J Med 323:1523–1530
11. Alba A, Khan A, Lee M (1981) Mouth IPPV for sleep. Rehab Gazette 24:47–49
12. Ellis ER, Bye PTB, Bruderer JW, Sullivan CE (1987) Treatment of respiratory failure during sleep in patients with neuromuscular disease. Am Rev Respir Dis 135:148–152
13. Mayer LS, Kerby GR, Whitman RA, Shivers-Smith C (1990) Continued evaluation of a new nasal device for administration of continuous positive airway pressure. Am Rev Respir Dis 141(S):A864
14. Simonds AK, Cramer D, Wedzicha J (1991) Nasal plugs (Adams circuit) for the delivery of CPAP and non-invasive intermittent positive pressure ventilation. Thorax (in press)
15. Sullivan CE, Berthon-Jones M, Issa FG, Eves L (1981) Reversal of obstructive sleep apnoea by continuous positive airway pressure applied through the nares. Lancet 1:862–865
16. Carroll N, Branthwaite MA (1988) Intermittent positive pressure ventilation by nasal mask: technique and applications. Intensive Care Med 14:115–117
17. Elliott MW, Mulvey D, Moxham J, Green M, Branthwaite MA (1991) Intermittent positive pressure ventilation by nasal mask diminishes inspiratory muscle activity in patients with COPD. Am Rev Respir Dis (in press)
18. Waldhorn RE, Robinson R, Murthy R, Jennings C (1990) Nasal intermittent positive pressure ventilation (NIPPV) with bi-level positive airway pressure (BiPAP) in acute and chronic respiratory failure. Am Rev Respir Dis 141(S):A238
19. Simonds AK, Elliott MW (1991) Use of the BiPAP ventilator for non-invasive ventilation: advantages and limitations. Am Rev Respir Dis (in press)
20. Spencer GT (1977) Respiratory insufficiency in scoliosis: clinical management and home care. In: Zorab PA (ed) Scoliosis. Academic Press, London, pp 315–328
21. Libby DM, Briscoe WA, Boyce B, Smith JP (1982) Acute respiratory failure in scoliosis or kyphosis. Prolonged survival and treatment. Am J Med 73:532–538
22. Goldstein RS, Molotiu N, Skrastins R, et al (1987) Reversal of sleep-induced hypoventilation and chronic respiratory failure by nocturnal negative pressure ventilation in patients with restrictive ventilatory impairment. Am Rev Respir Dis 135:1049–1055
23. Sawicka EH, Loh L, Branthwaite MA (1988) Domiciliary ventilatory support: an analysis of outcome. Thorax 43:31-35
24. Simonds AK, Sawicka EH, Carroll N, Branthwaite MA (1988) Use of negative pressure ventilation to facilitate the return of spontaneous ventilation. Anaesthesia 43:216–219
25. Samuels MP, Southall DP (1989) Negative extrathoracic pressure in treatment of respiratory failure in infants and young children. Br Med J 299:1253–1257
26. Shapiro SH, Martin JG, Gray-Donald K, et al (1989) A randomized clinical trial of negative pressure ventilation in patients with severe COPD. Am Rev Respir Dis 139(S):A516
27. Cooper CB, Harris ND, Howard P (1988) Physiological changes during external negative pressure ventilation in hypercapnic chronic obstructive airways disease. Thorax 43:P232
28. Cropp AA, DiMarco F (1987) Effects of intermittent negative pressure ventilation on respiratory muscle function in patients with COPD. Am Rev Respir Dis 135:1056–1061

29. Gutierrez M, Beroiza T, Contrera F, et al (1988) Weekly cuirass ventilation improves blood gases and inspiratory muscle strengths in patients with chronic airflow limitation and hypercarbia. Am Rev Respir Dis 138:617–623
30. Zibrak JD, Hill NS, Federman EC, Kwa SL, O'Donnell C (1988) Evaluation of intermittent long term negative-pressure ventilation in patients with severe COPD. Am Rev Respir Dis 138:1515–1518
31. Celli B, Lee H, Criner G, et al (1989) Controlled trial of external negative pressure ventilation in patients with severe chronic airflow limitation. Am Rev Respir Dis 140:1251–1256
32. Rochester DF, Braun NMT, Laine S (1977) Diaphragmatic energy expenditure in chronic respiratory failure. The effect of assisted ventilation with body respirators. Am J Med 63:223–232
33. Braun NMT, Marino W (1982) Effect of daily intermittent rest of respiratory muscles in patients with severe chronic airflow limitation (CAL). Chest 85:59S
34. Levy RD, Martin JG, Bradley TD, Macklem PT, Newman SL (1986) Effects of negative pressure ventilators on ventilation in normal subjects during sleep. Am Rev Respir Dis 133:A168
35. Rodenstein DO, Cuttitta G, Stanescu DC (1988) Ventilatory and diaphragmatic EMG changes during negative-pressure ventilation in healthy subjects. J Appl Physiol 64:2272–2278
36. Dubois F, Société de Pneumologie d'Ile-de-France, National Trial Group (1990) Negative pressure ventilation improves respiratory muscle strength and dyspnea in patients with severe chronic obstructive pulmonary disease (COPD). Am Rev Respir Dis 141(S):A37
37. Rochester DF (1988) Does respiratory muscle rest relieve fatigue or incipient fatigue? Am Rev Respir Dis 138:516–517
38. Ambrosino N, Montagna MD, Nava S, et al (1990) Short term effect of intermittent negative pressure ventilation in COPD patients with respiratory failure. Eur Respir J 3:502–508
39. Scano G, Gigliotti F, Duranti R, Spinelli A, Gorini M, Schiavina M (1990) Changes in ventilatory muscle function with negative pressure ventilation in COPD. Chest 97:322–327
40. Lisboa C, Contreras G, Barros M, Cruz E (1990) Which chronic airflow limitation patients benefit from intermittent negative pressure ventilation? Am Rev Respir Dis 141(S):A322
41. Elliott MW, Steven MH, Phillips GD, Branthwaite MA (1990) Non-invasive mechanical ventilation for acute respiratory failure. Br Med J 300:358–360
42. Goutorbe F, Robert D, Leger P, Jennequin J (1990) Acute failure of chronic respiratory insufficiency treated by nasal mechanical ventilation. Am Rev Respir Dis 141(S):A36
43. Muir JF, Benhamou D, Heliot P, Girault C, Callonnec F, Portier F (1990) Management of acute respiratory failure (ARF) in elderly patients with nasal intermittent positive pressure ventilation (NIPPV). Am Rev Respir Dis 141(S):A237
44. Berghauser Pont HG, van Kesteren RG, Rutgers MR (eds) (1990) Respiratory insufficiency in neuromuscular diseases: report of an international workshop. EAMDA, Baarn, The Netherlands
45. Ellis ER, McCauley VB, Mellis C, Sullivan CE (1987) Treatment of alveolar hypoventilation in a six-year-old girl with intermittent positive pressure ventilation through a nose mask. Am Rev Respir Dis 136:188–191
46. Heckmatt JZ, Loh L, Dubowitz (1990) Night-time nasal ventilation in neuromuscular disease. Lancet 1:579–582
47. Udwadia ZF, Steven M, Miller SJ, Simonds AK (1991) Value of non-invasive nasal positive pressure ventilation in weaning intubated patients from conventional intermittent positive pressure ventilation. Eur Respir J (in press)
48. Kerby GR, Mayer LS, Pingleton SK (1987) Nocturnal positive pressure ventilation via nasal mask. Am Rev Respir Dis 135:738–740
49. Bach JR, Alba A, Mosher R, DeLaubier A (1987) Intermittent positive pressure ventilation via nasal access in the management of respiratory insufficiency. Chest 92:168–170
50. Leger P, Madelon J, Jennequin J, Gerard M, Robert D (1987) Non-invasive home IPPV via nasal mask in nocturnal ventilator dependent patients with musculoskeletal disorders: an efficient alternative to tracheostomy. Am Rev Respir Dis 135(S):A193
51. Carroll N, Branthwaite MA (1988) Control of nocturnal hypoventilation by nasal intermittent positive pressure ventilation. Thorax 43:349–353

52. Simonds AK, Elliott MW, Carroll N, Branthwaite MA (1991) Longterm nasal intermittent positive pressure ventilation: clinical, physiological and economic outcome. Am Rev Respir Dis (in press)
53. Branthwaite MA (1989) Mechanical ventilation at home. Br Med J 298:1409
54. Robert D, Gerard M, Leger P, et al (1983) Domiciliary ventilation by tracheostomy for chronic respiratory failure. Rev Fr Mal Resp 11:923–936
55. Elliott M, Carroll M, Wedzicha J, Branthwaite M (1990) Nasal positive pressure ventilation can be used successfully at home to control nocturnal hypoventilation in COPD. Am Rev Respir Dis 141(S):A322
56. Elliott MW, Carroll M, Simonds AK, Wedzicha JA, Branthwaite MA (1991) Domiciliary nasal ventilation improves sleep and daytime blood gas tensions in patients with COPD. Am Rev Respir Dis (in press)
57. Strumpf DA, Carlisle CC, Millman RP, Erickson AD, Grattan LA, Hill NS (1990) Therapy of severe COPD with nocturnal nasal positive pressure ventilation. Am Rev Respir Dis 141(S):A322
58. Cooper CB, Waterhouse J, Howard P (1987) Twelve year clinical study of patients with hypoxic cor pulmonale given long term domiciliary oxygen therapy. Thorax 42:105–110
59. Carrey Z, Gottfried SB, Levy D (1990) Ventilatory muscle support in respiratory failure with nasal positive pressure ventilation. Chest 97:150–158
60. Elliott MW, Mulvey DA, Moxham J, Green M, Branthwaite M (1991) Domiciliary nocturnal nasal intermittent positive pressure ventilation in COPD: an analysis of mechanisms underlying changes in arterial blood gas tensions. Eur J Respir Dis (in press)

Airway Pressure Release Ventilation and BIPAP

J.J. Rouby

Introduction

Pressure release ventilation is a new mode of ventilatory support in which intermittent CPAP release provides mechanical assistance to alveolar ventilation. It differs from intermittent positive pressure ventilation (IPPV) and inspiratory pressure support as far as pressure changes throughout the respiratory cycle: during these two modes, either a preset tidal volume (VT) or a preset inspiratory pressure are delivered by the ventilator to the patient and, as a consequence, airway pressure increases during the inspiratory phase; during pressure release ventilation, passive exhalation of the respiratory system follows CPAP release and is associated with a marked decrease in airway pressure, the pressure re-increasing during the next respiratory cycle. Because of the limitation of the increase in peak airway pressure, the risk of pulmonary barotrauma is theoretically reduced.

There are two different types of pressure release ventilation:

1. Airway Pressure Release Ventilation (APRV), initially proposed by Downs et al. in the United States [1], during which entire alveolar ventilation is ensured by preset periodical CPAP releases.
2. Bi Positive Airway Pressure (BIPAP), advocated by our group, in which the patient's alveolar ventilation is partially assisted by a pressure release applied every 2, 3, 4, 5 or 6 spontaneous expirations, the patient being connected to a mechanical ventilator. This ventilatory mode is now provided by mechanical ventilators which offer the possibility of associating a small pressure support level (<5 cm H_2O) in order to antagonize the extra-work of breathing due to the endotracheal tube and the ventilatory circuits [2].

Airway Pressure Release Ventilation (APRV)

APRV can be delivered using a modified oxygen-powered venturi CPAP system [8]. Two additionnal valves have been added on the expiratory circuit: a second threshold resistor valve and a release valve connected to a timer. According to the position of the release valve, two different CPAP levels can be applied: high CPAP when the release valve is closed, low CPAP when the release valve is open. The frequency of CPAP release can be modified through a timer. APRV has been shown to ensure normal alveolar ventilation in paralyzed dogs under general anesthesia [3]. In animals without acute respiratory failure (ARF), CPAP was released from 8 cm H_2O to zero, 20 times per minute. In animals with oleic acid lung injury, CPAP was released from 15–20 cm H_2O to 5 cm H_2O, 20 times per minute. When compared with continuous positive pressure ventilation (CPPV), APRV was associated with a significant reduction in peak airway pressure, although both ventilatory modes were compared at the same level of mean airway pressure. Since high peak airway pressure seems to be involved in mechanical ventilation-induced lung damage [4–6], APRV could contribute to decrease the incidence of pulmonary barotrauma. In contrast, there is no difference between APRV and conventional ventilation in terms of hemodynamics: arterial pressure, heart rate, cardiac output and cardiac filling pressures are identical when both ventilatory modes are compared at the same level of mean airway pressure [3, 7].

It is also possible to superimpose APRV on patient's or animal's spontaneous breathing activity [7, 8]. If 20 APRV breaths per minute are insufficient to prevent spontaneous ventilatory efforts, high CPAP is increased to obtain a larger airway pressure release gradient, and consequently, a higher VT [8]. The APRV rate is then reduced to maintain an airway pressure release time shorter than one-half of the respiratory cycle. However, since spontaneous respiratory rate can markedly vary with time, the APRV rate has to be frequently adjusted in order to avoid discoordination between CPAP release and spontaneous respiratory activity. In anesthetized animals with drug-induced respiratory depression in whom the use of CPAP is constantly associated with alveolar hypoventilation and hypercarbia, APRV enables a normalization of alveolar ventilation without increasing peak airway pressure [8]. It must be pointed out that intermittent CPAP release does not alter arterial oxygenation in presence of ARF [8].

Bi Positive Airway Pressure (BIPAP)

Technical Aspects

In contrast to APRV, the pressure release frequency depends on patient's spontaneous respiratory frequency. The patient is connected to a normal conventional mechanical ventilator which can provide BIPAP. Inspiratory efforts are detected through a trigger, the sensitivity of which can be set from -0.5 cm H_2O to -3 cm H_2O. Two levels of CPAP are applied by changing the PEEP level every 2, 3, 4, 5 or 6 spontaneous expirations. As a consequence, no discoordination occurs between patient's spontaneous breaths and pressure release.

One of the commercially-available ventilator which provides BIPAP is the CESAR ventilator (Taema, CFPO France). In this ventilator, the PEEP valve, which is completely original, technologically-speaking, is connected to a central microprocessor which periodically changes the PEEP level. The following parameters can be set on the ventilator: the superior PEEP level, the amount of PEEP release and the PEEP release frequency. In addition, pressure support can be combined with BIPAP, and a pressure support of 5 cm H_2O can be superimposed to each spontaneous inspiration to antagonize the extra-work of breathing due to the respiratory cicuits (Fig. 1) [2]. One advantage of this new ventilatory mode is that ventilatory assistance depends on the patient's spontaneous respiratory rate: the more rapid

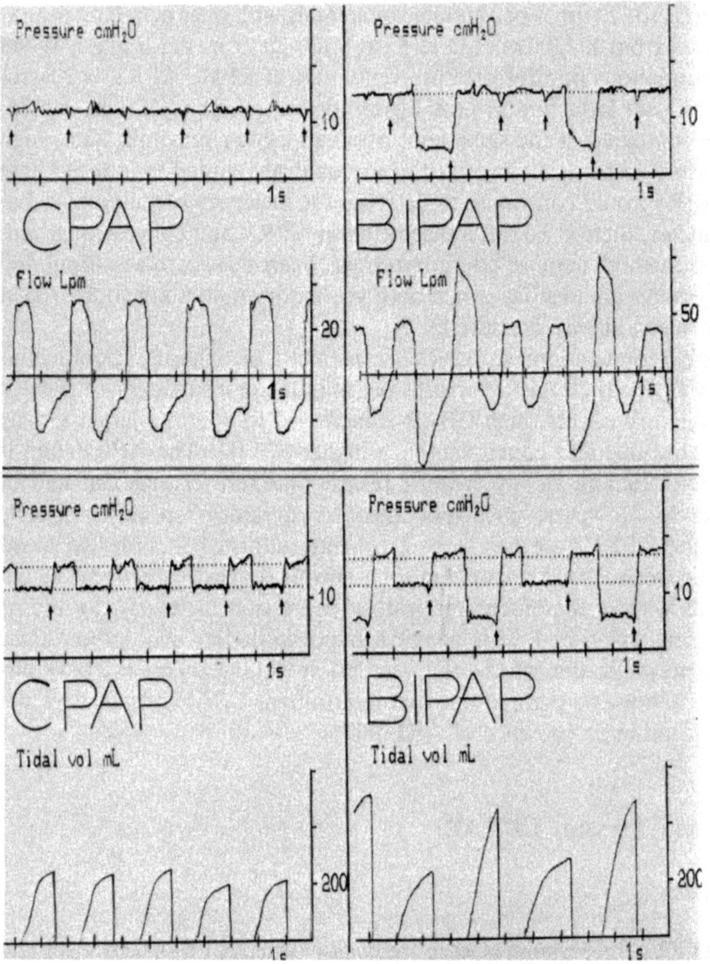

Fig. 1. Simultaneous recordings of airway pressure, gas flow and expired tidal volume in a patient during CPAP and BIPAP (Cesar Ventilator, Taema France). In the *upper part* of the figure, CPAP and BIPAP are administered without pressure support. Each arrow indicates patient's spontaneous inspiratory efforts. During CPAP, a PEEP of 12 cm H_2O is applied and the tidal volume is around 150 ml. During BIPAP, a PEEP of 15 cm H_2O is applied and released to 5 cm H_2O every 3 respiratory cycles. Change in the PEEP level induces an increase in expiratory flow and consequently an increase in expired tidal volume (450 ml). In the *lower part* of the figure, CPAP and BIPAP are administred with a pressure support of 5 cm H_2O. Tidal volumes increase (200 ml) and respiratory frequency decreases because the patient's respiratory work of breathing decreases

the patient's respiratory frequency, the greater the ventilatory assistance. It mut be pointed out that the patient's connection to a ventilator provides the possibility of continuously monitoring VT, airway pressure, gas flow and respiratory frequency. In the CESAR ventilator, these useful respiratory parameters are continuously displayed on a monitoring screen, and each 72 h, parameter trend can be reviewed.

Pathophysiology

During BIPAP, tidal volume varies according to CPAP changes. CPAP release, which always occurs during expiration, is followed by a marked increase in the expired tidal volume due to the sudden reduction of lung volume (Fig. 1). During the next expiration, lung volume is re-established at the precedent level without any phenomenon of gas trapping, via the reestablishing of the initial PEEP level. During BIPAP, functional residual capacity changes according to PEEP changes (Fig. 2).

It is important to differentiate "spontaneous VT" generated by the patient's spontaneous breathing activity at the superior CPAP level, from "assisted VT" generated by CPAP release. "Spontaneous VT" increases with the pressure support level and the patient's spontaneous inspiratory activity, and decreases when static respiratory compliance is reduced [9]. "Assisted VT" is influenced by the amount of CPAP release, the patient's spontaneous inspiratory activity and the static respiratory compliance. For a given respiratory compliance, the greater the amount of PEEP release, the greater the "assisted VT". For a given amout of PEEP release, the "assisted VT" increases when the preceding patient's inspiratory effort increases. Because of the variability of patient's spontaneous inspiratory activity, "spontaneous" as well as "assisted" VT vary from one cycle to another although airway pressure remains remarkably constant. Since in clinical practice, esophageal pressure, which indirectly reflects spontaneous inspiratory activity, is not routinely monitored, the presence or the absence of VT changes with time, provides information concerning the patient's spontaneous breathing activity.

When compared to pressure support ventilation, BIPAP enables a significant

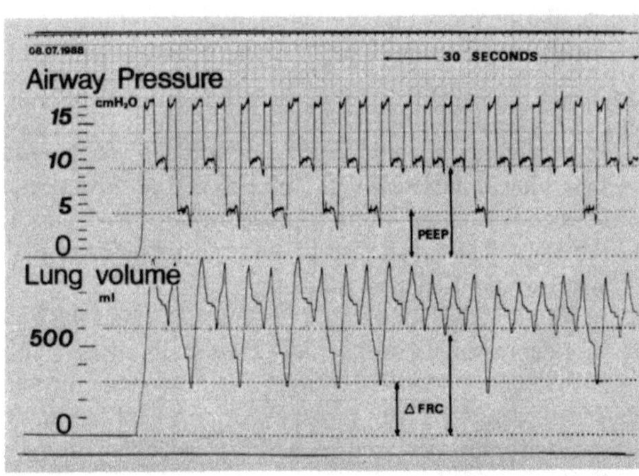

Fig. 2. Simultaneous changes in airway pressure and lung volume in a patient under BIPAP (Cesar Ventilator). PEEP is released from 11 to 5 cm H_2O and an inspiratory pressure support of 6 cm H_2O is applied. On the left part of the recording, PEEP is changed every 2 spontaneous respiratory cycles and on the right part of the recording, every 5 spontaneous respiratory cycles. Increase in lung volume above apneic functional residual capacity (Δ FRC) changes with pressure release from 600 ml to 300 ml. Δ FRC changes are not modified by decreasing the rate of pressure release

decrease in peak airway pressure, which never exceeds the superior PEEP level more than the pressure support used [10]. In contrast, respiratory frequency is lower during pressure support ventilation. Respiratory effects of changing pressure release frequency depend on the patient's initial clinical status: in non-sedated patients able to produce efficient spontaneous breathing, the decrease in pressure release frequency induces an increase in patient's "spontaneous VT", whereas minute ventilation and alveolar ventilation remain unchanged [3]. In contrast, in patients with central respiratory depression or chest wall mechanical impairment, the reduction in pressure release frequency is associated with a decrease in minute ventilation, leading to alveolar hypoventilation and hypercarbia.

Clinical Indications of Pressure Release Ventilation

Pressure release ventilation can be applied to paralyzed patients - APRV - or to spontaneously breathing patients - BIPAP -. The use of pressure release ventilation in a spontaneously breathing patient requires several technical conditions. First, pressure release should always be synchronized with patient's expiration, to avoid abrupt increase in airway pressure during an expiratory effort which creates a feeling of discomfort. Second, this ventilatory mode should be integrated in a conventional ventilator in order to monitor usual respiratory parameters. Third, the PEEP level shoud be automatically changed according to the patient's respiratory frequency; therefore, the PEEP valve is to be modified to be commanded by the microprocessor. Fourth, because BIPAP is a ventilatory mode during which a patient connected to a ventilator spontaneously breathes, the possibility of adding a small amount of pressure support should exist. Finally, as with any ventilatory mode, alarms should be present on main respiratory parameters such as respiratory frequency, tidal volume, peak airway pressure and minute ventilation.

What are the clinical indications of pressure release ventilation?

1. In paralyzed patients, APRV is associated with a reduction in peak airway pressure when compared with conventional positive pressure ventilation [7]. No difference was to be found in any of the other hemodynamic and respiratory parameters. The advantage of APRV in paralyzed patients appears limited to its effect on peak airway pressure.
2. In spontaneously-breathing patients with mild ARF, but without central respiratory depression or mechanical chest wall impairment, we found that CPAP and BIPAP gave identical results on hemodynamic and respiratory parameters. When compared with pressure support ventilation, CPAP and BIPAP were associated with increased respiratory frequency and lower peak airway pressure. In this population of patients, when switching CPAP for BIPAP, minute ventilation and respiratory rate did not change. A significant reduction in "spontaneous VT" occurred, suggesting that a significant part of the patient's alveolar ventilation was supported by PEEP release (Fig. 3). Therefore, in this category of critically ill patients, the advantage of BIPAP over CPAP could be a reduction of the patient's respiratory work of breathing. In critically ill patients with circulatory shock and/or severe ARF, BIPAP is most often not clinically toler-

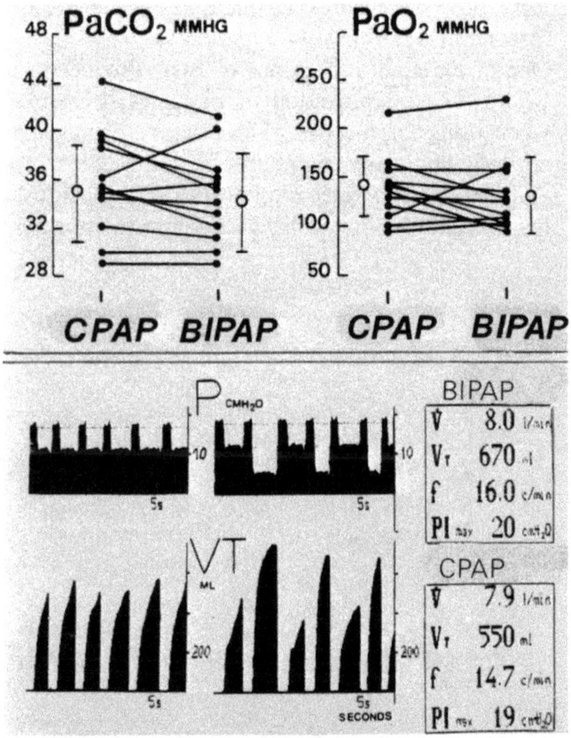

Fig. 3. Comparative effects of CPAP and BIPAP on gas exchange, airway pressure (P) and expired tidal volume (VT) in 12 non-sedated critically ill patients with mild acute respiratory failure (Cesar ventilator, inspiratory pressure of 5 cm H_2O, mean airway pressure of 10 cm H_2O, FIO_2 0.6, $PaCO_2$, PaO_2, minute Ventilation ($\dot{V}$), respiratory frequency (f) and peak airway pressure (PI max) are similar in both modes). In the lower part of the figure, an illustrative example of one of the patients is shown: during BIPAP (PEEP change from 12 to 5 cm H_2O every 2 spontaneous respiratory cycles), "assisted tidal volume" is around 670 ml, and "spontaneous tidal volumes" are around 400 ml, whereas during CPAP tidal volumes vary between 500 and 600 ml. Because of the pressure release induced ventilatory assistance, the patient reduces his own contribution to minute ventilation during BIPAP

ated in the absence of intravenous sedation: a high respiratory rate persists, despite the ventilatory assistance provided by BIPAP, and the patient becomes progressively exhausted. One possibility then, is to sedate the patient in order to decrease the respiratory rate and to maintain BIPAP as long as the patient is still able to trigger the flow.

3. BIPAP does offer significant advantages in patients with mechanical chest wall impairment or drug induced central respiratory depression. In such situations, CPAP invariably results in inadequate alveolar ventilation leading to increased respiratory rate and hypercarbia and imposing CPPV. BIPAP enables the continuation of spontaneous ventilatory mode, by partially assisting alveolar ventilation through pressure release. As long as the patient is able to trigger inspira-

tory flow, its ensures adequate gas exchange, without increasing peak airway pressure [11].

- One of the main indications of BIPAP concerns agitated patients with ARF in whom the administration of narcotics or benzodiazepines is necessary. Even when using large doses of respiratory depressant agents, the vast majority of critically ill patients maintain a certain degree of spontaneous inspiratory activity and are able to trigger inspiratory flow. When using CPAP, patient's VT is too low, respiratory frequency remains in the normal range, and $PaCO_2$ increases.

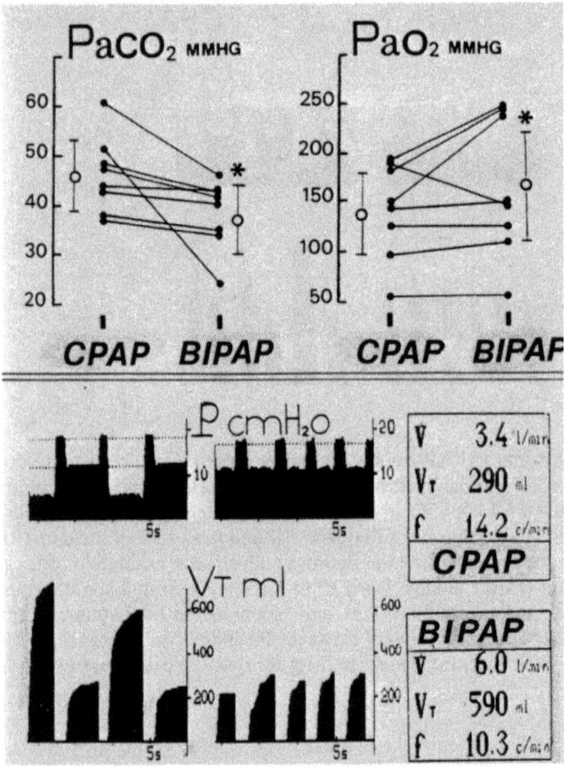

Fig. 4. Comparative effects on $PaCO_2$ and PaO_2 (FIO_2:0.6) of CPAP and BIPAP in 8 critically ill patients with ARF receiving intravenous narcotics because of agitation. All patients are ventilated with a Cesar Ventilator and both ventilatory modes are compared at the same level of mean airway pressure (12 cm H_2O), using a trigger sensitivity of -0.5 cm H_2O and an inspiratory pressure support of 5 cm H_2O. Under CPAP, 6 patients have a $PaCO_2$ above 40 mm Hg. In each individual, BIPAP (PEEP change every 2 spontaneous respiratory cycles) decreases $PaCO_2$. Simultaneously, PaO_2 increases in 7 of the 8 patients ($p<0.05$). In the lower part of the figure, comparative effects of CPAP and BIPAP on airway pressure (P) and expired tidal volume (V_T) are shown in one patient. CPAP is associated with a low minute ventilation ($\dot{V}$), with an expired V_T of 290 ml, a respiratory frequency of 14 bpm and a $PaCO_2$ of 61 mm Hg. BIPAP increases minute ventilation to 6 l/min, reduces respiratory frequency to 10 bpm, whereas "spontaneous tidal volume" remains around 300 ml. The increase in minute ventilation due to "assisted tidal volume" (around 600 ml) enables a decrease in $PaCO_2$ from 61 to 45 mm Hg. (From [11] with permission)

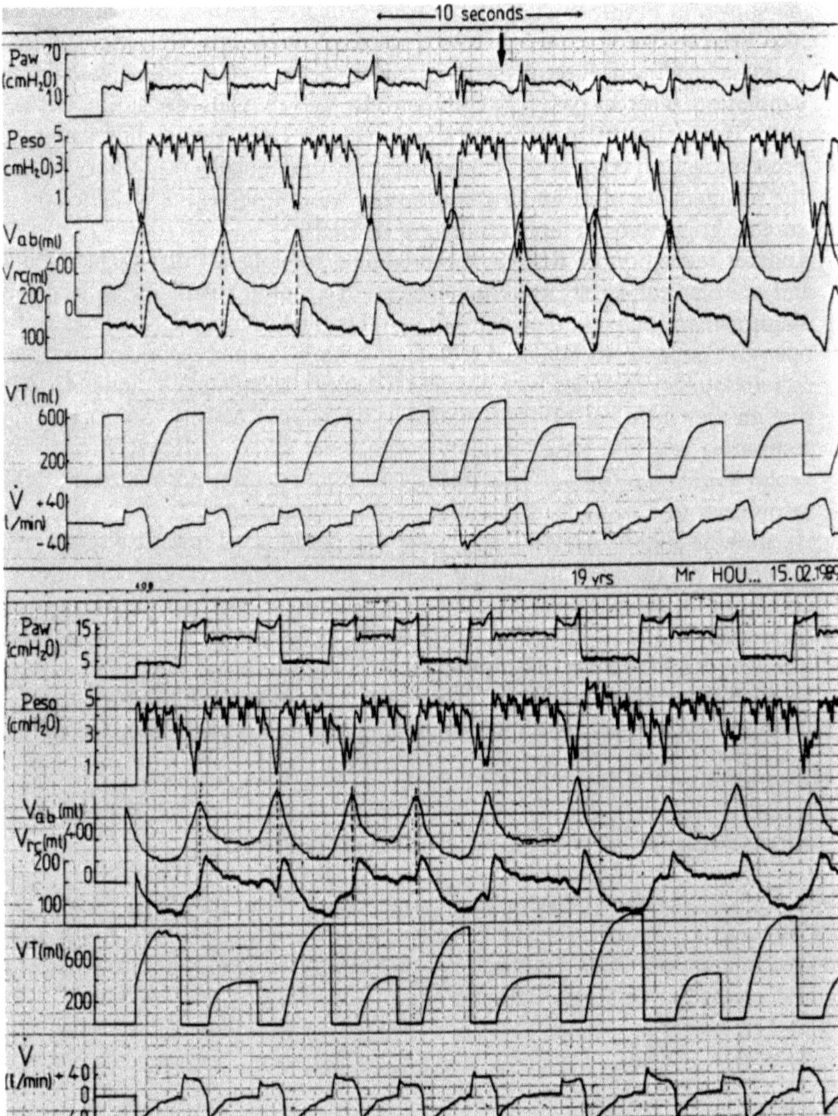

Fig. 5. Simultaneous recording of airway pressure (Paw), esophageal pressure (Peso), abdominal and rib cage contributions to tidal volume (Vab and Vrc), expired tidal volume (V_T) and gas flow ($\dot{V}$) in a critically ill patient with a traumatic C_7 quadraplegia. In the upper part of the figure CPAP (PEEP: 13 cm H_2O) is applied with (left part of the recordings) or without (right part of the recordings after the arrow) pressure support of 5 cm H_2O. In the lower part of the figure, BIPAP is applied (superior level of PEEP: 12 cm H_2O, PEEP release every 2 expirations, pressure support of 5 cm H_2O). The paradoxical wall motion is obvious during CPAP without pressure support (vertical dashed lines), is reduced during CPAP with pressure support of 5 cm H_2O and disappears during BIPAP. Simultaneously, a significant decrease in esophageal pressure variation is observed, suggesting a diminution of patient's respiratory work

As shown in Fig. 4, the use of BIPAP normalizes $PaCO_2$. Similar results have also been shown in experimental anesthetized dogs with ARF [8]. The marked increase in VT which results from pressure release enables an increase in minute ventilation, whereas patient's "spontaneous VT" remains low during CPAP and BIPAP. Finally, BIPAP in critically ill patients receiving potent respiratory depressant agents, enables the continuation of spontaneous respiratory mode and the maintenance of mean airway pressure, without increasing peak airway pressure as in pressure support ventilation or CPPV.

- Another indication of BIPAP is represented by critically ill patients with ARF and mechanical chest wall impairment. Tetraplegic patients with persisting diaphragmatic activity, patients with peripheral neuromuscular disease, and postoperative patients with marked reduction in lung volumes secondary to large thoracoabdominal incisions, are unable to achieve adequate VT under CPAP, although they have persisting spontaneous inspiratory activity. Hypercarbia, high respiratory rate and fatigue rapidly occur under CPAP. BIPAP, by assisting alveolar ventilation through intermittent pressure releases, normalizes $PaCO_2$ and respiratory rate without increasing peak airway pressure.
- As show in Fig. 5, BIPAP can reverse the paradoxical inward displacement of the chest wall observed in multiple trauma patients with cervical cord injury. The correction of the chest wall distorsion is due to the fact that CPAP changes induce passive and, consequently, synchronous movements of thoracic and abdominal compartments. Therefore, BIPAP appears as an interesting alternative ventilatory mode for patients with cervical cord injury and also for patients with mobile flail chest showing thoracoabdominal paradoxical wall motion.

Contraindications of Pressure Release Ventilation

The contraindications of APRV and BIPAP are those of PEEP. Patients with COPD and increased bronchial resistance develop intrinsic PEEP under pressure release ventilation which can lead to severe overdistention, pulmonary barotrauma and decreased alveolar ventilation.

References

1. Downs JB, Stock MC (1987) Airway pressure release ventilation: a new concept in ventilatory support. Crit Care Med 15:459–461
2. Brochard L, Rua F, Lorino H, Lemaire F, Harf A (1988) The extra-work of breathing due to the endotracheal tube is abolished during inspiratory pressure support breathing. Am Rev Respir Dis 137:A64
3. Stock MC, Downs JB, Deborah A, Frolicher BS (1987) Airway pressure release ventilation. Crit Care Med 15:462–466
4. Parker JC, Townsley MI, Rippe B, Taylor AE, Thigpen J (1984) Increased microvascular permeability in dog lungs due to high peak airway pressures. J Appl Physiol 57:1809–1816
5. Dreyfuss D, Basset G, Soler P, Soumon G (1985) Intermittent positive-pressure hyperventilation with high inflation pressures produces pulmonary microvascular injury in rats. Am Rev Respir Dis 132:880–884

6. Kolobow T, Moretti MP, Fumagalli R, et al (1988) Severe impairment in lung function induced by peak airway pressure during mechanical ventilation. Am Rev Respir Dis 135:312–315
7. Garner W, Downs JB, Stock C, Rasanen J (1988) Airway pressure release ventilation (APRV). A human trial. Chest 94:779–781
8. Rasanen J, Downs JB, Stock MC (1988) Cardiovascular effects of conventional positive pressure ventilation and airway pressure release ventilation. Chest 93:911–915
9. Rouby JJ, Jawish D, Andreev A, Arthaud M, Viars P (1989) Déterminants du volume courant en aide inspiratoire. Ann Fr Anesth Réan 8:R253
10. Jawish D, Rouby JJ, Andreev A, Arthaud M, Poete P, Viars P (1989) Aide inspiratoire, ventilation spontanée avec pression expiratoire positive et ventilation spontanée avec pression positive variable: une étude comparative randomisée. Ann Fr Anesth Rean 8:R255
11. Vrillon M, Rouby JJ, Andreev A, Jawish D, Ben Ameur M, Viars P (1990) Intermittent Mandatory Pressure Release Ventilation (IMPRV) in patients with acute respiratory failure. Anesthesiology 73:A255

Subject Index

MIX
Papier aus verantwortungsvollen Quellen
Paper from responsible sources
FSC® C105338

If you have any concerns about our products,
you can contact us on
ProductSafety@springernature.com

In case Publisher is established outside the EU,
the EU authorized representative is:
Springer Nature Customer Service Center GmbH
Europaplatz 3, 69115 Heidelberg, Germany

Printed by Libri Plureos GmbH
in Hamburg, Germany